D1571509

D1571510

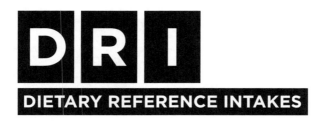

Calcium
Vitamin D

Committee to Review Dietary Reference Intakes for Vitamin D and Calcium
Food and Nutrition Board

A. Catharine Ross, Christine L. Taylor, Ann L. Yaktine, and
Heather B. Del Valle, *Editors*

INSTITUTE OF MEDICINE
OF THE NATIONAL ACADEMIES

THE NATIONAL ACADEMIES PRESS
Washington, D.C.
www.nap.edu

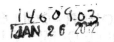

THE NATIONAL ACADEMIES PRESS   **500 Fifth Street, N.W.**   **Washington, DC 20001**

NOTICE: The project that is the subject of this report was approved by the Governing Board of the National Research Council, whose members are drawn from the councils of the National Academy of Sciences, the National Academy of Engineering, and the Institute of Medicine. The members of the committee responsible for the report were chosen for their special competences and with regard for appropriate balance.

This study was supported by Contract No. 4500196976 between the National Academy of Sciences and Health Canada; Contract No. 59-0204-8-155 between the National Academy of Sciences and the U.S. Department of Agriculture, Agriculture Research Service; Contract No. CNPP-08-0001 between the National Academy of Sciences and the U.S. Department of Agriculture (Center for Nutrition Policy and Promotion); Contract No. W81XWH-09-1-0288 between the National Academy of Sciences and the U.S. Department of the Army; Contract No. HHSF223200811157P between the National Academy of Sciences and the U.S. Department of Health and Human Services, Food and Drug Administration; Contract No. N01-OD-4-2139 between the National Academy of Sciences and the U.S. Department of Health and Human Services (National Institutes of Health); Contract No. HHSP223200800002T between the National Academy of Sciences and the U.S. Department of Health and Human Services (Office of Disease Prevention and Health Promotion). Any opinions, findings, conclusions, or recommendations expressed in this publication are those of the author(s) and do not necessarily reflect the view of the organizations or agencies that provided support for this project.

Library of Congress Cataloging-in-Publication Data

Dietary reference intakes for calcium and vitamin D / Committee to Review Dietary Reference Intakes for Vitamin D and Calcium, Food and Nutrition Board ; A. Catharine Ross ... [et al.], editors.
  p. ; cm.
  Includes bibliographical references and index.
  ISBN 978-0-309-16394-1 (hardcover : alk. paper) — ISBN 978-0-309-16395-8 (pdf) 1. Calcium in the body. 2. Vitamin D in the body. 3. Calcium in human nutrition. 4. Vitamin D in human nutrition. 5. Dietary supplements. I. Ross, A. Catharine. II. Institute of Medicine (U.S.). Committee to Review Dietary Reference Intakes for Vitamin D and Calcium.
  [DNLM: 1. Calcium, Dietary. 2. Vitamin D. 3. Nutrition Policy. 4. Nutritional Requirements. QU 130]
  QP535.C2D54 2011
  612.3'99—dc22
                            2011004590

Additional copies of this report are available from the National Academies Press, 500 Fifth Street, N.W., Lockbox 285, Washington, DC 20055; (800) 624-6242 or (202) 334-3313 (in the Washington metropolitan area); Internet, http://www.nap.edu.

For more information about the Institute of Medicine, visit the IOM home page at: **www.iom.edu.**

Suggested citation: IOM (Institute of Medicine). 2011. *Dietary Reference Intakes for Calcium and Vitamin D.* Washington, DC: The National Academies Press.

"Knowing is not enough; we must apply.
Willing is not enough; we must do."

—Goethe

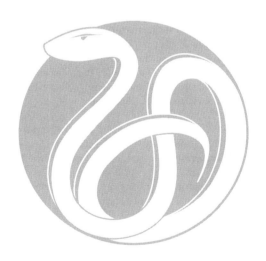

INSTITUTE OF MEDICINE
OF THE NATIONAL ACADEMIES

Advising the Nation. Improving Health.

THE NATIONAL ACADEMIES
Advisers to the Nation on Science, Engineering, and Medicine

The **National Academy of Sciences** is a private, nonprofit, self-perpetuating society of distinguished scholars engaged in scientific and engineering research, dedicated to the furtherance of science and technology and to their use for the general welfare. Upon the authority of the charter granted to it by the Congress in 1863, the Academy has a mandate that requires it to advise the federal government on scientific and technical matters. Dr. Ralph J. Cicerone is president of the National Academy of Sciences.

The **National Academy of Engineering** was established in 1964, under the charter of the National Academy of Sciences, as a parallel organization of outstanding engineers. It is autonomous in its administration and in the selection of its members, sharing with the National Academy of Sciences the responsibility for advising the federal government. The National Academy of Engineering also sponsors engineering programs aimed at meeting national needs, encourages education and research, and recognizes the superior achievements of engineers. Dr. Charles M. Vest is president of the National Academy of Engineering.

The **Institute of Medicine** was established in 1970 by the National Academy of Sciences to secure the services of eminent members of appropriate professions in the examination of policy matters pertaining to the health of the public. The Institute acts under the responsibility given to the National Academy of Sciences by its congressional charter to be an adviser to the federal government and, upon its own initiative, to identify issues of medical care, research, and education. Dr. Harvey V. Fineberg is president of the Institute of Medicine.

The **National Research Council** was organized by the National Academy of Sciences in 1916 to associate the broad community of science and technology with the Academy's purposes of furthering knowledge and advising the federal government. Functioning in accordance with general policies determined by the Academy, the Council has become the principal operating agency of both the National Academy of Sciences and the National Academy of Engineering in providing services to the government, the public, and the scientific and engineering communities. The Council is administered jointly by both Academies and the Institute of Medicine. Dr. Ralph J. Cicerone and Dr. Charles M. Vest are chair and vice chair, respectively, of the National Research Council.

www.national-academies.org

COMMITTEE TO REVIEW DIETARY REFERENCE INTAKES FOR VITAMIN D AND CALCIUM

Reviewers

This report has been reviewed in draft form by individuals chosen for their diverse perspectives and technical expertise, in accordance with procedures approved by the National Research Council's Report Review Committee. The purpose of this independent review is to provide candid and critical comments that will assist the institution in making its published report as sound as possible and to ensure that the report meets institutional standards for objectivity, evidence, and responsiveness to the study charge. The review comments and draft manuscript remain confidential to protect the integrity of the deliberative process. We wish to thank the following individuals for their review of this report:

Stephanie A. Atkinson, Department of Pediatrics, McMaster University, Hamilton, Ontario, Canada

Dennis M. Black, Division of Clinical Trials and Multicenter Studies, University of California, San Francisco

Edward M. Brown, Brigham and Women's Hospital and Harvard Medical School, Boston, MA

Lenore M. Buckley, School of Medicine, Virginia Commonwealth University

Bess Dawson-Hughes, Bone Metabolism Laboratory, Jean Mayer Human Nutrition Research Center, Tufts University, Boston, MA

James C. Fleet, Department of Foods and Nutrition, Purdue University, West Lafayette, IN

Richard David Granstein, Department of Dermatology, Weill Cornell Medical College, Ithaca, NY

Susan Harris, Bone Metabolism Laboratory, Jean Mayer Human Nutrition Research Center, Tufts University, Boston, MA

Robert P. Heaney, Creighton University Medical Center, Omaha, NE

Janet C. King, University of California at Berkeley and Davis, Children's Hospital Oakland Research Institute, Oakland

Michal Leora Melamed, Department of Medicine and Department of Epidemiology and Population Health, Albert Einstein College of Medicine, Bronx, NY

Robert L. Modlin, University of California, Los Angeles

Ann Prentice, MRC Human Nutrition Research, Elsie Widdowson Laboratory, Cambridge, United Kingdom

Connie M. Weaver, Department of Foods and Nutrition, Purdue University, West Lafayette, IN

Walter C. Willett, Department of Nutrition, Harvard School of Public Health, Boston, MA

Although the reviewers listed above have provided many constructive comments and suggestions, they were not asked to endorse the conclusions or recommendations nor did they see the final draft of the report before its release. The review of this report was overseen by **Irwin H. Rosenberg**, Friedman School of Nutrition Science and Policy, Tufts University, and **Enriqueta C. Bond**, Burroughs Wellcome Fund (retired). Appointed by the National Research Council and Institute of Medicine, they were responsible for making certain that an independent examination of this report was carried out in accordance with institutional procedures and that all review comments were carefully considered. Responsibility for the final content of this report rests entirely with the authoring committee and the institution.

Preface

It has been an honor to chair this committee tasked with reviewing Dietary Reference Intake (DRI) values for calcium and vitamin D. In this preface, I would like, first and foremost, to thank those persons without whose help this report would not have been possible. I also would like to comment briefly on the nature of the task we had at hand, and how our committee proceeded, from its first meeting in 2009 to the final stage of its report.

The work of our committee was preceded by three important papers and reports. At a time when interest in vitamin D had reached new heights, and many various claims for benefits were reported, health professionals in the governments of the United States and Canada worked together to address the question: Since the 1997 IOM report on DRIs, including vitamin D, is there sufficient new evidence on this micronutrient to warrant a new DRI study? The publication from this group, "Dietary reference intakes for vitamin D: justification for a review of the 1997 values"[1] concluded that there were sufficient new data to warrant a reevaluation. In funding the DRI review for vitamin D, the sponsors also judged that calcium should be reviewed as well, given its interrelationship with vitamin D. I thank the many individuals from the U.S. and Canadian governments who put into motion the processes that led to this report. Moreover, understanding that

---

[1]Yetley, E. A., D. Brule, M. C. Cheney, C. D. Davis, K. A. Esslinger, P. W. Fischer, K. E. Friedl, L. S. Greene-Finestone, P. M. Guenther, D. M. Klurfeld, M. R. L'Abbe, K. Y. McMurry, P. E. Starke-Reed and P. R. Trumbo. 2009. Dietary reference intakes for vitamin D: justification for a review of the 1997 values. American Journal of Clinical Nutrition 89(3): 719-27.

a review of the literature would be a tremendous undertaking by itself, this group also commissioned an independent systematic review of the literature on vitamin D and health outcomes for the use of this DRI committee, and intended to update an earlier systematic review on vitamin D and bone health. The systematic review carried out by Dr. Joseph Lau and his colleagues at the Tufts Evidence-based Practice Center, and a preceding systematic review led by Dr. Ann Cranney of the University of Ottawa, both greatly aided the work of the current committee.

In the Statement of Task, the sponsors requested that our report be developed using a risk assessment framework. Such a framework is not one that committee members would naturally have been familiar with at the outset, and some readers of this report may also wonder, "What is that?" The process is discussed and diagrammed in the report in Chapter 1 and referred to throughout. We were greatly helped in adhering to the risk assessment approach by Christine Taylor, Ph.D., Study Director for this DRI study, whose previous background paper, "Framework for DRI Development,"[2] provided us with a much-needed understanding of the uses of risk assessment and the steps in conducting it that we would follow. Chris' insights, as well as her discipline, good humor, and willingness to engage over and over in discussions to obtain a broad understanding and consensus were very much at the heart of the committee's process. I thank her for being the amazing study director she has been. Our committee's work also benefited from the excellent research and support of Ann Yaktine, Ph.D., Heather Del Valle, and Heather Breiner. Linda Meyers, Ph.D., Director, Food and Nutrition Board, kept a watchful eye on our progress and willingly provided guidance as needed. The committee never lacked for exceptionally well-qualified, rigorous, hardworking, professional, and friendly support from the FNB staff, and I sincerely thank each one of them.

It may be of interest to briefly comment on the committee's approach, and how work evolved during its deliberations. The development of IOM reports is a consensus process. Thus, throughout we worked together, dividing specific tasks according to expertise but making sure that discussions proceeded and decisions were always made as a group. During this time, research did not stand still; not a week passed without new publications on these nutrients. We spent a good deal of effort, and staff performed invaluable service for us, in arraying new data, comparing aspects of study design, etc. The committee worked not only at the scheduled committee meetings, but also in a myriad of working groups by conference calls and emails. It was important to keep firmly in mind that DRIs are values meant for im-

---

[2]Taylor, C. L. 2008. Framework for DRI Development: Components "Known" and Components "To Be Explored." Washington, DC.

proving public health—the health of the *general population* of the United States and Canada. They provide recommendations for adequate and safe daily intakes of nutrients consumed over *many* years, possibly a lifetime, not just for days, weeks, months, or a year. Thus, the need for sound, causal evidence to make the evidence-based recommendations in this report was always at the forefront of our thinking and deliberations. The terms *causality, dose–response, evidence-based, totality of evidence, uncertainty, caveats* were often on the committee minds and prominent in our discussions. On some points, we consulted with experts, whom we thank for generously providing their input in response to our needs, sometimes on quite short notice. New data on the intakes of vitamin D and calcium in the United States and Canada arrived from the Centers for Disease Control and Prevention and Health Canada just as we needed them, and here I would like to thank the persons in these organizations who worked diligently to make these new intake data available for the committee's use. As DRI values evolved, we thought carefully about the implications of these recommendations for practitioners and decision makers in public health and policy who will use this report in their work, and for special populations in both the United States and Canada. Lastly, we considered research recommendations, linking our recommendations to knowledge gaps identified while using the risk assessment framework. This, of course, was a future-directed activity, and we hope that our recommendations will clarify the types of research and resulting new information that will make determining DRIs for calcium and vitamin D easier and more accurate in the future.

Throughout, the committee members worked together with common purpose and always amicably, even when viewpoints differed, and this made working on this study a remarkable experience for all of us. I sincerely thank all the members of the committee for sharing their expertise and greatly enriching the development of this report.

Finally, it is important to acknowledge the many people who assisted the committee with its work and who provided technical input and invaluable perspectives through a variety of venues ranging from white papers to participation in workshops and public information gathering meetings. Foremost, the committee is grateful to Dr. Hector DeLuca, who served as a tireless consultant and generously offered his wisdom and considerable experience to the committee. Many discussions were enriched by his input. Others who provided scientific evaluations and background information for the committee include: Dr. David Bushinsky, Dr. Thomas Carpenter, Dr. Gary Curhan, Dr. Gordon Guyatt, Dr. Craig Langman, Dr. Dwight Towler, and Dr. Susan Whiting. The committee is deeply appreciative of the heroic efforts of those who worked long hours to provide the committee timely national data on calcium and vitamin D intake as well as measures of serum 25-hydroxyvitamin D concentrations, specifically the

National Center for Health Statistics (Mr. Clifford Johnson, Dr. Lester R. Curtin, and Dr. Te-Ching Chen), the U.S. Department of Agriculture (Ms. Alanna Moshfegh and Ms. Joanne Holden), the National Cancer Institute (Dr. Kevin Dodd), and Statistics Canada (Mrs. Jeanine Bustros, Mr. Didier Garriguet, Mr. Christopher Oster, and Miss Dawn Warner). Also, invaluable and illuminating analytical assistance was provided by statisticians at Cornell University, Dr. Francoise Vermeylen and Dr. Shamil Sadigov. Finally, the committee wishes to thank the sponsors of this report for their support and without whom there would not have been the opportunity to carry out this important study.

A. Catharine Ross, *Chair*
Committee to Review Dietary Reference
Intakes for Vitamin D and Calcium

Contents

SUMMARY TABLES

*Appendixes B through K are not printed in this book, but can be found on the CD at the back of the book or online at http://www.nap.edu.

Summary

Calcium and vitamin D are undoubtedly essential nutrients for the human body. The key questions are: What processes can these nutrients affect in terms of desirable health outcomes, and how much of each nutrient is needed to achieve the effect?

During the past 10 years, there has been increasing interest in the possibility of enhanced roles for vitamin D in human health. A number of researchers in the scientific community have suggested relationships between vitamin D intake and health outcomes ranging from cancer prevention to increased immunity; others have suggested possible roles in preventing diabetes or preeclampsia during pregnancy. The media have also taken an interest, and public expectations have been raised. At the same time, physicians have been ordering blood tests that seem to suggest, based on use of criteria that have yet to be validated, that many in our North American population are vitamin D deficient. For calcium, there is concern that some may not be obtaining sufficient amounts given the foods they eat. Calcium has been increasingly added to foods, and calcium supplement use, particularly among older persons, is widespread. There is controversy concerning levels of nutrient intake, and at times the concept that "more is better" emerges. However, for both calcium and vitamin D, there is another underlying question: How much is too much?

Against this backdrop, the Institute of Medicine (IOM) was requested by the U.S. and Canadian governments to conduct a review of data pertaining to calcium and vitamin D requirements and to identify Dietary Reference Intakes (DRIs) based on current scientific evidence about the roles of calcium and vitamin D in human health. The DRIs, as nutrient reference values, are used by various stakeholders, ranging from those who set national nutrition policy to health practitioners in community settings. Such reference values specify, for normal, healthy persons, an average daily requirement for the nutrient, known as the Estimated Average Requirement (EAR). They also identify levels of intake that are likely to meet the needs of about 97.5 percent of the population (the Recommended Dietary Allowance, or RDA). Further, they include a Tolerable Upper Intake Level (UL) above which the potential for harm increases.

THE COMMITTEE AND ITS CHARGE

The two governments requested that the IOM conduct a study to assess current data and to update as appropriate the DRIs for vitamin D and calcium. The study was to include consideration of chronic disease indicators (e.g., reduction in risk of cancer or diabetes) and other (non-chronic disease) indicators/outcomes, and to assess the ability of each to serve as the basis for specifying adequate intake or excess intake. The final DRI indicators were to be selected based on the strength and quality of the evidence.

To carry out the request, the IOM established an ad hoc consensus committee of 14 scientists. The committee met eight times, held a public workshop and open sessions to gather information and receive input on the nature of the available data, maintained a website that accepted comments and data from stakeholders, conducted a review of existing data, and developed a report that included the specification of DRI values. Committee members had expertise in the areas of vitamin D and calcium or a related topic area, with specific expertise related to pregnancy and reproductive nutrition, pediatrics and infant nutrition, minority health and health disparities, cellular metabolism, toxicology and risk assessment, dermatology, immunology, endocrinology, skeletal health, oncology, cardiovascular health, epidemiology; nutrition monitoring, and biostatistics. Three members of the committee had served on other DRI committees.

DRI CONTEXT FOR COMMITTEE'S WORK

This report marks the first DRI review since the completion of the 1997-2004 DRIs, which in contrast with their predecessors were based on a different approach to respond to expanded uses of the values and newer understandings of the role of nutrients. The DRIs now incorporate the statistical concept of a distribution, including the distributions of requirements and intakes. The major components of the DRIs are shown in Box S-1.

The first DRIs, contained in six volumes, are now used in both the United States and Canada. The governments of these two countries have

> ## BOX S-1
> ## Dietary Reference Intake Components*
>
> *Estimated Average Requirement (EAR):* Reflects the estimated median requirement and is particularly appropriate for applications related to planning and assessing intakes for groups of persons.
>
> *Recommended Dietary Allowance (RDA):* Derived from the EAR and meets or exceeds the requirement for 97.5 percent of the population.
>
> *Tolerable Upper Intake Level (UL):* As intake increases above the UL, the potential risk of adverse effects may increase. The UL is the highest average daily intake that is likely to pose no risk of adverse effects to almost all individuals in the general population.
>
> *Adequate Intake (AI):* Used when an EAR/RDA cannot be developed; average intake level based on observed or experimental intakes.
>
> ---
>
> *Also, Acceptable Macronutrient Distribution Range (AMDR): An intake range for an energy source associated with reduced risk of chronic disease.

also supported a recent evaluation of the DRI development process, which has informed the approach used to develop this report. The evaluation pointed to the need for enhanced "transparency" about the decisions made, more clarification about uncertainties in the values, and use of a risk assessment framework to organize the scientific assessments. Risk assessment encompasses a series of decision steps and anticipates the need to address uncertainties through documentation and the use of expert judgment.

THE COMMITTEE'S APPROACH AND
EXAMINATION OF DATA

To set the stage for its review, the committee gathered background information on the metabolism and physiology of calcium and vitamin D (Chapters 2 and 3). It then identified those relationships that could potentially serve as indicators for establishing nutrient reference values for adequate intakes of the nutrients. To ensure comprehensiveness, the committee included relationships that appeared marginal by standard scientific principles as well as those suggested to be of interest by stakeholders. Box S-2 lists these potential indicators in alphabetical order. The close inter-relationship between calcium and vitamin D often resulted in potential indicators being relevant to both nutrients.

Chapter 4 provides the committee's review of potential indicators,

BOX S-2
Potential Indicators of Health Outcomes for Nutrient
Adequacy for Calcium and Vitamin D

Cancer/neoplasms
- All cancers
- Breast cancer
- Colorectal cancer/colon polyps
- Prostate cancer

Cardiovascular diseases and hypertension
Diabetes (type 2) and metabolic syndrome (obesity)
Falls
Immune responses
- Asthma
- Autoimmune disease
  - Diabetes (type 1)
  - Inflammatory bowel and Crohn's disease
  - Multiple sclerosis
  - Rheumatoid arthritis
  - Systemic lupus erythematosus
- Infectious diseases
  - Tuberculosis
  - Influenza/upper respiratory infections

Neuropsychological functioning
- Autism
- Cognitive function
- Depression

Physical performance*
Preeclampsia of pregnancy and other non-skeletal reproductive outcomes
Skeletal health (commonly bone health)
- Serum 25-hydroxyvitamin D, as intermediate
- Parathyroid hormone, as intermediate
- Calcium absorption
- Calcium balance
- Bone mineral content/bone mineral density
- Fracture risk
- Rickets/osteomalacia

---

*In the discussions related to review of potential indicators, physical performance is considered together with falls.

based on literature identified by the committee and incorporating the systematic evidence-based reviews from the Agency for Healthcare Research and Quality (AHRQ). In sum, with the exception of measures related to bone health, the potential indicators examined are currently not supported by evidence that could be judged either convincing or adequate in terms of cause and effect, or informative regarding dose–response relationships for determining nutrient requirements. Outcomes related to cancer/neoplasms, cardiovascular disease and hypertension, diabetes and metabolic syndrome, falls and physical performance, immune functioning and autoimmune disorders, infections, neuropsychological functioning, and preeclampsia could not be linked reliably with calcium or vitamin D intake and were often conflicting. Although data related to cancer risk and vitamin D are potentially of interest, a relationship between cancer incidence and vitamin D (or calcium) nutriture is not adequately and causally demonstrated at present; indeed, for some cancers, there appears to be an increase in incidence associated with higher serum 25-hydroxyvitamin D (25OHD) concentrations or higher vitamin D intake. The role of vitamin D related to falls and physical performance, cardiovascular disease, autoimmune disorders, and immune functioning has also received considerable attention, and remains unresolved. These potential roles of vitamin D are currently best described as hypotheses of emerging interest, and the conflicting nature of available evidence cannot be used to establish health benefits with any level of confidence. In contrast, the evidence surrounding bone health provides a reasonable and supportable basis to allow this indicator to be used for DRI development.

In making its conclusions about potential indicators other than bone health, the committee noted the observation previously highlighted by others tasked with examining the evolution of evidence for nutrient and disease relationships: that evidence about relationships between specific nutrients and a disease or health outcome remains typically elusive, for a number of reasons. These include the difficulty of isolating the effects of a single nutrient under investigation from the confounding effects of other nutrients and non-nutrient factors; the multi-factorial etiology of the chronic diseases the committee considered; the paucity of data from randomized controlled clinical trials, which typically provide the highest level of scientific evidence relevant for DRI development; and the mixed and inconclusive results from observational studies.

For indicators associated with excess intakes of calcium and vitamin D, a process similar to that for reference values for adequacy was undertaken and potential indicators of excess intake were identified (see Box S-3). The ULs serve as a measure for chronic intake of a free-living, unmonitored population. They are not specified for clinical research; it may be appro-

---

BOX S-3
Potential Indicators of Adverse Outcomes for
Excess Intake of Calcium and Vitamin D

Calcium
- Hypercalcemia
- Hypercalciuria
- Vascular and soft tissue calcification
- Nephrolithiasis (kidney stones)
- Prostate cancer
- Interactions with iron and zinc
- Constipation

Vitamin D
- Intoxication and related hypercalcemia and hypercalciuria
- Serum calcium
- Measures in infants: retarded growth, hypercalcemia
- Emerging evidence for all-cause mortality, cancer, cardiovascular risk, falls and fractures

---

priate to conduct clinical research with doses exceeding the UL, as long as there is monitoring and the protocol is carefully considered.

KEY CHALLENGES

Beyond the challenge of limited data and the resulting uncertainties, the study faced two additional challenges. The first is that vitamin D, an essential nutrient, is also synthesized in the skin following exposure to sunlight. Thus, the examination of data is complicated by the confounding factors this introduces. Further, vitamin D requirements could not address the level of sun exposure because public health concerns about skin cancer preclude this possibility. There have not been studies to determine whether ultraviolet B (UVB)–induced vitamin D synthesis can occur without increased risk of skin cancer. The best approach was to estimate vitamin D requirements under conditions of minimal sun exposure.

Second, vitamin D when activated functions as a hormone and is regulated by metabolic feedback loops. The intertwining of the effects of vitamin D and calcium represents an extreme case of nutrient–nutrient inter-relationships. Indeed, many studies administered these nutrients together rather than separately. For this reason, distinguishing the health outcomes for one nutrient versus the other was challenging.

THE COMMITTEE'S OUTCOMES

An assumption in developing the DRIs for calcium is that they are predicated on intakes that meet requirements for vitamin D; similarly, DRIs for vitamin D rest on the assumption of intakes that meet requirements for calcium.

Dietary Reference Intakes for Calcium

DRIs for calcium were established as EARs and RDAs except for infants up to 12 months of age for whom AIs were specified. The DRIs for calcium are shown in Table S-1.

TABLE S-1 Calcium Dietary Reference Intakes by Life Stage (amount/day)

Life Stage Group	AI	EAR	RDA	UL
Infants				
0 to 6 mo	200 mg	—	—	1,000 mg
6 to 12 mo	260 mg	—	—	1,500 mg
Children				
1–3 y	—	500 mg	700 mg	2,500 mg
4–8 y	—	800 mg	1,000 mg	2,500 mg
Males				
9–13 y	—	1,100 mg	1,300 mg	3,000 mg
14–18 y	—	1,100 mg	1,300 mg	3,000 mg
19–30 y	—	800 mg	1,000 mg	2,500 mg
31–50 y	—	800 mg	1,000 mg	2,500 mg
51–70 y	—	800 mg	1,000 mg	2,000 mg
> 70 y	—	1,000 mg	1,200 mg	2,000 mg
Females				
9–13 y	—	1,100 mg	1,300 mg	3,000 mg
14–18 y	—	1,100 mg	1,300 mg	3,000 mg
19–30 y	—	800 mg	1,000 mg	2,500 mg
31–50 y	—	800 mg	1,000 mg	2,500 mg
51–70 y	—	1,000 mg	1,200 mg	2,000 mg
> 70 y	—	1,000 mg	1,200 mg	2,000 mg
Pregnancy				
14–18 y	—	1,100 mg	1,300 mg	3,000 mg
19–30 y	—	800 mg	1,000 mg	2,500 mg
31–50 y	—	800 mg	1,000 mg	2,500 mg
Lactation				
14–18 y	—	1,100 mg	1,300 mg	3,000 mg
19–30 y	—	800 mg	1,000 mg	2,500 mg
31–50 y	—	800 mg	1,000 mg	2,500 mg

NOTE: AI = Adequate Intake; EAR = Estimated Average Requirement; RDA = Recommended Dietary Allowance; UL = Tolerable Upper Intake Level.

The EARs and RDAs relied primarily upon calcium balance studies for persons 1 to 50 years of age. The effect of menopause on bone resulted in specifying different EARs and RDAs for women and men 51 to 70 years of age. After the age of 70 years, the effects of aging on bone loss resulted in EARs and RDAs that are the same for men and women. The AIs for infants are based on the calcium content of human milk. There is no evidence that calcium requirements are different for pregnant and lactating females compared with their non-pregnant or non-lactating counterparts.

The ULs for calcium for adults are based on data related to the incidence of kidney stones, largely from work conducted with postmenopausal women who use calcium supplements. Newer data from a feeding study provided evidence of intake levels among infants not associated with elevated calcium excretion, and allowed derivation of a UL for infants. The UL for children and adolescents 9 to 18 years of age gives consideration to the pubertal growth spurt and increases the UL as compared with that for children 1 to 8 years of age.

Dietary Reference Intakes for Vitamin D

DRI values for vitamin D (Table S-2) were established as EARs and RDAs for all life stage groups except infants up to 12 months of age for which an AI was specified. These reference values assume minimal sun exposure.

Measures of serum 25OHD level serve as a reflection of total vitamin D exposure—from food, supplements, and synthesis. Although serum 25OHD level cannot be considered a validated health outcome surrogate, it allowed comparison of intake or exposure with health outcomes. Newer data also allowed the simulation of a requirement distribution based on serum 25OHD concentrations. A level of 40 nmol/L (16 ng/mL) was consistent with the intended nature of an average requirement, in that it reflects the desired level for a population median—it meets the needs of approximately half the population. Moreover, benefit for most in the population is associated with serum 25OHD levels of approximately 50 nmol/L (20 ng/mL), making this level a reasonable estimate for a value akin to "coverage" for nearly all the population. Available data were used to link specified serum levels of 25OHD with total intakes of vitamin D under conditions of minimal sun exposure in order to estimate DRIs.

For children and adolescents 1 to 18 years of age, EARs and RDAs are specified on the basis of serum 25OHD concentrations of 40 and 50 nmol/L (16 and 20 ng/mL), respectively. Likewise this approach was used for young adults and adults from 19 through 50 years of age and was supported by data on osteomalacia. The EAR for persons older than 50 years of age is the same as that for younger adults, as the simulated requirement

TABLE S-2 Vitamin D Dietary Reference Intakes by Life Stage (amount/day)

Life Stage Group	AI	EAR	RDA	UL
Infants				
0 to 6 mo	400 IU (10 µg)	—	—	1,000 IU (25 µg)
6 to 12 mo	400 IU (10 µg)	—	—	1,500 IU (38 µg)
Children				
1–3 y	—	400 IU (10 µg)	600 IU (15 µg)	2,500 IU (63 µg)
4–8 y	—	400 IU (10 µg)	600 IU (15 µg)	3,000 IU (75 µg)
Males				
9–13 y	—	400 IU (10 µg)	600 IU (15 µg)	4,000 IU (100 µg)
14–18 y	—	400 IU (10 µg)	600 IU (15 µg)	4,000 IU (100 µg)
19–30 y	—	400 IU (10 µg)	600 IU (15 µg)	4,000 IU (100 µg)
31–50 y	—	400 IU (10 µg)	600 IU (15 µg)	4,000 IU (100 µg)
51–70 y	—	400 IU (10 µg)	600 IU (15 µg)	4,000 IU (100 µg)
> 70 y	—	400 IU (10 µg)	800 IU (20 µg)	4,000 IU (100 µg)
Females				
9–13 y	—	400 IU (10 µg)	600 IU (15 µg)	4,000 IU (100 µg)
14–18 y	—	400 IU (10 µg)	600 IU (15 µg)	4,000 IU (100 µg)
19–30 y	—	400 IU (10 µg)	600 IU (15 µg)	4,000 IU (100 µg)
31–50 y	—	400 IU (10 µg)	600 IU (15 µg)	4,000 IU (100 µg)
51–70 y	—	400 IU (10 µg)	600 IU (15 µg)	4,000 IU (100 µg)
> 70 y	—	400 IU (10 µg)	800 IU (20 µg)	4,000 IU (100 µg)
Pregnancy				
14–18 y	—	400 IU (10 µg)	600 IU (15 µg)	4,000 IU (100 µg)
19–30 y	—	400 IU (10 µg)	600 IU (15 µg)	4,000 IU (100 µg)
31–50 y	—	400 IU (10 µg)	600 IU (15 µg)	4,000 IU (100 µg)
Lactation				
14–18 y	—	400 IU (10 µg)	600 IU (15 µg)	4,000 IU (100 µg)
19–30 y	—	400 IU (10 µg)	600 IU (15 µg)	4,000 IU (100 µg)
31–50 y	—	400 IU (10 µg)	600 IU (15 µg)	4,000 IU (100 µg)

NOTE: AI = Adequate Intake; EAR = Estimated Average Requirement; IU = International Units; RDA = Recommended Dietary Allowance; UL = Tolerable Upper Intake Level.

distribution suggested no effect due to age. However, there is notable variability around these estimates in the case of bone health for older persons. This suggests that the assumption about the variance associated with coverage for 97.5 percent of the population should be greater for this older group than for the younger group. Therefore, the RDA value for persons older than 70 years of age was increased to a level greater than the two standard deviations used for other groups. In fact, available data provide more information about maximal population coverage than they do about average requirements for these life stage groups. The factors taken into account included changes in bone density and fracture risk. For infants, an AI was established based on evidence that maintaining serum 25OHD levels in the range of 40 to 50 nmol/L (16 to 20 ng/mL) was desirable, coupled with observational data suggesting that 400 International Units (IU) (10 µg) per day was adequate to maintain this level.

The ULs for vitamin D were especially challenging because available data have focused on very high levels of intake that cause intoxication and little is known about the effects of chronic excess intake at lower levels. The committee examined the existing data and followed an approach that would maximize public health protection. The observation that 10,000 IU (250 µg) of vitamin D per day was not associated with classic toxicity served as the starting point for adults; this value was corrected for uncertainty by taking into consideration emerging data on adverse outcomes (e.g., all-cause mortality), which appeared to present at intakes lower than those associated with classic toxicity and at serum 25OHD concentrations previously considered to be at the high end of physiological values. Possible ethnic/racial differences were taken into account as well. The UL for adults is used for 9 to 18 years olds, but is "scaled down" for children 1 to 8 years of age. Earlier studies remain the best basis for ULs for infants.

DIETARY INTAKE ASSESSMENT

Calcium remains a nutrient of concern given that median calcium intakes from foods in both the United States and Canada are close to the EAR values for most groups. In particular, girls 9 to 18 years of age are falling below desirable intakes when only food sources of calcium are considered, as are women over the age of 50 years. Available data from the United States on the total intake of calcium when dietary supplements are considered suggest that older women have noticeably increased calcium intakes with supplement. For girls, the increase in intake attributable to supplement use is small. No life stage groups exceeded the UL for calcium when foods alone were considered. However, when supplement use was taken into account (United States only), women at the 95th percentile of calcium intake appeared to be at risk for exceeding the UL. The data underscore the possible need to modestly increase calcium intake among older girls; among older women, a high calcium intake from supplements may be concerning.

Although daily median vitamin D intake from foods in both countries for all life stage groups was below the established reference value, these data should be considered in light of the average serum 25OHD concentrations. U.S. serum 25OHD concentrations on average were well above 40 nmol/L (16 ng/mL), the level established as consistent with an intake equivalent to the EAR; in fact, all mean serum 25OHD concentrations were above 50 nmol/L (20 ng/mL). In the case of serum 25OHD concentrations from Canadian surveys, mean serum 25OHD levels for all life stage groups were at or above 60 nmol/L (24 ng/mL). The fact that these values are higher for the Canadian than for the U.S. population may be in part due to differences in assay methodologies used.

IMPLICATIONS AND SPECIAL CONCERNS

The final risk assessment step is risk characterization, which highlights implications of the DRI outcomes and special concerns including the population segments shown in Box S-4. The nature and extent of the risk associated with these population segments vary.

Uncertainties

On balance, the uncertainties surrounding the DRI values for calcium are less than those for vitamin D because the evidence base is considerably larger for calcium, and the physiology and metabolism of calcium are better understood. The following key issues were identified as introducing uncertainty into DRI values for calcium and vitamin D, as based on bone health outcomes:

- The tendency for study protocols to administer a combination of calcium and vitamin D, reducing the opportunity to ascertain effects of each nutrient independently;
- The lack of data examining the responses and health outcomes

---

BOX S-4
Population Segments and Conditions of Interest

Adiposity
Persons living at upper latitudes in North America
Persons who experience reduced vitamin D synthesis from sun exposure
- Dark skin (including immigrant groups and exclusively breast-fed infants)
- Use of sunscreen
- Indoor environments and institutionalized older persons
Alternative diets or changes in dietary patterns
- Dairy and animal product exclusion
- Changes in dietary patterns of indigenous Canadian populations
Use of calcium supplements
Oral contraceptive use
Premature infants
Interaction between vitamin D and prescription drugs

---

from graded doses of calcium or vitamin D intake so as to elucidate dose–response relationships;

- The interaction between calcium and vitamin D to the extent that it would appear that adequate calcium intake greatly diminishes the need for vitamin D relative to bone health outcomes;
- The unique situation in which a nutrient (vitamin D) is physiologically managed by the body as a hormone, introducing a myriad of variables and feedback loops related to its health effects;
- The paucity of data and resulting uncertainty concerning sun exposure, which confounds the interpretation of dose–response data for intakes of vitamin D. This, coupled with the apparent contribution of sun exposure to overall vitamin D nutriture in North American populations, leads to an inability to characterize and integrate sun exposure with dietary intake recommendations as much as may be appropriate, given the concern for skin cancer risk reduction. Thus, for individuals who experience sun exposure, the uncertainty of the DRI is greater than for those who do not;
- The lack of clarity concerning the validity of the serum 25OHD measure as a biomarker of effect;
- The variability surrounding measures of serum 25OHD concentrations owing to different methodologies used;
- The evidence of the non-linear nature of the relationship between serum 25OHD concentrations and total intake of vitamin D, suggesting that lower levels of intake have more impact on serum 25OHD concentrations than previously believed and that higher intakes may have less impact;
- The limited number of long-term clinical trials related to calcium and vitamin D intake and health outcomes; and
- The need to set ULs based on limited data in order to ensure public health protection.

For vitamin D, the challenges introduced by issues of sun exposure are notable. This nutrient is unique in that it functions as a hormone and the body has the capacity to synthesize it. However, concerns about skin cancer risk preclude incorporating the effects of sun exposure in the DRI process. At this time, the only solution is to proceed on the basis of the assumption of minimal sun exposure and set reference values assuming that all of the vitamin D comes from the diet. This is a markedly cautious approach given that the vast majority of North Americans obtain at least some vitamin D from inadvertent or intentional sun exposure. Therefore, the estimated intake data for vitamin D cannot stand alone as a basis for broad public health action. Rather, national policy should consider intake data in the context of measures of serum 25OHD, a well-established biomarker of total vitamin D exposure (endogenous synthesis and diet including supplements). Although estimates of vitamin D intake appear to be less than needed to meet requirements, the serum 25OHD data available—when coupled with the committee's assessment of serum 25OHD levels consistent with EAR and RDA values—suggest that requirements are being met for most if not all persons in both countries. Moreover, the possibility of risk for subpopulations of concern due to reduced synthesis of vitamin D, such as persons with dark skin or older persons in institutions, is minimized given the assumption of minimal sun exposure as a basis for the DRIs.

CONCLUSIONS ABOUT VITAMIN D DEFICIENCY IN THE UNITED STATES AND CANADA

Serum levels of 25OHD have been used as a measure of adequacy for vitamin D, as they reflect intake from the diet coupled with the amount contributed by cutaneous synthesis. The cut-point levels of serum 25OHD intended to specify deficiency for the purposes of interpreting laboratory analyses and for use in clinical practice are not specifically within the charge to this committee. However, the committee noted with some concern that serum 25OHD cut-points defined as indicative of deficiency for vitamin D have not undergone a systematic, evidence-based development process.

From this committee's perspective, a considerable over-estimation of the levels of vitamin D deficiency in the North American population now exists due to the use by some of cut-points for serum 25OHD levels that greatly exceed the levels identified in this report as consistent with the available data. Early reports specified a serum 25OHD concentration of at least 27.5 nmol/L (11 ng/mL) as an indicator of vitamin D adequacy from birth through 18 years of age, and a concentration of at least 30 nmol/L (12 ng/mL) as an indicator of vitamin D adequacy for adults 19 to 50 years of age. In recent years, others have suggested different cut-points as determinants of deficiency and what has been termed "insufficiency." In the current literature, these include values ranging from less than 50 nmol/L (20 ng/mL) to values above 125 nmol/L (50 ng/mL). Use of higher than appropriate cut-points for serum 25OHD levels would be expected to artificially increase the estimates of the prevalence of vitamin D deficiency.

The specification of cut-points for serum 25OHD levels has serious ramifications not only for the conclusions about vitamin D nutriture and nutrition public policy, but also for clinical practice. At this time, there is no central body that is responsible for establishing such values for clinical use. This committee's review of data suggests that persons are at risk of deficiency relative to bone health at serum 25OHD levels of below 30 nmol/L (12 ng/mL). Some, but not all, persons are potentially at risk for inadequacy at serum 25OHD levels between 30 and 50 nmol/L (12 and 20 ng/mL). Practically all persons are sufficient at serum 25OHD levels of at least 50 nmol/L (20 ng/mL). Serum 25OHD concentrations above 75 nmol/L (30 ng/mL) are not consistently associated with increased benefit. There may be reason for concern at serum 25OHD levels above 125 nmol/L (50 ng/mL). Given the concern about high levels of serum 25OHD as well as the desirability of avoiding mis-classification of vitamin D deficiency, there is a critical public health and clinical practice need for consensus cut-points for serum 25OHD measures relative to vitamin D deficiency as well as excess. The current lack of evidence-based consensus guidelines is problematic and of concern because individuals with serum 25OHD levels above 50 nmol/L (20 ng/mL) may at times be classified as deficient and treated with high-dose supplements of vitamin D containing many times the levels of intake recommended by this report.

Closing Remarks

At this time, the scientific data available indicate a key role for calcium and vitamin D in skeletal health and provide a sound basis for DRIs. The data do not, however, provide compelling evidence that either nutrient is causally related to extra-skeletal health outcomes or that intakes greater than those established in the DRI process have benefits for health. The last chapter of this report specifies the research needs and reflects an urgent and worthwhile agenda. If carried out, this research will assist greatly in clarifying DRIs for vitamin D and calcium in the future.

1

Introduction

For more than half a century, specification of the quantities of nutri-ents needed to meet human requirements—dietary reference values—has been carried out at the national level in the United States and Canada. Reference values known in the United States as Recommended Dietary Allowances (RDAs) and in Canada as Recommended Nutrient Intakes (RNIs) were used well into the 1990s (IOM, 2008). They were established primarily to set nutrition and health policy (IOM, 2008) and have found broad application in government programs ranging from standards for school meals to the basis for food fortification. They have also been used to counsel individuals about dietary intake. Over the years, both govern-ments have funded on-going updates and reviews of these reference values.

In 1994, in response to important changes in the nutrition field as well as the recognition that for many nutrients the single-value RDA or RNI did not meet the expanding needs for nutrient reference values, the Institute of Medicine (IOM) in Washington, DC, began an initiative to develop a new, broader set of values known as the Dietary Reference Intakes or DRIs (IOM, 2008). The U.S. and Canadian governments have jointly supported this initiative, and the resulting DRIs are now used in both countries. As a result of the initiative, the DRIs as reference values now

- Include an estimate of an average (or median) requirement as well as an estimate of an intake level that meets, and in turn exceeds, the needs of most (97.5 percent) of the population;
- Include upper levels of intake to ensure no harm from nutrient intake;

- Incorporate chronic disease indicators when the data allow; and
- Highlight concepts of probability and risk for defining reference values.

With this new model as a backdrop, the IOM in 1997 issued the first set of DRIs. The nutrients included in the first of what became a series of DRI reports were: calcium, phosphorus, magnesium, vitamin D, and fluoride (IOM, 1997). Therefore, the 1997 DRIs for calcium and vitamin D—the nutrients that are the topic of this 2010 review—have been in existence for 13 years. In 2008, the U.S. and Canadian governments made the decision that there were now sufficient new data to warrant funding another study of the DRIs for vitamin D (Yetley et al., 2009). They included calcium in this study because of its close inter-relationship with vitamin D. A 14-member ad hoc expert committee was convened by the IOM in 2009 to take on this task; its work was to be completed by 2010. Committee members had general expertise in the areas of vitamin D and calcium or a closely related topic area, with specific expertise related to endocrinology, bone and skeletal health, immunology, oncology, dermatology, cardiovascular health, pregnancy and reproductive nutrition, pediatrics and infant nutrition, epidemiology, cellular metabolism, toxicology and risk assessment, nutrition monitoring, biostatistics, and minority health and health disparities. Three members of the committee had served on other DRI committees.

The current consideration of the DRIs for vitamin D and calcium takes place at a time when the interest in vitamin D is enormous. This vitamin—with its hormone-related activities—has received much media attention and has been the subject of countless publications and lay press reporting of its benefits for an array of health outcomes. Concerns about widespread vitamin D deficiency in North American populations are often expressed. This committee's focus was, first, to review objectively the existing evidence concerning the benefits and health outcomes associated with vitamin D as well as calcium, using the well-established scientific principles for judging the quality and relevance of data from intervention as well as observational studies. The members of the committee next integrated the available data and, within the context of the risk assessment approach for establishing DRIs, carried out activities to specify DRIs for calcium and vitamin D. The reference values established in 1997 were noted by the committee, but they were not binding on the committee's work.

THE TASK

The charge to the committee was to assess current relevant data and update, as appropriate, the DRIs for vitamin D and calcium. The review was to include consideration of chronic disease indicators (e.g., reduction in risk of cancer) and other (non-chronic disease) indicators and health outcomes. The definitions of these terms are discussed below. Consistent with the framework for DRI development, the indicators to assess adequacy and excess intake were to be selected based on the strength and quality of the evidence and their demonstrated public health significance, taking into consideration sources of uncertainty in the evidence. Further, the committee deliberations were to incorporate, as appropriate, systematic evidence-based reviews of the literature.

Specifically, in carrying out its work, the committee was to:

- Review evidence on indicators to assess adequacy and indicators to assess excess intake relevant to the general North American population, including groups whose needs for or sensitivity to the nutrient may be affected by particular conditions that are widespread in the population such as obesity or age-related chronic diseases. Special groups under medical care whose needs or sensitivities are affected by rare genetic disorders or diseases and their treatments were to be excluded;
- Consider systematic evidence-based reviews, including those made available by the sponsors as well as others, and carefully document the approach used by the committee to carry out any of its own literature reviews;
- Regarding selection of indicators upon which to base DRI values for adequate intake, give priority to selecting indicators relevant to the various age, gender, and life stage groups that will allow for the determination of an Estimated Average Requirement (EAR);
- Regarding selection of indicators upon which to base DRI values for upper levels of intake, give priority to examining whether a critical adverse effect can be selected that will allow for the determination of a so-called benchmark intake;
- Update DRI values, as appropriate, using a risk assessment approach that includes (1) identification of potential indicators to assess adequacy and excess intake, (2) selection of the indicators of adequacy and excess intake, (3) intake-response assessment, (4) dietary intake assessment, and (5) risk characterization.
- Identify research gaps to address the uncertainties identified in the process of deriving the reference values and evaluating their public health implications.

THE DIETARY REFERENCE INTAKE FRAMEWORK

The framework for DRI development has been described by others (IOM, 2006, 2008; Taylor, 2008) and will be outlined here to set the context for this report. The original framework for DRIs was put in place in 1994 (IOM, 1994), and the reviews of nutrients were completed in 2004. During the 4-year period between 2004 and 2008, it was the subject of discussions concerning its needed improvements as well as it successes (IOM, 2008). The present DRI effort described in this report for vitamin D and calcium is the first to be issued since the 2004 to 2008 evaluative discussions.

In developing and enhancing the DRI framework, two goals were identified. The first is that the framework should ensure and foster transparency of the decision-making process. The second goal is that the framework should anticipate the need to make decisions in the face of limited data and, in turn, offer options for making scientific judgments. Scientific judgment in the face of limited data is important, given the interest in protecting public health and the reality that "no decision is not an option"—that is, a science-based judgment is more useful than no recommendation at all. In other words, the framework must operate under conditions of uncertainty.

The framework that has evolved for DRI development is increasingly recognized as akin to that developed in other fields and referred to as *risk assessment*. Risk assessment is a component of risk analysis, a process for managing situations where public health interventions and monitoring come into play. It analyzes and controls the "risks" that may be experienced by a population of interest (Taylor, 2008). In the case of DRI development, the "risk" is nutrient intakes that are too low or too high. Although the terminology associated with the discipline of risk analysis may at times be unfamiliar to those in the nutrition field, the discipline's structure and application are a good match for DRI development (Taylor, 2008).

Risk analysis, as considered generically for all fields of study, typically is described as including three components: risk assessment, risk management, and risk communication. These are often illustrated as overlapping circles. The component known as *risk assessment* has received attention as an organizing scheme for the DRI study committee review process, and is described separately in a section below. Overall, however, the basic assumptions underlying all of risk analysis are relevant to DRI development. At its most basic, risk analysis is predicated on the assumption that *scientific deliberations should be organized in a manner that meets user/sponsor needs while maintaining the scientific integrity of the assessment* (NRC, 1983). Further, the following general assumptions of risk analysis relate directly to the overall development of DRIs, particularly concerning scientific judgments when uncertainties and limited data exist (Taylor, 2008):

- *Failure to provide a reference value ("no decision") is often not a viable option from the perspective of protecting public health.* It is better to offer those operating in the public health arena an informed decision based on the best available scientific expertise and judgment, even if not perfect or very precise, than to offer no information, which by default provides no guidance for evaluating or dealing with the current situation.

- *Available datasets are often incomplete*, and scientific uncertainties must be dealt with through use of scientific judgment and judicious, transparent documentation.
- Meeting the scientific needs of users/sponsors requires a framework for ensuring *understanding of the needs* and a *useful presentation* of the scientific assessments, as well as the *independence* of the scientific evaluations and protection of the scientific reviewers from undue stakeholder influence.

Finally, the DRI framework recognizes the considerable utility in organizing and rating the available data through the use of systematic reviews (Taylor, 2008; Russell et al., 2009), which are now a well-established process in many fields of medicine. However, unlike a systematic review of a medical intervention, a systematic review for the relationship between nutrient intake and a health outcome is much broader. In contrast with focused clinical interventions, most nutrients have direct and indirect effects on a wide range of health outcomes and could potentially reduce the risk of chronic diseases. In turn, the breadth of outcomes—and thus research that needs to be assessed—is greater than that for a medical intervention; as a result, considerable care is required in formulating and prioritizing the key questions to be addressed (Chung et al., 2010).

Definition of Dietary Reference Intakes

The DRIs are comprised of several reference values that relate to the concept of a distribution of requirements and a distribution of intakes. These different values are tools for assessing and planning diets and are most applicable for use with groups of people because the exact nutritional requirements of an individual cannot be known. The application of DRI nutrient reference values for these general purposes is wide and diverse. They range from use by federal government agencies in making national nutrition policy or developing federal nutrition and food assistance programs, to work at the local level in assessing diets of groups and individuals. Public health protection and promotion is the common interest. Further, DRIs address nutrients in foods overall. Because people structure diets primarily by selecting individual foods as opposed to selecting a set of nutrients, an important role of government and related advisory groups has been the task of translating quantitative nutrient reference values into food-based recommendations for the generally healthy U.S. and Canadian populations. That was not the task of this committee for whom the focus has been the quantitative nutrient requirements and upper levels of intake.

Currently, the mainstays of DRI development are the EAR, and the Tolerable Upper Intake Level, or UL (also referred to at times as Upper Levels of Intake). The RDA is to be derived from the EAR and reflects an estimate of an intake that meets the needs of 97.5 percent of the population's requirements. It is not a target intended to be met by all individuals, and intakes below the RDA cannot be assumed to be inadequate because the RDA by definition exceeds the actual requirements of all but 2 to 3 percent of the population. The Adequate Intake (AI) was originally incorporated into the framework to address the inevitable uncertainties associated with specifying requirements for infants, given the challenges in obtaining sufficient information for this group, but has expanded to include use when available data for any life stage group are too limited to establish a requirement. The AI is the subject of some debate, given that it does not appear to readily "fit" into the probability assumptions for DRI use (Taylor, 2008). There are also other reference values, as described in other IOM documents (IOM, 2006), but as these are not relevant to this report, they are not described here.

Estimated Average Requirement

The EAR is the average daily nutrient intake level that is estimated to meet the nutrient needs of half of the healthy individuals in a life stage or gender group. Although the term "average" is used, the EAR is actually an estimated *median* requirement (IOM, 2006). Therefore, by definition, the EAR exceeds the needs of half of the population and is less than the needs of the other half (Taylor, 2008).

The 1994 to 2004 DRI process placed emphasis on the distribution of requirements for a population, rather than focusing on a single value constructed to "cover" the great majority of the population, as had been the case in earlier efforts (Taylor, 2008). This, along with the development of newer methodologies for assessing and planning adequate intakes for groups, made the EAR a central reference value, along with the UL. The 10 years of DRI development moved the process from a black-and-white cutoff in the form of an RDA to consideration of a probability model. Doing so made it clear that there is a distribution of requirements in the population (Taylor, 2008).

The EAR itself presents little controversy as an expressed reference value. Beyond the question of how to handle EAR estimation in the face of limited data, most of the issues that surround EAR development are related to the uncertainty surrounding the value and ensuring appropriate discussions about the variation in requirements. A challenge lies in obtaining adequate data to allow a reasonable approximation of the variability in requirements and hence the distribution of the requirement among individuals (Taylor, 2008).

Recommended Dietary Allowance

The RDA is calculated from the EAR. It is dependent upon estimating the variance around the EAR and reflects a point estimate defined generally as two standard deviations above the EAR (Taylor, 2008). Although some refer to this reference value as "the requirement plus a safety factor," this is potentially misleading in that it underplays the importance of the variability around the median. The RDA is intended to reflect the EAR plus two standard deviations.

This RDA calculation starts with the assumption that the distribution of a nutrient requirement is generally normal. However, this is not the case for a number of nutrients. There is also the need to describe the variance around the EAR. Such data are usually limited; when the variance is not known, the coefficient of variation is assumed, commonly as 10 percent. There is concern expressed by some that RDAs cannot be considered to be scientifically derived because too often the variance around the EAR cannot be determined precisely from the available data, and is therefore unknown, and the assumptions made about the variance may be inappropriate (Taylor, 2008).

The estimation of the RDA results in a value that is above the intake required for about 97.5 percent of the population. The RDA thus exceeds the requirements of nearly all members of the life stage group. Current guidance (IOM, 2000a, 2003) stipulates that the RDA is useful for some applications with individuals, but it is not appropriate when working with groups of persons for the purposes of assessing and planning for nutrient intake (Taylor, 2008).

Adequate Intake

The possibility of the AI—except for reference values for infants—was not considered when the DRI framework was first developed in 1994 (IOM, 2008). The AIs emerged as a result of the deliberations of the early study committees during the implementation of the initial DRI process. When the available data were judged lacking for the purposes of estimating an EAR, an AI was set. The value was seen as filling the gap that would have existed had no value been issued (Taylor, 2008).

The AI is defined as a value based on observed or experimentally determined estimates of nutrient intake by a group of people who are apparently healthy and assumed to be maintaining an adequate nutritional state. Examples of adequate nutritional states include normal growth, maintenance of normal levels of nutrients in plasma, and other aspects of nutritional well-being or general health. The AI is obviously derived differently from the EAR/RDA, and a distribution of requirements cannot be offered.

Tolerable Upper Intake Level

As intake increases above the UL, the potential risk of adverse effects may increase; it is a level above which the risk for harm begins to increase. The UL is the highest average daily nutrient intake level likely to pose no risk of adverse health effects for nearly all people in a particular group. The need to set a UL grew out of two major trends; increased fortification of foods with nutrients and the use of dietary supplements by more people in larger doses (IOM, 2006).

The UL is not a recommended level of intake, but rather the highest intake level that can be tolerated without the possibility of causing adverse effects in most people. The value applies to chronic daily intake among free-living persons in the community (IOM, 2006). It has often been misused as a determination of levels to be allowed in controlled clinical trials. However, ULs are not defined to fit this purpose, and higher levels may be approved for controlled research purposes if there is a rationale for the levels to be used and if monitoring and other safety precautions are put in place. Rather, the UL is meant for public health protection. The biggest challenge in establishing ULs is the paucity of data indicating the effects of chronic intakes of high levels of nutrients. Experimental animal data as well as observational data are useful and relevant under these circumstances.

Applications of DRIs

The application of the DRIs in real world settings has been the subject of detailed IOM reports (IOM, 2000a, 2003). The EAR is the foundation of DRI development and is relevant to the planning and assessing of diets as they relate to population groups. The EAR is a reference value often important to the government sponsors of the report who may use requirement distributions to set national food policy, establish criteria for food programs, and make decisions about the adequacy of the food supply.

An individual's nutrient requirement cannot be readily determined, and the use of DRIs for the purposes of assessing and planning diets of individuals is challenging. If an individual's daily intake is typically below the

EAR, there is likely a need for improved intake. If daily intake is typically between the EAR and the RDA, there is probably a need for improvement because the probability of adequacy, although more than 50 percent, is less than 97.5 percent. However, intakes below the RDA cannot be assumed to be inadequate because the RDA by definition exceeds the actual requirements of all but 2 to 3 percent of the population; many with intakes below the RDA may be meeting their individual requirements (IOM, 2006).

Life Stage Groups

The DRIs are expressed on the basis of reference values for a number of different life stage groups. These life stages have been stipulated generally on the basis of variations in the requirements of all the nutrients under review. A recent IOM report (IOM, 2006) described these general groupings as follows.

Infancy

Infancy covers the first 12 months of life and is divided into two 6-month intervals. In this report infancy is designated as 0 to 6 months (meaning from birth to 5.9 months or about the first 182 days of life) and as 6 to 12 months (meaning from 6.0 months to 11.9 months or approximately the second 182 days of life). Intake is relatively constant during the first 6 months after birth. That is, as infants grow, they ingest more food; however, on a body-weight basis their intake remains the same. During the second 6 months of life, growth rate slows. As a result, total daily nutrient needs on a body-weight basis may be less than those during the first 6 months of life (IOM, 2005). In general, special consideration was not given to possible variations in physiological need during the first month after birth or to the intake variations that result from differences in milk volume and nutrient concentration during early lactation (IOM, 2005). Specific recommended intakes to meet the needs of formula-fed infants are not set as part of the DRI process.

Children: Ages 1 Through 3 Years

In terms of height, toddlers experience a faster growth rate compared with older children, and this distinction provides the biological basis for establishing separate recommended intakes for 1- to 3-year-olds compared with 4- to 8-year-olds. However, data on which to base DRIs for toddlers are often sparse; in many cases, DRIs must be derived by extrapolating data taken from the studies of infants or adults.

Children: Ages 4 Through 8 Years

During early childhood, children ages 4 through 8 or 9 years (the latter depending on the onset of puberty in each gender) undergo major changes in growth rate and endocrine status. For many nutrients, a reasonable number of data have been available on nutrient intake, and various criteria for adequacy serve as the basis for nutrient reference values for this group. For nutrients that lack data on the requirements of children in this age group, the nutrient reference values must be based on extrapolations from other life stage groups.

Children/Adolescence: Ages 9 Through 13 Years and 14 Through 18 Years

The adolescent years are divided into two categories. Several conclusions support the biological appropriateness of creating two adolescent age groups within the DRI framework (IOM, 2006):

- The mean age of onset of breast development for white girls in North America is 10 years; this is a physical marker for the beginning of increased estrogen secretion (in African American girls, onset is about a year earlier, for unknown reasons).
- The female growth spurt begins before the onset of breast development, thereby supporting the grouping of 9 through 13 years.
- The mean age of onset of testicular development in boys is 10.5 through 11 years.
- The male growth spurt begins 2 years after the start of testicular development, thereby supporting the grouping of 14 through 18 years.

Young Adulthood and Middle Age: Ages 19 Through 30 Years and 31 Through 50 Years

Adulthood was divided into two age groups, in part due to consumption of higher nutrient intakes during early adulthood compared with later in life. Mean energy expenditure decreases from ages 19 through 50 years, and nutrient needs related to energy metabolism may also decrease (IOM, 2006).

Older Adults: Ages 51 Through 70 Years and Over 70 Years

The age period of 51 through 70 years spans active work years for most adults. After age 70, people of the same age increasingly display different levels of physiological functioning and physical activity (IOM, 2000b). Age-related declines in nutrient absorption and kidney function also may occur.

Pregnancy and Lactation

Unique changes in physiology and nutrition needs occur during pregnancy and lactation. For the DRI framework, consideration is often given to the following factors:

- The needs of the fetus during pregnancy and the production of milk during lactation;
- Adaptations to increased nutrient demand, such as increased absorption and greater conservation of many nutrients; and
- Net loss of nutrients due to physiological mechanisms, regardless of intake.

Owing to the last two factors, for some nutrients there may not be a basis for setting reference values for pregnant or lactating women that differ from the values set for other women of comparable age.

Indicators for DRI Development

Indicators for DRIs are defined as the health outcomes that serve as the basis for estimating a nutrient requirement. Within the fields of biology and medicine, the term "indicators" has been defined differently and in some cases the definition may not be the same used for DRI purposes. In the case of indicators for DRIs, they can take various forms and many different indicators have been used in the more than 15 years of DRI experience (Taylor, 2008). The term in other settings encompasses what are variously referred to as *endpoints, surrogates, biomarkers,* or *risk factors.* Additionally, the term *clinical outcome,* also referred to as *health outcome,* is used to refer to the ultimate measurable effect of interest for nutrients, which is, of course, an indicator. Other measures preceding the occurrence of a clinical outcome can be predictive of the clinical outcome itself, although this is not necessarily the case and they must be validated before this can be assumed.

The term *biomarker,* like the term indicator, is defined differently within different fields of study. In the field of nutrition it is often referred to in the same way in which this report uses the term indicator. In order for them to equate, however, the biomarker must be causally related to the outcome indicator. Important terms in common parlance are *biomarker of exposure* and *biomarkers of effect.* The former is a validated measure that can be relied upon to reflect intake or exposure in the case of nutrients. A biomarker of effect is an indicator and can be relied upon to be causally related to and predictive of the health outcome of interest.

The guiding principles for selecting indicators as they are used in DRI development is that they must be feasible, valid, reproducible, sensitive, and specific (WHO, 2006). As pointed out by others (WHO, 2006), they must, however, be used intelligently and appropriately. In addition to causal association, general characteristics of indicators for DRI development include the following:

- Changes in the indicator are plausibly related to changes in the risk of an adverse health outcome.
- Changes in the indicator are usually outside the homeostatic range.
- Changes in the indicator are generally associated with adverse sequelae.
- Measurement of the indicator can be accomplished accurately and is reproducible between laboratories.

DRI Risk Assessment

Beginning in the 1990s, the process of risk assessment formally entered into DRI development as the basis for the model for establishing ULs for nutrients (IOM, 1998). However, the risk assessment organizing scheme is as applicable to the activities focused on requirements for ensuring nutritional benefit (i.e., the EAR) as it is to establishing ULs. Risk assessment reflects a flexible, objective scientific scheme for making transparent and accountable decisions, whatever the indicator of interest. It is applied across a range of disciplines and has been generically described as shown in Figure 1-1.

The word "risk" causes some in the nutrition field difficulty, in that it does not seem appropriate to link the benefits of nutrient intake to the concept of "risk," despite the ultimate purpose of reducing the risk for intakes too low to provide the health benefits (Taylor, 2008). Other risk assessment terminology may also seem inappropriate, such as the decision steps labeled as "hazard identification" and "hazard characterization," as well as the final step of "risk characterization." Nonetheless, the approach that has evolved for estimating EARs rests on a sequence of decisions that are similar to those specified within generic risk assessment (Taylor, 2008).

Given that the DRI development process couples the considerations for nutrient adequacy with those for excess intakes, there are advantages to applying the same organizing scheme for both ULs and EARs. For instance, incorporating the same general decision-making process to derive both adequate and excess intakes allows side-by-side comparisons of the process as it progresses. This could be of value in identifying unintended conse-

Key Topic Areas	Key Activities

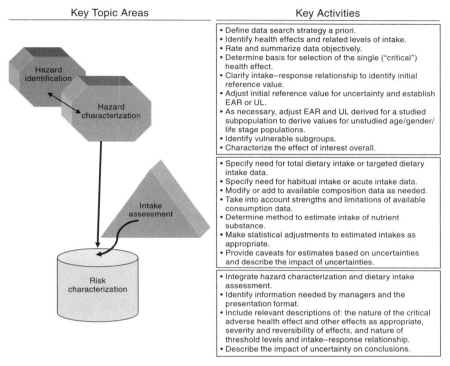

Hazard identification / Hazard characterization	• Define data search strategy a priori. • Identify health effects and related levels of intake. • Rate and summarize data objectively. • Determine basis for selection of the single ("critical") health effect. • Clarify intake–response relationship to identify initial reference value. • Adjust initial reference value for uncertainty and establish EAR or UL. • As necessary, adjust EAR and UL derived for a studied subpopulation to derive values for unstudied age/gender/ life stage populations. • Identify vulnerable subgroups. • Characterize the effect of interest overall.
Intake assessment	• Specify need for total dietary intake or targeted dietary intake data. • Specify need for habitual intake or acute intake data. • Modify or add to available composition data as needed. • Take into account strengths and limitations of available consumption data. • Determine method to estimate intake of nutrient substance. • Make statistical adjustments to estimated intakes as appropriate. • Provide caveats for estimates based on uncertainties and describe the impact of uncertainties.
Risk characterization	• Integrate hazard characterization and dietary intake assessment. • Identify information needed by managers and the presentation format. • Include relevant descriptions of: the nature of the critical adverse health effect and other effects as appropriate, severity and reversibility of effects, and nature of threshold levels and intake–response relationship. • Describe the impact of uncertainty on conclusions.

FIGURE 1-1 The four generic steps of risk assessment.
SOURCE: Modified from WHO (2006).

quences or inconsistencies among the various DRI development activities. One example is the procedures used for extrapolation relative to EAR and UL values. Study committees would likely notice potential incompatibilities if the evaluations for both adequate and excess intakes were compared in a side-by-side risk assessment framework. Additionally, as the methodological challenges in the studies used to evaluate risks are likely to be associated with both inadequate and excess intakes, a consistent framework for analyzing both is logical (Taylor, 2008).

The steps associated with risk assessment, as applied in this report on vitamin D and calcium, are briefly described below.

Step 1: "Hazard Identification" or Indicator Review and Selection

An initial starting point for this report—as for all deliberations based on risk assessment—is the identification and review of the potential indicators to be used in developing the DRIs. Based on this review, the indicators to be used are selected. As described within the DRI framework, this step of indicator identification (or hazard identification) is outlined as follows.

- **Literature reviews and interpretation** Subject-appropriate and well-done systematic evidence-based reviews as well as other relevant scientific reports and findings serve as a basis for deliberations and development of findings and recommendations for the nutrient under study. De novo literature reviews carried out as part of the study are well documented, including, but not limited to, information on search criteria, inclusion/exclusion criteria, study quality criteria, summary tables, and study relevance to the task at hand consistent with generally accepted methodology used in the systematic review process.
- **Identification of indicators to assess adequacy and excess intake** Based on results from literature reviews and information gathering activities, the evidence is examined for potential indicators related to adequacy for requirements and the effects of excess intakes of the substance of interest. Chronic disease outcomes are taken into account. The approach includes a full consideration of all relevant indicators, identified for each age, gender, and life stage group for the nutrients under study as data allow.
- **Selection of indicators to assess adequacy and excess intake** Consistent with the general approach, indicators are selected based on the strength and quality of the evidence and their demonstrated public health significance, taking into consideration sources of uncertainty in the evidence. They are in consideration of the state of the science and public health ramifications within the context of the current science. The strengths and weaknesses of the evidence for the identified indicators of adequacy and adverse effects are documented.

*Step 2: "Hazard Characterization" or Intake-Response
Assessment and Specification of Reference Values*

The intake–response (more commonly referred to as dose–response) relationships for the selected indicators of adequacy and excess are specified to the extent the available data allow. If the available information is insufficient, then appropriate statistical modeling techniques or other appropriate approaches that allow for the construction of intake-response curves from a variety of data sources are used. In some instances, most notably for the derivation of UL relative to excess intake, it is necessary to make use of specified levels or thresholds in the absence of the ability to describe a dose–response relationship, specifically a no observed effect level or a lowest observed effect level. Further, the levels of intake determined for adequacy and excess are adjusted as required, appropriate, and feasible by uncertainty factors, variance in requirements, nutrient interactions, bioavailability and bioequivalence, and scaling or extrapolation.

Step 3: Intake Assessment

Consistent with risk assessment approaches, after the reference value is established, based on the information derived from scientific studies, an assessment of the current intake of (or exposure to) the nutrient of interest is carried out in preparation for the risk characterization step. That is, the known "exposure" to the substance (or the known intake in the case of nutrients) is examined in light of the reference value established. Where information is available, an assessment of biochemical and clinical measures of nutritional status for all age, gender, and life stage groups can be a useful adjunct.

Step 4: "Risk Characterization" or Discussion of Implications and Special Concerns

Risk characterization is a hallmark of the risk assessment approach. For DRI purposes, it includes an integrated discussion of the public health implications of the DRIs and how the reference values may need to be adjusted for special vulnerable groups within the normal population. As appropriate, discussions on the certainty/uncertainty associated with the reference values are included as well as ramifications of the committee's work that the committee has identified as relevant to its risk assessment tasks.

THE APPROACH

The committee began its task in early 2009 and held a total of eight meetings through 2010. Committee members first reviewed the documents concerning the DRI framework (IOM, 2006, 2008; Taylor, 2008) so that members were well versed in the context of their work related to reference values. One of the committee's first activities was to open a website where anyone could submit data or comments to the committee concerning vitamin D and calcium. Any information that was available to the public could be considered by the committee. During its first meeting, the committee made plans for a 1-day public workshop so that information could be presented and explained to the committee, and questions asked of stakeholders.

In order to set the stage for its review, the committee gathered current background information on the metabolism of calcium and vitamin

D, including life stage differences in metabolism (Chapters 2 and 3). This information may be helpful to those less familiar with the biology and physiology of the two nutrients that are the subject of this report.

Consistent with the risk assessment approach, the committee then initiated the first step of risk assessment in Chapter 4—that is, the work to identify potential indicators. As described in Chapter 4, it reviewed the evidence related to those relationships that could potentially serve as the indicators for establishing DRIs. In order to ensure comprehensiveness, the committee included, as potential indicators, relationships that appeared marginal by standard scientific principles, as well as those suggested to be of interest by stakeholders.

An important set of analyses for the committee's work was the evidence-based reviews on vitamin D (and vitamin D in combination with calcium) carried out by the Agency for Healthcare Research and Quality (AHRQ) (Cranney et al., 2007; Chung et al., 2009). These are referred to throughout the report as AHRQ-Ottawa and AHRQ-Tufts, respectively, at times without a specific reference citation. The methods and results chapters from AHRQ-Ottawa and AHRQ-Tufts are included in their entirety in the appendix section of this report. These large, comprehensive analyses were prepared by AHRQ at the request of the U.S. and Canadian governments and were conducted independently from this committee's work. They provided valuable in-depth information on the quality of the available studies and the overall nature of the database for DRI development for vitamin D and to a lesser extent for calcium.

The AHRQ-Ottawa and AHRQ-Tufts analyses represent the current thinking on approaches to developing dietary reference values in which expansive and at times conflicting bodies of evidence must be arrayed and evaluated in as objective a manner as possible. The key to ensuring the relevance of such analyses to the DRIs as well as their rigor and objectivity is to integrate subject matter experts with methodologists at the planning stages of the systematic reviews. Although the importance of evidence synthesis in medicine was recognized in the 1970s, its widespread use has taken place more recently, especially with the concern that the judgments and opinions of experts could be inadvertently biased (Moher and Tricco, 2008). The questions identified for the analysis must be reflective of the physiological and biological issues, and the inclusion/exclusion criteria must be agreed upon and specified a priori. As described by Moher and Tricco (2008), the four main components of the relevant questions are (1) the population or problem; (2) the intervention, the independent variable, or exposure; (3) the comparators; and (4) the dependent variable or outcomes of interest. The movement to systematic reviews in the nutrition field has been the subject of discussion recently and has been called out as particularly relevant for nutrient reference value development (Russell et al., 2009). Their utility is their ability to analyze objectively the available data; their strength derives from including subject matter experts in the planning stages and in the review stages as well. The specific approach used for each of the AHRQ analyses is described in the methodologies section of each (Appendixes C and D) and includes the itemization of the questions asked for the analysis.

It is important to underscore that systematic reviews array much but not all of the data and can assist a DRI committee in identifying relevant indicators. But they do not and cannot establish nutrient reference values, nor do they replace the rigorous integration process and exercise of scientific judgment that characterizes DRI development. That process remains within the purview of the committee.

The committee actively identified other relevant studies not included in the AHRQ analyses or that were published after the close of the AHRQ analyses. These were included in the data consideration. Information from the committee's open sessions as well as the work of committee consultants was also used. In this way, a totality of the body of evidence was established and carefully examined by the committee.

At the close of the literature review process, the committee selected the best indicators to serve as the basis of the DRI values (in Chapter 4). As shown in Chapter 5, the committee then moved to Step 2 in risk assessment, which was to consider the intake-response (or dose–response) relationships based on the available literature. The information identified in Chapter 4 underpins the conclusions reached in Chapter 5. As a result of these discussions, the committee specified first for the purposes of adequacy (EARs, RDAs, and AIs; Chapter 5) and then for preventing excess intakes (ULs; Chapter 6). Step 3 in risk assessment followed, during which the committee performed an intake assessment using current national survey data from the United States and Canada (Chapter 7). For vitamin D, consideration was given to the measures of serum 25OHD concentrations available from national surveys.

In the final step, Step 4, the committee outlined the implications of its work and discussed population segments of interest (Chapter 8). Medical conditions that may relate to special calcium or vitamin D nutriture are specifically outside the scope of the work for this committee and are not addressed in this report. However, a few prevalent clinical groups (e.g., premature infants) are mentioned briefly in Chapter 8. Finally, consistent with its charge, the committee identified research needs for the further development of DRIs for calcium and vitamin D (Chapter 9). Appendix A contains a glossary of terms, acronyms, and abbreviations. With the exception of the Summary and the tables that present the DRIs, this report expresses quantities of calcium as milligrams (mg) and quantities of vitamin D as International Units (IU). In some venues vitamin D is expressed as micrograms (μg) for which 1 μg is equivalent to 40 IU. Serum levels of

25-hydroxyvitamin D are expressed as nanomoles per liter (nmol/L), but are also often expressed elsewhere as nanograms per milliliter (ng/mL). Values expressed as nmol/L are divided by the conversation factor of 2.5 to obtain the equivalent measure in ng/mL. The Summary and the tables presenting the DRIs express vitamin D using µg as well as IU and express serum 25OHD levels using ng/mL as well as nmol/L.

In sum, Chapters 2 and 3 as developed provide background information about the basic biology of calcium and vitamin D for the readers of this report, but they are not central to the risk assessment process that forms the foundation for this report. The risk assessment approach begins with Chapter 4, which reflects a literature review and evaluation concerning potential indicators for development of DRIs for adequacy; at the close of the chapter, the indicator to be used for the development of DRIs for adequacy is identified. Chapters 5 through 8 contain discussions related to the other steps of risk assessment as specified in the generic model with Chapter 5 providing the reference values related to adequacy of calcium and vitamin D. Chapter 6 overviews the literature related to adverse events and specifies the ULs. Appendix B lists special issues of interest identified by the sponsors of this report and taken into account during committee deliberations.

Finally, it should be noted that this report is not intended to critique or reevaluate the specific conclusions arrived at in the 1997 DRI report related to calcium and vitamin D. This would not be appropriate given the closed nature of those deliberations as well as the specific charge to this committee, which was to review the state of the data currently and come to its own conclusions about DRI values. When necessary to clarify this committee's conclusions, and as relevant to set these new reference values in context, mention is made of the 1997 report.

REFERENCES

Chung, M., E. M. Balk, S. Ip, J. Lee, T. Terasawa, G. Raman, T. Trikalinos, A. H. Lichtenstein and J. Lau. 2010. Systematic review to support the development of nutrient reference intake values: challenges and solutions. American Journal of Clinical Nutrition 92(2): 273-6.

Chung M., E. M. Balk, M. Brendel, S. Ip, J. Lau, J. Lee, A. Lichtenstein, K. Patel, G. Raman, A. Tatsioni, T. Terasawa and T. A. Trikalinos. 2009. Vitamin D and Calcium: A Systematic Review of Health Outcomes. Evidence Report No. 183 (Prepared by the Tufts Evidence-based Practice Center under Contract No. HHSA 290-2007-10055-I.) AHRQ Publication No. 09-E015. Rockville, MD: Agency for Healthcare Research and Quality.

Cranney A., T. Horsley, S. O'Donnell, H. A. Weiler, L. Puil, D. S. Ooi, S. A. Atkinson, L. M. Ward, D. Moher, D. A. Hanley, M. Fang, F. Yazdi, C. Garritty, M. Sampson, N. Barrowman, A. Tsertsvadze and V. Mamaladze. 2007. Effectiveness and Safety of Vitamin D in Relation to Bone Health. Evidence Report/Technology Assessment No. 158 (Prepared by the University of Ottawa Evidence-based Practice Center (UO-EPC) under Contract No. 290-02-0021). AHRQ Publication No. 07-E013. Rockville, MD: Agency for Healthcare Research and Quality.

IOM (Institute of Medicine). 1994. How Should the Recommended Dietary Allowances Be Revised? Washington, DC: National Academy Press.

IOM. 1997. Dietary Reference Intakes for Calcium, Phosphorus, Magnesium, Vitamin D, and Fluoride. Washington, DC: National Academy Press.

IOM. 1998. Dietary Reference Intakes: A Risk Assessment Model for Establishing Upper Intake Levels for Nutrients. Washington, DC: National Academy Press.

IOM. 2000a. Dietary Reference Intakes: Applications in Dietary Assessment. Washington, DC: National Academy Press.

IOM. 2000b. Dietary Reference Intakes for Vitamin C, Vitamin E, Selenium, and Carotenoids. Washington, DC: National Academy Press.

IOM. 2003. Dietary Reference Intakes: Applications in Dietary Planning. Washington, DC: The National Academies Press.

IOM. 2005. Dietary Reference Intakes for Water, Potassium, Sodium, Chloride, and Sulfate. Washington, DC: The National Academies Press.

IOM. 2006. Dietary Reference Intakes: The Essential Guide to Nutrient Requirements. Washington, DC: The National Academies Press.

IOM. 2008. The Development of DRIs 1994-2004: Lessons Learned and New Challenges: Workshop Summary. Washington, DC: The National Academies Press.

Moher, D. and A. C. Tricco. 2008. Issues related to the conduct of systematic reviews: a focus on the nutrition field. American Journal of Clinical Nutrition 88(5): 1191-9.

NRC (National Research Council). 1983. Risk Assessment in the Federal Government: Managing the Process. Washington, DC: National Academy Press.

Russell, R., M. Chung, E. M. Balk, S. Atkinson, E. L. Giovannucci, S. Ip, A. H. Lichtenstein, S. T. Mayne, G. Raman, A. C. Ross, T. A. Trikalinos, K. P. West, Jr. and J. Lau. 2009. Opportunities and challenges in conducting systematic reviews to support the development of nutrient reference values: vitamin A as an example. American Journal of Clinical Nutrition 89(3): 728-33.

Taylor, C. L. 2008. Framework for DRI Development: Components "Known" and Components "To Be Explored. " Washington, DC.

WHO (World Health Organization). 2006. A Model for Establishing Upper Levels of Intake for Nutrients and Related Substances: A Report of a Joint FAO/WHO Technical Workshop on Food Nutrient Risk Assessment. Geneva, Switzerland: World Health Organization.

Yetley, E. A., D. Brule, M. C. Cheney, C. D. Davis, K. A. Esslinger, P. W. Fischer, K. E. Friedl, L. S. Greene-Finestone, P. M. Guenther, D. M. Klurfeld, M. R. L'Abbe, K. Y. McMurry, P. E. Starke-Reed and P. R. Trumbo. 2009. Dietary reference intakes for vitamin D: justification for a review of the 1997 values. American Journal of Clinical Nutrition 89(3): 719-27.

2

Overview of Calcium

INTRODUCTION

Calcium as a nutrient is most commonly associated with the formation and metabolism of bone. Over 99 percent of total body calcium is found as calcium hydroxyapatite $(Ca_{10}[PO_4]_6[OH]_2)$ in bones and teeth, where it provides hard tissue with its strength. Calcium in the circulatory system, extracellular fluid, muscle, and other tissues is critical for mediating vascular contraction and vasodilatation, muscle function, nerve transmission, intracellular signaling, and hormonal secretion. Bone tissue serves as a reservoir for and source of calcium for these critical metabolic needs through the process of bone remodeling.

Calcium metabolism is regulated in large part by the parathyroid hormone (PTH)–vitamin D endocrine system, which is characterized by a series of homeostatic feedback loops. The rapid release of mineral from the bone is essential to maintain adequate levels of ionized calcium in serum. During vitamin D deficiency states, bone metabolism is significantly affected as a result of reduced active calcium absorption. This leads to increased PTH secretion as the calcium sensing receptor in the parathyroid gland senses changes in circulating ionic calcium. Increased PTH levels induce enzyme activity (1α-hydroxylase) in the kidney, which converts vitamin D to its active hormonal form, calcitriol. In turn, calcitriol stimulates enhanced calcium absorption from the gut. Not surprisingly, the interplay between the dynamics of calcium and vitamin D often complicates the interpretation of data relative to calcium requirements, deficiency states, and excess intake.

SOURCES OF CALCIUM

Ingested calcium comes from food sources and dietary supplements. In this report dietary calcium refers to both food sources and supplements combined (although some researchers reserve the term dietary calcium to mean only food sources) and is most often referred to as total calcium intake for clarity. With more than one-half of the U.S. population (Bailey et al., 2010)—and between 24 and 60 percent of Canadians (2004 Canadian Community Health Survey, personal communication, D. Brulé, Health Canada, April 29, 2010)—reporting use of dietary supplements of some type, dietary supplements must be taken into account when considering the sources of calcium in the diet and, in turn, estimating total calcium intake. Current estimates from 2003 to 2006 indicate that the median total intake of calcium from all sources for persons > 1 year of age ranges from 918 to 1,296 mg/day, depending upon life stage (Bailey et al., 2010). Only small amounts of calcium are contributed by water, depending upon geographic location. Chapter 7 of this report contains an assessment of quantitative calcium intake in the U.S. and Canadian populations.

Food

Calcium is classically associated with dairy products; milk, yogurt, and cheese are rich sources of calcium, providing the major share of calcium from foods in the general diet in the United States and Canada. In the United States, an estimated 72 percent of calcium comes from milk, cheese and yogurt and from foods to which dairy products have been added (e.g., pizza, lasagna, dairy desserts). The remaining calcium comes from vegetables (7 percent); grains (5 percent); legumes (4 percent); fruit (3 percent); meat, poultry, and fish (3 percent); eggs (2 percent); and miscellaneous foods (3 percent).[1] Similar data from Canada are not currently available.

Fortification with calcium for a number of foods that do not naturally contribute calcium—such as orange juice, other beverages, and ready-to-eat cereals—is becoming commonplace in the United States (Calvo et al., 2004; Rafferty et al., 2007; Poliquin et al., 2009). These practices challenge the ability of national food composition databases, such as those maintained by U.S. Department of Agriculture (USDA), to keep abreast of these newer products and may result in some underestimation of actual calcium intake from food sources. However, for those persons who choose such foods, total calcium intake is increased.

---

[1] U.S. Department of Agriculture/Economic Research Service Nutrient Availability Data (2009). Available online at http://www.ers.usda.gov/Data/FoodConsumption/Nutrient AvailIndex.htm. Accessed October 19, 2010.

Dietary Supplements

Among the U.S. population, about 43 percent of all persons—but almost 70 percent of older women—reported calcium intake from supplements, based on a national survey conducted between 2003 and 2006 (Bailey et al., 2010). When calcium from supplement use is taken into account based on these survey data, the average intake increases by about 7 percent for males and 14 percent for females. However, this is not a meaningful snapshot of the effect of supplement use, because non-users of supplements are averaged with users, meaning that the effect is much more skewed than can be reflected by a mean estimate. Similar data are not available for Canada, but the frequency of use data show that 48 to 82 percent of Canadians reported taking a calcium supplement within the previous 30 days (2004 Canadian Community Health Survey, personal communication, D. Brulé, Health Canada, April 29, 2010).

The most common forms of supplemental calcium are calcium carbonate and calcium citrate.[2] The bioavailability of the calcium in these forms is discussed below in the section titled "Other Factors Related to Calcium Nutriture." Generally fewer tablets of calcium carbonate are required to achieve given dose of elemental calcium because calcium carbonate generally provides 40 percent elemental calcium, compared with 21 percent for calcium citrate. Thus, costs tend to be lower with calcium carbonate (Heaney et al., 2001; Keller et al., 2002) than with calcium citrate, and compliance may be higher among patients who do not want to take (or have difficulty swallowing) multiple pills. Chewable calcium carbonate supplements are also available. However, compared with calcium citrate, calcium carbonate is more often associated with gastrointestinal side effects, including constipation, flatulence, and bloating (Straub, 2007). Calcium citrate is less dependent than calcium carbonate on stomach acid for absorption (Hunt and Johnson, 1983; Recker, 1985; Straub, 2007) and thus can be taken without food. It is useful for individuals with achlorhydria, inflammatory bowel disease, or absorption disorders or who are taking histamine-2 receptor blockers or proton pump inhibitors; for residents of long-term care facilities where calcium supplements are not given with meals; and for others whose schedules preclude taking supplements with food (Bo-Linn et al., 1984; Carr and Shangraw, 1987; Straub, 2007). Calcium can compete or interfere with the absorption of iron, zinc, and magnesium. For this reason, persons with known deficiencies of these other minerals who require calcium supplementation usually take calcium supplements between meals (Straub, 2007).

---

[2]Other forms of calcium dietary supplements include lactate, gluconate, glucoheptonate, and hydroxyapatite; their relevance for life stage groups may vary.

METABOLISM OF CALCIUM

Absorption

Calcium is absorbed by active transport (transcellularly) and by passive diffusion (paracellularly) across the intestinal mucosa. Active transport of calcium is dependent on the action of calcitriol and the intestinal vitamin D receptor (VDR). This transcellular mechanism is activated by calcitriol and accounts for most of the absorption of calcium at low and moderate intake levels. Transcellular transport occurs primarily in the duodenum where the VDR is expressed in the highest concentration, and is dependent on up-regulation of the responsive genes including the calcium transport protein called transient receptor potential cation channel, vanilloid family member 6 or TRPV6 (Li et al., 1993; Xue and Fleet, 2009). These features—up-regulation of VDR and TRPV6—are most obvious during states in which a high efficiency of calcium absorption is required.

Passive diffusion or paracellular uptake involves the movement of calcium between mucosal cells and is dependent on luminal:serosal electrochemical gradients. Passive diffusion occurs more readily during higher calcium intakes (i.e., when luminal concentrations are high) and can occur throughout the length of the intestine (Ireland and Fordtran, 1973). However, the permeability of each intestinal segment determines passive diffusion rates. The highest diffusion of calcium occurs in the duodenum, jejunum, and ileum (Weaver and Heaney, 2006b).

From a recent series of controlled metabolic studies undertaken by the USDA, mean calcium absorption (also referred to as "fractional calcium absorption," which is the percentage of a given dose of calcium that is absorbed) in men and non-pregnant women—across a wide age range— has been demonstrated to be approximately 25 percent of calcium intake (Hunt and Johnson, 2007). Mean urinary loss averages 22 percent and fecal loss 75 percent of total calcium intake, with minor losses from sweat, skin, hair, etc. In general, mean calcium absorption and calcium intake are directly related (Heaney et al., 1975; Gallagher et al., 1980; Hunt and Johnson, 2007). However, fractional calcium absorption varies inversely with calcium intake when the intake is very low (Malm, 1958; Spencer et al., 1969; Ireland and Fordtran, 1973). For example, when calcium intake was lowered from 2,000 to 300 mg, healthy women increased their fractional whole body retention of ingested calcium, an index of calcium absorption, from 27 percent to about 37 percent (Dawson-Hughes et al., 1993). This type of adaptation occurs within 1 to 2 weeks and is accompanied by a decline in serum calcium concentration and a rise in serum PTH and calcitriol concentrations (see section below titled "Homeostatic Regulation of Calcium"). The fraction of calcium absorbed rises adaptively as intake is lowered. However, this rise is not sufficient to offset the loss in absorbed calcium that occurs as a result of the lower intake of calcium—however modest that decrease may be—and thus net calcium absorption is reduced.

Fractional calcium absorption varies during critical periods of life. In infancy, it is high at approximately 60 percent, although the range is large (Fomon and Nelson, 1993; Abrams et al., 1997). Calcium absorption in newborns is largely passive and facilitated by the lactose content of breast milk (Kocian et al., 1973; Kobayashi et al., 1975). As the neonate ages, passive absorption declines and calcitriol-stimulated active intestinal calcium absorption becomes more important (Ghishan et al., 1980; Halloran and DeLuca, 1980; Ghishan et al., 1984).

A recent preliminary report on breast-fed infants in the first 2 months of life (Hicks et al., 2010) reported calcium absorption of approximately 33.7 ± 2.0 mg/100 kcal. In an earlier study using stable isotopes (Abrams et al., 1997), calcium absorption was measured in 14 breast milk–fed infants who were 5 through 7 months of age at the time of the study. Mean absorption was 61 ± 23 percent of intake when approximately 80 percent of the calcium intake was from human milk (IOM, 1997). There was no significant relationship between calcium intake from solid foods and the fractional calcium absorption from human milk. This finding suggests that calcium from solid foods does not negatively affect the bioavailability of calcium from human milk (IOM, 1997). Using measured urinary calcium and estimates of endogenous excretion, net retention of calcium was calculated to be 68 ± 38 mg/day for those infants. Abrams (2010) concluded that in infancy, based on calcium intakes that vary from as low as 200 mg/day in exclusively breast-fed infants in the early months of life to 900 mg/day in older formula-fed infants receiving some solids, calcium absorption depends primarily on the level of intake. The author reported that the absorption fraction can range from somewhat above 60 percent with lower intakes to about 30 percent with higher intakes. As the infant transitions into childhood, fractional calcium absorption declines, only to rise again in early puberty, a time when modeling of the skeleton is maximal. Abrams and Stuff (1994) found fractional absorption in white girls with a mean calcium intake of about 931 mg/day to average 28 percent before puberty, 34 percent during early puberty (the age of the growth spurt), and 25 percent 2 years after early puberty. Fractional absorption remains about 25 percent in young adults. In 155 healthy men and women between 20 and 75 years of age, mean calcium absorption was 24.9 ± 12.4 percent of total intake (Hunt and Johnson, 2007). During pregnancy, calcium absorption doubles (Kovacs and Kronenberg, 1997; Kovacs, 2001). Metabolic status also influences calcium absorption such that severe obesity is associated with higher calcium absorption and dieting reduces the fractional calcium absorption by 5 percent (Cifuentes et al., 2002; Riedt et al., 2006).

With aging and after menopause, fractional calcium absorption has been reported to decline on average by 0.21 percent per year after 40 years of age (Heaney et al., 1989). Nordin et al. (2004) and Aloia et al. (2010) also reported decreased absorption with age. There are early reports of an inverse correlation between age and calcium absorption in women (Avioli et al., 1965), and several studies have indicated that despite an increase in circulating levels of calcitriol in older women, which would be anticipated to increase calcium uptake, fractional calcium absorption was unaffected (Bullamore et al., 1970; Alevizaki et al., 1973; Gallagher et al., 1979; Tsai et al., 1984; Eastell et al., 1991; Ebeling et al., 1992). Thus, although calcium absorption (active calcium transport) has been reported to decrease with age, it is challenging to take this factor into consideration given that calcium intake must be very high to have a significant effect on calcium uptake via the passive absorption.

Homeostatic Regulation of Calcium

Maintaining the level of circulating ionized calcium within a narrow physiological range is critical for the body to function normally, and control of serum calcium levels is maintained through an endocrine system—a system of glands that secrete hormones and is characterized by controlling factors and feedback mechanisms—that includes a major role for vitamin D metabolites, principally calcitriol, and PTH. Calcium balance within the body is closely linked to the hormonal actions of calcitriol. The vitamin D-related endocrine system that maintains serum calcium levels is discussed in Chapter 3 but is also summarized below and illustrated in Figure 2-1.

The vitamin D metabolic system forms the basis of the calcium homeostatic mechanism in mammals. Total calcium concentration in serum is tightly regulated to remain between 8.5 and 10.5 mg/dL (2.12 and 2.62 mmol/L). If this level deviates slightly, the calcium sensing receptor of the parathyroid gland signals the secretion of PTH, which functions as a calcium sensor. PTH then stimulates the kidney to produce calcitriol, the hormonal form of vitamin D, as well as to activate bone resorption, which will increase extracellular calcium levels. Calcitriol acts in an endocrine manner on the intestine, bone, and kidney to raise serum calcium levels; it also acts on the intestine and, to some extent, the kidneys to raise serum phosphorus levels. As the serum calcium level rises, the feedback mechanism causes the calcium sensing receptor to be turned off and PTH secretion to drop. If there is an overshoot in serum calcium levels, the "C" cells (parafollicular) cells of the thyroid gland secrete calcitonin, which can block bone calcium resorption, helping to keep serum calcium levels in the normal range. Calcitriol, through its receptor, also provides feedback relative to suppressing the production and release of PTH, commonly referred

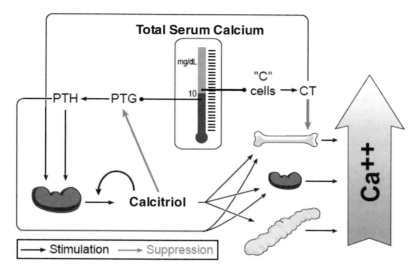

FIGURE 2-1 Endocrine feedback system that maintains serum calcium levels: Involvement of vitamin D and parathyroid hormone (PTH).
NOTE: CT = calcitonin; PTG = parathyroid gland.
SOURCE: Reprinted with permission from Hector DeLuca.

to as PTH suppression. Not shown in the figure is that calcitriol is also directly controlled by the serum phosphorus level; a high serum phosphorus level suppresses the formation of calcitriol, whereas a low level stimulates it.

Excretion

Calcium leaves the body mainly in urine and feces, but also in other body tissues and fluids, such as sweat. Calcium excretion in the urine is a function of the balance between the calcium load filtered by the kidneys and the efficiency of reabsorption from the renal tubules. Nearly 98 percent of filtered calcium (i.e., glomerular filtrate) is reabsorbed by either passive or active processes occurring at four sites in the kidney, each contributing to maintaining neutral calcium balance. Seventy percent of the filtered calcium is reabsorbed passively in the proximal tubule. Active calcium transport is regulated by the calcium sensing receptor located in the ascending loop of Henle, where, in response to high calcium levels in the extracellular fluid, active reabsorption in the loop is blocked through actions of the calcium sensing receptor. In contrast, when the filtered calcium load is low, the calcium sensing receptor is activated, and a greater fraction of the filtered calcium is reabsorbed. In the distal tubule, the ion channels known as transient receptor potential cation channel, vanilloid family member 5 or TRPV5 control active calcium transport and this process is regulated by calcitriol and estradiol (Hoenderop et al., 2000). Finally, the collecting duct also can participate in passive calcium transport, although the relative percentage of total calcium reabsorption in the collecting duct is low. Overall, a typical daily calcium loss for a healthy adult man or woman via renal excretion is 5 mmol/day (Weaver and Heaney, 2006a).

Calcium is excreted through the feces as unabsorbed intestinal calcium and is shed in mucosal cells and secretions including saliva, gastric juices, pancreatic juice, and bile. Endogenous fecal calcium losses are approximately 2.1 mg/kg per day in adults and about 1.4 mg/kg per day in children (Abrams et al., 1991). These intestinal losses as well as minor losses in sweat are referred to collectively as endogenous calcium excretion. Endogenous calcium excretion, in contrast to urinary excretion, does not change appreciably with aging (Heaney and Recker, 1994).

PTH can be a major determinant of urinary calcium excretion; during states of low calcium intake, secondary increases in PTH levels result in reduced urinary calcium excretion. Impaired renal function due to aging paradoxically reduces calcium loss due to impaired filtration, but there is also a secondary increase in PTH levels due to reduced phosphate clearance. However, renal 1α-hydroxylase activity declines with impaired renal function, so the net result is calcium loss from the kidney, but also reduced active transport of calcium from the intestine.

Excess Intake

Although excess intake of calcium is almost never due to calcium intake from foods, the use of calcium supplements (including the voluntary fortification of a range of foods that are not naturally sources of calcium) has increased (Ricci et al., 1998; Riedt et al., 2005), and excess calcium intake may occur as a result of high intake from calcium supplements. Excess calcium intake can result in adverse effects. Calcium plays a major role in the metabolism of virtually every cell in the body and interacts with a large number of other nutrients, and as a result, disturbances of calcium metabolism may give rise to a variety of adverse effects (IOM, 1997). A review of the considerations related to adverse effects from excess calcium ingestion can be found in Chapter 6, which focuses on the establishment of Tolerable Upper Intake Levels (ULs).

FUNCTIONS AND PHYSIOLOGICAL ACTIONS OF CALCIUM

Calcium is an integral component of the skeleton, and the skeleton provides a reservoir of calcium for other essential calcium-dependent functions throughout the body. The skeleton serves at least three main functions. First, calcium, as part of the mineral hydroxyapatite, deposited into the organic matrix of the skeleton, is critical for its structure and is necessary for tissue rigidity, strength, and elasticity. This function allows for normal movement and exercise. Second, the skeleton functions as a source of minerals and alkali and therefore is critical for overall mineral homeostasis. The skeleton is the principal depot for calcium, containing 98 percent of total body calcium. It can be called on repeatedly, through the processes of bone formation and resorption (referred to as remodeling, as discussed below), to maintain circulating levels of calcium at a constant level. While the same qualitative processes apply to skeletal calcium metabolism across the life cycle, there are quantitative differences by age and hormonal status. These life cycle differences for skeletal growth and remodeling are discussed in a section below. Excessive calcium resorption can compromise the integrity and strength of the skeletal tissues. Third, the marrow cavity of bone serves as a major site for the development of hematopoietic cells and as a major compartment of the immune system. Several of the cell types involved in bone remodeling originate in the bone marrow compartment. Stromal or connective tissue cells are found in the bone marrow; at one time, these were thought to be inert, but they are now considered multi-potent stem cells that can become either fat or bone cells under the influence of specific differentiation factors (Muruganandan et al., 2009).

A principal physiological function of calcium apart from its role in maintaining the skeleton, is as an essential intracellular messenger in cells and tissues throughout the body. Although this pool of calcium is quantitatively small, the ionized calcium present in the circulatory system, extracellular fluid, muscle, and other tissues, is critical for mediating vascular contraction and vasodilatation, muscle function, nerve transmission, and hormonal secretion. Ionized calcium is the most common signal transduction element in biology, owing to its ability to reversibly bind to proteins and to complex with anions such as citrate and bicarbonate (Weaver and Heaney, 2006b).

Bone Formation and Remodeling

Bone is composed of a mineral compartment, predominantly calcium hydroxyapatite and an organic matrix, osteoid, composed principally of collagen and non-collagenous proteins and growth factors. The relative contributions of the mineralized and organic compartments depend on the age of the individual; in general, 50 to 70 percent of bone is mineral, 20 to 40 percent is organic matrix, and the rest is water and lipid. The organic matrix is critical for both the structural and functional components of the skeleton, providing elasticity and contributing to regenerative and remodeling properties. Much of the organic matrix is composed of type I collagen fibrils that are organized in such a manner that strength and elasticity are combined. Numerous non-collagenous proteins are also present in the organic matrix. Some of them, such as osteocalcin and matrix GLA protein, contain γ-carboxyglutamate, an amino acid with high affinity for calcium that is required for proper mineralization of the matrix (see below). The role of phosphate in bone development should not be overlooked. As described below, first phosphorus is laid down during the mineralization process, and then calcium binds to it. Calcitriol stimulates the uptake of both calcium and phosphorus from the intestine.

Development

The skeleton develops through a process of either intramembranous or endochondral bone formation, depending on location and function. Intramembranous bone formation is the predominant process in the skull, whereas endochondral bone formation occurs in long bone and the axial skeleton. Intramembranous bone is formed by direct differentiation of mesenchymal precursors into osteoblasts, cells of the fibroblast–stromal lineage that produce bone matrix proteins and synthesize a lattice for subsequent mineralization. In contrast, during endochondral bone formation chondrocytic differentiation occurs first, leading to a soft cartilaginous infrastructure. The cartilage then becomes calcified, and the provisional calcified cartilage is subsequently replaced by bone. This occurs by vascular invasion, which allows entry of hematopoietic precursors and osteoclasts, macrophage-like cells that originate from the monocyte–macrophage lineage, which remove apoptotic chondrocytes and cartilage (Provot and Schipani, 2007). New bone is formed by osteoblasts. Osteoblastogenesis follows chondrogenesis after release of growth factors from terminally differentiated chondrocytes. The first bone formed is woven and relatively unorganized. However, through osteoclastic modeling that bone is replaced by lamellar bone, which is highly organized and provides the strength necessary to support soft tissue (Yang and Yang, 2008).

Endochondral bone formation allows for linear development of the growth plate as well as periosteal expansion, which ultimately results in a longer and thicker bone. Mineralization is the final stage in terminal differentiation of the osteoblast and occurs through a complex process whereby ion deposition is followed by crystal formation between the collagen fibrils. This occurs because of undersaturation of calcium hydroxyapatite in the extracellular fluid and the binding of calcium to non-collagenous proteins in the matrix (Favus, 2008). Initially, phosphate drives the mineralization by being laid down in bone as hydroxyapatite; the negative charge of hydroxyapatite then causes calcium to avidly bind to it. In states of phosphorus deficiency, unmineralized osteoid persists despite adequate calcium intake. Bone mechanical properties are then influenced by the distribu-

> ## BOX 2-1
> ## Bone Remodeling Terms and Definitions
>
> - Cortical bone: One of two types of bone; makes up the outer part of all skeletal structures (nearly 80 percent of the skeleton); is dense and compact with a slow turnover rate and is highly resistant to bending and torsion.
> - Trabecular bone: Second of the two bone types; found inside of long bones, vertebrae, pelvis, and other large flat bones; is less dense than cortical bone and has a higher turnover rate.
> - Osteoblast: A type of bone cell that is responsible for the production of bone and bone formation.
> - Osteoclast: A type of bone cell that resorbs bone using acid and enzymes.
> - Bone remodeling: Process that occurs throughout the lifetime that results from the pairing action of osteoclasts (breaking down) and osteoblasts (building up), which replaces damaged bone with new material.
> - Bone modeling: A similar process to remodeling, except that new bone is formed at a location different from the site of resorption, such as during times of growth.
>
> SOURCE: Hadjidakis and Androulakis, 2006.

tion, size, and density of the apatite crystals. Too much or too little mineral can lead to impaired bone strength; the former makes the bone too brittle, whereas the latter makes the bone too ductile and weak.

Remodeling

Calcium balance is preserved within the non-bone tissues of the body, because adult bone constantly undergoes remodeling through bone resorption, mainly by osteoclasts and bone formation mainly by osteoblasts.[3] Terminology associated with remodeling is shown in Box 2-1. In adults, virtually all of the human skeleton is remodeled over a 10-year cycle, although trabecular bone turns over more readily. In contrast, bone formation incorporates calcium into the matrix, and this process requires significant time

---

[3]Not all calcium enters the skeleton through bone formation or leaves the skeleton through bone resorption, as discussed by Parfitt (2003). Moreover, during lactation and in response to other acute demands for calcium, osteocytes have been shown to resorb the matrix surrounding them and then to restore it after the stress is over (Teti and Zallone, 2009).

and energy. Overall calcium balance is maintained at the skeletal level by opposing actions of bone cells. Skeletal remodeling occurs in microscopic elements of bone referred to as remodeling units or basic multicellular units, which contain the osteoblasts (bone-resorbing cells) and osteoclasts (bone-forming cells). Old osteoblasts then become osteocytes entombed within the bone matrix after mineralization.

The axial and appendicular skeletons are composed of both cortical and trabecular bone. The hard outer shell of bone is cortical, which is remodeled less frequently, but is important for strength and periosteal expansion during puberty and with aging. The trabecular compartment is bathed by bone marrow and is remodeled much more frequently, which is in part due to a much greater surface area and the existence of marrow elements that are in close proximity to the endosteal surface of bone (which contribute progenitor cells for eventual remodeling).

Physical activity—or more specifically mechanical loading—is a critical component of skeletal homeostasis. It is thought that osteocytes in cortical bone sense changes in gravitational forces and elaborate growth factors that initiate remodeling. Unloading of the skeleton in cases such as bed rest or weightlessness (space travel) is associated with a profound uncoupling of remodeling, such that bone resorption is dramatically increased, whereas bone formation is suppressed. These changes cause rapid bone loss and are a major problem for long-term spaceflight. Loading of the skeleton by mechanical means (e.g., weight-bearing exercise such as running, walking, or jumping) can promote bone formation, particularly in early childhood and adolescence, although it has benefits later in life as well.

Concept of Normal, Healthy Bone Accretion

Bone is a dynamic tissue; it is metabolically active, responding to both genetically determined and environmental stimuli that ultimately determine its composition and structural integrity. Bone modeling describes events that occur primarily during growth resulting in increased bone size and modification of its shape in response to genetic determinants and mechanical loading. Bone remodeling occurs in response to stimulation by surface-dependent factors initiated by damage or mechanical loading. It includes bone resorption and deposition but does not alter the size or shape of bone (reviewed in Seeman, 2009).

Although the role of genetic and environmental factors in bone modeling and remodeling has long been debated in the literature, genetics remains the chief determinant of bone mass, which, in turn, is the determinant of bone strength (Krall and Dawson-Hughes, 1993; Jouanny et al., 1995; Jones and Nguyen, 2000; Sigurdsson et al., 2008; Perez-Lopez et al., 2010). Given uncertainties in understanding the cumulative impact of genetic and environmental influences on bone mass across life stages, the question of whether attainment of maximal, optimal, or "peak" bone mass can be achieved on a lasting basis through dietary manipulation and/or use of supplements has not been completely resolved.

A 2-year longitudinal multiethnic study (Abrams et al., 2000) of changes in calcium absorption, bone accretion, and markers of bone growth in pre-pubertal girls (7 to 8 years of age) maintained on a calcium intake of 1,200 mg/day found a significant increase in calcium use associated with pubertal development. The increase paralleled markers of bone formation; supporting the hypothesis that calcium intake during the early to late pubertal stage influences peak rates of calcium gain in bone during pubertal development. An earlier study followed pre-pubertal males and females (mean age 8.5 years) for 18 months after calcium supplementation and also found gains in bone mineral content (BMC) and bone area of the lumbar spine; however, the increases in bone accretion disappeared after supplements were withdrawn (Lee et al., 1996). In a longer-term randomized clinical trial, Matkovic et al. (2005) evaluated the effects of calcium supplementation on bone accretion in the transition from childhood into early adulthood. This study found significant increases in bone accretion for total bone density, distal and proximal radius, and metacarpal indexes after 4 years of supplementation; by 7 years, however, only the proximal radius and metacarpal indexes still showed significantly increased bone accretion over non-supplemented controls.

These findings corroborate a role for calcium intake and skeletal size; however, they also suggest that bone accretion diminishes during skeletal consolidation in late adolescence, and attainment of a peak bone mass was transient for some skeletal sites, even though the study subjects continued calcium supplementation through year 7. When considered together, these studies support an increase in skeletal size and mineralization that occurs with calcium supplementation, but fail to show consistently that BMC is retained over the long term, particularly after supplementation is withdrawn.

Effect of Menopause

Studies of bone histomorphometry (Recker et al., 2004) and markers of bone remodeling (Uebelhart et al., 1990) indicate that bone remodeling is accelerated in the perimenopausal and postmenopausal periods. The span of 5 to 10 years surrounding menopause is characterized by a decrease in estrogen production and an increase in resorption of calcium from bone (Stevenson et al., 1981; Riggs, 2002; Masse et al., 2005; Finkelstein et al., 2008), resulting in a marked decrease in bone density. For example, Ebeling et al. (1996) measured changes in markers of bone mineral density (BMD) in a cohort of 281 women who were 45–57 years of age, and found the BMD in lumbar spine and femoral neck was decreased by 20 percent in perimenopausal and postmenopausal women compared with premeno-pausal women. The bone loss is most rapid in the early years of menopause, and then approximately 6 to 7 years postmenopause the loss continues at a slower rate (Pouilles et al., 1995)

The bone loss associated with menopause results from uncoupling in the bone remodeling units, such that resorption of bone is greater than formation of new bone. Over time, such changes lead to skeletal fragility and decreased bone mass. Some cohort studies demonstrate that acceler-ated bone loss is an independent risk factor for fracture, such that the combination of low bone mass and high rates of bone turnover markedly increase the potential for a future fracture (Garnero et al., 1996). Bone remodeling in postmenopausal osteoporosis includes changes in osteoid thickness, surface area, and volume. Parfitt et al. (1995) determined that defective osteoblast recruitment in women with osteoporosis resulted in decreased osteoid thickness, a characteristic of osteoporosis.

Considerable variability exists among women regarding the effects of menopause on bone loss, and such effects vary according to body mass index and ethnicity (Finkelstein et al., 2008). The effect of estrogen/ progesterone treatment on preventing bone loss and reducing fracture risk is well established. However, the use of such therapy has declined as a result of recent reports of adverse non-skeletal effects. Because rapid bone loss occurs after estrogen treatment is discontinued (Gallagher et al., 2002), the potential impact on subsequent fracture rates is of interest but remains unclear.

Skeletal Disorders

Rickets and Osteomalacia

Rickets is the term for the end-stage condition in infants and children that begins with suboptimal bone mineralization at the growth plate and progresses with associated physiological perturbations that include second-ary hyperparathyroidism, hypocalcemia, and hypophosphatemia leading to irreversible changes in skeletal structure. The disease is a disorder of the growth apparatus of bone in which growth cartilage fails to mature and mineralize normally. Because the bone is undermineralized it is also soft and ductile, and this leads to bowing of the limbs, widening and compres-sion of the ends of the long bones, etc. The similar condition of osteoma-lacia (defective mineralization of bone and softening of bone) also occurs, and is seen in adults as well as children. Although these conditions are commonly associated with inadequate vitamin D exposure, each can also result from calcium (or phosphorus) deficiency. Rickets and osteomalacia due to a lack of calcium in the diet cannot be corrected by increasing levels of calcitriol (i.e., the active form of vitamin D also referred to as 1,25–dihyroxyvitamin D).

Rickets   In rickets, during prolonged deficiency of calcium (and phosphate), the body increases PTH to prevent hypocalcemia by causing osteoclastic absorption of the bone. This, in turn, causes the bone to become progressively weaker, resulting in rapid osteoblastic activity. The osteoblasts produce large amounts of organic bone matrix, osteoid, which does not become calcified (Guyton and Hall, 2001). Consequently, the newly formed, uncalcified osteoid gradually takes the place of other bone that is being reabsorbed. During the later stages of rickets, the serum calcium level falls precipitously, and tetany (neuromuscular spasm) develops. In infants and young children, a long-standing calcium intake deficiency, in association with suboptimal vitamin D exposure, can produce rickets. Indeed, in experimental animals and in humans with extremely low vitamin D levels, genetic absence of calcitriol (vitamin D–dependent rickets [VDDR] type I), or genetic absence of the vitamin D receptor (VDDR type II), the use of increased calcium supplementation or calcium infusions will prevent and treat rickets. These observations indicate that the primary cause of rickets is inadequate delivery of calcium to the bone surface, not a defect in osteoblast function. In other words, the primary role for vitamin D and calcitriol in regulating skeletal homeostasis is indirectly accomplished by stimulating the intestinal absorption of calcium and phosphorus.

The clinical symptoms of rickets include stunted growth and bowing of the extremities. A serum 25-hydroxyvitamin D (25OHD) level of less than 27 to 30 nmol/L is not diagnostic of the disease but is associated with an increased risk for developing rickets (Specker et al., 1992).

Osteomalacia   In osteomalacia, as seen in adults, the newly deposited bone matrix fails to mineralize adequately. Poor calcium intake is associated with secondary increases in PTH in an attempt to compensate for low serum calcium levels. The secondary hyperparathyroidism of calcium deficiency states is associated with increased bone resorption and suppression of bone formation. As a result, older adults who have calcium-poor diets and very low vitamin D levels may develop not only osteoporosis, as described below (i.e., a reduction in bone mass), but also osteomalacia (a reduction in mineral within the bone matrix). Osteomalacia is actually the clinical syndrome of undermineralization of bone associated with muscle weakness, bone pain, and fractures. The characteristic histological feature of osteomalacia is unmineralized matrix, which is often represented experimentally as the ratio of osteoid volume to bone volume. Ultimately, reductions in mineralization lead to impaired bone strength and significant softening of the skeleton. The calcium levels in the blood of patients with osteomalacia are often normal despite the undermineralization of bone, underscoring the importance of maintaining the blood calcium level over maintaining the mineralization of the skeleton. However, serum phosphorus levels are frequently low, PTH concentrations are 5 to 10 times the normal levels, and there is an increased level of alkaline phosphatase together with increased markers of bone turnover. Bone scans often indicate dramatically increased skeletal uptake by resident osteoblasts. As recognized by Parfitt et al. (1995) and illustrated by the histological classification scheme used for osteomalacia, what clinicians generally recognize as osteomalacia is the end-stage results from a prolonged severe deficiency of calcium and/or vitamin D. During the earliest stages (preosteomalacia), there exists a calcium-deficient state, even though the osteoid thickness, mineralization lag time, and osteoid volume are still normal. Subsequently, more dramatic changes occur including a greater increase in osteoid thickness, and impaired mineralization.

Osteomalacia is estimated to be present in about 4 to 5 percent of general medical and geriatric patients (Anderson, 1961; Stacey and Daly, 1989; Campbell et al., 1994). However, the clinical syndrome of bone pain, muscle weakness, and impaired bone mineralization is much less frequently recognized. In the face of severe osteoporosis, the diagnosis of osteomalacia can only be made by bone biopsy, usually using the method of double tetracycline labeling, demonstrating impaired mineralization of the skeleton (Villareal et al., 1991; Chapuy et al., 1992; Komar et al., 1993). In fact, osteomalacia is noted histologically in the bones of 20 to 40 percent of first-time hip fracture patients (Jenkins et al., 1973; Aaron et al., 1974; Sokoloff, 1978). These results suggest that these individuals may be presenting with a mixture of osteoporosis and osteomalacia. This clinical scenario can be related to both nutrient insufficiency and the coincidental progression of age-related bone loss.

Osteoporosis and Fractures

Osteoporosis is a skeletal disorder associated with aging and characterized by compromised bone strength due to reduced bone mass and reduced bone quality. Reduced bone mass—as measured by low BMD—increases bone fragility and, in turn, predisposes a person to an increased risk of fracture, notably at the vertebrae, hip, and forearm (NIH Consensus Development Panel on Osteoporosis Prevention, Diagnosis, and Therapy, 2001). As shown in Figure 2-2, the relationship between BMD measures and the incidence of fractures is notable. Overall, osteoporosis-related morbidity and mortality, as well as health care costs, are a significant public health concern (NIH Consensus Development Panel on Osteoporosis Pre-

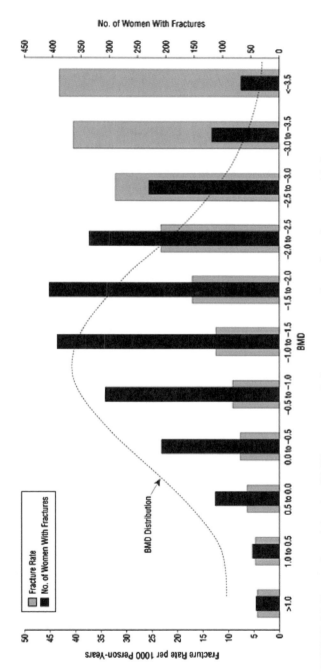

FIGURE 2-2 Bone mineral density (BMD), osteoporotic fracture rate, and number of women with fractures.

SOURCE: Siris et al. (2004). *Archives of Internal Medicine* 164(10): 1108-12. Copyright © 2004 American Medical Association. All rights reserved.

vention, Diagnosis, and Therapy, 2001). Osteoporosis is most commonly associated with women, but the condition also occurs in men.

Menopause can initiate osteoporosis through elevated bone remodeling, which occurs characteristically in postmenopausal women. Remodeling activity, although designed to repair weakened bone, actually makes it temporarily weaker when remodeling is excessive. It can lead to enhanced skeletal fragility (Heaney, 2003). Although it is unclear to what extent calcium intake can mitigate such bone loss, inadequate calcium intake can exacerbate the situation.

Men experience age-related bone loss as well, although not due to menopause. This, in turn, can result in osteoporosis. However, the incidence of fracture risk increases some 5 to 10 years later in men than it does in women (Tuck and Datta, 2007).

CALCIUM ACROSS THE LIFE CYCLE

The body's need for calcium relative to skeletal growth and remodeling varies by life stage. The major physiological activities include bone accretion during skeletal growth and maintenance of bone mass after growth is completed. Later in adult life, net calcium is lost from the body when bone formation no longer keeps up with bone resorption. For all life stages highlighted below, specific studies and conclusions are detailed in Chapter 4.

Infancy

At full-term birth, the human infant has accrued about 26 to 30 g of calcium, most of which is in the skeleton. When calcium transfer from the placenta ceases at birth, the newborn infant is dependent on dietary calcium. Calcium deposition into bone occurs at a proportionately higher rate during the first year of life than during other periods. Breast-fed infants absorb about 55 to 60 percent of the calcium in human milk (Abrams et al., 1997). Formula-fed infants receive more calcium than breast-fed infants because formula contains nearly double the calcium of breast milk. However, fractional calcium absorption is lower in formula-fed infants, averaging about 40 percent among different formula types (Abrams et al., 2002). Studies to establish the level of calcium provided by human milk are long-standing in nature, and little information has emerged to change the conclusions of earlier analyses. Although the composition of milk varies significantly from the start to the end of each feed, the average calcium concentration of milk produced in total for each feeding remains relatively constant over the months of lactation, with an estimated value of 259 ± 59 mg/L at 30 days, followed by a small decrease during the second 6 months. This estimate is based on the average concentrations found in several studies from the United States and the United Kingdom, as summarized in Atkinson et al. (1995). Variations in milk calcium content have been found between population groups. For example, in comparison with the above data from the United States, milk calcium concentrations have been found to be lower (by approximately 20 mg/100 mL at 5 months of lactation) in mothers from the Gambia, but this difference appears to be genetic and not due to differences in total intake of calcium (Prentice et al., 1995; IOM, 1997).

Relative to the average amount of milk consumed by infants, there are three key studies based on weighing full-term infants before and after feeding (Butte et al., 1984; Allen et al., 1991; Heinig et al., 1993). While it has been noted that the volume of intake is somewhat lower during the first month of life than in subsequent months (Widdowson, 1965; Southgate et al., 1969; Lonnerdal, 1997) and that a number of factors contribute to variability in intake, an estimate of 780 mL/day is reasonable based on the data from the three test weighing studies. Therefore, given an intake of milk estimated to be 780 mL/day from the infant weighing studies and the average content of 259 ± 59 mg of calcium per liter, the intake of calcium for infants fed exclusively human milk is estimated to be 202 mg/day.

Childhood and Adolescence

Calcium deposition into bone is an ongoing process throughout childhood and into adolescence, reaching maximal accretion during the pubertal growth spurt. Measures of bone density in adolescent girls indicate that about 37 percent of total skeletal bone mass is achieved between pubertal stages 2 (mean age 11 years) and 4 (mean age 15 years), with an average daily calcium accretion rate of 300 to 400 mg/day (Matkovic et al., 1994). For growing children, bone modeling (i.e., formation over resorption) is the predominant skeletal process promoting longitudinal extension of the growth plate and periosteal expansion. Modeling requires mineralization; hence, calcium requirements are increased, particularly during neonatal and pubertal growth spurts. Approximately 40 percent of total skeletal bone mass is acquired within a relatively short window of 3 to 5 years, when gonadal steroids and growth hormone secretion are maximal (Weaver and Heaney, 2006b). During this time, bone formation far outpaces resorption and longitudinal growth, and consolidation of bone occurs. The most recent estimate of average calcium accretion is 92 to 210 mg/day calcium in 9- to 18-year-old boys and girls (Vatanparast et al., 2010), and bone calcium accretion can peak at 300 to 400 mg/day (Bailey et al., 2000).

During this developmental period, calcium absorption is maximal and variation in calcium intake accounts for 12 to 15 percent of the variance in calcium retention for both boys and girls. Increases in total calcium transiently enhance bone mass (Lee et al., 1996; Matkovic et al., 2005). These effects disappear during or after cessation of increased calcium intake; final bone mass, measured in randomized trials of calcium supplementation during this period, did not differ between controls and calcium-supplemented individuals (Matkovic et al., 2005). However, this period of bone accretion determines adult bone mass, which, in turn, is a significant predictor of fracture risk late in life.

Young Adults

After puberty and throughout most of adulthood, bone formation and resorption are balanced. During this period, bone mass is consolidated, and calcium requirements are relatively stable. Peak bone mass, the maximum amount of bone that can be accumulated, is reached in early adulthood (Bonjour et al., 1994). The ability to attain peak bone mass is affected by genetic background and by lifestyle factors such as physical activity and total calcium intake. Specific skeletal sites have been found to reach peak bone mass at different ages, and bone mineral accretion has been reported to continue slowly into the third decade of life (Recker et al., 1992). Bone is a dynamic tissue, and a number of clinical studies suggest that increasing bone mass early in life has a transient effect, but does not confer protection against later bone loss and osteoporosis (Gafni and Baron, 2007). The calcium content of bone at maturity is approximately 1,200 g in women and 1,400 g in men (Ilich and Kerstetter, 2000; Anderson, 2001). In men, this level remains relatively constant until the onset of age-related bone loss later in life. In women, the level remains relatively constant until the onset of menopause. Although bone mass generally remains at a plateau during reproductive years, some studies have suggested that mean bone mass gradually reaches a plateau and then declines slowly with age.

Older Adults

Age-related bone loss, in both men and women, results when bone remodeling becomes uncoupled and bone resorption exceeds bone formation. However, the pathogenesis of bone loss is a multi-faceted process. The roles and interactions of various hormonal, genetic, and other factors in bone loss and risk for decreased bone health are not yet clear. Moreover, the ability of increased calcium intake to overcome the effects of bone loss related to menopause or normal aging continues to be debated.

In postmenopausal women, estrogen loss increases the rate of bone remodeling, characterized by an imbalance between osteoclast and osteoblast activity, resulting in irreversible bone loss (Riggs et al., 1998; Seeman, 2003). Estrogen loss can further accelerate bone loss through its effect on decreased absorption of calcium and increased urinary loss of calcium (Nordin et al., 2004). Evidence suggests that remodeling in women becomes imbalanced just prior to, during, and immediately after menopause, when the rate of bone loss becomes more rapid. However, the rate of bone loss as a result of menopause varies greatly depending upon a number of factors, including genetics, body composition, other hormonal changes and endogenous production of estradiol.

The effects of lower estrogen levels on calcium balance continue to be debated. However, the principal effect of estrogen deficiency on the skeleton is increased bone resorption. The range of bone loss in the 7 to 10 years around the onset of menopause can range from 3 to 7 percent annually (Kenny and Prestwood, 2000). In women over age 65, the rate of bone loss slows again to 0.5 to 2 percent per year (Greenspan et al., 1994). Later in menopause—and in men over 70 years of age—if reduced calcium intake occurs, it contributes to a secondary form of hyperparathyroidism, which serves as a compensatory mechanism to maintain extracellular calcium balance. This compensation results in accelerated bone resorption, leading to a net loss of bone mass under these conditions.

For men over 65 years of age, the loss of bone is about 1 to 2 percent per year (Orwoll et al., 1990; Hannan et al., 1992). Additionally, reduced glomerular filtration rate is another factor associated with aging that affects renal conservation of calcium in both men and women (Goldschmied et al., 1975) and also leads to secondary hyperparathyroidism, which can cause significant bone loss. This is underscored by patients with renal disease who have renal osteodystrophy, now referred to as chronic kidney disease–mineral disorder (Demer and Tintut, 2010; Peacock, 2010).

Pregnancy and Lactation

Pregnancy

The fetal need for calcium is met by maternal physiological changes, primarily through increased calcium absorption. There is currently debate about whether calcium is also mobilized from maternal skeleton, as discussed in Chapter 4. In any case, calcium is actively transported across the placenta from mother to fetus, an essential activity to mineralizing the fetal skeleton. Calcium accretion in the developing fetus is low until the third trimester of pregnancy when the fetus requires about 200 to 250 mg/day calcium to sustain skeletal growth (Givens and Macy, 1933; Trotter and Hixon, 1974). Intestinal calcium absorption of the mother doubles beginning early in pregnancy—even though there is little calcium transfer to the embryo at this stage (Heaney and Skillman, 1971; Kovacs and Kronenberg, 1997)—and continues through late pregnancy (Kent et al., 1991). Overall, relatively few studies have examined the effect of calcium supplementation on either fetal or maternal outcomes.

Maternal serum calcium falls during pregnancy (Pedersen et al., 1984), but this is likely not important from a physiological perspective in that it reflects the fall in serum albumin caused by plasma volume expansion and therefore does not imply calcium deficiency. Reports indicate that the concentration of ionized calcium remains normal during pregnancy (Frolich et al., 1992; Seely et al., 1997).

Pregnant women consuming moderate (800 to 1,000 mg/day [Gertner et al., 1986; Allen et al., 1991]) to high (1,950 mg/day [Cross et al., 1995]) levels of calcium are often hypercalciuric due to increased intestinal calcium absorption (i.e., absorptive hypercalciuria), and as such pregnancy itself can be a risk factor for kidney stones.

Within the developing human fetus, calcium metabolism is regulated differently from that of its mother. Serum calcium, ionized calcium, and phosphorus are raised above the maternal values, while PTH and calcitriol are low. The high calcium and phosphorus as well as the low levels of PTH all contribute to suppression of the renal 1α-hydroxylase and maintenance of low levels of calcitriol.

In adolescents, whose skeleton is still growing, pregnancy could theoretically reduce peak bone mass and increase the long-term risk of osteoporosis. Although most cross-sectional studies comparing BMD in teens early post-partum to never-pregnant teens (reviewed by Kovacs and Kronenberg, 1997) suggest that BMD or bone mass after adolescent pregnancy is not adversely affected, a few smaller associational studies report that adolescent age at first pregnancy is associated with lower BMD in the adult (Sowers et al., 1985, 1992; Fox et al., 1993). Chantry et al. (2004) analyzed data from the Third National Health and Nutrition Examination Survey (NHANES III) on BMD as measured by dual-energy X-ray absorptiometry (DXA) for 819 women ages 20 to 25 years and found that women pregnant as adolescents had the same BMD as nulliparous women and women pregnant as adults.

Lactation

Breast milk calcium content is homeostatically regulated, and maternal calcium intake does not appear to alter the breast milk calcium content (Kalkwarf et al., 1997; Jarjou et al., 2006). Generally, human breast milk will provide two to three times the amount of calcium to the infant during 6 months of lactation as the pregnant woman will have provided to the fetus during the preceding 9 months of pregnancy. To meet the calcium demands of pregnancy, key physiological changes in the female will also occur, but the adaptations differ from those that take place during pregnancy

(Kovacs and Kronenberg, 1997; Kalkwarf, 1999; Prentice, 2003; Kovacs, 2005, 2008; Kovacs and Kronenberg, 2008). Maternal bone resorption is markedly up-regulated (Specker et al., 1994; Kalkwarf et al., 1997), and it appears that most of the calcium present in milk derives from the maternal skeleton. Maternal BMD can decline 5 to 10 percent during the 2- to 6-month time period of exclusive breastfeeding. However, it normally returns to baseline during the 6 to 12 months post-weaning (Kalkwarf, 1999). Thus, in the long term, a history of lactation does not appear to increase the risk of low BMD or osteoporosis.

The physiological responses appear to be similar for lactating adolescents. In fact, an analysis using NHANES III data compared BMD from DXA measures in 819 women ages 20 to 25 years (Chantry et al., 2004), and found that young women who had breast-fed as adolescents had higher BMD than those who had not breast-fed, even after controlling for obstetrical variables. This suggests that the normal loss of BMD during lactation and the post-lactation recovery occurs in adolescents as well.

BONE MASS MEASURES ASSOCIATED WITH CALCIUM

Several key bone mass measures are commonly used in the context of calcium nutriture and related health outcomes. The accumulation and level of bone mass can be determined using the calcium balance method or, alternatively, the measurement of BMC or BMD based on DXA. The latter method relies on the assumption that about 32 percent of the measured bone mineral is calcium (Ellis et al., 1996; Ma et al., 1999). These methods are described below.

Calcium Balance

Calcium balance (positive, neutral, or negative) is the measure derived by taking the difference between the total intake and the sum of the urinary and endogenous fecal excretion. Balance studies embody a metabolic approach to examining the relationship between calcium intake and calcium retention and are based on the assumption that the body retains the amount of calcium that is needed. As such, measures of calcium balance (or of "calcium retention") can reflect conditions of bone accretion, bone maintenance, or bone loss. Calcium balance analyses involve measuring as precisely as possible the intake and the output of calcium. Output is usually reflected by urine and fecal calcium; sweat calcium is not usually measured, but its inclusion adds to the precision of the estimates. Calcium balance studies are expensive and require considerable subject cooperation owing to the prolonged stays in metabolic wards. Measures of calcium balance have limitations and are generally cross–sectional in nature, and their precision is difficult to ascertain. However, if well conducted, they provide valuable information on calcium requirements relative to the typical intake of the population under study. Long-term balance studies for calcium are generally not carried out because of the difficult study protocol. Calcium balance can also be estimated by using stable isotopes to trace the amount of calcium absorbed, usually in infants from a single feeding (Abrams, 2006).

Calcium balance outcomes that are *positive* are indicative of calcium accretion and are sometimes referred to as net calcium retention; *neutral* balance suggests maintenance of bone, and *negative* balance indicates bone loss. The relevance of the calcium balance state varies depending upon developmental stage. Infancy through late adolescence are characterized by positive calcium balance. In female adolescents and adults, even within the normal menstrual cycle, there are measurable fluctuations in calcium balance owing to the effects of fluctuating sex steroid levels and other factors on the basal rates of bone formation and resorption. Later in life, menopause and age-related bone loss lead to a net loss as a result of calcium due to enhanced bone resorption.

In the 1997 IOM report that focused on calcium DRIs (IOM, 1997), metabolic studies of calcium balance were used to obtain data on the relationship between calcium intakes and retention, from which a non-linear regression model was developed; from this was derived an intake of calcium that would be adequate to attain a predetermined *desirable* calcium retention.[4] The approach used in 1997 was a refinement of an earlier approach suggested to determine the point at which additional calcium does not significantly increase calcium retention, called the *plateau intake* (Spencer et al., 1984; Matkovic and Heaney, 1992).

The balance studies included in the 1997 IOM report (IOM, 1997) met

---

[4]A footnote to the 1997 IOM report (IOM, 1997) explains the decision not to base considerations on maximal calcium retention: The 1997 committee intended to use a recently described statistical model (Jackman et al., 1997) to estimate an intake necessary to support maximal calcium retention and from which to derive an EAR, and did so in the pre-publication of the report. In the original paper by Jackman et al. (1997), an estimate was made of the lowest level of calcium intake that was statistically indistinguishable from 100 percent maximal retention in some individuals. However, the Standing Committee on the Scientific Evaluation of Dietary Reference Intakes (DRI Committee) reviewed the approach in the pre-publication of the report and adopted a different interpretation of the data for the purpose of establishing an AI. The 1997 committee was subsequently advised that there were both statistical and biological concerns with the application of the percent maximal retention model (presented in Appendix E of the 1997 IOM report [IOM, 1997]). The final print of the 1997 report retained the statistical model described by Jackman et al. (1997), but applied it to determine, from the same calcium balance data as was used in the pre-publication report, an estimate of the calcium intake that is sufficient to achieve a defined, desirable level of calcium retention specific to the age groups considered.

criteria that included the following: subjects had a wide range of calcium intakes, as variability in retention increases at higher intakes; the balance studies were initiated at least 7 days after starting the diet in order for subjects to approach a steady state, as observed by Dawson-Hughes et al. (1988); and, where possible, the adult balance studies included were only for subjects who were consuming calcium at their usual intakes, unless otherwise indicated. By selecting studies conducted on such subjects, the 1997 committee concluded that it obviated the concern about whether the *bone remodeling transient* (i.e., the temporary alteration in the balance between bone formation and bone resorption) might introduce bias in the calcium retentions observed (IOM, 1997). Such selection was not possible in studies in children who were randomized to one of two calcium intakes. However, in children, the impact of the bone remodeling transient related to changing intake is overshadowed by their rapid and constantly changing rates of calcium accretion (i.e., their modeling and remodeling rates are not in steady state, even without an intake change).

For the 1997 DRI development (IOM, 1997), the non-linear regression model describing the relationship between calcium intake and retention was solved to obtain a predetermined *desirable* calcium retention that was specific for each age group. According to the report, the major limitation of the data available was that bone mineral accretion during growth had not yet been studied over a wide range of calcium intakes. Overall, the committee expressed concern about the uncertainties in the methods inherent in balance studies.

Specifics about calcium balance studies that relate to DRI development are provided in Chapter 4, but, as background the recent work of Hunt and Johnson (2007) offers some remedy for the uncertainties surrounding the precision of balance studies. Hunt and Johnson (2007) examined data from 155 subjects—men and women between the ages of 20 and 75 years—who took part in 19 feeding studies conducted at one site (Grand Forks Human Nutrition Research Unit) between 1976 and 1995 in a metabolic unit under carefully controlled conditions.

In their overall analysis, the relationship between intake and output was examined by fitting random coefficient models. Rather than model calcium retention compared with calcium intake by using the Jackman et al. (1997) model, as was done in the 1997 DRI report (IOM, 1997), Hunt and Johnson (2007) modeled output rather than retention to avoid confounding in the precision of estimates that would be caused by including intake as a component of the dependent variable. In the Hunt and Johnson (2007) analysis, the data summary did not show non-linearity and therefore did not justify the use of a more complex non-linear model. The authors noted that the coefficients of the 1997 approach appeared to be greatly influenced by data points above the 99th percentile of daily calcium intake and pointed out that the data in their model reflected typical calcium intake between the 5th and approximately 95th percentiles for all boys and men 9 or more years of age, and between the approximately 25th and greater than 99th percentiles for all girls and women 9 or more years of age.

Hunt and Johnson (2007) also pointed out that most (but not all) studies with adults that indicate a positive influence of high total calcium in reducing the rate of bone remodeling were confounded by the presence of vitamin D as an experimental co-variable. In their study, the metabolic diets were similar to the estimated median intake of vitamin D by free-living young women. In short, the analysis may provide a reasonable approach for extracting meaningful data from calcium balance studies that are often confounded by multiple dietary factors. At this point, factorial methods should be briefly noted as the determination of calcium requirements has also made use of a factorial approach as noted in the 1997 DRI report (IOM, 1997). The factorial approach allows the estimate of an intake level that achieves the measured levels of calcium accretion/retention. The method combines estimates of losses of calcium via its main routes in apparently healthy individuals and then assumes that these losses represent the degree to which calcium intake, as corrected by estimated absorption, is required to balance these losses. The weakness in this method is that it is unusual for all of the necessary measurements to be obtained within a single study. Therefore, most calculations using the factorial approach are compiled from data in different studies and thus in different subjects; this can introduce considerable variation and confound the outcomes. This approach, as carried out in the 1997 IOM report on DRIs for calcium and vitamin D (IOM, 1997), where the interest was in desirable retention, is illustrated in Table 2-1.

Bone Mineral Content and Bone Mineral Density

BMC is the amount of mineral at a particular skeletal site, such as the femoral neck, lumbar spine, or total body. BMC is correctly a three-dimensional measurement, but when it is commonly measured by DXA, a cross-section of bone is analyzed, and the two-dimensional output is a real BMD (i.e., BMC divided by the area of the scanned region). True measurements of BMC (volumetric BMD) can be determined non-invasively by computed tomography. Throughout this report, the term "BMD" generally means areal BMD unless specified as volumetric BMD. Most importantly, any of these measures are strong predictors of fracture risk (IOM, 1997). Bone density studies can be considered to reflect average intakes of calcium over a long period of time. When available, such data likely provide

TABLE 2-1 1997 DRI Factorial Approach for Determining Calcium Requirements During Peak Calcium Accretion in White Adolescents

	Number of Observations	Female Calcium Requirements (mg/day)	Number of Observations	Male Calcium Requirements (mg/day)
Peak calcium accretion	507	212[a]	471	282[a]
Urinary losses	28	106[b]	14	127[c]
Endogenous fecal calcium	14	112[d]	3	108[e]
Sweat Losses		55[f]		55[f]
Total		485		572
Total adjusted for absorption[g]		1,276		1,505

[a]Martin et al. (1997) using peak BMC velocity.
[b]Greger et al. (1978); Weaver et al. (1995).
[c]Matkovic (1991).
[d]Wastney et al. (1996) for mean age 13 years on calcium intakes of 1,330 mg/day.
[e]Abrams et al. (1992).
[f]Taken from Peacock (1991) who adjusted the adult data of Charles et al. (1983) for body weight.
[g]Absorption is 38% for mean age 13 years on calcium intakes of 1,330 mg/day (Wastney et al., 1996).

a better snapshot of long-term calcium intake than does the combination of accretion/retention data.

In children, change in BMC is a useful indicator of calcium retention; change in BMD is less suitable, because it overestimates mineral content as a result of changes in skeletal size from growth (IOM, 1997). In adults, with their generally stable skeletal size, changes in either BMD or BMC are useful measures. In the context of longitudinal calcium intervention trials that measure change in BMC, the measures can provide data on the long-term impact of calcium intake not only on the total skeleton, but also on skeletal sites that are subject to osteoporotic fracture (IOM, 1997). However, because DXA does not distinguish between calcium that is within bone and calcium on the surface (e.g., osteophytes, calcifications in other tissues) or within blood vessels (e.g., calcified aorta), an increase in BMC or BMD, particularly in the spine, may result in false positive readings suggesting high bone mass (Banks et al., 1994).

In DXA, fan beam dual-energy X-ray beams are used to measure bone mass, with correction for overlying soft tissue. Data are converted to BMC and the area represented is measured. The BMD measurement is annotated in grams of mineral per square centimeter. BMC represents the amount of mineral in a volume of bone without consideration of total body size. It is thus independent of growth. The DXA method is also limited by excessive soft tissue as present in massively obese individuals. Dual-energy computed tomography measurements, which are much more expensive and require larger X-ray doses can provide density as well as volumetric determinants and are useful for estimating the entire mineral component.

Direct estimation of calcium balance in older adults by BMD is highly dependent on other factors besides calcium intake, such as serum levels of estrogen and PTH, intake of other nutrients (e.g., phosphorus and sodium), as well as adequate intestinal absorption and normal kidney function. Indeed, bone remodeling is not directly regulated by calcium, although it can suppress PTH-induced increases in bone resorption under certain conditions. Circumstances that enhance bone resorption, such as estrogen deficiency, or glucocorticoid use, alter the organic matrix and reduce the thickness and density of trabeculae, independent of calcium intake. In short, density measurements do not directly reflect calcium stores.

OTHER FACTORS RELATED TO CALCIUM NUTRITURE

As described above, not all calcium consumed is absorbed once it enters the gut. In general, the efficiency of calcium absorption is in reverse proportion to the amount of calcium consumed at any one time. Other factors also affect the amount of calcium available to the body.

Bioavailability of Calcium

Humans absorb about 30 percent of the calcium present in foods, but this varies with the type of food consumed. Bioavailability is generally increased when calcium is well solubilized and inhibited in the presence of agents that bind calcium or form insoluble calcium salts. The absorption of calcium is about 30 percent from dairy and fortified foods (e.g., orange juice, tofu, soy milk) and nearly twice as high from certain green vegetables (bok choy, broccoli, and kale). If a food contains compounds that bind calcium or otherwise interfere with calcium absorption, such as oxalic acid and phytic acid, then the food source is considered to be a poor source of calcium. Foods with high levels of oxalic acid include spinach, collard greens, sweet potatoes, rhubarb, and beans. Among the foods high in phytic acid are fiber-containing whole-grain products and wheat bran, beans, seeds, nuts, and soy isolates. The extent to which these compounds affect calcium absorption varies, and food combinations affect overall absorption efficiency. Eating spinach with milk at the same time reduces the absorption of the calcium in the milk (Weaver and Heaney, 1991); in contrast, wheat products (with the exception of wheat bran) do not appear to have a negative impact on calcium absorption (Weaver et al., 1991).[5] Vegan sources of calcium may be less bioavailable and, in turn, problematic for ensuring adequate calcium intake (Weaver, 2009).

The calcium salts most commonly used as supplements or food fortificants exhibit similar absorbability when tested in pure chemical form (Rafferty et al., 2007), but the absorbability of calcium from pharmaceutical preparations can fall short of predictions from studies of pure salts (Weaver and Heaney, 2006a). Calcium citrate appears to be better absorbed than calcium carbonate (Harvey et al., 1988); when they are taken with food, however, some researchers (Heaney et al., 1999), but not all (Heller et al., 2000), suggest comparable bioavailability of the two forms of calcium.

Factors in the Diet

Protein

Protein intake stimulates acid release in the stomach, and this, in turn, enhances calcium absorption. However, it has long been known that protein also increases urinary calcium excretion. The effect of protein on calcium retention and hence bone health has been controversial (IOM, 1997). Several observational and clinical studies have examined the effect of high-protein diets on bone (Shapses and Sukumar, 2010). Over a 4-year period in the Framingham Osteoporosis Study (Hannan et al., 2000), a higher protein intake (84 to 152 g/day), was positively associated with change in femoral neck and spine BMD (Shapese and Sukumar, 2010). Additionally, NHANES II suggested a positive association between femoral neck BMD and total protein intake (> 75 g/day) (Kerstetter et al., 2000; Shapses and Sukumar, 2010). In contrast, some epidemiological studies suggest that high protein diets reduce bone mass; this has been attributed to a higher acid load, leading to a buffering response by the skeleton and greater urinary calcium excretion. A recent meta-analysis (Darling et al., 2009) concluded that there is a small benefit of protein for bone health, but the benefit may not necessarily translate into reduced fracture risk in the long term. Shapses and Sukumar (2010) suggested that the currently available data would lead to the conclusion that there is a beneficial effect of increasing protein intake on bone in older individuals who normally have a habitually low intake of protein.

---

[5]Available online at http://ods.od.nih.gov/factsheets/calcium/ (accessed July 23, 2010).

Foods and Food Components

Sodium and potassium in the diet may also affect calcium nutriture. High intakes of sodium increase urinary calcium excretion. In contrast, adding more potassium to a high-sodium diet might help decrease calcium excretion, particularly in postmenopausal women (Sellmeyer et al., 2002; IOM, 2005).

Alcohol intake can affect calcium nutriture by reducing calcium absorption (Hirsch and Peng, 1996), although the amount of alcohol required to cause an effect and whether moderate alcohol consumption is helpful or harmful to bone are unknown.

Caffeine from coffee and tea modestly increases calcium excretion and reduces absorption (Heaney and Recker, 1982; Bergman et al., 1990). Two studies have indicated that caffeine intake (two to three or more cups of coffee per day) will result in bone loss, but only in individuals with low milk or low total calcium intake (Barrett-Connor et al., 1994; Harris and Dawson-Hughes, 1994).

Phosphate is also of interest. Food phosphate is a mixture of inorganic and organic forms, and there is no evidence that its absorption efficiency varies with dietary intake. A portion of phosphorus absorption is due to saturable, active transport facilitated by calcitriol. However, fractional phosphorus absorption is virtually constant across a broad range of intakes suggesting that absorption occurs primarily by a passive, concentration-dependent process. Several observational studies have suggested that the consumption of carbonated soft drinks with high levels of phosphate is associated with reduced bone mass and increased fracture risk, but it is likely that the effect is due to replacing milk with soda, rather than to phosphorus itself (Calvo, 1993; Heaney and Rafferty, 2001).

REFERENCES

Aaron, J. E., J. C. Gallagher, J. Anderson, L. Stasiak, E. B. Longton, B. E. Nordin and M. Nicholson. 1974. Frequency of osteomalacia and osteoporosis in fractures of the proximal femur. Lancet 1(7851): 229-33.

Abrams, S. A., J. B. Sidbury, J. Muenzer, N. V. Esteban, N. E. Vieira and A. L. Yergey. 1991. Stable isotopic measurement of endogenous fecal calcium excretion in children. Journal of Pediatric Gastroenterology and Nutrition 12(4): 469-73.

Abrams, S. A., N. V. Esteban, N. E. Vieira, J. B. Sidbury, B. L. Specker and A. L. Yergey. 1992. Developmental changes in calcium kinetics in children assessed using stable isotopes. Journal of Bone and Mineral Research 7(3): 287-93.

Abrams, S. A. and J. E. Stuff. 1994. Calcium metabolism in girls: current dietary intakes lead to low rates of calcium absorption and retention during puberty. American Journal of Clinical Nutrition 60(5): 739-43.

Abrams, S. A., J. Wen and J. E. Stuff. 1997. Absorption of calcium, zinc, and iron from breast milk by five- to seven-month-old infants. Pediatric Research 41(3): 384-90.

Abrams, S. A., K. C. Copeland, S. K. Gunn, C. M. Gundberg, K. O. Klein and K. J. Ellis. 2000. Calcium absorption, bone mass accumulation, and kinetics increase during early pubertal development in girls. Journal of Clinical Endocrinology and Metabolism 85(5): 1805-9.

Abrams, S. A., I. J. Griffin and P. M. Davila. 2002. Calcium and zinc absorption from lactose-containing and lactose-free infant formulas. American Journal of Clinical Nutrition 76(2): 442-6.

Abrams, S. A. 2006. Building bones in babies: can and should we exceed the human milk-fed infant's rate of bone calcium accretion? Nutrition Reviews 64(11): 487-94.

Abrams, S. A. 2010. Calcium absorption in infants and small children: methods of determination and recent findings. Nutrients 2(4): 474-80.

Alevizaki, C. C., D. G. Ikkos and P. Singhelakis. 1973. Progressive decrease of true intestinal calcium absorption with age in normal man. Journal of Nuclear Medicine 14(10): 760-2.

Allen, J. C., R. P. Keller, P. Archer and M. C. Neville. 1991. Studies in human lactation: milk composition and daily secretion rates of macronutrients in the first year of lactation. American Journal of Clinical Nutrition 54(1): 69-80.

Aloia, J. F., D. G. Chen, J. K. Yeh and H. Chen. 2010. Serum vitamin D metabolites and intestinal calcium absorption efficiency in women. American Journal of Clinical Nutrition 92(4): 835-40.

Anderson, J. 1961. Metabolic diseases affecting the locomotor system. III. Investigations of biochemical changes in osteomalacia and osteoporosis. Annals of Physical Medicine 6: 1-9.

Anderson, J. J. 2001. Calcium requirements during adolescence to maximize bone health. Journal of the American College of Nutrition 20(2 Suppl): 186S-91S.

Atkinson, S. A., B. P. Alston-Mills, B. Lonnerdal, M. C. Neville and M. P. Thompson. 1995. Major minerals and ionic constituents of human and bovine milk. In *Handbook of Milk Composition*, edited by R. J. Jensen. San Diego, CA: Academic Press. Pp. 593-619.

Avioli, L. V., J. E. McDonald and S. W. Lee. 1965. The influence of age on the intestinal absorption of 47-Ca absorption in post-menopausal osteoporosis. Journal of Clinical Investigation 44(12): 1960-7.

Bailey, D. A., A. D. Martin, H. A. McKay, S. Whiting and R. Mirwald. 2000. Calcium accretion in girls and boys during puberty: a longitudinal analysis. Journal of Bone and Mineral Research 15(11): 2245-50.

Bailey, R. L., K. W. Dodd, J. A. Goldman, J. J. Gahche, J. T. Dwyer, A. J. Moshfegh, C. T. Sempos and M. F. Picciano. 2010. Estimation of total usual calcium and vitamin D intake in the United States. Journal of Nutrition 140(4): 817-22.

Banks, L. M., B. Lees, J. E. MacSweeney and J. C. Stevenson. 1994. Effect of degenerative spinal and aortic calcification on bone density measurements in post-menopausal women: links between osteoporosis and cardiovascular disease? European Journal of Clinical Investigation 24(12): 813-7.

Barrett-Connor, E., J. C. Chang and S. L. Edelstein. 1994. Coffee-associated osteoporosis offset by daily milk consumption. The Rancho Bernardo Study. JAMA 271(4): 280-3.

Bergman, E. A., L. K. Massey, K. J. Wise and D. J. Sherrard. 1990. Effects of dietary caffeine on renal handling of minerals in adult women. Life Sciences 47(6): 557-64.

Bo-Linn, G. W., G. R. Davis, D. J. Buddrus, S. G. Morawski, C. Santa Ana and J. S. Fordtran. 1984. An evaluation of the importance of gastric acid secretion in the absorption of dietary calcium. Journal of Clinical Investigation 73(3): 640-7.

Bonjour, J. P., G. Theintz, F. Law, D. Slosman and R. Rizzoli. 1994. Peak bone mass. Osteoporosis International 4(Suppl 1): 7-13.

Bullamore, J. R., R. Wilkinson, J. C. Gallagher, B. E. Nordin and D. H. Marshall. 1970. Effect of age on calcium absorption. Lancet 2(7672): 535-7.

Butte, N. F., C. Garza, E. O. Smith and B. L. Nichols. 1984. Human milk intake and growth in exclusively breast-fed infants. Journal of Pediatrics 104(2): 187-95.

Calvo, M. S. 1993. Dietary phosphorus, calcium metabolism and bone. Journal of Nutrition 123(9): 1627-33.

Calvo, M. S., S. J. Whiting and C. N. Barton. 2004. Vitamin D fortification in the United States and Canada: current status and data needs. American Journal of Clinical Nutrition 80(6 Suppl): 1710S-6S.

Campbell, S. B., D. J. Macfarlane, S. J. Fleming and F. A. Khafagi. 1994. Increased skeletal uptake of Tc-99m methylene diphosphonate in milk-alkali syndrome. Clinical Nuclear Medicine 19(3): 207-11.

Carr, C. J. and R. F. Shangraw. 1987. Nutritional and pharmaceutical aspects of calcium supplementation. American Pharmacy NS27(2): 49-50, 54-7.

Chantry, C. J., P. Auinger and R. S. Byrd. 2004. Lactation among adolescent mothers and subsequent bone mineral density. Archives of Pediatrics and Adolescent Medicine 158(7): 650-6.

Chapuy, M. C., M. E. Arlot, F. Duboeuf, J. Brun, B. Crouzet, S. Arnaud, P. D. Delmas and P. J. Meunier. 1992. Vitamin D3 and calcium to prevent hip fractures in the elderly women. New England Journal of Medicine 327(23): 1637-42.

Charles, P., F. T. Jensen, L. Mosekilde and H. H. Hansen. 1983. Calcium metabolism evaluated by 47Ca kinetics: estimation of dermal calcium loss. Clinical Science (London) 65(4): 415-22.

Cifuentes, M., A. B. Morano, H. A. Chowdhury and S. A. Shapses. 2002. Energy restriction reduces fractional calcium absorption in mature obese and lean rats. Journal of Nutrition 132(9): 2660-6.

Cross, N. A., L. S. Hillman, S. H. Allen, G. F. Krause and N. E. Vieira. 1995. Calcium homeostasis and bone metabolism during pregnancy, lactation, and postweaning: a longitudinal study. American Journal of Clinical Nutrition 61(3): 514-23.

Darling, A. L., D. J. Millward, D. J. Torgerson, C. E. Hewitt and S. A. Lanham-New. 2009. Dietary protein and bone health: a systematic review and meta-analysis. American Journal of Clinical Nutrition 90(6): 1674-92.

Dawson-Hughes, B., D. T. Stern, C. C. Shipp and H. M. Rasmussen. 1988. Effect of lowering dietary calcium intake on fractional whole body calcium retention. Journal of Clinical Endocrinology and Metabolism 67(1): 62-8.

Dawson-Hughes, B., S. Harris, C. Kramich, G. Dallal and H. M. Rasmussen. 1993. Calcium retention and hormone levels in black and white women on high- and low-calcium diets. Journal of Bone and Mineral Research 8(7): 779-87.

Demer, L. and Y. Tintut. 2010. The bone-vascular axis in chronic kidney disease. Current Opinion in Nephrology and Hypertension 19(4): 349-53.

Eastell, R., A. L. Yergey, N. E. Vieira, S. L. Cedel, R. Kumar and B. L. Riggs. 1991. Interrelationship among vitamin D metabolism, true calcium absorption, parathyroid function, and age in women: evidence of an age-related intestinal resistance to 1,25-dihydroxyvitamin D action. Journal of Bone and Mineral Research 6(2): 125-32.

Ebeling, P. R., M. E. Sandgren, E. P. DiMagno, A. W. Lane, H. F. DeLuca and B. L. Riggs. 1992. Evidence of an age-related decrease in intestinal responsiveness to vitamin D: relationship between serum 1,25-dihydroxyvitamin D3 and intestinal vitamin D receptor concentrations in normal women. Journal of Clinical Endocrinology and Metabolism 75(1): 176-82.

Ebeling, P. R., L. M. Atley, J. R. Guthrie, H. G. Burger, L. Dennerstein, J. L. Hopper and J. D. Wark. 1996. Bone turnover markers and bone density across the menopausal transition. Journal of Clinical Endocrinology and Metabolism 81(9): 3366-71.

Ellis, K. J., R. J. Shypailo, A. Hergenroeder, M. Perez and S. Abrams. 1996. Total body calcium and bone mineral content: comparison of dual-energy X-ray absorptiometry with neutron activation analysis. Journal of Bone and Mineral Research 11(6): 843-8.

Favus, M. J. 2008. Mineral and bone homeostasis. In *Cecil Medicine, 23rd Edition*, edited by L. Goldman and D. Ausiello. Philadelphia, PA: Saunders Elsevier. Pp. 1871-8.

Finkelstein, J. S., S. E. Brockwell, V. Mehta, G. A. Greendale, M. R. Sowers, B. Ettinger, J. C. Lo, J. M. Johnston, J. A. Cauley, M. E. Danielson and R. M. Neer. 2008. Bone mineral density changes during the menopause transition in a multiethnic cohort of women. Journal of Clinical Endocrinology and Metabolism 93(3): 861-8.

Fomon, S. J. and S. E. Nelson. 1993. Calcium, phosphorus, magnesium, and sulfur. In *Nutrition of Normal Infants*, edited by S. J. Fomon. St. Louis: Mosby-Year Book, Inc. Pp. 192-216.

Fox, K. M., J. Magaziner, R. Sherwin, J. C. Scott, C. C. Plato, M. Nevitt and S. Cummings. 1993. Reproductive correlates of bone mass in elderly women. Study of Osteoporotic Fractures Research Group. Journal of Bone and Mineral Research 8(8): 901-8.

Frolich, A., M. Rudnicki, T. Storm, N. Rasmussen and L. Hegedus. 1992. Impaired 1,25-dihydroxyvitamin D production in pregnancy-induced hypertension. European Journal of Obstetrics, Gynecology, and Reproductive Biology 47(1): 25-9.

Gafni, R. I. and J. Baron. 2007. Childhood bone mass acquisition and peak bone mass may not be important determinants of bone mass in late adulthood. Pediatrics 119(Suppl 2): S131-6.

Gallagher, J. C., B. L. Riggs, J. Eisman, A. Hamstra, S. B. Arnaud and H. F. DeLuca. 1979. Intestinal calcium absorption and serum vitamin D metabolites in normal subjects and osteoporotic patients: effect of age and dietary calcium. Journal of Clinical Investigation 64(3): 729-36.

Gallagher, J. C., B. L. Riggs and H. F. DeLuca. 1980. Effect of estrogen on calcium absorption and serum vitamin D metabolites in postmenopausal osteoporosis. Journal of Clinical Endocrinology and Metabolism 51(6): 1359-64.

Gallagher, J. C., P. B. Rapuri, G. Haynatzki and J. R. Detter. 2002. Effect of discontinuation of estrogen, calcitriol, and the combination of both on bone density and bone markers. Journal of Clinical Endocrinology and Metabolism 87(11): 4914-23.

Garnero, P., E. Hausherr, M. C. Chapuy, C. Marcelli, H. Grandjean, C. Muller, C. Cormier, G. Breart, P. J. Meunier and P. D. Delmas. 1996. Markers of bone resorption predict hip fracture in elderly women: the EPIDOS Prospective Study. Journal of Bone and Mineral Research 11(10): 1531-8.

Gertner, J. M., D. R. Coustan, A. S. Kliger, L. E. Mallette, N. Ravin and A. E. Broadus. 1986. Pregnancy as state of physiologic absorptive hypercalciuria. American Journal of Medicine 81(3): 451-6.

Ghishan, F. K., J. T. Jenkins and M. K. Younoszai. 1980. Maturation of calcium transport in the rat small and large intestine. Journal of Nutrition 110(8): 1622-8.

Ghishan, F. K., P. Parker, S. Nichols and A. Hoyumpa. 1984. Kinetics of intestinal calcium transport during maturation in rats. Pediatric Research 18(3): 235-9.

Givens, M. H. and I. G. Macy. 1933. The chemical composition of the human fetus. Journal of Biological Chemistry 102(1): 7-17.

Goldschmied, A., B. Modan, R. A. Greenberg, S. Zurkowski and M. Modan. 1975. Urinary calcium excretion in relation to kidney function in the adult. Journal of the American Geriatrics Society 23(4): 155-60.

Greenspan, S. L., L. A. Maitland, E. R. Myers, M. B. Krasnow and T. H. Kido. 1994. Femoral bone loss progresses with age: a longitudinal study in women over age 65. Journal of Bone and Mineral Research 9(12): 1959-65.

Greger, J. L., P. Baligar, R. P. Abernathy, O. A. Bennett and T. Peterson. 1978. Calcium, magnesium, phosphorus, copper, and manganese balance in adolescent females. American Journal of Clinical Nutrition 31(1): 117-21.

Guyton, A. C. and J. E. Hall, Eds. (2001). *Textbook in Medical Physiology, 10th Edition.* Philadelphia, PA: W.B. Saunders.

Hadjidakis, D. J. and I. I. Androulakis. 2006. Bone Remodeling. Annals of the New York Academy of Sciences 1092(Women's Health and Disease: Gynecologic, Endocrine, and Reproductive Issues): 385-96.

Halloran, B. P. and H. F. DeLuca. 1980. Calcium transport in small intestine during pregnancy and lactation. American Journal of Physiology 239(1): E64-8.

Hannan, M. T., D. T. Felson and J. J. Anderson. 1992. Bone mineral density in elderly men and women: results from the Framingham Osteoporosis Study. Journal of Bone and Mineral Research 7(5): 547-53.

Hannan, M. T., K. L. Tucker, B. Dawson-Hughes, L. A. Cupples, D. T. Felson and D. P. Kiel. 2000. Effect of dietary protein on bone loss in elderly men and women: the Framingham Osteoporosis Study. Journal of Bone and Mineral Research 15(12): 2504-12.

Harris, S. S. and B. Dawson-Hughes. 1994. Caffeine and bone loss in healthy postmenopausal women. American Journal of Clinical Nutrition 60(4): 573-8.

Harvey, J. A., M. M. Zobitz and C. Y. Pak. 1988. Dose dependency of calcium absorption: a comparison of calcium carbonate and calcium citrate. Journal of Bone and Mineral Research 3(3): 253-8.

Heaney, R. P. and T. G. Skillman. 1971. Calcium metabolism in normal human pregnancy. Journal of Clinical Endocrinology and Metabolism 33(4): 661-70.

Heaney, R. P., P. D. Saville and R. R. Recker. 1975. Calcium absorption as a function of calcium intake. Journal of Laboratory and Clinical Medicine 85(6): 881-90.

Heaney, R. P. and R. R. Recker. 1982. Effects of nitrogen, phosphorus, and caffeine on calcium balance in women. Journal of Laboratory and Clinical Medicine 99(1): 46-55.

Heaney, R. P., R. R. Recker, M. R. Stegman and A. J. Moy. 1989. Calcium absorption in women: relationships to calcium intake, estrogen status, and age. Journal of Bone and Mineral Research 4(4): 469-75.

Heaney, R. P. and R. R. Recker. 1994. Determinants of endogenous fecal calcium in healthy women. Journal of Bone and Mineral Research 9(10): 1621-7.

Heaney, R. P., M. S. Dowell and M. J. Barger-Lux. 1999. Absorption of calcium as the carbonate and citrate salts, with some observations on method. Osteoporosis International 9(1): 19-23.

Heaney, R. P., M. S. Dowell, J. Bierman, C. A. Hale and A. Bendich. 2001. Absorbability and cost effectiveness in calcium supplementation. Journal of the American College of Nutrition 20(3): 239-46.

Heaney, R. P. and K. Rafferty. 2001. Carbonated beverages and urinary calcium excretion. American Journal of Clinical Nutrition 74(3): 343-7.

Heaney, R. P. 2003. Is the paradigm shifting? Bone 33(4): 457-65.

Heinig, M. J., L. A. Nommsen, J. M. Peerson, B. Lonnerdal and K. G. Dewey. 1993. Energy and protein intakes of breast-fed and formula-fed infants during the first year of life and their association with growth velocity: the DARLING Study. American Journal of Clinical Nutrition 58(2): 152-61.

Heller, H. J., L. G. Greer, S. D. Haynes, J. R. Poindexter and C. Y. Pak. 2000. Pharmacokinetic and pharmacodynamic comparison of two calcium supplements in postmenopausal women. Journal of Clinical Pharmacology 40(11): 1237-44.

Hicks, P. D., K. M. Hawthorne, J. Marunyzy, C. Berseth, J. Heubi and S. A. Abrams. 2010. Similar calcium status is present in infants fed formula with and without prebiotics. Presented at Pediatric Academic Societies (PAS). Vancouver, British Columbia.

Hirsch, P. E. and T. C. Peng. 1996. Effects of alcohol on calcium homeostasis and bone. In *Calcium and Phosphorus in Health and Disease*, edited by J. Anderson and S. Garner. Boca Raton, FL: CRC Press.

Hoenderop, J. G., D. Muller, M. Suzuki, C. H. van Os and R. J. Bindels. 2000. Epithelial calcium channel: gate-keeper of active calcium reabsorption. Current Opinion in Nephrology and Hypertension 9(4): 335-40.

Hunt, J. N. and C. Johnson. 1983. Relation between gastric secretion of acid and urinary excretion of calcium after oral supplements of calcium. Digestive Diseases and Sciences 28(5): 417-21.

Hunt, C. D. and L. K. Johnson. 2007. Calcium requirements: new estimations for men and women by cross–sectional statistical analyses of calcium balance data from metabolic studies. American Journal of Clinical Nutrition 86(4): 1054-63.

Ilich, J. Z. and J. E. Kerstetter. 2000. Nutrition in bone health revisited: a story beyond calcium. Journal of the American College of Nutrition 19(6): 715-37.

IOM (Institute of Medicine). 1997. *Dietary Reference Intakes for Calcium, Phosphorus, Magnesium, Vitamin D, and Fluoride*. Washington, DC: National Academy Press.

IOM. 2005. *Dietary Reference Intakes for Water, Potassium, Sodium, Chloride, and Sulfate*. Washington, DC: The National Academies Press.

Ireland, P. and J. S. Fordtran. 1973. Effect of dietary calcium and age on jejunal calcium absorption in humans studied by intestinal perfusion. Journal of Clinical Investigation 52(11): 2672-81.

Jackman, L. A., S. S. Millane, B. R. Martin, O. B. Wood, G. P. McCabe, M. Peacock and C. M. Weaver. 1997. Calcium retention in relation to calcium intake and postmenarcheal age in adolescent females. American Journal of Clinical Nutrition 66(2): 327-33.

Jarjou, L. M., A. Prentice, Y. Sawo, M. A. Laskey, J. Bennett, G. R. Goldberg and T. J. Cole. 2006. Randomized, placebo-controlled, calcium supplementation study in pregnant Gambian women: effects on breast-milk calcium concentrations and infant birth weight, growth, and bone mineral accretion in the first year of life. American Journal of Clinical Nutrition 83(3): 657-66.

Jenkins, D. H., J. G. Roberts, D. Webster and E. O. Williams. 1973. Osteomalacia in elderly patients with fracture of the femoral neck. A clinico-pathological study. Journal of Bone and Joint Surgery. British Volume 55(3): 575-80.

Jones, G. and T. V. Nguyen. 2000. Associations between maternal peak bone mass and bone mass in prepubertal male and female children. Journal of Bone and Mineral Research 15(10): 1998-2004.

Jouanny, P., F. Guillemin, C. Kuntz, C. Jeandel and J. Pourel. 1995. Environmental and genetic factors affecting bone mass. Similarity of bone density among members of healthy families. Arthritis & Rheumatism 38(1): 61-7.

Kalkwarf, H. J., B. L. Specker, D. C. Bianchi, J. Ranz and M. Ho. 1997. The effect of calcium supplementation on bone density during lactation and after weaning. New England Journal of Medicine 337(8): 523-8.

Kalkwarf, H. J. 1999. Hormonal and dietary regulation of changes in bone density during lactation and after weaning in women. Journal of Mammary Gland Biology and Neoplasia 4(3): 319-29.

Keller, J. L., A. J. Lanou and N. D. Barnard. 2002. The consumer cost of calcium from food and supplements. Journal of the American Dietetic Association 102(11): 1669-71.

Kenny, A. M. and K. M. Prestwood. 2000. Osteoporosis. Pathogenesis, diagnosis, and treatment in older adults. Rheumatic Diseases Clinics of North America 26(3): 569-91.

Kent, G. N., R. I. Price, D. H. Gutteridge, K. J. Rosman, M. Smith, J. R. Allen, C. J. Hickling and S. L. Blakeman. 1991. The efficiency of intestinal calcium absorption is increased in late pregnancy but not in established lactation. Calcified Tissue International 48(4): 293-5.

Kerstetter, J. E., A. C. Looker and K. L. Insogna. 2000. Low dietary protein and low bone density. Calcified Tissue International 66(4): 313.

Kobayashi, A., S. Kawai, Y. Obe and Y. Nagashima. 1975. Effects of dietary lactose and lactase preparation on the intestinal absorption of calcium and magnesium in normal infants. American Journal of Clinical Nutrition 28(7): 681-3.

Kocian, J., I. Skala and K. Bakos. 1973. Calcium absorption from milk and lactose-free milk in healthy subjects and patients with lactose intolerance. Digestion 9(4): 317-24.

Komar, L., J. Nieves, F. Cosman, A. Rubin, V. Shen and R. Lindsay. 1993. Calcium homeostasis of an elderly population upon admission to a nursing home. Journal of the American Geriatrics Society 41(10): 1057-64.

Kovacs, C. S. and H. M. Kronenberg. 1997. Maternal-fetal calcium and bone metabolism during pregnancy, puerperium, and lactation. Endocrine Reviews 18(6): 832-72.

Kovacs, C. S. 2001. Calcium and bone metabolism in pregnancy and lactation. Journal of Clinical Endocrinology and Metabolism 86(6): 2344-8.

Kovacs, C. S. 2005. Calcium and bone metabolism during pregnancy and lactation. Journal of Mammary Gland Biology and Neoplasia 10(2): 105-18.

Kovacs, C. S. 2008. Vitamin D in pregnancy and lactation: maternal, fetal, and neonatal outcomes from human and animal studies. American Journal of Clinical Nutrition 88(2): 520S-8S.

Kovacs, C. S. and H. M. Kronenberg. 2008. Pregnancy and lactation. In *Primer on the Metabolic Bone Diseases and Disorders of Mineral Metabolism, 7th Edition*, edited by C. J. Rosen. Washington, DC: ASBMR Press. Pp. 90-5.

Krall, E. A. and B. Dawson-Hughes. 1993. Heritable and life-style determinants of bone mineral density. Journal of Bone and Mineral Research 8(1): 1-9.

Lee, W. T., S. S. Leung, D. M. Leung and J. C. Cheng. 1996. A follow-up study on the effects of calcium-supplement withdrawal and puberty on bone acquisition of children. American Journal of Clinical Nutrition 64(1): 71-7.

Li, X. Q., V. Tembe, G. M. Horwitz, D. A. Bushinsky and M. J. Favus. 1993. Increased intestinal vitamin D receptor in genetic hypercalciuric rats. A cause of intestinal calcium hyperabsorption. Journal of Clinical Investigation 91(2): 661-7.

Lonnerdal, B. 1997. Effects of milk and milk components on calcium, magnesium, and trace element absorption during infancy. Physiological Reviews 77(3): 643-69.

Ma, R., K. J. Ellis, S. Yasumura, R. J. Shypailo and R. N. Pierson, Jr. 1999. Total body-calcium measurements: comparison of two delayed-gamma neutron activation facilities. Physics in Medicine and Biology 44(6): N113-8.

Malm, O. J. 1958. Calcium requirement and adaptation in adult men. Scandinavian Journal of Clinical and Laboratory Investigation 10(Suppl 36): 1-290.

Martin, A. D., D. A. Bailey, H. A. McKay and S. Whiting. 1997. Bone mineral and calcium accretion during puberty. American Journal of Clinical Nutrition 66(3): 611-5.

Masse, P. G., J. Dosy, J. L. Jougleux, M. Caissie and D. S. Howell. 2005. Bone mineral density and metabolism at an early stage of menopause when estrogen and calcium supplement are not used and without the interference of major confounding variables. Journal of the American College of Nutrition 24(5): 354-60.

Matkovic, V. 1991. Calcium metabolism and calcium requirements during skeletal modeling and consolidation of bone mass. American Journal of Clinical Nutrition 54(1 Suppl): 245S-60S.

Matkovic, V. and R. P. Heaney. 1992. Calcium balance during human growth: evidence for threshold behavior. American Journal of Clinical Nutrition 55(5): 992-6.

Matkovic, V., T. Jelic, G. M. Wardlaw, J. Z. Ilich, P. K. Goel, J. K. Wright, M. B. Andon, K. T. Smith and R. P. Heaney. 1994. Timing of peak bone mass in Caucasian females and its implication for the prevention of osteoporosis. Inference from a cross–sectional model. Journal of Clinical Investigation 93(2): 799-808.

Matkovic, V., P. K. Goel, N. E. Badenhop-Stevens, J. D. Landoll, B. Li, J. Z. Ilich, M. Skugor, L. A. Nagode, S. L. Mobley, E. J. Ha, T. N. Hangartner and A. Clairmont. 2005. Calcium supplementation and bone mineral density in females from childhood to young adulthood: a randomized controlled trial. American Journal of Clinical Nutrition 81(1): 175-88.

Muruganandan, S., A. A. Roman and C. J. Sinal. 2009. Adipocyte differentiation of bone marrow-derived mesenchymal stem cells: cross talk with the osteoblastogenic program. Cellular and Molecular Life Sciences 66(2): 236-53.

NIH Consensus Development Panel on Osteoporosis Prevention Diagnosis and Therapy. 2001. Osteoporosis prevention, diagnosis, and therapy. JAMA 285(6): 785-95.

Nordin, B. E., J. M. Wishart, P. M. Clifton, R. McArthur, F. Scopacasa, A. G. Need, H. A. Morris, P. D. O'Loughlin and M. Horowitz. 2004. A longitudinal study of bone-related biochemical changes at the menopause. Clinical Endocrinology 61(1): 123-30.

Orwoll, E. S., S. K. Oviatt, M. R. McClung, L. J. Deftos and G. Sexton. 1990. The rate of bone mineral loss in normal men and the effects of calcium and cholecalciferol supplementation. Annals of Internal Medicine 112(1): 29-34.

Parfitt, A. M., A. R. Villanueva, J. Foldes and D. S. Rao. 1995. Relations between histologic indices of bone formation: implications for the pathogenesis of spinal osteoporosis. Journal of Bone and Mineral Research 10(3): 466-73.

Parfitt, A. M. 2003. Misconceptions (3): calcium leaves bone only by resorption and enters only by formation. Bone 33(3): 259-63.

Peacock, M. 1991. Calcium absorption efficiency and calcium requirements in children and adolescents. American Journal of Clinical Nutrition 54(Suppl 1): 261S-5S.

Peacock, M. 2010. Calcium metabolism in health and disease. Clinical Journal of the American Society of Nephrology 5(Suppl 1)1: S23-30.

Pedersen, E. B., P. Johannesen, S. Kristensen, A. B. Rasmussen, K. Emmertsen, J. Moller, J. G. Lauritsen and M. Wohlert. 1984. Calcium, parathyroid hormone and calcitonin in normal pregnancy and preeclampsia. Gynecologic and Obstetric Investigation 18(3): 156-64.

Perez-Lopez, F. R., P. Chedraui and J. L. Cuadros-Lopez. 2010. Bone mass gain during puberty and adolescence: deconstructing gender characteristics. Current Medicinal Chemistry 17(5): 453-66.

Poliquin, S., L. Joseph and K. Gray-Donald. 2009. Calcium and vitamin D intakes in an adult Canadian population. Canadian Journal of Dietetic Practice & Research 70(1): 21-7.

Pouilles, J. M., F. Tremollieres and C. Ribot. 1995. Effect of menopause on femoral and vertebral bone loss. Journal of Bone and Mineral Research 10(10): 1531-6.

Prentice, A., L. M. Jarjou, T. J. Cole, D. M. Stirling, B. Dibba and S. Fairweather-Tait. 1995. Calcium requirements of lactating Gambian mothers: effects of a calcium supplement on breast-milk calcium concentration, maternal bone mineral content, and urinary calcium excretion. American Journal of Clinical Nutrition 62(1): 58-67.

Prentice, A. 2003. Micronutrients and the bone mineral content of the mother, fetus and newborn. Journal of Nutrition 133(5 Suppl 2): 1693S-9S.

Provot, S. and E. Schipani. 2007. Fetal growth plate: a developmental model of cellular adaptation to hypoxia. Annals of the New York Academy of Sciences 1117: 26-39.

Rafferty, K., G. Walters and R. P. Heaney. 2007. Calcium fortificants: overview and strategies for improving calcium nutriture of the U.S. population. Journal of Food Science 72(9): R152-8.

Recker, R. R. 1985. Calcium absorption and achlorhydria. New England Journal of Medicine 313(2): 70-3.

Recker, R. R., K. M. Davies, S. M. Hinders, R. P. Heaney, M. R. Stegman and D. B. Kimmel. 1992. Bone gain in young adult women. JAMA 268(17): 2403-8.

Recker, R., J. Lappe, K. M. Davies and R. Heaney. 2004. Bone remodeling increases substantially in the years after menopause and remains increased in older osteoporosis patients. Journal of Bone and Mineral Research 19(10): 1628-33.

Ricci, T. A., H. A. Chowdhury, S. B. Heymsfield, T. Stahl, R. N. Pierson, Jr. and S. A. Shapses. 1998. Calcium supplementation suppresses bone turnover during weight reduction in postmenopausal women. Journal of Bone and Mineral Research 13(6): 1045-50.

Riedt, C. S., M. Cifuentes, T. Stahl, H. A. Chowdhury, Y. Schlussel and S. A. Shapses. 2005. Overweight postmenopausal women lose bone with moderate weight reduction and 1 g/day calcium intake. Journal of Bone and Mineral Research 20(3): 455-63.

Riedt, C. S., R. E. Brolin, R. M. Sherrell, M. P. Field and S. A. Shapses. 2006. True fractional calcium absorption is decreased after Roux-en-Y gastric bypass surgery. Obesity (Silver Spring) 14(11): 1940-8.

Riggs, B. L., W. M. O'Fallon, J. Muhs, M. K. O'Connor, R. Kumar and L. J. Melton, 3rd. 1998. Long-term effects of calcium supplementation on serum parathyroid hormone level, bone turnover, and bone loss in elderly women. Journal of Bone and Mineral Research 13(2): 168-74.

Riggs, B. L. 2002. Endocrine causes of age-related bone loss and osteoporosis. Novartis Foundation Symposium 242: 247-59; discussion 260-4.

Seely, E. W., E. M. Brown, D. M. DeMaggio, D. K. Weldon, and S. W. Graves. 1997. A prospective study of calciotropic hormones in pregnancy and post partum: reciprocal changes in serum intact parathyroid hormone and 1,25-dihydroxyvitamin D. American Journal of Obstetrics and Gynecology 176(1 Pt 1): 214-7.

Seeman, E. 2003. Reduced bone formation and increased bone resorption: rational targets for the treatment of osteoporosis. Osteoporosis International 14(Suppl 3): S2-8.

Seeman, E. 2009. Bone modeling and remodeling. Critical Reviews in Eukaryotic Gene Expression 19(3): 219-33.

Sellmeyer, D. E., M. Schloetter and A. Sebastian. 2002. Potassium citrate prevents increased urine calcium excretion and bone resorption induced by a high sodium chloride diet. Journal of Clinical Endocrinology and Metabolism 87(5): 2008-12.

Shapses, S. A. and D. Sukumar. 2010. Protein intake during weight loss: effects on bone. In Nutritional Aspects of Osteoporosis, edited by P. Burckhardt, B. Dawson-Hughes and C. M. Weaver. London: Springer. Pp. 9-16.

Sigurdsson, G., B. V. Halldorsson, U. Styrkarsdottir, K. Kristjansson and K. Stefansson. 2008. Impact of genetics on low bone mass in adults. Journal of Bone and Mineral Research 23(10): 1584-90.

Siris, E. S., Y. T. Chen, T. A. Abbott, E. Barrett-Connor, P. D. Miller, L. E. Wehren and M. L. Berger. 2004. Bone mineral density thresholds for pharmacological intervention to prevent fractures. Archives of Internal Medicine 164(10): 1108-12.

Sokoloff, L. 1978. Occult osteomalacia in American (U.S.A.) patients with fracture of the hip. American Journal of Surgical Pathology 2(1): 21-30.

Southgate, D. A., E. M. Widdowson, B. J. Smits, W. T. Cooke, C. H. Walker and N. P. Mathers. 1969. Absorption and excretion of calcium and fat by young infants. Lancet 1(7593): 487-9.

Sowers, M., R. B. Wallace and J. H. Lemke. 1985. Correlates of forearm bone mass among women during maximal bone mineralization. Preventive Medicine 14(5): 585-96.

Sowers, M. R., M. K. Clark, B. Hollis, R. B. Wallace and M. Jannausch. 1992. Radial bone mineral density in pre- and perimenopausal women: a prospective study of rates and risk factors for loss. Journal of Bone and Mineral Research 7(6): 647-57.

Specker, B. L., M. L. Ho, A. Oestreich, T. A. Yin, Q. M. Shui, X. C. Chen and R. C. Tsang. 1992. Prospective study of vitamin D supplementation and rickets in China. Journal of Pediatrics 120(5): 733-9.

Specker, B. L., N. E. Vieira, K. O. O'Brien, M. L. Ho, J. E. Heubi, S. A. Abrams and A. L. Yergey. 1994. Calcium kinetics in lactating women with low and high calcium intakes. American Journal of Clinical Nutrition 59(3): 593-9.

Spencer, H., I. Lewin, J. Fowler and J. Samachson. 1969. Influence of dietary calcium intake on Ca47 absorption in man. American Journal of Medicine 46(2): 197-205.

Spencer, H., L. Kramer, M. Lesniak, M. De Bartolo, C. Norris and D. Osis. 1984. Calcium requirements in humans. Report of original data and a review. Clinical Orthopedics Related Research (184): 270-80.

Stacey, J. and C. Daly. 1989. Osteomalacia in the elderly: biochemical screening in general practice. Irish Medical Journal 82(2): 72-3.

Stevenson, J. C., G. Abeyasekera, C. J. Hillyard, K. G. Phang, I. MacIntyre, S. Campbell, P. T. Townsend, O. Young and M. I. Whitehead. 1981. Calcitonin and the calcium-regulating hormones in postmenopausal women: effect of oestrogens. Lancet 1(8222): 693-5.

Straub, D. A. 2007. Calcium supplementation in clinical practice: a review of forms, doses, and indications. Nutrition in Clinical Practice 22(3): 286-96.

Teti, A. and A. Zallone. 2009. Do osteocytes contribute to bone mineral homeostasis? Osteo-cytic osteolysis revisited. Bone 44(1): 11-6.

Trotter, M. and B. B. Hixon. 1974. Sequential changes in weight, density, and percentage ash weight of human skeletons from an early fetal period through old age. Anatomical Record 179(1): 1-18.

Tsai, K. S., H. Heath, 3rd, R. Kumar and B. L. Riggs. 1984. Impaired vitamin D metabolism with aging in women. Possible role in pathogenesis of senile osteoporosis. Journal of Clinical Investigation 73(6): 1668-72.

Tuck, S. P. and H. K. Datta. 2007. Osteoporosis in the aging male: treatment options. Clinical Intervention Aging 2(4): 521-36.

Uebelhart, D., E. Gineyts, M. C. Chapuy and P. D. Delmas. 1990. Urinary excretion of pyri-dinium crosslinks: a new marker of bone resorption in metabolic bone disease. Bone and Mineral 8(1): 87-96.

Vatanparast, H., D. A. Bailey, A. D. Baxter-Jones and S. J. Whiting. 2010. Calcium require-ments for bone growth in Canadian boys and girls during adolescence. British Journal of Nutrition: 1-6.

Villareal, D. T., R. Civitelli, A. Chines and L. V. Avioli. 1991. Subclinical vitamin D deficiency in postmenopausal women with low vertebral bone mass. Journal of Clinical Endocrinol-ogy and Metabolism 72(3): 628-34.

Wastney, M. E., J. Ng, D. Smith, B. R. Martin, M. Peacock and C. M. Weaver. 1996. Differences in calcium kinetics between adolescent girls and young women. American Journal of Physiology 271(1 Pt 2): R208-16.

Weaver, C. M. and R. P. Heaney. 1991. Isotopic exchange of ingested calcium between labeled sources. Evidence that ingested calcium does not form a common absorptive pool. Calci-fied Tissue International 49(4): 244-7.

Weaver, C. M., R. P. Heaney, B. R. Martin and M. L. Fitzsimmons. 1991. Human calcium absorption from whole-wheat products. Journal of Nutrition 121(11): 1769-75.

Weaver, C. M., B. R. Martin, K. L. Plawecki, M. Peacock, O. B. Wood, D. L. Smith and M. E. Wastney. 1995. Differences in calcium metabolism between adolescent and adult fe-males. American Journal of Clinical Nutrition 61(3): 577-81.

Weaver, C. and R. Heaney. 2006a. Chapter 9: Food sources, supplements, and bioavailability. In *Calcium in Human Health*, edited by C. Weaver and R. Heaney. Totowa, NJ: Humana Press. Pp. 129-44.

Weaver, C. M. and R. Heaney. 2006b. Calcium. In *Modern Nutrition in Health and Disease, 10th Edition*, edited by M. E. Shils, M. Shike, A. C. Ross, B. Cabellero and R. J. Cousins. Baltimore, MD: Lippincott Williams & Wilkins.

Weaver, C. M. 2009. Should dairy be recommended as part of a healthy vegetarian diet? Point. American Journal of Clinical Nutrition 89(5): 1634S-7S.

Widdowson, E. M. 1965. Absorption and excretion of fat, nitrogen, and minerals from "filled" milks by babies one week old. Lancet 2(7422): 1099-105.

Xue, Y. and J. C. Fleet. 2009. Intestinal vitamin D receptor is required for normal calcium and bone metabolism in mice. Gastroenterology 136(4): 1317-27, e1-2.

Yang, Y. C. and C. Y. Yang. 2008. The influence of residual stress on the shear strength between the bone and plasma-sprayed hydroxyapatite coating. Journal of Materials Science. Materials in Medicine 19(3): 1051-60.

3

Overview of Vitamin D

INTRODUCTION

Vitamin D, first identified as a vitamin early in the 20th century, is now recognized as a prohormone. A unique aspect of vitamin D as a nutrient is that it can be synthesized by the human body through the action of sunlight. These dual sources of vitamin D make it challenging to develop dietary reference intake values.

Vitamin D, also known as calciferol, comprises a group of fat-soluble seco-sterols. The two major forms are vitamin D_2 and vitamin D_3. Vitamin D_2 (ergocalciferol) is largely human-made and added to foods, whereas vitamin D_3 (cholecalciferol) is synthesized in the skin of humans from 7-dehydrocholesterol and is also consumed in the diet via the intake of animal-based foods. Both vitamin D_3 and vitamin D_2 are synthesized commercially and found in dietary supplements or fortified foods. The D_2 and D_3 forms differ only in their side chain structure. The differences do not affect metabolism (i.e., activation), and both forms function as prohormones. When activated, the D_2 and D_3 forms have been reported to exhibit identical responses in the body, and the potency related to the ability to cure vitamin D–deficiency rickets is the same (Fieser and Fieser, 1959; Jones et al., 1998; Jurutka et al., 2001). Experimental animal studies have indicated that vitamin D_2 is less toxic than vitamin D_3, but this has not been demonstrated in humans.

The activation steps involved in converting vitamin D from the diet and cutaneous synthesis are illustrated in Figure 3-1. Vitamin D, in either the D_2 or D_3 form, is considered biologically inactive until it undergoes two

75

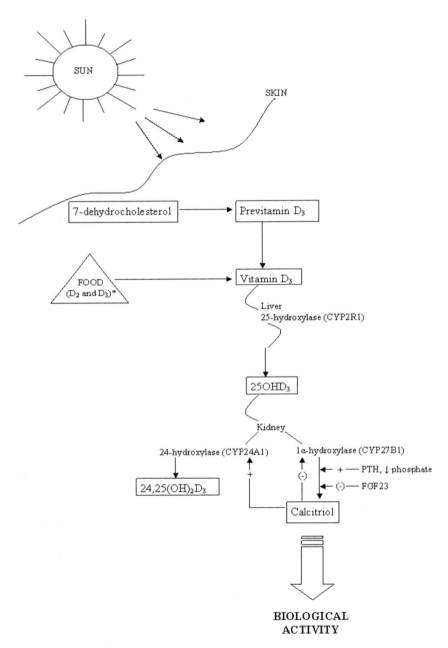

FIGURE 3-1 Overview of vitamin D synthesis, intake, and activation.

enzymatic hydroxylation reactions. The first takes place in the liver, mediated by the 25-hydroxylase (most likely cytochrome P450 2R1 [CYP2R1]) which forms 25-hydroxyvitamin D (hereafter referred to as 25OHD). The second reaction takes place in the kidney, mediated by 1α-hydroxylase (CYP27B1), which converts 25OHD to the biologically active hormone, calcitriol (1,25-dihydroxyvitamin D). The 1α-hydroxylase gene is also expressed in several extra-renal tissues, but its contribution to calcitriol formation in these tissues is unknown. 25OHD, the precursor of calcitriol, is the major circulating form of vitamin D; it circulates bound to a specific plasma carrier protein, vitamin D binding protein (DBP). DBP also transports vitamin D and calcitriol.

The renal synthesis of calcitriol is tightly regulated by two counteracting hormones, with up-regulation via parathyroid hormone (PTH) and down-regulation via fibroblast-like growth factor-23 (FGF23) (Galitzer et al., 2008; Bergwitz and Juppner, 2010). Low serum phosphorus levels stimulate calcitriol synthesis, whereas high serum phosphorus levels inhibit it. Following its synthesis in the kidney, calcitriol binds to DBP to be transported to target organs. The biological actions of calcitriol, involve regulation of gene expression at the transcriptional level, and are mediated through binding to a vitamin D receptor (VDR), located primarily in the nuclei of target cells (Jones et al., 1998; Jurutka et al., 2001). Additional hydroxylation reactions, such as that mediated by CYP24A1, as shown in Figure 3-1, result in more polar metabolites with greatly reduced or no apparent biological activity.

The classical actions of vitamin D—which by itself is inactive—are due to the functions of the active metabolite, calcitriol. These actions take the form of the regulation of serum calcium and phosphate homeostasis and, in turn, the development and maintenance of bone health (DeLuca, 1988; Reichel et al., 1989; Jones et al., 1998). Non-classical functions are less well elucidated. VDRs are found fairly ubiquitously throughout the body in tissues not involved with calcium and phosphate homeostasis, and the presence of VDRs in these tissues implies that calcitriol may play a more general role or that ligands other than calcitriol can activate the VDR. Furthermore, the specific vitamin D–responsive elements (VDREs), considered the hallmark of vitamin D action, are present in a large number of human genes involved in a wide range of classical and non-classical roles, such as the regulation of cell proliferation, cell differentiation, and apoptosis. It has been suggested that calcitriol exerts immunomodulatory and anti-proliferative effects through autocrine and paracrine pathways (Adams and Hewison, 2008). These wide-ranging actions of calcitriol have further been hypothesized to play a potential role in preventive or therapeutic action in cancer (Masuda and Jones, 2006) and chronic conditions such as auto-immune conditions (including type 1 diabetes), cardiovascular disease, and infections (Holick et al., 2007).

Outside of the biological forms of vitamin D, a number of analogues based on the vitamin D structure have been synthesized for use as potential pharmacological agents. These are not, however, dietary or biosynthesized compounds; rather, they are designed for specific applications in research or clinical treatment. Examples of synthetic analogues that have gained importance in clinical medicine are briefly mentioned below.

The term vitamin D is generally used in this report to refer to both the D_2 and D_3 forms as well as their metabolites, although the two forms are distinguished when necessary for clarification (see Box 3-1 for definitions). Vitamin D levels in the diet—from foods and supplements—are expressed in International Units (IU), but may be expressed elsewhere in micrograms (µg). The biological activity of 1 µg of vitamin D is equivalent to 40 IU. Owing to the frequency with which serum 25OHD levels are included in this report text, the levels are expressed only as nanomoles per liter (nmol/L). As shown in Box 3-1, the nanomoles per liter measure can be converted to nanograms per milliliter (ng/mL) by dividing by a factor of 2.5.

BOX 3-1
Terms and Conversions Used in Reference to Vitamin D

Terms:
Vitamin D—also referred to as *calciferol*
Vitamin D$_2$—also referred to as *ergocalciferol*
Vitamin D$_3$—also referred to as *cholecalciferol*

25OHD—25-hydroxyvitamin D also referred to as *calcidiol* or *calcifediol;* indicates no distinction between D_2 and D_3 forms. When relevant, forms are distinguished as **25OHD$_2$** and **25OHD$_3$**
Calcitriol—1,25-dihydroxyvitamin D$_3$ (Note: *Ercalcitriol*—refers to 1,25-dihydroxyvitamin D$_2$, but in this report, the term "calcitriol" will be used for both)
24,25(OH)$_2$D—24,25-dihydroxyvitamin D

IU = International Unit is a measurement based on biological activity or effect; 1 IU of vitamin D is defined as the activity of 0.025 µg of cholecalciferol in bioassays with rats and chicks.

Conversions for Vitamin D$_3$:
[sources] 40 IU = 1 µg
[serum] 2.5 nmol/L = 1 ng/mL

SOURCES OF VITAMIN D

Diet

The dietary sources of vitamin D include food and dietary supplements; therefore, "total vitamin D intake" reflects the combined dietary contribution from foods and supplements. There are a few naturally occurring food sources of vitamin D. These include fatty fish, fish liver oil, and egg yolk. Some foods are, however, fortified with vitamin D. After vitamin D was recognized as important for the prevention of rickets in the 1920s (Steenbock and Black, 1924), vitamin D fortification of some foods was initiated on a voluntary basis.

In the United States, fluid milk is voluntarily fortified with 400 IU per quart (or 385 IU/L) of vitamin D (U.S. regulations do not specify the form) (FDA, 2009). In Canada, under the Food and Drug Regulation,[1] fortification of fluid milk and margarine with vitamin D is mandatory. Fluid milk must contain 35–45 IU vitamin D per 100 mL and margarine, 530 IU per 100 g. In addition, fortified plant-based beverages must contain vitamin D in an amount equivalent to fluid milk. In analyses conducted in the 1980s and early 1990s, a significant portion of milk samples in the United States were found to contain less than the specified amount of vitamin D (Tanner et al., 1988). Holick et al. (1992) found that 62 percent of milk sampled from five eastern states contained less than 80 percent and 10 percent contained more than 120 percent of the amount of vitamin D stated on the label. Chen et al. (1993) reported similar findings. A more recent report on vitamin D–fortified milk sampled in New York State over a period of 4 years showed that an average of only 47.7 percent of samples fell within the range of acceptable levels of vitamin D fortification (Murphy et al., 2001). However, recent surveys from the U.S. Department of Agriculture (USDA) indicate that these problems have been corrected. In a presentation to this committee, Byrdwell (2009) reported that a USDA survey of milk samples taken in 2007 from 24 locations across the United States showed that most samples had vitamin D levels within the range of 400 to 600 IU/quart.

In Canada, Faulkner et al. (2000) surveyed milk samples and found that 20 percent of skim milk, 40 percent of 2 percent fat milk, and 20 percent of whole milk, contained the recommended level of vitamin D. Samples collected by the Canadian Food Inspection Agency from 1999 through 2009 and analyzed for vitamin D indicated that during the last 4 years of sample collection, 47 to 69 percent were within the range specified by regulation (personal communication, S. Brooks, Health Canada, April

---

[1]Available online at http://laws.justice.gc.ca/PDF/Regulation/C/C.R.C.,_c._870.pdf (accessed July 23, 2010).

30, 2010). In addition, over the past 5 years, the average vitamin D content of analyzed milk samples fell within this range. Over time, manufacturers in the United States have added vitamin D to other foods, and the food industry is increasingly marketing foods fortified with vitamin D (Yetley, 2008). Based on data from a U.S. Food and Drug Administration (FDA) survey that provides information on the labels of processed, packaged food products in the United States, Yetley (2008) reported that almost all fluid milks, approximately 75 percent of ready-to-eat breakfast cereals, slightly more than half of all milk substitutes, approximately one-quarter of yogurts, and approximately 8 to 14 percent of cheeses, juices, and spreads are fortified with vitamin D in the U.S. market. Many product labels included in the survey indicated that the form of added vitamin D was vitamin D_3. However, some milk substitutes are fortified with vitamin D_2. Cereal labels did not specify the form of added vitamin D. Levels of vitamin D ranged from 40 IU per regulatory serving for cereals and cheeses to 60 IU per regulatory serving for spreads and 100 IU per regulatory serving for fluid milk. Several food categories had within-category ranges of 40 to 100 IU of vitamin D per regulatory serving. Serum vitamin D and 25OHD have low penetrance into breast milk, together comprising 40 to 50 IU of antirachitic activity per liter, most of which is contributed by 25OHD (Leerbeck and Sondergaard, 1980; Hollis et al., 1981; Reeve et al., 1982; Specker et al., 1985). Data from the USDA report the vitamin D content of human milk to be 4.3 IU/100 kcal.[2] However, the vitamin D biological activity may be higher than the analyzed values, because human milk contains small amounts of 25OHD in addition to vitamin D_3 (Reeve et al., 1982); further, the biological activity of 25OHD is approximately 50 percent higher than that of vitamin D (Blunt et al., 1968).

The FDA has established that infant formula must contain 40 to 100 IU of vitamin D per 100 kcal.[3] Commercial infant formulas contain approximately 60 IU of vitamin D per 100 kcal, as estimated by the USDA food composition database,[4] and Yetley (2008) reported that commercial milk-based infant formulas collected between 2003 and 2006 contained 87

---

[2]USDA National Nutrient Database for Standard Reference Release 23. NBD No. 01107. Milk, human, mature, fluid. Available online at http://www.ars.usda.gov/Services/docs.htm?docid=8964 (accessed August 3, 2010).

[3]USDA National Nutrient Database for Standard Reference Release 23. NBD No. 03946. Infant formula, ROSS, SIMILAC LACTOSE FREE ADVANCE, ready-to-feed, with ARA and DHA; and NDB no. 03815. Infant formula, MEAD JOHNSON, ENFAMIL LIPIL, with iron, ready-to-feed, with ARA and DHA. Available online at http://www.ars.usda.gov/main/site_main.htm?modecode=12-35-45-00 (accessed April 28, 2010).

[4]Available online at http://www.nal.usda.gov/fnic/foodcomp/search/ (accessed March 16, 2010).

to 184 percent of label declarations. In Canada, infant formula is required by regulation to contain between 40 and 80 IU of vitamin D per 100 kcal.

In recent years, dietary supplements containing vitamin D have become more common and have been more frequently consumed. The form of vitamin D used in supplement products can be either vitamin D_2 or vitamin D_3. It would appear from informal observations of the market place that manufacturers are increasingly switching from vitamin D_2 to vitamin D_3, and some are increasing the vitamin D content of their products. Traditionally, many marketed dietary supplements have contained 400 IU per daily dose, but levels in supplements have been increasing. In the United States, vitamin D can now be found in multi-vitamin/multi-mineral formulations as well as a single supplement in a range of dosage levels, including 1,000 to 5,000 IU of vitamin D_3 per dose and even up to 50,000 IU of vitamin D_2 per dose. In Canada, dosage levels of vitamin D above 1,000 IU are obtainable only with a prescription.

Information about current national survey estimates of the intake of vitamin D from foods and supplements can be found in Chapter 7.

Synthesis in the Skin

Vitamin D_3 is synthesized in human skin from 7-dehydrocholesterol following exposure to ultraviolet B (UVB) radiation with wavelength 290 to 320 nm.[5] The process of UVB-mediated conversion of 7-dehydrocholesterol to the previtamin D_3 form and subsequent thermal isomerization to vitamin D_3 occurring in the epidermis is illustrated in Figure 3-2.

The production of vitamin D_3 in skin is a function of the amount of UVB radiation reaching the dermis as well as the availability of 7-dehydrocholesterol (Holick, 1995). As such, the level of synthesis is influenced by a number of factors, as described below in the section entitled "Measures Associated with Vitamin D: Serum 25OHD," including season of the year, skin pigmentation, latitude, use of sunscreen, clothing, and amount of skin exposed. Age is also a factor, in that synthesis of vitamin D declines with increasing age, due in part to a fall in 7-dehydrocholesterol levels and due in part to alterations in skin morphology (MacLaughlin and Holick, 1985).

Toxic levels of vitamin D do not occur from prolonged sun exposure. Thermal activation of previtamin D_3 in the skin gives rise to multiple non–vitamin D forms, such as lumisterol, tachysterol and others (Holick et al., 1981; Webb et al., 1989), as illustrated in Figure 3-2; this limits the

---

[5]The chemical processes that lead to the formation of vitamin D_3 from its precursor are non-enzymatic and can take place ex vivo and in organic solvents, as well as in vivo. Therefore, vitamin D_3 can also be synthesized commercially.

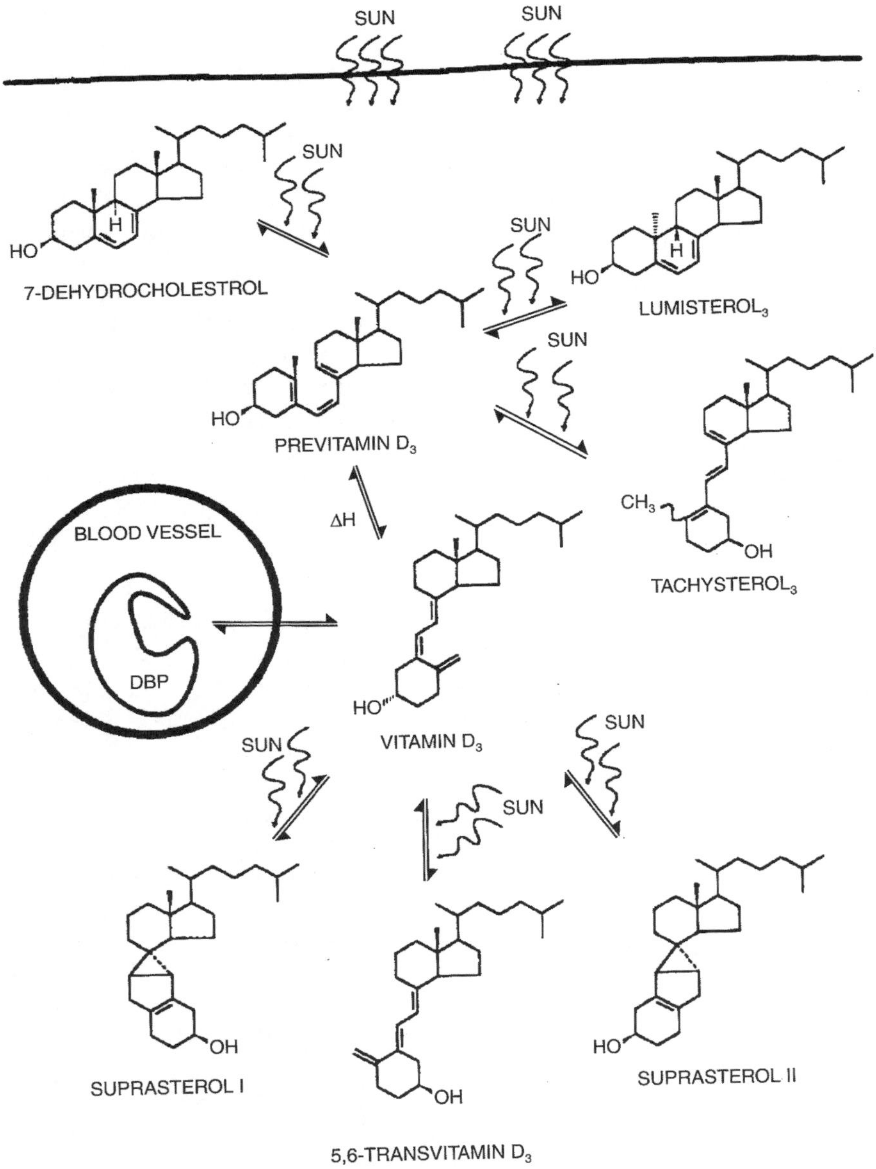

FIGURE 3-2 Photochemical events that lead to the production and regulation of vitamin D_3 (cholecalciferol) in the skin.

NOTE: DBP = vitamin D binding protein.

SOURCE: Holick (1994). Reprinted with permission from the *American Journal of Clinical Nutrition* (1994, volume 60, pages 619-630), American Society for Nutrition.

formation of vitamin D_3 itself. Vitamin D_3 can also be converted to nonactive forms.

The absolute percentage of circulating 25OHD that arises from cutaneous synthesis versus oral intake of vitamin D in the free-living North American population cannot be clearly specified. Individuals living at Earth's poles during winter months and submariner crew members with very limited or no measurable UVB exposure have detectable levels of 25OHD in blood, arising from dietary sources and likely from previously synthesized and stored vitamin D. This topic is further explored in the section below that focuses on serum 25OHD.

METABOLISM OF VITAMIN D

Absorption

Owing to its fat-soluble nature, dietary vitamin D (either D_2 or D_3) is absorbed with other dietary fats in the small intestine (Haddad et al., 1993; Holick, 1995). The efficient absorption of vitamin D is dependent upon the presence of fat in the lumen, which triggers the release of bile acids and pancreatic lipase (Weber, 1981, 1983). In turn, bile acids initiate the emulsification of lipids, pancreatic lipase hydrolyzes the triglycerides into monoglycerides and free fatty acids, and bile acids support the formation of lipid-containing micelles, which diffuse into enterocytes. Early studies demonstrated that radiolabeled vitamin D_3 appeared almost exclusively in the lymphatics and in the chylomicron fraction of plasma; as well, subjects with impaired bile acid release or pancreatic insufficiency both demonstrated significantly reduced absorption of vitamin D (Thompson et al., 1966; Blomstrand and Forsgren, 1967; Compston et al., 1981). Subsequently, other clinical and experimental animal studies confirmed that vitamin D is most efficiently absorbed when consumed with foods containing fat (Weber, 1981; Johnson et al., 2005; Mulligan and Licata, 2010) and, conversely, that a weight-loss agent that blocks fat absorption also impairs the absorption of vitamin D (James et al., 1997; McDuffie et al., 2002). The optimal amount of fat required for maximal absorption of vitamin D has not been determined.

Within the intestinal wall, vitamin D, cholesterol, triglycerides, lipoproteins, and other lipids are packaged together into chylomicrons. Importantly, while a fraction of newly absorbed intestinal vitamin D is also transported along with amino acids and carbohydrates into the portal system to reach the liver directly, the main pathway of vitamin D uptake is incorporation into chylomicrons that reach the systemic circulation via the lymphatics. Chylomicron lipids are metabolized in peripheral tissues that express lipoprotein lipase, but particularly in adipose tissue and skeletal muscle, which are rich in this enzyme. During hydrolysis of the chylomicron triglycerides, a fraction of the vitamin D contained in the chylomicron can be taken up by these tissues. Uptake into adipose tissue and skeletal muscle accounts for the rapid postprandial disappearance of vitamin D from plasma and probably also explains why increased adiposity causes sequestering of vitamin D and is associated with lower 25OHD levels (Jones, 2008). What remains of the original chylomicron after lipolysis is a chylomicron remnant, a cholesterol-enriched, triglyceride-depleted particle that still contains a fraction of its vitamin D content.

Metabolism to the Active Hormonal Form

Vitamin D, regardless of origin, is an inactive prohormone and must first be metabolized to its hormonal form before it can function. Once vitamin D enters the circulation from the skin or from the lymph, it is cleared by the liver or storage tissues within a few hours. The processes that follow are illustrated in Figure 3-3. Vitamin D is converted in the liver to 25OHD, a process carried out by a CYP enzyme that has yet to be fully defined but is likely CYP2R1 (Cheng et al., 2003). The crystal structure of CYP2R1 has been determined with vitamin D in the active site, and the enzyme has been shown to metabolize both vitamin D_2 and vitamin D_3 equally efficiently (Strushkevich et al., 2008). There is little, if any, feedback regulation of this enzyme. A large genome-wide association study of factors that might be determinants of the circulating 25OHD levels identified the human chromosomal 11p15 locus of CYP2R1 as a significant determinant, whereas the loci of the other enzymes purported to have 25-hydroxylase activity (e.g., CYP27A1 and CYP3A4) were not identified (Wang et al., 2010). The other determinants of serum 25OHD besides CYP2R1 have been reported to be DBP (also known as Gc protein), which has six common phenotypes (Laing and Cooke, 2005) as well as 7-dehydrocholesterol reductase and CYP24A1. Increasing intake of vitamin D results in higher blood levels of 25OHD, although perhaps not in a linear manner (Stamp et al., 1977; Clements et al., 1987).

At this point, 25OHD bound to DBP circulates in the blood stream and, when calcitriol is required due to a lack of calcium (or lack of phosphate), 25OHD is 1α-hydroxylated in the kidney to form calcitriol, the active form, by the 1α-hydroxylase enzyme (also known as CYP27B1) (Tanaka and DeLuca, 1983). This metabolic step is very tightly regulated by blood calcium and phosphate levels through PTH and the phosphaturic hormone, FGF23, and constitutes the basis of the vitamin D endocrine system that is central to maintaining calcium and phosphate homeostasis (see discussion below on functions and physiological actions). FGF23 acts by reducing the expression of renal sodium–phosphate transporters and reducing serum calcitriol levels.

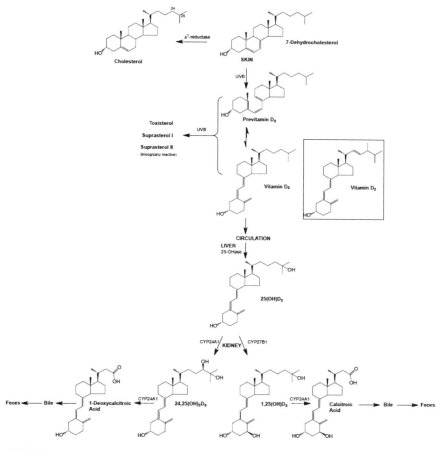

FIGURE 3-3 The metabolism of vitamin D$_3$ from synthesis/intake to formation of metabolites. The process is the same for vitamin D$_2$ once it enters the circulation.
NOTE: CYP = cytochrome P450 (a large and diverse group of enzymes).
SOURCE: Reprinted with permission from Hector DeLuca.

Production of the CYP27B1 enzyme is stimulated by PTH, which is secreted in response to a lack of calcium. It is also stimulated by the hypophosphatemic action of FGF23 on renal phosphate excretion, but to a lesser extent. When PTH is suppressed, or FGF23, produced by osteocytes, is stimulated, 1α-hydroxylation is markedly reduced (Liu et al., 2007; Quarles, 2008). Furthermore, calcitriol can act as a suppressor of CYP27B1, although the mechanism is not fully understood.

Calcitriol has its strongest metabolic activity in inducing its own destruction by stimulating the 24-hydroxylase enzyme (now known as CYP24A1;

Figure 3-1) (Jones et al., 1998). The enzyme CYP24A1 is found in all target tissues and is induced in response to calcitriol interacting with the VDR. CYP24A1 is largely responsible for the metabolic degradation of calcitriol and its precursor, 25OHD, and its deletion in the mouse results in 50 percent lethality at weaning and an inability to efficiently clear the active form of vitamin D (Masuda et al., 2005). CYP24A1 carries out a series of reactions resulting ultimately in production of calcitroic acid from calcitriol and 1-desoxycalcitroic acid from $24,25(OH)_2D$, the major metabolite of 25OHD. These products are excreted through the bile into the feces (Jones et al., 1998); very little is eliminated through the urine (Kumar et al., 1976). The active forms of vitamin D_2 are also catabolized by CYP24A1 into a series of biliary metabolites, somewhat analogous to those of vitamin D_3.

As described above, all naturally occurring vitamin D compounds interact with DBP. Calcitriol and vitamin D have significantly lower affinity for this protein than does 25OHD. Whereas vitamin D has an average lifetime in the body of approximately 2 months, 25OHD has a lifetime of 15 days, and calcitriol has a lifetime measured in hours (Jones et al., 1998). Aside from these key elements in vitamin D metabolism, more than 30 other metabolites have been found, including the 3-epi series of vitamin D compounds (DeLuca and Schnoes, 1983; Siu-Caldera et al., 1999). Their importance seems minimal and need not be discussed here.

Although the route of catabolism between $1\alpha,25(OH)_2D_2$ and $1\alpha,25(OH)_2D_3$ differs beyond the initial 24-hydroxylation step, because 24-hydroxylation is primarily a deactivation step (Brommage and DeLuca, 1985; Horst et al., 1986; Lohnes and Jones, 1992; Jones et al., 1998), the rate of this initial step should be the important indicator of the loss of biological action. Comparisons of initial rate kinetics of the 24-hydroxylase enzyme (CYP24A1) activity toward $1\alpha,25(OH)_2D_2$ and $1\alpha,25(OH)_2D_3$ and their precursors suggest that the rates of inactivation by CYP24A1 in vitro are virtually identical (Jones et al., 2009; Urushino et al., 2009). Although side-chain hydroxylation of $1\alpha,25(OH)_2D_2$ represents the primary route of metabolism in the target cell, clearance of the metabolic products in vivo is complicated by additional non-specific liver CYPs (e.g., CYP3A4) (Gupta et al., 2004, 2005) that are inducible by $1\alpha,25(OH)_2D_3$ in certain extra-hepatic tissues (Thompson et al., 2002) and also Phase II enzymes, including uridine diphosphate–glucuronosyl transferases, which are known to subject vitamin D metabolites to glucuronidation (LeVan et al., 1981; Hashizume et al., 2008). The pharmacokinetic consequence of the sum of these catabolic systems, as shown in studies in rats, is a slightly reduced half-life for $1\alpha,25(OH)_2D_2$ compared with $1\alpha,25(OH)_2D_3$ (Knutson et al., 1997).

There are reports that vitamin D_2 and vitamin D_3 are differentially susceptible to these non-specific inactivating modifications, such as those occurring in the liver in response to a variety of drugs. These enzymes include the liver and intestinal CYPs that are known to metabolize vitamin D compounds differently, such as CYP27A1, which 25-hydroxylates vitamin D_3 and 24-hydroxylates vitamin D_2 (Guo et al., 1993), and CYP3A4, which 24- and 25-hydroxylates vitamin D_2 substrates more efficiently than vitamin D_3 substrates (Gupta et al., 2004, 2005) and 23R- and 24S-hydroxylates $1\alpha,25(OH)_2D_3$ (Xu et al., 2006); the latter enzyme has recently been shown to be selectively induced by $1\alpha,25(OH)_2D$ in the intestine (Thompson et al., 2002; Xu et al., 2006). Both CYP27A1 and CYP3A4 are known to have significantly lower Michaelis-Menten constants (K_m values) for $25OHD_3$ compared with CYP2R1 (Guo et al., 1993; Sawada et al., 2000), in the micromole per liter range; this questions their physiological but not their pharmacological relevance. Recent work (Helvig et al., 2008; Jones et al., 2009) has shown that both human intestinal microsomes and recombinant CYP3A4 protein break down $1\alpha,25(OH)_2D_2$ at a significantly faster rate than $1\alpha,25(OH)_2D_3$, suggesting that this non-specific CYP might limit vitamin D_2 action preferentially in target cells, where it is expressed and when the substrate is in the pharmacological dose range. The same type of mechanism involving differential induction of non-specific CYPs may underlie the occasional reports of co-administered drug classes, such as anticonvulsants (Christiansen et al., 1975; Tjellesen et al., 1985; Hosseinpour et al., 2007), causing accelerated degradation of one vitamin D form over the other.

Storage

Adipose tissue stores of vitamin D probably represent "non-specific" stores sequestered because of the hydrophobic nature of vitamin D, but the extent to which the processes of accumulation or mobilization are regulated by normal physiological mechanisms remains unknown at this time. Rosenstreich et al. (1971) first identified adipose tissue as the primary site of vitamin D accumulation from experiments in which radiolabeled vitamin D was administered to vitamin D–deficient rats. Tissue levels of radioactivity measured during vitamin D repletion and during a subsequent period of deprivation showed that adipose tissue acquired the greatest quantity of radioactive compound and had the slowest rate of release. Work by Liel et al. (1988) suggested that there was enhanced uptake and clearance of vitamin D by adipose tissue in obese subjects compared with those of normal weights. Similarly, Wortsman et al. (2000) concluded that in obese subjects, vitamin D was stored in adipose tissue and not released when needed. Finally, Blum et al. (2008) found that, in elderly subjects supplemented with 700 IU of vitamin D per day, for every additional 15 kg of weight above "normal" at baseline, the mean adjusted change in 25OHD level was approximately 10 nmol/L lower after 1 year of supplementation.

The authors estimated that in order for subjects with body mass indexes (BMIs) above the normal range to obtain an increase in serum 25OHD level similar to that of subjects with weight in the normal range, an additional 17 percent increase in vitamin D above the administered dose of 700 IU/day would be needed for every 10 kg increase in body weight above baseline in their study population.

The implication of these studies is that vitamin D deposited in fat tissue is not readily available, and obese individuals may require larger than usual doses of vitamin D supplements to achieve a serum 25OHD level comparable to that of their normal weight counterparts. In support of the hypothesis that vitamin D is stored in adipose tissues, weight reduction studies show that serum 25OHD levels rise when obese individuals lose body fat (Riedt et al., 2005; Zitterman et al., 2009; Tzotzas et al., 2010). Conclusive statements regarding changes in serum 25OHD levels after gastric bypass surgery cannot be made, as a result of confounding factors, such as weight change, possible malabsorption, and diet. There is evidence of a rise in serum 25OHD levels after surgery (Mahdy et al., 2008; Aasheim et al., 2009; Goldner et al., 2009; Bruno et al., 2010), as well as evidence that there is no change after surgery (Riedt et al., 2006; Fleischer et al., 2008; Valderas et al., 2009). Gehrer et al. (2010) indicated that serum 25OHD levels decrease after gastric bypass surgery, although the quality of the methods used is questionable.

Excretion

As described previously, the products of vitamin D metabolism are excreted through the bile into the feces, and very little is eliminated through the urine. This is in part due to renal reuptake of vitamin D metabolites bound to DBP, as mediated by the cubilin–megalin receptor system (Willnow and Nykjaer, 2005).

Excess Intake

Excess intake of vitamin D—but not sun exposure, which is associated with a series of thermal and photoisomerization reactions (see Figure 3-2) —can lead to a state of vitamin D "intoxication" or "hypervitaminosis D." Chemically synthesized vitamin D became available late in the third decade of the 20th century; reports of vitamin D intoxication were first found from 1928 to 1932 and continued throughout most of the 20th century (DeLuca, 2009). The condition of hypervitaminosis D leads to hypercalcemia and eventually to soft tissue calcification and resultant renal and cardiovascular damage (DeLuca, 1974). In the case of animal models, at necropsy, vitamin D–intoxicated rats show widespread calcification of organs and tissues.

The form of the vitamin implicated in the intoxication is 25OHD (Vieth, 1990; Jones, 2008). In fact, it has been shown in dietary supplementation studies using the CYP27B1 knockout mouse, which is incapable of making calcitriol, sufficiently high concentrations of serum levels of 25OHD can cause changes in vitamin D–dependent general expression even in the absence of calcitriol (Rowling et al., 2007; Fleet et al., 2008).

FUNCTIONS AND PHYSIOLOGICAL ACTIONS OF VITAMIN D

Calcium and Phosphate Homeostasis

The dominant function of vitamin D in its hormonal form (calcitriol or 1,25-dihydroxyvitamin D) is the elevation of plasma calcium and phosphate levels, which are required for mineralization of bone (DeLuca, 1979b; Holick, 1996). Furthermore, the elevation of plasma calcium to normal levels is also required for the functioning of the neuromuscular junction as well as vasodilatation, nerve transmission, and hormonal secretion.

Calcitriol—functioning as part of the endocrine system for maintaining serum calcium levels as outlined in Chapter 2—elevates plasma ionized calcium levels to the normal range by three different mechanisms (see Figure 2-1 in Chapter 2). The first mechanism, which does not require PTH, is the well-established role of calcitriol in stimulating intestinal calcium absorption throughout the entire length of the intestine, although its greatest activity is in the duodenum and jejunum. It is clear that calcitriol directly stimulates intestinal calcium and, independently, phosphate absorption.

In the second mechanism, calcitriol plays an essential role in the mobilization of calcium from bone, a process requiring PTH (Garabedian et al., 1972; Lips, 2006). It induces the formation and activation of the osteoclast to function in the mobilization of calcium from bone, as discussed in Chapter 2. In short, calcitriol facilitates the formation of osteoclasts by stimulating the secretion of a protein called receptor activator for nuclear factor κ B (RANK) ligand, which, in turn, is responsible for osteoclastogenesis and bone resorption (Suda et al., 1992; Yasuda et al., 2005).

In the third mechanism, calcitriol together with PTH stimulates the renal distal tubule reabsorption of calcium, ensuring retention of calcium by the kidney when calcium is needed (Sutton et al., 1976; Yamamoto et al., 1984). These well-known functions dominate vitamin D physiology and many of the functional proteins involved in these processes have been identified, although the exact molecular mechanisms of all of these systems have yet to be elucidated.

Thus, overall, calcitriol acts on the intestine, bone, and kidney as described above, and as illustrated in Figure 2-1 in Chapter 2, to elevate serum calcium levels, closing the calcium loop. As serum calcium levels rise, PTH secretion drops. If serum calcium levels become too high, the parafollicular cells ("C" cells) of the thyroid secrete calcitonin, which blocks calcium resorption from bone and helps to keep calcium levels in the normal range. Calcitriol, through its receptor, the VDR, suppresses parathyroid gene expression and parathyroid cell proliferation, providing important feedback loops that reinforce the direct action of increased serum calcium levels (Slatopolsky et al., 1984; Silver et al., 1986).

Not shown in Figure 2-1 in Chapter 2 is the mechanism of action of vitamin D in regulating serum phosphorus levels, certain aspects of which remain obscure. What is known is that (1) a deficiency of phosphate stimulates CYP27B1 to produce more calcitriol, which in turn stimulates phosphate absorption in the small intestine; and (2) calcitriol can also induce the secretion of FGF23 by osteocytes in bone, which results in phosphate excretion in the kidney (Liu et al., 2008), as well as feedback on vitamin D metabolism.

Other Actions

It is noteworthy that the VDR is present in the nucleus of many tissues that are not involved in the regulation of calcium and phosphate metabolism. For example, the VDR has been clearly described in epidermal keratinocytes, in activated T cells of the immune system, in antigen-presenting cells, in macrophages and monocytes, and in cytotoxic T cells. Gene array studies in many cells and tissues show that calcitriol regulates several hundred genes throughout the body or as much as 5 percent of the human genome (Pike et al., 2008). However, exactly how calcitriol functions in these tissues and the physiological consequences are not clearly known.

Likewise, the importance of the paracrine or autocrine synthesis of calcitriol under non-disease conditions is unclear. The 1α-hydroxylase (CYP27B1) gene has been reported to be expressed in many extra-renal tissues (Hewison et al., 2007). In some cases, this is based upon in vitro production of calcitriol by cell lines as a consequence of culture conditions, but it also includes detection of the messenger ribonucleic acid (mRNA) transcript or protein for CYP27B1 in tissues in vivo (Hewison et al., 2007). There is no doubt that the kidney is physiologically the overwhelming site of production of calcitriol for the circulation, as chronic kidney disease or nephrectomy results in a significant fall in the serum calcitriol level (Martinez et al., 1995). The contribution of calcitriol to the maternal circulation stemming from production by the placenta is not clearly known; based on a case report for an anephric patient, it appears that the placenta produces calcitriol, but its contribution to the maternal circulation is low (Turner et al., 1988). The pregnancy-related rise in calcitriol is due to up-regulation of the enzymes in the maternal kidney (Kovacs and Kronenberg, 1997). However, there may be other extra-renal 1α-hydroxylation sites that can act as intracrine systems primarily involved in regulation of cell or tissue growth: skin, gastrointestinal tract, or glandular tissue, such as prostate and breast (Diesing et al., 2006). In mice missing the *Vdr* gene (*Vdr*-null), calcitriol and the VDR play a role in lactational physiology; there is accelerated mammary development during pregnancy, but delayed involution of the mammary tissue after lactation (Zinser and Welsh, 2004). Extra-renal CYP27B1 may be up-regulated during inflammation (Ma et al., 2004; Liu et al., 2008) or down-regulated in cancerous tissue proliferation (Bises et al., 2004; Wang et al., 2004). Furthermore, extra-renal production of calcitriol is clearly found in certain pathological diseases, including granulomatous conditions such as sarcoidosis, lymphoma, and tuberculosis (Adams et al., 1989), which can be associated with hypercalcemia. If sarcoidosis is left untreated, the extra-renally produced calcitriol can enter the circulation, resulting in hypercalciuria and eventually hypercalcemia.

There is emerging evidence that calcitriol plays a role in the immune system that has not yet been clearly described. Exogenous calcitriol can suppress autoimmune diseases, but with hypercalcemia as an important side effect (DeLuca and Cantorna, 2001). It has been shown that the local conversion of 25OHD into calcitriol in monocytes or macrophages results in an increase in cellular immunity by stimulating the production of cathelicidin, an anti-microbial peptide capable of killing bacteria, particularly *Mycobacterium tuberculosis* (Liu et al., 2006). Recently, Stubbs et al. (2010) showed that renal dialysis patients treated with high-dose vitamin D_3 develop a population of immune cells with increased CYP27B1, VDR, and cathelicidin expression, although the role of these cells in vivo is unknown. Ironically, calcitriol has an opposite effect on the adaptive immune (B and T cell function) response. Calcitriol generally inhibits T helper cell proliferation and B cell immunoglobulin production. In contrast, calcitriol promotes the proliferation of immunosuppressive regulatory T cells and their accumulation at sites of inflammation (Penna et al., 2007).

A role for vitamin D in carcinogenesis evolved initially from in vitro studies as cell culture approaches became more widely available for the evaluation of the mechanisms of action of vitamin D and its metabolites (Masuda and Jones, 2006). The active hormone, calcitriol, was shown to consistently inhibit the growth of cancer cells and promote differentiation in vitro by regulating multiple pathways (Deeb et al., 2007; Kovalenko et al., 2010). Additional studies documented the presence of the VDR in a wide array of cancer cell types. Vitamin D orchestrates cell cycle progression via alterations in key regulators such as cyclin-dependent kinases, retinoblastoma protein phosphorylation, and repression of the proto-oncogene myc as well as by modulating growth factor receptor-mediated signaling pathways (Koga et al., 1988; Kawa et al., 1996; Campbell et al., 1997; Xie et al., 1997; Yanagisawa et al., 1999; Sundaram et al., 2000; Gaschott and Stein, 2003; Li et al., 2004). In addition, calcitriol restores or enhances pro-apoptotic effects in cancer cells by several possible pathways, including repression of several pro-survival proteins such as Bc12 and telomerase reverse transcriptase and by activating pro-apoptotic proteins Bax and μ-calpain (James et al., 1996; Diaz et al., 2000; Jiang et al., 2004; Kumagai et al., 2005). Evidence also supports an anti-angiogenic effect of vitamin D. Vascular endothelial growth factor (VEGF) expression by cancer cells is suppressed and endothelial cell responses to VEGF are inhibited by vitamin D, an observation supported by in vivo xenograft studies (Mantell et al., 2000; Bao et al., 2006). The immunoregulatory effects of vitamin D may also have an impact on cancer biology. Inflammation is a critical early step in the carcinogenesis cascade for many cancers, and the ability of vitamin D to exhibit anti-inflammatory effects on cancer cells by down-regulating the pro-inflammatory pathways, such as cyclooxygenase-2, may contribute to cancer inhibition (Moreno et al., 2005). In contrast, the role of vitamin D in cancer immunosurveillance of nascent or established cancers remains to be defined.

The encouraging in vitro findings, tempered with concerns about hypercalcemia, led to the development of many vitamin D analogues in the hope of retaining anti-cancer activity, but without increasing serum calcium, for the pharmacological therapy of cancer, as recently reviewed (Beer and Myrthue, 2004; Masuda and Jones, 2006; Trump et al., 2010).

Vitamin D_2 Versus Vitamin D_3

Vitamins D_2 and D_3, as described previously, differ only in their side chain structure. Physiological responses to both forms of the vitamin include regulation of calcium and phosphate homeostasis and regulation of cell proliferation and cell differentiation of specific cell types, as described above. Qualitatively, vitamins D_2 and D_3 exhibit virtually identical biological responses throughout the body (i.e., through gene expression) that are mediated by the VDR (Jones et al., 1998; Jurutka et al., 2001).

Regarding the potency of the two forms of vitamin D, there are reports that certain animals, such as avian species and New World monkeys (Chen and Bosmann, 1964; Drescher et al., 1969), discriminate against vitamin D_2. However, it has been assumed for several decades that the two forms are essentially equipotent in humans (Christiansen et al., 1975). Recent reports involving human dietary studies have argued for (Trang et al., 1998; Armas et al., 2004) or against (Holick et al., 2008) a metabolic discrimination against vitamin D_2, compared with vitamin D_3. Part of the apparent conflict between these different studies (Trang et al., 1998; Armas et al.,

2004; Holick et al., 2008) is almost certainly due to differences in size and frequency of dose (which have ranged from 1,000 IU daily doses to 50,000 IU in a single dose); the differences reported suggest a difference in pharmacokinetic parameters between vitamin D_2 and vitamin D_3.

This debate runs parallel to the suggestion that vitamin D_2 is less toxic than its vitamin D_3 counterpart. Experimental animal data from a number of mammalian species ranging from rodents to primates (Roborgh and de Man, 1959, 1960; Hunt et al., 1972; Sjoden et al., 1985; Weber et al., 2001), support the concept that the D_2 form is less toxic than D_3, but there is no evidence available in humans. Nonetheless, the implication of these diverse studies in several mammalian species is that vitamin D_2 compounds may show differences in pharmacokinetics that manifest as lower toxicity from high doses.

There is considerable evidence that most of the steps involved in the metabolism and actions of vitamin D_2 and vitamin D_3 are identical (Jones et al., 1998). The identification of the series of vitamin D_3 metabolites in the late 1960s and early 1970s was followed by the identification of their vitamin D_2 counterparts: $25OHD_2$, $1\alpha,25(OH)_2D_2$, and $24,25(OH)_2D_2$ (Suda et al., 1969; Jones et al., 1975, 1979, 1980a). Noteworthy here is the fact that the structural features unique to the vitamin D_2 side chain did not preclude either the 25- or 1α-hydroxylation steps in activation of the molecule or the first step of inactivation, namely 24-hydroxylation. Studies have also shown that the steps in the specific vitamin D signal transduction cascade do not appear to discriminate discernibly between the two vitamin D homologues at the molecular level (e.g., binding to the transport protein, DBP [Hay and Watson, 1977; Jones et al., 1980a] or binding to the receptor, VDR [Jones et al., 1980b; Reinhardt et al., 1989]). Overall, it can be concluded that specific signal transduction systems designed to respond to vitamin D_3 respond to physiological doses of vitamin D_2 equally well.

At this time, firm conclusions about different effects of the two forms of vitamin D cannot be drawn; however, it would appear that at low doses, D_2 and D_3 are equivalent, but at high doses, D_2 is less effective than D_3. In essence, the potency of the two forms (as judged by the dose required to cure rickets) is assumed to be the same (Park, 1940). Differences in toxicity for humans, as judged by the dose to cause hypervitaminosis D, are unclear, but there is evidence from experimental animal data to suggest that D_2 is less toxic than D_3.

Skeletal Disorders

Vitamin D deficiency results in inadequate mineralization of the skeleton. Commonly referred to as rickets in children and osteomalacia in adults, this disorder has been described in Chapter 2 relative to calcium.

Vitamin D deficiency is characterized by aberrations in the mineralization of the bone. In children, the deficiency results in rickets (see also Chapter 2), in which the cartilage fails to mature and mineralize normally. Rickets is characterized by widening at the end of the long bones, rachitic rosary, deformations in the skeleton, including craniotabes and deformities of the lower limbs, known as bowed legs and knocked knees. In adults, the deficiency of vitamin D leads to osteomalacia in which the newly deposited bone matrix fails to mineralize adequately, and there are wide unmineralized bone matrix (osteoid) seams.

Vitamin D–dependent rickets type I (VDDR I) is an autosomal recessive trait that results in abnormally low calcitriol levels but normal serum 25OHD levels. The mutation in VDDR I affects the 1α-hydroxylase enzyme and leads to impaired intestinal calcium absorption and the resulting rickets (Fraser et al., 1973). VDDR I manifests in the first year after birth and is treated with calcitriol. Supplemental calcium and phosphate are usually not needed. The second disorder is vitamin D–dependent rickets type II (VDDR II), which results in hypocalcemia, tetany, convulsions, alopecia, and rickets. VDDR II is also an autosomal recessive trait, resulting from a mutation in the *Vdr* gene, which can appear in the second year after birth or go unrecognized until adulthood.

VITAMIN D ACROSS THE LIFE CYCLE

Overall, vitamin D's role at different life stages is less clearly age-related than that of calcium, and also less well understood, with numerous gaps in basic information. Although some aspects of vitamin D nutrition and physiology have been found to differ with life stage, most of the functions of vitamin D are quite consistent across life stages from infancy and childhood, to adolescence, adulthood, and old age. For all life stages highlighted below, specific studies and conclusions are detailed in Chapter 4.

Infancy

Healthy skeletal development in infancy requires adequate intakes of vitamin D as well as calcium. Inadequate vitamin D intake during periods of growth leads to development of vitamin D deficiency rickets, which when it occurs in North American populations typically manifests around 20 months of age (DeLucia et al., 2003). If rickets is diagnosed early, vitamin D therapy can cure it, but not if skeletal deformities are severe and growth plates have started to mature in puberty (DeLuca, 1979a). Infants at risk for developing rickets include those who are exclusively breast-fed, because vitamin D and 25OHD are normally present at low levels in breast milk (Bachrach et al., 1979; Ward et al., 2007). Health Canada currently recommends that exclusively breast-fed infants receive a supplement of vitamin D,[6] and the American Academy of Pediatrics guidelines support supplementation of breastfeeding infants with vitamin D (Gartner and Greer, 2003). Commercial infant formula contains vitamin D, as discussed previously in this chapter.

Childhood and Adolescence

This life stage is characterized by bone accretion. During the rapid growth phase of adolescence, almost 50 percent of the adult skeletal mass will be accumulated. The onset of puberty stimulates increased metabolism of 25OHD levels to calcitriol (Aksnes and Aarskog, 1982) and subsequent increased calcium intestinal absorption, decreased urinary calcium excretion, and greater calcium deposition into bone (Wastney et al., 1996). Information on relationships between 25OHD levels and optimal intestinal absorption of calcium or risk for rickets or fracture in children and adolescents is lacking, although Abrams et al. (2005) found evidence for an indirect relationship between low serum 25OHD and increased calcium absorption in young adolescents. Although a recent set of systematic reviews (Cranney et al., 2007; Chung et al., 2009), to be discussed in Chapter 4, did not report specifically on bone mass for this age group in relation to vitamin D nutriture, the reviews suggested the possibility of a relationship between serum levels of 25OHD and bone mineral density (BMD) in adolescents. A recent analysis of vitamin D intake and BMD in male and female adolescents and adults ages 13 to 36 years found positive correlations between vitamin D intake and bone density from adolescence into adulthood among male but not female subjects (van Dijk et al., 2009).

Adults

The life stages associated with younger adults, covering several decades, are characterized by a need for adequate nutrition for bone maintenance. The bone is constantly undergoing remodeling, and the maintenance of normal bone density reduces the risk of skeletal disorders ranging from osteomalacia to the onset of osteoporotic fractures later in life. It is also the time of pregnancy and lactation for some female members of this population.

Older adults, especially those characterized as frail, may have poor dairy and vitamin D intake, decreased sun exposure, reduced dermal conversion of 7-dehydrocholesterol to vitamin D_3 and secondary hyperparathy-

---

[6]Available online at http://www.hc-sc.gc.ca/fn-an/nutrition/infant-nourisson/vita_d_supp-eng.php (accessed September 1, 2010).

roidism, all of which contribute to increased risk for poor bone health and osteoporotic fractures. As discussed below, there is inconsistent evidence as to whether intestinal absorption of vitamin D declines with age. In women, bone loss occurs as a result of the decreased estrogen levels that accompany menopause. As aging continues, both men and women experience age-related bone loss. As is the case for calcium intake, it is not well established whether and to what extent intakes of vitamin D may mitigate the bone loss.

Pregnancy and Lactation

The role of vitamin D in pregnancy and fetal development is the focus of current attention. However, at present the role of vitamin D is not clear, and there are very few data by which to examine the questions surrounding the effect of the nutrient on pregnancy and lactation. Animal studies and inferential human data do not readily elucidate a specific function in fetal development, especially with respect to formation and mineralization of the fetal skeleton. Calcitriol levels increase during pregnancy, but factors other than vitamin D appear to stimulate the increased calcium absorption. Although a number of avenues are still being explored, the bulk of the evidence suggests that calcium is moved from the mother to the fetus without requiring calcitriol.

Breast milk is not normally a significant source of vitamin D for the infant and remains unchanged with supplementation at least up to 2,000 IU/day. Existing evidence suggests that vitamin D nutriture does not appear to affect the maternal processes of bone resorption that occur during lactation, nor its restoration post-lactation.

MEASURES ASSOCIATED WITH VITAMIN D: SERUM 25OHD

Serum 25OHD level is widely considered as a marker of vitamin D nutriture, and consideration of serum 25OHD measures for the purposes of nutrient reference value development has generated notable interest. There is agreement that circulating serum 25OHD levels are currently the best available indicator of the net incoming contributions from cutaneous synthesis *and* total intake (foods and supplements) (Davis et al., 2007; Brannon et al., 2008; Davis, 2008). Thus, the serum 25OHD level may function as a *biomarker of exposure*; it is a reflection of the supply of vitamin D to the body and can be a useful adjunct to examining the intake level of vitamin D if the confounders and the measure's variability depending upon a range of variables are kept in mind. However, what is not clearly established is the extent to which 25OHD levels serve as a *biomarker of effect*. That is, there is some question as to whether levels of 25OHD relate to health outcomes via a causal pathway and can serve as predictors of such outcomes.

Research recommendations in the previous Dietary Reference Intake (DRI) review of vitamin D (IOM, 1997), as well as an Institute of Medicine (IOM) workshop on DRI research needs (IOM, 2007), called for studies to evaluate the intake requirements for vitamin D as related to optimal circulating 25OHD concentrations across life stage and race/ethnicity groups of U.S. and Canadian populations, taking into account variability in UVB radiation exposures. The issue of the role of serum 25OHD concentrations was also identified by the sponsors of this current study on vitamin D and calcium DRIs as central to the development of DRIs for vitamin D (Yetley et al., 2009). Much in the way of this information gap for serum 25OHD concentrations has not yet been addressed. Nonetheless, measures of serum 25OHD are important considerations in developing DRI values for vitamin D intake. The sections below highlight factors affecting serum 25OHD level and methodologies for its measurement. It is important to note that these discussions refer to 25OHD, not to calcitriol (i.e., 1,25-dihydroxyvitamin D). Calcitriol, the active hormonal form of the nutrient, has not been used typically as a measure associated with vitamin D nutriture or as an intermediate related to health outcomes. Calcitriol is not useful as such a measure, for several reasons. Its half-life is short (hours), its formation is not directly regulated by vitamin D intake, its levels are regulated by other factors (such as serum PTH), and, even in the presence of severe vitamin D deficiency the calcitriol level may be normal or even elevated as a result of up-regulation of the 1α-hydroxylase enzyme.

Factors Affecting Serum 25OHD Levels

Dietary Intake (Foods and Supplements)

Available literature demonstrates that serum 25OHD levels increase in response to increased vitamin D intake, although overall it can be concluded that the relationship is non-linear rather than linear. Factors that may affect the relationship between vitamin D intake and serum 25OHD levels are not entirely clear, and the reliability of such measures may be less than desirable. Moreover, there remains debate over the equivalence of vitamins D_2 and D_3 in the diet (Armas et al., 2004; Rapuri et al., 2004; Vieth, 2004), although it has been assumed that they are 25-hydroxylated at similar rates (see previous discussion of functions and physiological actions of vitamin D).

As part of the 2007 Agency for Healthcare Research and Quality (AHRQ) systematic review (Cranney et al., 2007, 2008), referred to hereafter as AHRQ-Ottawa, exploratory meta-regression analysis was conducted of 16 trials in adults, which suggested an association between vitamin D dose and serum 25OHD concentrations. The analysis found that for each additional 100 IU of vitamin D_3, serum 25OHD concentrations rose by 1 to 2 nmol/L. Trials varied in their use of vitamin D_2 or vitamin D_3. A few of the studies reported different effects of vitamin D_2 and vitamin D_3 on serum 25OHD levels. Although the later AHRQ-Tufts analysis (Chung et al., 2009) did not identify newer (compared with AHRQ-Ottawa) randomized controlled trials related to intake of vitamin D and serum 25OHD levels, it did graphically evaluate the net changes in serum 25OHD concentrations against the doses of vitamin D supplementation using data from the trials in adults. The analysis confirmed the relationship between increasing doses of vitamin D and increasing net change in serum 25OHD concentrations in both adults and children, but it also concluded that the dose–response relationships differ depending upon study participants' baseline serum 25OHD levels (≤ 40 vs. > 40 nmol/L) and duration of the supplementation (≤ 3 vs. > 3 months).

In a recent study conducted by Smith et al. (2009), personnel stationed in the Antarctic in winter months (and thus presumed to obtain vitamin D from food and supplements only) were given graded doses of 400, 1,000, or 2,000 IU of vitamin D_3 per day for 5 months. Baseline levels of serum 25OHD rose from approximately 44 nmol/L to 57, 63, and 71 nmol/L, respectively, representing a change in 25OHD levels of 13, 19, or 27 nmol/L. Evident in this study is the continuing fall in 25OHD level in the "no pill" group (to 34 nmol/L) of men who were deprived of sunlight and received approximately 250 to 350 IU of vitamin D (which included foods and any non-study supplements) per day. A possible complicating factor in interpreting these data is that the subjects were consuming diets with a vitamin D content that ranged from 241 to 356 IU/day, in addition to the graded doses of vitamin D from administered supplements, although the amounts of vitamin D obtained from foods (or non-study supplements) were not significantly different between treatment groups. Therefore, any effect of these sources of vitamin D on serum levels would have been consistent between treatment groups.

Another study of serum 25OHD response to total intake under conditions of minimal sun exposure used two populations based in Cork, Ireland (51°N), and Coleraine, Northern Ireland (55°N). The study estimated the dose of vitamin D required to maintain 25OHD levels above certain chosen cutoff values (i.e., 25.0, 37.5, 50.0, and 80.0 nmol/L) during the winter months (Cashman et al., 2008). The researchers found that serum 25OHD levels that ranged between 65.7 and 75.9 nmol/L in late fall fell in all groups receiving 200, 400, and 600 IU of vitamin D_3 per day, as well as in the placebo group, in winter. The decrease in the 600 IU/day group was minimal, from 75.9 to 69.0 nmol/L. Cashman et al. (2008) went on to plot the serum 25OHD levels attained after 5 months versus the estimated total vitamin D intake (approximately 0 to 1,400 IU/day) in 215 individuals, as shown in Figure 3-4. They concluded that, in these two populations at 51°N and 55°N, the wintertime intake required to achieve 25OHD cutoff levels of 37.5, 50.0, and 80.0 nmol/L were 796, 1,120, and 1,644 IU/day, respectively.

Importantly, the relationship between vitamin D intake and serum 25OHD response appears not to be linear, given evidence that increasing serum 25OHD level above 50 nmol/L requires more vitamin D intake than does increasing serum 25OHD levels when the starting point is less than 50 nmol/L (Aloia et al., 2008). Factors such as baseline serum 25OHD level in the population may be relevant. Further, there have been reports that the rise in serum 25OHD levels for a given dose tends to stabilize by week 6 (Harris and Dawson-Hughes, 2002; Holick et al., 2008) and that it does

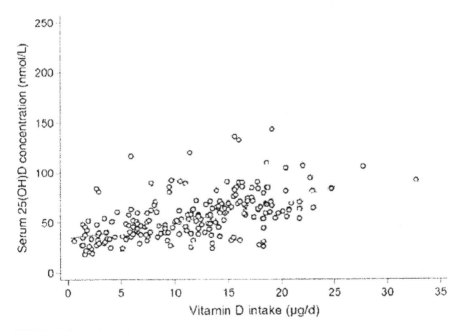

FIGURE 3-4 The relationship between serum 25-hydroxyvitamin D concentrations (in late winter 2007) and total vitamin D intake (dietary and supplemental) in 20- to 40-year-old healthy persons (*n* = 215) living at northern latitudes (51°N and 55°N).

SOURCE: Cashman et al. (2008). Reprinted with permission from the *American Journal of Clinical Nutrition* (2008, 88, 1535-42), American Society for Nutrition.

not vary with age at least up to 80 years of age (Harris and Dawson-Hughes, 2002; Cashman et al., 2008, 2009).

Sun Exposure

The cutaneous synthesis of vitamin D, and in turn its contribution to the concentration of serum 25OHD, is initially dependent upon the presence of 7-dehydrocholesterol in the skin. However, many variables can affect the cutaneous synthesis of vitamin D, making it difficult to estimate an average amount of vitamin D and, in turn, serum 25OHD levels that are produced by sun exposure in North America. There is, however, agreement that sun exposure is a significant source of the circulating serum 25OHD in summer for many North Americans, and is notably reduced as a contributor in the winter months. Early work from Webb et al. (1988, 1989) as well as a letter from Holick et al. (1989) have outlined the role of sunlight in regulating cutaneous synthesis of the vitamin and have implicated factors in vitamin D_3 synthesis in the skin to include aging, melanin pigmentation, season of the year, latitude, and use of sunscreen. Matsuoka et al. (1992) has discussed the role of clothing in preventing synthesis.

The 2007 AHRQ-Ottawa systematic review (Cranney et al., 2007) noted that the few available randomized clinical trials conducted between 1982 and the time of the analysis, which focused on the effect of UVB radiation on serum 25OHD level revealed little information about the impact of age, ethnicity, skin pigmentation, BMI, or latitude on serum 25OHD levels. However, UVB exposure increased serum 25OHD levels in vitamin D–deficient and –sufficient subjects with mean increases ranging from 15 to 42 nmol/L.

The difference in seasonal contributions to serum 25OHD level from sun exposure is discussed first. Next, factors affecting the synthesis of vitamin D—and, in turn, the levels of 25OHD in serum—are outlined.

Effect of season on circulating serum 25OHD level   Sunlight exposure as a source of cutaneous synthesis of vitamin D is subject to a number of limitations. For example, excess exposure can lead to photo-degradation as a regulatory mechanism to avoid toxicity (Chen et al., 2007). In addition, latitude, time of exposure, and season all affect cutaneous synthesis, depending on the ability of UV rays to stimulate vitamin D production. Differences in seasonal exposure can vary by as much as 6 months at extreme northern and southern latitudes (Lucas et al., 2005; Kull et al., 2009).

A number of studies have examined serum 25OHD levels in different seasons. Van der Mei et al. (2007) compared cross–sectional data from men and women less than 60 years of age living in Australia and concluded that season was a strong determinant of serum 25OHD concentrations. Berry et al. (2009) examined white adults ages 20 to 60 years living in the United Kingdom (UK) at latitude 53°N. In this study, women were found to have higher average serum 25OHD levels than men in both summer and winter (9 and 20 percent higher, respectively). In a study of young adults of diverse ethnic backgrounds living in Toronto, Gozdik et al. (2009) found that in winter, serum 25OHD levels of individuals with East and South Asian backgrounds were significantly lower than those of individuals with European ancestry. Kull et al. (2009) measured seasonal variance of 25OHD levels in adults ages 25 to 70 years living in Estonia in northern Europe, where dairy products are not fortified with vitamin D. During the winter, 73 percent of the study population had 25OHD levels that were below 50 nmol/L, and 8 percent had levels that were below 25 nmol/L, compared with 29 percent and 1 percent, respectively, during the summer. Rapuri et al. (2002) examined white, black, and Hispanic women 65 to 77 years of age in Omaha and reported mean serum 25OHD levels of 68 nmol/L in February and 86 nmol/L in August. These studies, despite variations in age, gender, and ethnicity, all suggest that seasonal change can affect cutaneous vitamin D synthesis. The winter low serum 25OHD concentrations and the summer high serum 25OHD concentrations from these studies are summarized in Table 3-1.

Although there are variations in the available data as well as a number of unknowns that may influence such values, they suggest a seasonal change in serum 25OHD concentrations between the winter nadir and the summer zenith of approximately 25 nmol/L. Free-living individuals in the latitudes studied appear to experience an approximately one-third seasonal increase in their circulating serum 25OHD levels as they moved from the winter months to the summer months.

The 25 nmol/L change in serum 25OHD level would appear to be similar in magnitude to change experienced by subjects given 2,000 IU/day in the Antarctic study (Smith et al., 2009). Although these data suggest that average cutaneous synthesis during the summer in northern latitudes equates to 2,000 IU/day, this may be a questionable conclusion given the many variables that come into play, ranging from feedback mechanisms to skin pigmentation to baseline levels of 25OHD. For example, recent work from Olds et al. (2008) suggested a curvilinear relationship between sun exposure and serum 25OHD levels, as well as variation depending upon initial concentrations of 7-dehydrocholesterol levels. At lower doses, vitamin D_3 production rises immediately in response to UV exposure, whereas at higher doses, the rate of production is lower and reaches an earlier plateau.

Effect of skin pigmentation on synthesis   The presence of melanin in the epidermal layer is responsible for skin pigmentation. A number of

TABLE 3-1 Winter Low 25OHD Levels and Summer High 25OHD Levels Around the World

Location (Latitude)	Winter Baseline	Summer High
Toronto, Canada[a] 43°N	35 nmol/L	50 nmol/L[b]
Tasmania, Australia[c] 43°S	40 nmol/L	62 nmol/L
Estonia, northern Europe[d] 59°N	44 nmol/L	59 nmol/L
Salford/Manchester, UK[e] 53°N	46 nmol/L	71 nmol/L
Geelong region, Australia[c] 38°S	57 nmol/L	93 nmol/L
Omaha, USA[f] 41°N	68 nmol/L	86 nmol/L

[a]Gozdik et al., 2009.
[b]high value recorded in autumn.
[c]van der Mei et al., 2007.
[d]Kull et al., 2009.
[e]Berry et al., 2009.
[f]Rapuri et al., 2002.

recent studies have reinforced the relationship of skin pigmentation to the capacity to produce vitamin D_3 after UV exposure, but the results are not all consistent. Armas et al. (2007) studied the incremental change in serum 25OHD levels in individuals with average 25OHD baseline levels of 52 nmol/L and with different skin pigmentation who were exposed to different daily doses of 20 to 80 mJ/cm^2 of UVB light three times per week for 4 weeks on 90 percent of their skin surface area. The work suggested that for individuals at the lighter pigmentation scale,[7] exposed to similar UVB doses (20 to 80 mJ/cm^2) resulted in twice the increase in serum 25OHD concentration compared with individuals at the opposite extreme (i.e., 62 vs. 32 nmol/L change) (Armas et al., 2007) (see modeled representation in Figure 3-5). However, other studies have shown that the response to UV dose is non-linear and dependent on genetic factors (Snellman et al., 2009), duration and dose rate of UV exposure, and baseline serum 25OHD levels (Bogh et al., 2010).

Another population study of 237 subjects at a single geographical location (Toronto, 43°N) also explored the effect of skin pigmentation on

---

[7]L*=70; the lightest skin tone of northern Europeans.

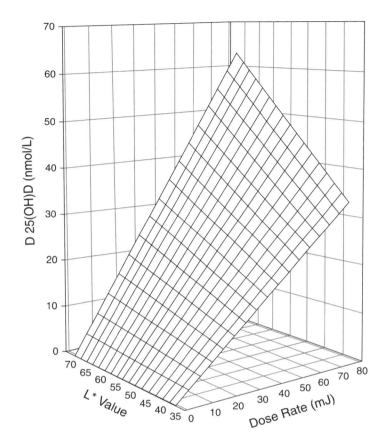

FIGURE 3-5 Three-dimensional scatter-plot of 4-week change in serum 25OHD concentration above baseline expressed as a function of both basic skin lightness (L*) and UVB dose rate. Surface is hyperboloid, plotting equation 1, and was fitted to data using least squares regression methods.

NOTE: Equation 1 is $z = b * x * y$, where z is the induced increase in serum 25OHD level from baseline (in nmol/L); x is UVB dose (in mJ/cm² per session); y is skin lightness (expressed as the L* score value from the reflective meter); and b is the sole parameter to be fitted.

SOURCE: Reprinted with permission from Robert Heaney.

25OHD synthesis (Gozdik et al., 2009). The mean serum 25OHD levels in Canadians of European, East Asian, and South Asian ancestry were 71.7, 44.6, and 33.9 nmol/L, respectively, in late fall; and 51.6, 28.1, and 26.5 nmol/L, respectively, in the winter. The authors found that differences between the three subgroups were strongly associated with skin pigmentation as well as amount of time spent outdoors and total vitamin D intake. A recent study of 182 individuals in Denmark, screened in January and February and selected to reflect wide ranges of baseline 25OHD levels and skin pigmentation, found that the increase in 25OHD levels after UVB exposure was inversely correlated with skin pigmentation as well as with baseline 25OHD (Bogh et al., 2010).

A number of small studies have reported serum 25OHD levels to be consistently lower in persons with darker skin pigmentation, and data from NHANES suggest that serum 25OHD levels are highest in whites, lowest in non-Hispanic blacks, and intermediate in Hispanic groups (Looker et al., 2008). Overall, there is considerable evidence that darker skin pigmentation is associated with a smaller increase in serum 25OHD concentration for a given amount of UVB exposure.

Effect of latitude on synthesis   Early on, in vitro methods, such as exposure of sealed vials of 7-dehydrocholesterol to UVB radiation under "idealized conditions" at various geographical locations, were used to assess the effect of latitude, time of day, and season on the rate of vitamin D production (Webb et al., 1988). However, this approach cannot completely simulate the in vivo conditions in the body, where many factors serve to regulate this process. Furthermore, although the measurement of vitamin D concentrations in a mixture of irradiation products is analytically simple, vitamin D_3 levels in human serum are rarely used to estimate cutaneous synthesis of the vitamin, in part because of the transient nature of this blood parameter and the difficulty of measuring the low levels in serum (Holick, 1988; Hollis, 2008). Nevertheless, Holick and colleagues used a serum vitamin D_3 assay to augment in vitro methodology and suggested that, at latitudes above 43°N, cutaneous synthesis contributes little serum 25OHD to the system in the winter months between October and March in North America (Webb et al., 1988; Matsuoka et al., 1989).

More recent data may call into question current assumptions about the effect of latitude. In fact, Kimlin et al. (2007), using computer modeling, concluded that it may no longer be correct to assume that vitamin D levels in populations follow latitude gradients. Indeed, the relationship between UVB penetration and latitude is complex, as a result of differences in, for example, the height of the atmosphere (50 percent less at the poles), cloud cover (more intense at the equator than at the poles), and ozone cover. The duration of sunlight in summer versus winter is another factor contributing to the complexity of the relationship. Geophysical surveys have shown that UVB penetration over 24 hours, during the summer months at Canadian north latitudes when there are many hours of sunlight, equals or exceeds UVB penetration at the equator (Lubin et al., 1998). Consequently, there is ample opportunity during the spring, summer, and fall months in the far north for humans (as well as animals that serve as food sources) to form vitamin D_3 and store it in liver and fat. These factors may explain why latitude alone does not consistently predict the average serum 25OHD level of a population.

Effect of sunscreen on synthesis   Sunscreens are used to protect the skin from ultraviolet A (UVA) and UVB waveband exposure that is associated with deoxyribonucleic acid (DNA) damage—the same UVB exposure that is needed for vitamin D synthesis. Experimental studies suggest that sunscreens can decrease cutaneous vitamin D synthesis (Misra et al., 2008). However, emerging evidence suggests that although sunscreens are effective, many may not actually be blocking UVB because they are improperly or inadequately applied. Thus, sunscreen use may not actually diminish vitamin D synthesis in real world use, although further study is needed to verify its actual impact (Diehl and Chiu, 2010; Springbett et al., 2010).

Other variables affecting synthesis   A number of other variables can impede sun exposure and thus inhibit cutaneous vitamin D synthesis. Clothing is an effective barrier to sun exposure and the UVB waveband, but the effectiveness of sun blocking depends on the thickness or weave of the fabric (Diehl and Chiu, 2010). Likewise, ethnic practices, such as extensive skin coverage with clothing, urban environments that reduce or block sunlight, air pollution, and cloud cover that reduces solar penetration can variously reduce sun exposure. In contrast, high altitude reduces the atmospheric protection against UVB waveband and can increase risk for sun damage as well as increase vitamin D synthesis (Misra et al., 2008). There may be a role for measures of physical activity in affecting vitamin D synthesis, although many covariates may be relevant, and some have suggested that genetics can account for some of the differences in synthesis of serum 25OHD.

Confounders Affecting Serum 25OHD Concentrations

Adiposity   Interpreting data on serum 25OHD concentrations in obese and overweight persons is particularly challenging. Data from NHANES showed lower circulating levels of 25OHD among young adult obese non-Hispanic white women compared with their leaner counterparts; the relationship appeared to be weaker among non-Hispanic blacks. Differences in physical activity levels partially explain these differences (Looker, 2005, 2007). However, overweight and obese persons in NHANES also reported lower use of dietary supplements than did leaner persons of the same age or gender group (Radimer et al., 2004; Picciano et al., 2007), suggesting that lower dietary exposures could also contribute to the lower serum 25OHD levels in obese and overweight people.

Sequestration of vitamin D into fat likely also plays a significant role in reducing the amount that can be presented to the liver for 25-hydroxylation. As noted previously, vitamin D is absorbed with fat as part of chylomicrons and is taken up first by peripheral tissues that express lipoprotein lipase, especially adipose tissue and skeletal muscle. This pathway predicts that increased adiposity should lead to lower serum 25OHD levels and, conversely, that weight loss should reduce peripheral sequestration and enable higher 25OHD levels. Consistent with this, not only does increasing adiposity correlate with lower 25OHD levels, but also a few studies of modest weight loss have found the circulating 25OHD levels to increase despite no increased intake of vitamin D from diet or sunlight exposure (Riedt et al., 2005; Reinehr et al., 2007; Zittermann et al., 2009; Tzotzas et al., 2010). The measured increase in serum 25OHD levels in overweight and obese individuals was about 1.5 nmol/L for a 100 IU/day vitamin D intake over 12 months (Sneve et al., 2008; Zittermann et al., 2009). Others found that obese subjects show a lower rise in serum 25OHD levels in response to both oral vitamin D intake and UVB exposure (Wortsman et al., 2000) or in a retrospective analysis in response to 700 IU/day vitamin D_3 supplementation (Blum et al., 2008). It is interesting that in severely obese individuals after malabsorptive gastric bypass surgery, vitamin D supplementation resulted in a marked rise in serum 25OHD level of approximately 3 nmol/100 IU intake when the dose was 800 to 2,000 IU/day, but only a 1 nmol/L rise when intake was increased to 5,000 IU/day (Goldner et al., 2009).

African American ancestry Serum 25OHD levels are lower in African Americans compared with light-skinned population groups (Looker et al., 2008), yet the risk for fracture is lower for African Americans than for other ethnic groups (Aloia, 2008). It should be noted, however, that there is a wide range of variability among individuals of any race or ethnicity (Aloia, 2008). Serum 25OHD levels in African Americans and whites have been shown to be similarly responsive to vitamin D supplementation at 40°N latitude (equivalent to Philadelphia or Indianapolis), increasing by 1 to 2 nmol/L per 100 IU/day at a dose of 3,440 IU/day (Aloia et al., 2008), although at doses below 2,000 IU/day, serum 25OHD levels do not increase above 50 nmol/L in African American girls (Talwar et al., 2007). The significance of maintaining a higher serum 25OHD level in African Americans is not understood at this time because of a lack of evidence on extra-skeletal effects of vitamin D.

Size and frequency of dose Dosing of vitamin D daily, weekly, or monthly has been tested, and there are reports of annual dosing as well. The results of a study by Chel et al. (2008) suggested that daily (600 IU/day) and weekly doses of vitamin D will increase serum 25OHD levels more than monthly doses, but Ish-Shalom et al. (2008) using a dose of 1,500 IU/day found no difference due to timing of the doses. Ish-Shalom et al. (2008) suggested that the attenuated response to monthly dose in the Chel et al. (2008) study may have been due to poor compliance with a powdered monthly supplement compared with pills used for their daily and weekly doses. An alternative explanation is that only a lower (Chel et al., 2008) and not a higher (Ish-Shalom et al., 2008) dose is influenced by timing of the vitamin D supplement. Thus far, studies suggest that weekly and daily dosing give similar serum 25OHD responses.

Assays for Serum 25OHD

Serum 25OHD comprises the sum of $25OHD_2$ and $25OHD_3$. Because of the widespread use of both vitamin D_2 and vitamin D_3 in the United States and Canada, analysts must measure both $25OHD_2$ and $25OHD_3$ in order to provide the total 25OHD level in serum. This is in contrast to the situation in Europe where there has been a tradition of using only vitamin D_3 and where commercial methods that purport to measure only $25OHD_3$ are available.

In North America, several assay types are currently in use, each with strengths and weaknesses (Makin et al., 2010). The two most common types of assays are

- Antibody-based methods, which use a kit or an automated clinical chemistry platform; and
- Liquid chromatography (LC)-based methods, which use automated equipment featuring either UV or mass spectrometric (MS)-detection.

As discussed below, both these methods are equivalent in terms of measuring the physiologically relevant parameter (total 25OHD level in serum), but there remains controversy over the performance of these assays in clinical and research laboratories. Moreover, reports in the literature for serum 25OHD measures should be interpreted with care, taking into account the type of assay employed, use of automation, year of analysis, and context of the analysis.

Overview of Assay Methodology

Assays for total 25OHD level in serum have existed for four decades since the metabolite was first discovered (Blunt et al., 1968). The earliest assays were competitive protein-binding assays (CPBAs), based upon the ability of either $25OHD_2$ or $25OHD_3$ to displace $[^3H]25OHD_3$ from the plasma binding protein, DBP (Belsey et al., 1971; Haddad and Hahn,

1973). These assays incorporated extraction, chromatographic purification, and detection steps, but the assays were laborious and not easily simplified, owing to the presence of co-extracted interfering substances. They therefore fell out of favor. Non-chromatographic CPBA assays tended to read erroneously high, and some data from this period (1970s) are viewed as extremely questionable for this reason.

In the late 1970s LC-based assays emerged that used refined extraction and chromatographic steps with some form of fixed- or variable-wavelength UV detector to measure the distinctive native absorbance of the vitamin D metabolites with λmax at 265 nm (Jones, 1978; Horst et al., 1979). These allowed for the separate estimation of 25OHD$_2$ and 25OHD$_3$ from serum samples. This type of assay has undergone much refinement over the years, with improvements in LC, improved automation, or the introduction of diode-array UV detectors that minimize the chance of picking up interfering substances (Lensmeyer et al., 2006). Although these assays require expensive equipment as well as sequential sample analysis, which make them somewhat time-consuming, they are still popular with a minority of analysts.

In the early to late 1980s, antibody-based assays were introduced, which use a proprietary antibody to a vitamin D molecular antigen, usually with a truncated vitamin D side chain. They are therefore devoid of the features that allow the resultant antibody to distinguish between 25OHD$_2$ and 25OHD$_3$ (Hollis and Napoli, 1985); this is of value, but at the expense of detecting other minor metabolites. Consequently, antibody-based methods measure only total 25OHD in serum. Various commercial assays differ because of the nature of the antibody used, some claiming an advantage that they do not discriminate between 25OHD$_2$ and 25OHD$_3$ (Hollis and Napoli, 1985), whereas others in fact do underestimate the 25OHD$_2$ pool and therefore provide correction factors to compensate for high 25OHD$_2$ content. Over the past decade, antibody-based 25OHD assays have become automated into a multiwell plate-format and the increased throughput has made them extremely popular. It is important to note that the majority of the data collected over the past 20 to 30 years have been analyzed using antibody-based assays.

Recently, LC-based assays have also undergone a radical transformation with the replacement of the UV detection step by a "universal detector" in the form of a tandem mass spectrometer (LC-MS/MS) (Jones and Makin, 2000). LC-MS/MS assays allow the analyst to discriminate between 25OHD$_2$ and 25OHD$_3$ and other serum lipids by their unique molecular masses and mass fragments. Accordingly, these methods measure 25OHD$_2$ and 25OHD$_3$, and therefore total 25OHD (Makin et al., 2010). Because these methods use short LC retention times, automated robotic extraction and LC separation steps, and computerized MS systems, they can be made relatively operator-free and provide high throughput. Further, their potential advantages also include high specificity, high sensitivity, and better repro-ducibility (< 10 percent). The consensus among analysts is that LC-MS/MS assays will become the "gold standard" for assay performance in the future.

Thus, a variety of methods are available to determine serum 25OHD levels, each with its advantages and disadvantages that must be considered in evaluating the data arising from them.

Assay Performance Concerns

The methodologies used over four decades of assaying 25OHD levels in serum have each presented technical problems. These include, first, CPBA assays without chromatography that read high because of poorly defined "interferences" (Morris and Peacock, 1976; Stamp et al., 1976). Second, some LC-MS/MS assays with short LC run times read high be-cause they cannot resolve 3-epi-25OHD$_3$, an isomer found in abundance in neonatal samples (Singh et al., 2006). Third, some antibody-based as-says, particularly some of the automated versions, fail to recover or detect, and therefore underestimate 25OHD$_2$ (Carter et al., 2004). Fourth, some antibody-based assays overestimate values by detecting further metabolites of 25OHD (e.g., 24,25[OH]$_2$D and 26,23-lactone) particularly those found in hypervitaminotic D situations (i.e., 25OHD > 250 nmol/L) (Jones et al., 1987); and some antibody-based methods are sensitive to exogenous inter-ferences such as the presence of dilutants (ethanol, non-human serum) used in quality control materials (Phinney, 2009). Thus, no assay is free from problems, and performance must be monitored vigilantly.

Performance has been a concern of analysts and clinicians in the vita-min D field for some time. Inter-laboratory comparisons have been con-ducted and published for two decades and suggest an unacceptable degree of variability in the different results (Jongen et al., 1984, 1989). This has led to the creation of external quality assurance schemes, such as the Vitamin D External Quality Assurance Scheme or DEQAS[8] (Charing Cross Hospital, London, UK), similar to those used in other areas of clinical chemistry. Since its inception in the early 1990s, DEQAS has grown steadily, such that it now serves as a quarterly monitor of performance of analysts and 25OHD analytical methods for approximately 700 laboratories worldwide (Carter et al., 2010). Although initially DEQAS used gas chromatography-mass spectrometry (GC-MS) as its "gold standard," more recently it has adopted an all-laboratory trimmed mean (ALTM) as the value it uses to judge per-formance. Using ALTM, DEQAS has served as an early-warning system for method and operator biases that have alerted the commercial kit manu-facturers to modify their products or steps in their procedures or withdraw their kits. DEQAS has published performance characteristics (precision,

---

[8]Available online at http://www.deqas.org/ (accessed March 9, 2010).

accuracy, and variability) regularly over the past decade (Carter et al., 2004; Carter, 2009; Jones et al., 2009). These publications have been augmented by other independent method comparisons (Glendenning et al., 2006; Lensmeyer et al., 2006; Roth et al., 2008).

In brief, these performance reports suggest some method biases in terms of accuracy and precision as well as variability as high as 15 to 20 percent. However, some skilled analysts can perform better than this with a coefficient of variation less than 10 percent. The recent introduction of the National Institute of Standards and Technology (NIST) reference standards[9] calibrated using a "validated" LC-MS/MS method (Phinney, 2009) offers some hope that the variability of all methods can or will be improved in the future. Indeed, recent data suggest that an improvement is already occurring (Carter and Jones, 2009). At this time, however, serum 25OHD data in the literature must be viewed with care based upon the knowledge that they have been acquired using a variety of methods, each with its own shortcomings and subject to high variability.

Assay Shift and Drift: U.S. National Health and Nutrition Examination Survey

Recently, the National Center for Health Statistics (NCHS) posted an analytical note on its NHANES web page informing users about two issues that should be addressed when analyzing and using serum 25OHD data from NHANES.[10] The first involved making direct comparisons between serum 25OHD levels from NHANES III (1988 to 1994) and those from the 2000 to 2006 NHANES because of a reformulation of the DiaSorin radioimmunoassay (RIA) kit[11] that resulted in shifts in assay results between the two time periods. Second, the note also cautioned that the data from the 2000 to 2006 NHANES were likely affected by drifts in the assay performance (method bias and imprecision) over time. A standard reference material (SRM 972, Vitamin D in Human Serum) and calibration solution (SRM 2972, 25-Hydroxyvitamin D_2 and D_3 Calibration Solutions) are currently available from the NIST. The NCHS plans to incorporate use of this SRM into future measures of 25OHD in NHANES. The web page also indicates that guidance concerning a correction factor and data interpretation regarding this shift and drift will be forthcoming from the agency. In the case of the Canadian survey of 25OHD levels in the Canadian population, the analytical methods used to determine 25OHD concentrations were the

---

[9]Available online at http://ts.nist.gov/measurementservices/referencematerials/index.cfm (accessed March 15, 2010).

[10]Available online at http://www.cdc.gov/nchs/data/nhanes/nhanes3/VitaminD_analytic note.pdf (accessed March 17, 2010).

[11]DiaSorin Radio-immunoassay (RIA) (Stillwater, MN).

Diasorin total 25OHD (Liaison) kit[12] (personal communication, S. Brooks, Health Canada, December 18, 2009).

MEASURES ASSOCIATED WITH VITAMIN D: PARATHYROID HORMONE

PTH, which, as described above, plays a role in vitamin D metabolism, is also a known marker for bone resorption, based upon the bone manifestations of secondary hyperparathyroidism—increased bone turnover, increased rates of bone loss, osteoporosis, and increased risk of fractures. Serum PTH level has thus been explored and suggested as a measure indicative of adequate vitamin D nutriture, notably on the basis of the level of serum 25OHD at which serum PTH level rises or, alternatively, the level of serum 25OHD at which serum PTH level no longer declines. This measure is discussed more fully in Chapter 4.

REFERENCES

Aasheim, E. T., S. Bjorkman, T. T. Sovik, M. Engstrom, S. E. Hanvold, T. Mala, T. Olbers and T. Bohmer. 2009. Vitamin status after bariatric surgery: a randomized study of gastric bypass and duodenal switch. American Journal of Clinical Nutrition 90(1): 15-22.

Abrams, S. A., I. J. Griffin, K. M. Hawthorne, S. K. Gunn, C. M. Gundberg and T. O. Carpenter. 2005. Relationships among vitamin D levels, parathyroid hormone, and calcium absorption in young adolescents. Journal of Clinical Endocrinology and Metabolism 90(10): 5576-81.

Adams, J. S., R. L. Modlin, M. M. Diz and P. F. Barnes. 1989. Potentiation of the macrophage 25-hydroxyvitamin D-1-hydroxylation reaction by human tuberculous pleural effusion fluid. Journal of Clinical Endocrinology and Metabolism 69(2): 457-60.

Adams, J. S. and M. Hewison. 2008. Unexpected actions of vitamin D: new perspectives on the regulation of innate and adaptive immunity. National Clinical Practice Endocrinology Metabolism 4(2): 80-90.

Aksnes, L. and D. Aarskog. 1982. Plasma concentrations of vitamin D metabolites in puberty: effect of sexual maturation and implications for growth. Journal of Clinical Endocrinology and Metabolism 55(1): 94-101.

Aloia, J. F. 2008. African Americans, 25-hydroxyvitamin D, and osteoporosis: a paradox. American Journal of Clinical Nutrition 88(2): 545S-50S.

Aloia, J. F., M. Patel, R. Dimaano, M. Li-Ng, S. A. Talwar, M. Mikhail, S. Pollack and J. K. Yeh. 2008. Vitamin D intake to attain a desired serum 25-hydroxyvitamin D concentration. American Journal of Clinical Nutrition 87(6): 1952-8.

Armas, L. A., B. W. Hollis and R. P. Heaney. 2004. Vitamin D_2 is much less effective than vitamin D3 in humans. Journal of Clinical Endocrinology and Metabolism 89(11): 5387-91.

Armas, L. A., S. Dowell, M. Akhter, S. Duthuluru, C. Huerter, B. W. Hollis, R. Lund and R. P. Heaney. 2007. Ultraviolet-B radiation increases serum 25-hydroxyvitamin D levels: the effect of UVB dose and skin color. Journal of the American Academy of Dermatology 57(4): 588-93.

---

[12]DiaSorin Liaison (Stillwater, MN).

Bachrach, S., J. Fisher and J. S. Parks. 1979. An outbreak of vitamin D deficiency rickets in a susceptible population. Pediatrics 64(6): 871-7.

Bao, B. Y., J. Yao and Y. F. Lee. 2006. 1alpha, 25-dihydroxyvitamin D_3 suppresses interleukin-8-mediated prostate cancer cell angiogenesis. Carcinogenesis 27(9): 1883-93.

Beer, T. M. and A. Myrthue. 2004. Calcitriol in cancer treatment: from the lab to the clinic. Moleecular Cancer Therapy 3(3): 373-81.

Belsey, R., H. F. Deluca and J. T. Potts, Jr. 1971. Competitive binding assay for vitamin D and 25-OH vitamin D. Journal of Clinical Endocrinology and Metabolism 33(3): 554-7.

Bergwitz, C. and H. Juppner. 2010. Regulation of phosphate homeostasis by PTH, vitamin D, and FGF23. Annual Review of Medicine 61: 91-104.

Berry, J. L., A. R. Webb, R. Kift, M. Durkin, A. Vail, S. J. O'Brien and L. E. Rhodes. 2009. Should we, in the U.K. be taking vitamin D supplements during the winter? Presented at 14th Workshop on Vitamin D, October 4-8, 2009. Brugge, Belgium.

Bises, G., E. Kallay, T. Weiland, F. Wrba, E. Wenzl, E. Bonner, S. Kriwanek, P. Obrist and H. S. Cross. 2004. 25-hydroxyvitamin D_3-1alpha-hydroxylase expression in normal and malignant human colon. Journal of Histochemistry and Cytochemistry 52(7): 985-9.

Blomstrand, R. and L. Forsgren. 1967. Intestinal absorption and esterification of vitamin D_3-1,2-3H in man. Acta Chemica Scandinavica 21(6): 1662-3.

Blum, M., G. E. Dallal and B. Dawson-Hughes. 2008. Body size and serum 25 hydroxy vitamin D response to oral supplements in healthy older adults. Journal of the American College of Nutrition 27(2): 274-9.

Blunt, J. W., H. F. DeLuca and H. K. Schnoes. 1968. 25-hydroxycholecalciferol. A biologically active metabolite of vitamin D3. Biochemistry 7(10): 3317-22.

Bogh, M. K., A. V. Schmedes, P. A. Philipsen, E. Thieden and H. C. Wulf. 2010. Vitamin D production after UVB exposure depends on baseline vitamin D and total cholesterol but not on skin pigmentation. Journal of Investigative Dermatology 130(2): 546-53.

Brannon, P. M., E. A. Yetley, R. L. Bailey and M. F. Picciano. 2008. Vitamin D and health in the 21st century: an update. Proceedings of a conference held September 2007 in Bethesda, Maryland, USA. American Journal of Clinical Nutrition 88(2): 483S-592S.

Brommage, R. and H. F. DeLuca. 1985. Evidence that 1,25-dihydroxyvitamin D_3 is the physiologically active metabolite of vitamin D_3. Endocrine Reviews 6(4): 491-511.

Bruno, C., A. D. Fulford, J. R. Potts, R. McClintock, R. Jones, B. M. Cacucci, C. E. Gupta, M. Peacock and R. V. Considine. 2010. Serum markers of bone turnover are increased at six and 18 months after Roux-en-Y bariatric surgery: correlation with the reduction in leptin. Journal of Clinical Endocrinology and Metabolism 95(1): 159-66.

Byrdwell, W. C. 2009. Analysis of vitamin D in food control materials and fortified foods. Presented at the Committee to Review Dietary Reference Intakes for Vitamin D and Calcium Information-gathering Workshop, March 26, 2009. Washington, DC.

Campbell, M. J., E. Elstner, S. Holden, M. Uskokovic and H. P. Koeffler. 1997. Inhibition of proliferation of prostate cancer cells by a 19-nor-hexafluoride vitamin D_3 analogue involves the induction of p21waf1, p27kip1 and E-cadherin. Journal of Molecular Endocrinology 19(1): 15-27.

Carter, G. D., R. Carter, J. Jones and J. Berry. 2004. How accurate are assays for 25-hydroxyvitamin D? Data from the international vitamin D external quality assessment scheme. Clinical Chemistry 50(11): 2195-7.

Carter, G. D. 2009. 25-hydroxyvitamin D assays: the quest for accuracy. Clinical Chemistry 55(7): 1300-2.

Carter, G. D. and J. C. Jones. 2009. Use of a common standard improves the performance of liquid chromatography-tandem mass spectrometry methods for serum 25-hydroxyvitamin-D. Annals of Clinical Biochemistry 46(Pt 1): 79-81.

Carter, G. D., J. L. Berry, E. Gunter, G. Jones, J. C. Jones, H. L. Makin, S. Sufi and M. J. Wheeler. 2010. Proficiency testing of 25-hydroxyvitamin D (25-OHD) assays. Journal of Steroid Biochemistry and Molecular Biology 121(1-2): 176-9.

Cashman, K. D., T. R. Hill, A. J. Lucey, N. Taylor, K. M. Seamans, S. Muldowney, A. P. Fitzgerald, A. Flynn, M. S. Barnes, G. Horigan, M. P. Bonham, E. M. Duffy, J. J. Strain, J. M. Wallace and M. Kiely. 2008. Estimation of the dietary requirement for vitamin D in healthy adults. American Journal of Clinical Nutrition 88(6): 1535-42.

Cashman, K. D., J. M. Wallace, G. Horigan, T. R. Hill, M. S. Barnes, A. J. Lucey, M. P. Bonham, N. Taylor, E. M. Duffy, K. Seamans, S. Muldowney, A. P. Fitzgerald, A. Flynn, J. J. Strain and M. Kiely. 2009. Estimation of the dietary requirement for vitamin D in free-living adults ≥64 y of age. American Journal of Clinical Nutrition 89(5): 1366-74.

Chel, V., H. A. Wijnhoven, J. H. Smit, M. Ooms and P. Lips. 2008. Efficacy of different doses and time intervals of oral vitamin D supplementation with or without calcium in elderly nursing home residents. Osteoporosis International 19(5): 663-71.

Chen, P. S., Jr. and H. B. Bosmann. 1964. Effect of vitamins D2 and D3 on serum calcium and phosphorus in rachitic chicks. Journal of Nutrition 83: 133-9.

Chen, T. C., A. Shao, H. Heath, 3rd and M. F. Holick. 1993. An update on the vitamin D content of fortified milk from the United States and Canada. New England Journal of Medicine 329(20): 1507.

Chen, T. C., F. Chimeh, Z. Lu, J. Mathieu, K. S. Person, A. Zhang, N. Kohn, S. Martinello, R. Berkowitz and M. F. Holick. 2007. Factors that influence the cutaneous synthesis and dietary sources of vitamin D. Archives of Biochemistry and Biophysics 460(2): 213-7.

Cheng, J. B., D. L. Motola, D. J. Mangelsdorf and D. W. Russell. 2003. De-orphanization of cytochrome P450 2R1: a microsomal vitamin D 25-hydroxilase. Journal of Biological Chemistry 278(39): 38084-93.

Christiansen, C., P. Rodbro and O. Munck. 1975. Actions of vitamins D_2 and D_3 and 25-OHD_3 in anticonvulsant osteomalacia. British Medical Journal 2(5967): 363-5.

Chung M., E. M. Balk, M. Brendel, S. Ip, J. Lau, J. Lee, A. Lichtenstein, K. Patel, G. Raman, A. Tatsioni, T. Terasawa and T. A. Trikalinos. 2009. Vitamin D and calcium: a systematic review of health outcomes. Evidence Report No. 183. (Prepared by the Tufts Evidence-based Practice Center under Contract No. HHSA 290-2007-10055-I.) AHRQ Publication No. 09-E015. Rockville, MD: Agency for Healthcare Research and Quality.

Clements, M. R., M. Davies, D. R. Fraser, G. A. Lumb, E. B. Mawer and P. H. Adams. 1987. Metabolic inactivation of vitamin D is enhanced in primary hyperparathyroidism. Clinical Science (London) 73(6): 659-64.

Compston, J. E., A. L. Merrett, F. G. Hammett and P. Magill. 1981. Comparison of the appearance of radiolabelled vitamin D_3 and 25-hydroxy-vitamin D_3 in the chylomicron fraction of plasma after oral administration in man. Clinical Science (London) 60(2): 241-3.

Cranney A., T. Horsley, S. O'Donnell, H. A. Weiler, L. Puil, D. S. Ooi, S. A. Atkinson, L. M. Ward, D. Moher, D. A. Hanley, M. Fang, F. Yazdi, C. Garritty, M. Sampson, N. Barrowman, A. Tsertsvadze and V. Mamaladze. 2007. Effectiveness and safety of vitamin D in relation to bone health. Evidence Report/Technology Assessment No. 158 (Prepared by the University of Ottawa Evidence-based Practice Center [UO-EPC] under Contract No. 290-02-0021). AHRQ Publication No. 07-E013. Rockville, MD: Agency for Healthcare Research and Quality.

Cranney, A., H. A. Weiler, S. O'Donnell and L. Puil. 2008. Summary of evidence-based review on vitamin D efficacy and safety in relation to bone health. American Journal of Clinical Nutrition 88(2): 513S-9S.

Davis, C. D., V. Hartmuller, D. M. Freedman, P. Hartge, M. F. Picciano, C. A. Swanson and J. A. Milner. 2007. Vitamin D and cancer: current dilemmas and future needs. Nutrition Reviews 65(8 Pt 2): S71-4.

Davis, C. D. 2008. Vitamin D and cancer: current dilemmas and future research needs. American Journal of Clinical Nutrition 88(2): 565S-9S.

Deeb, K. K., D. L. Trump and C. S. Johnson. 2007. Vitamin D signalling pathways in cancer: potential for anticancer therapeutics. Nature Reviews Cancer 7(9): 684-700.

DeLuca, H. F. 1974. Vitamin D: the vitamin and the hormone. Federation Proceedings 33(11): 2211-9.

Deluca, H. F. 1979a. Vitamin D-resistant rickets. A prototype of nutritional management of a genetic disorder. Current Concepts in Nutrition 8: 3-32.

Deluca, H. F. 1979b. The transformation of a vitamin into a hormone: the vitamin D story. Harvey lectures 75: 333-79.

DeLuca, H. F. and H. K. Schnoes. 1983. Vitamin D: recent advances. Annual Review of Biochemistry 52: 411-39.

DeLuca, H. F. 1988. The vitamin D story: a collaborative effort of basic science and clinical medicine. FASEB Journal 2(3): 224-36.

DeLuca, H. F. and M. T. Cantorna. 2001. Vitamin D: its role and uses in immunology. FASEB Journal 15(14): 2579-85.

Deluca, H. F. 2009. Vitamin D toxicity. Paper prepared for the Committee to Review Dietary Reference Intakes for Vitamin D and Calcium. Washington, DC.

DeLucia, M. C., M. E. Mitnick and T. O. Carpenter. 2003. Nutritional rickets with normal circulating 25-hydroxyvitamin D: a call for reexamining the role of dietary calcium intake in North American infants. Journal of Clinical Endocrinology and Metabolism 88(8): 3539-45.

Diaz, G. D., C. Paraskeva, M. G. Thomas, L. Binderup and A. Hague. 2000. Apoptosis is induced by the active metabolite of vitamin D_3 and its analogue EB1089 in colorectal adenoma and carcinoma cells: possible implications for prevention and therapy. Cancer Research 60(8): 2304-12.

Diehl, J. W. and M. W. Chiu. 2010. Effects of ambient sunlight and photoprotection on vitamin D status. Dermatologic Therapy 23(1): 48-60.

Diesing, D., T. Cordes, D. Fischer, K. Diedrich and M. Friedrich. 2006. Vitamin D—metabolism in the human breast cancer cell line MCF-7. Anticancer Research 26(4A): 2755-9.

Drescher, D., H. F. Deluca and M. H. Imrie. 1969. On the site of discrimination of chicks against vitamin D. Archives of Biochemistry and Biophysics 130(1): 657-61.

Faulkner, H., A. Hussein, M. Foran and L. Szijarto. 2000. A survey of vitamin A and D contents of fortified fluid milk in Ontario. Journal of Dairy Science 83(6): 1210-6.

FDA (Food and Drug Administration). 2009. Agency Information Collection Activities; Submission for Office of Management and Budget Review; Comment Request; Food Labeling Regulations. Federal Register 74(201): 53743-6.

Fieser, L. F. and M. Fieser. 1959. Vitamin D. New York: Reinhold. Pp. 90-168.

Fleet, J. C., C. Gliniak, Z. Zhang, Y. Xue, K. B. Smith, R. McReedy and S. A. Adedokon. 2008. Serum metabolite profiles and target tissue gene expression define the effect of cholecalciferol intake on calcium metabolism in rats and mice. Journal of Nutrition 138(6): 1114-20.

Fraser, D., S. W. Kooh, H. P. Kind, M. F. Holick, Y. Tanaka and H. F. DeLuca. 1973. Pathogenesis of hereditary vitamin-D-dependent rickets. An inborn error of vitamin D metabolism involving defective conversion of 25-hydroxyvitamin D to 1 alpha,25-dihydroxyvitamin D. New England Journal of Medicine 289(16): 817-22.

Galitzer, H., I. Ben-Dov, V. Lavi-Moshayoff, T. Naveh-Many and J. Silver. 2008. Fibroblast growth factor 23 acts on the parathyroid to decrease parathyroid hormone secretion. Current Opinion in Nephrology and Hypertension 17(4): 363-7.

Garabedian, M., M. F. Holick, H. F. Deluca and I. T. Boyle. 1972. Control of 25-hydroxycholecalciferol metabolism by parathyroid glands. Proceedings of the National Academy of Sciences of the United States of America 69(7): 1673-6.

Gartner, L. M. and F. R. Greer. 2003. Prevention of rickets and vitamin D deficiency: new guidelines for vitamin D intake. Pediatrics 111(4 Pt 1): 908-10.

Gaschott, T. and J. Stein. 2003. Short-chain fatty acids and colon cancer cells: the vitamin D receptor—butyrate connection. Recent Results in Cancer Research 164: 247-57.

Gehrer, S., B. Kern, T. Peters, C. Christoffel-Courtin and R. Peterli. 2010. Fewer nutrient deficiencies after laparoscopic sleeve gastrectomy (LSG) than after laparoscopic Roux-Y-gastric bypass (LRYGB)—a prospective study. Obesity Surgery 20(4): 447-53.

Glendenning, P., M. Taranto, J. M. Noble, A. A. Musk, C. Hammond, P. R. Goldswain, W. D. Fraser and S. D. Vasikaran. 2006. Current assays overestimate 25-hydroxyvitamin D_3 and underestimate 25-hydroxyvitamin D_2 compared with HPLC: need for assay-specific decision limits and metabolite-specific assays. Annals of Clinical Biochemistry 43(Pt 1): 23-30.

Goldner, W. S., J. A. Stoner, E. Lyden, J. Thompson, K. Taylor, L. Larson, J. Erickson and C. McBride. 2009. Finding the optimal dose of vitamin D following Roux-en-Y gastric bypass: a prospective, randomized pilot clinical trial. Obesity Surgery 19(2): 173-9.

Gozdik, A., J. L. Barta, H. Wu, D. Cole, R. Vieth, S. Whiting and E. Parra. 2009. Seasonal changes in vitamin D status in healthy young adults of different ancestry in the greater Toronto area. Presented at the 14th Workshop on Vitamin D. October 4-8, 2009. Brugge, Belgium.

Guo, Y. D., S. Strugnell, D. W. Back and G. Jones. 1993. Substrate specificity of the liver mitochondrial cytochrome P-450, CYP-27, towards vitamin D and its analogs. Proceedings of the National Academy of Sciences of the United States of America 90: 8668-72.

Gupta, R. P., B. W. Hollis, S. B. Patel, K. S. Patrick and N. H. Bell. 2004. CYP3A4 is a human microsomal vitamin D 25-hydroxylase. Journal of Bone and Mineral Research 19(4): 680-8.

Gupta, R. P., Y. A. He, K. S. Patrick, J. R. Halpert and N. H. Bell. 2005. CYP3A4 is a vitamin D-24- and 25-hydroxylase: analysis of structure function by site-directed mutagenesis. Journal of Clinical Endocrinology and Metabolism 90(2): 1210-9.

Haddad, J. G., Jr. and T. J. Hahn. 1973. Natural and synthetic sources of circulating 25-hydroxyvitamin D in man. Nature 244(5417): 515-7.

Haddad, J. G., L. Y. Matsuoka, B. W. Hollis, Y. Z. Hu and J. Wortsman. 1993. Human plasma transport of vitamin D after its endogenous synthesis. Journal of Clinical Investigation 91(6): 2552-5.

Harris, S. S. and B. Dawson-Hughes. 2002. Plasma vitamin D and 25OHD responses of young and old men to supplementation with vitamin D_3. Journal of the American College of Nutrition 21(4): 357-62.

Hashizume, T., Y. Xu, M. A. Mohutsky, J. Alberts, C. Hadden, T. F. Kalhorn, N. Isoherranen, M. C. Shuhart and K. E. Thummel. 2008. Identification of human UDP-glucuronosyltransferases catalyzing hepatic 1alpha,25-dihydroxyvitamin D_3 conjugation. Biochemical Pharmacology 75(5): 1240-50.

Hay, A. W. and G. Watson. 1977. The binding of 25-hydroxycholecalciferol and 25-hydroxyergocalciferol to receptor proteins in a New World and an Old World primate. Comparative Biochemistry and Physiology. B: Comparative Biochemistry 56(2): 131-4.

Helvig C., D. Cuerrier, A. Kharebov, B. Ireland, J. Kim, K. Ryder and M. Petkovich. 2008. Comparison of 1,25-dihydroxyvitamin D2 and calcitriol effects in an adenine-induced model of CKD reveals differential control over serum calcium and phosphate. Journal of Bone and Mineral Research 23(S357).

Hewison, M., F. Burke, K. N. Evans, D. A. Lammas, D. M. Sansom, P. Liu, R. L. Modlin and J. S. Adams. 2007. Extra-renal 25-hydroxyvitamin D3-1alpha-hydroxylase in human health and disease. Journal of Steroid Biochemistry and Molecular Biology 103(3-5): 316-21.

Holick, M. F., J. A. MacLaughlin and S. H. Doppelt. 1981. Regulation of cutaneous previtamin D3 photosynthesis in man: skin pigment is not an essential regulator. Science 211(4482): 590-3.

Holick, M. F. 1988. Skin: site of the synthesis of vitamin D and a target tissue for the active form, 1,25-dihydroxyvitamin D_3. Annals of the New York Academy of Sciences 548: 14-26.

Holick, M. F., L. Y. Matsuoka and J. Wortsman. 1989. Age, vitamin D, and solar ultraviolet. Lancet 334(8671): 1104-5.

Holick, M. F., Q. Shao, W. W. Liu and T. C. Chen. 1992. The vitamin D content of fortified milk and infant formula. New England Journal of Medicine 326(18): 1178-81.

Holick, M. 1994. McCollum Award Lecture, 1994: vitamin D—new horizons for the 21st century. American Journal of Clinical Nutrition 60(4): 619-630.

Holick, M. F. 1995. Vitamin D: photobiology, metabolism, and clinical applications. In *Endocrinology, 3rd Edition*, edited by L. J. DeGroot, M. Besser, H. G. Burger et al. Philadelphia, PA: W. B. Saunders.

Holick, M. F. 1996. Vitamin D: photobiology, metabolism, mechanism of action, and clinical application. In *Primer on the Metabolic Bone Diseases and Disorders of Mineral Metabolism, 3rd Edition*, edited by M. J. Favus. Philadelphia, PA: Lippincott-Raven. Pp. 74-81.

Holick, M. F. 2008. Vitamin D and sunlight: strategies for cancer prevention and other health benefits. Clinical Journal of the American Society of Nephrology 3(5): 1548-54.

Holick, M. F., R. M. Biancuzzo, T. C. Chen, E. K. Klein, A. Young, D. Bibuld, R. Reitz, W. Salameh, A. Ameri and A. D. Tannenbaum. 2008. Vitamin D_2 is as effective as vitamin D_3 in maintaining circulating concentrations of 25-hydroxyvitamin D. Journal of Clinical Endocrinology and Metabolism 93(3): 677-81.

Hollis, B. W., B. A. Roos, H. H. Draper and P. W. Lambert. 1981. Vitamin D and its metabolites in human and bovine milk. Journal of Nutrition 111(7): 1240-8.

Hollis, B. W. and J. L. Napoli. 1985. Improved radioimmunoassay for vitamin D and its use in assessing vitamin D status. Clinical Chemistry 31(11): 1815-9.

Hollis, B. W. 2008. Measuring 25-hydroxyvitamin D in a clinical environment: challenges and needs. American Journal of Clinical Nutrition 88(2): 507S-10S.

Horst, R. L., R. M. Shepard, N. A. Jorgensen and H. F. DeLuca. 1979. The determination of the vitamin D metabolites on a single plasma sample: changes during parturition in dairy cows. Archives of Biochemistry and Biophysics 192(2): 512-23.

Horst, R. L., T. A. Reinhardt, C. F. Ramberg, N. J. Koszewski and J. L. Napoli. 1986. 24-hydroxylation of 1,25-dihydroxyergocalciferol. An unambiguous deactivation process. Journal of Biological Chemistry 261(20): 9250-6.

Hosseinpour, F., M. Ellfolk, M. Norlin and K. Wikvall. 2007. Phenobarbital suppresses vitamin D_3 25-hydroxylase expression: a potential new mechanism for drug-induced osteomalacia. Biochemical and Biophysical Research Communications 357(3): 603-7.

Hunt, R. D., F. G. Garcia and R. J. Walsh. 1972. A comparison of the toxicity of ergocalciferol and cholecalciferol in rhesus monkeys (Macaca mulatta). Journal of Nutrition 102(8): 975-86.

IOM (Institute of Medicine). 1997. *Dietary Reference Intakes for Calcium, Phosphorus, Magnesium, Vitamin D, and Fluoride.* Washington, DC: National Academy Press.

IOM. 2007. *Dietary Reference Intakes Research Synthesis: Workshop Summary.* Washington, DC: The National Academies Press.

Ish-Shalom, S., E. Segal, T. Salganik, B. Raz, I. L. Bromberg and R. Vieth. 2008. Comparison of daily, weekly, and monthly vitamin D_3 in ethanol dosing protocols for two months in elderly hip fracture patients. Journal of Clinical Endocrinology and Metabolism 93(9): 3430-5.

James, S. Y., A. G. Mackay and K. W. Colston. 1996. Effects of 1,25 dihydroxyvitamin D_3 and its analogues on induction of apoptosis in breast cancer cells. Journal of Steroid Biochemistry and Molecular Biology 58(4): 395-401.

James, W. P., A. Avenell, J. Broom and J. Whitehead. 1997. A one-year trial to assess the value of orlistat in the management of obesity. International Journal of Obesity and Related Metabolic Disorders 21(Suppl 3): S24-30.

Jiang, F., J. Bao, P. Li, S. V. Nicosia and W. Bai. 2004. Induction of ovarian cancer cell apoptosis by 1,25-dihydroxyvitamin D_3 through the down-regulation of telomerase. Journal of Biological Chemistry 279(51): 53213-21.

Johnson, J. L., V. V. Mistry, M. D. Vukovich, T. Hogie-Lorenzen, B. W. Hollis and B. L. Specker. 2005. Bioavailability of vitamin D from fortified process cheese and effects on vitamin D status in the elderly. Journal of Dairy Science 88(7): 2295-301.

Jones, G., H. K. Schnoes and H. F. DeLuca. 1975. Isolation and identification of 1,25-dihydroxyvitamin D_2. Biochemistry 14(6): 1250-6.

Jones, G. 1978. Assay of vitamins D_2 and D_3, and 25-hydroxyvitamins D_2 and D_3 in human plasma by high-performance liquid chromatography. Clinical Chemistry 24(2): 287-98.

Jones, G., A. Rosenthal, D. Segev, Y. Mazur, F. Frolow, Y. Halfon, D. Rabinovich and Z. Shakked. 1979. Isolation and identification of 24,25-dihydroxyvitamin D_2 using the perfused rat kidney. Biochemistry 18(6): 1094-11.

Jones, G., B. Byrnes, F. Palma, D. Segev and Y. Mazur. 1980a. Displacement potency of vitamin D_2 analogs in competitive protein-binding assays for 25-hydroxyvitamin D_3, 24,25-dihydroxyvitamin D_3, and 1,25-dihydroxyvitamin D_3. Journal of Clinical Endocrinology and Metabolism 50(4): 773-5.

Jones, G., H. K. Schnoes, L. Levan and H. F. Deluca. 1980b. Isolation and identification of 24-hydroxyvitamin D_2 and 24,25-dihydroxyvitamin D_2. Archives of Biochemistry and Biophysics 202(2): 450-7.

Jones, G., D. Vriezen, D. Lohnes, V. Palda and N. S. Edwards. 1987. Side-chain hydroxylation of vitamin D_3 and its physiological implications. Steroids 49(1-3): 29-53.

Jones, G., S. A. Strugnell and H. F. DeLuca. 1998. Current understanding of the molecular actions of vitamin D. Physiological Reviews 78(4): 1193-231.

Jones, G. and H. L. Makin. 2000. Vitamin Ds: metabolites and analogs. In *Modern Chromatographic Analysis of Vitamins, 3rd Edition*, edited by A. P. de Leenheer, W. E. Lambert and J. F. Van Bocxlaer. New York: Marcel Dekker.

Jones, G. 2008. Pharmacokinetics of vitamin D toxicity. American Journal of Clinical Nutrition 88(2): 582S-6S.

Jones, G., V. Byford, C. Helvig and M. Petkovich. 2009. Differential disposition of vitamin D_2 does not involve CYP24A1. Presented at 14th International Vitamin D Workshop, October 4-8, 2009. Brugge, Belgium.

Jongen, M. J., F. C. Van Ginkel, W. J. van der Vijgh, S. Kuiper, J. C. Netelenbos and P. Lips. 1984. An international comparison of vitamin D metabolite measurements. Clinical Chemistry 30(3): 399-403.

Jongen, M., W. J. van der Vijgh, J. C. Netelenbos, G. J. Postma and P. Lips. 1989. Pharmacokinetics of 24,25-dihydroxyvitamin D_3 in humans. Hormone and Metabolic Research 21(10): 577-80.

Jurutka, P. W., G. K. Whitfield, J. C. Hsieh, P. D. Thompson, C. A. Haussler and M. R. Haussler. 2001. Molecular nature of the vitamin D receptor and its role in regulation of gene expression. Reviews in Endocrinology and Metabloic Disorders 2(2): 203-16.

Kawa, S., K. Yoshizawa, M. Tokoo, H. Imai, H. Oguchi, K. Kiyosawa, T. Homma, T. Nikaido and K. Furihata. 1996. Inhibitory effect of 22β-oxa-1,25-dihydroxyvitamin D_3 on the proliferation of pancreatic cancer cell lines. Gastroenterology 110(5): 1605-13.

Kimlin, M. G., W. J. Olds and M. R. Moore. 2007. Location and vitamin D synthesis: is the hypothesis validated by geophysical data? Journal of Photochemistry and Photobiology. B, Biology 86(3): 234-9.

Knutson, J. C., L. W. LeVan, C. R. Valliere and C. W. Bishop. 1997. Pharmacokinetics and systemic effect on calcium homeostasis of 1 alpha,24-dihydroxyvitamin D_2 in rats. Comparison with 1 alpha,25-dihydroxyvitamin D_2, calcitriol, and calcipotriol. Biochemical Pharmacology 53(6): 829-37.

Koga, M., J. A. Eisman and R. L. Sutherland. 1988. Regulation of epidermal growth factor receptor levels by 1,25-dihydroxyvitamin D_3 in human breast cancer cells. Cancer Research 48(10): 2734-9.

Kovacs, C. S. and H. M. Kronenberg. 1997. Maternal-fetal calcium and bone metabolism during pregnancy, puerperium, and lactation. Endocrine Reviews 18(6): 832-72.

Kovalenko, P. L., Z. Zhang, M. Cui, S. K. Clinton and J. C. Fleet. 2010. 1,25 dihydroxyvitamin D-mediated orchestration of anticancer, transcript-level effects in the immortalized, nontransformed prostate epithelial cell line, RWPE1. BMC Genomics 11: 26.

Kull, M., Jr., R. Kallikorm, A. Tamm and M. Lember. 2009. Seasonal variance of 25-(OH) vitamin D in the general population of Estonia, a Northern European country. BMC Public Health 9: 22.

Kumagai, T., L. Y. Shih, S. V. Hughes, J. C. Desmond, J. O'Kelly, M. Hewison and H. P. Koeffler. 2005. 19-Nor-1,25(OH)2D2 (a novel, noncalcemic vitamin D analogue), combined with arsenic trioxide, has potent antitumor activity against myeloid leukemia. Cancer Research 65(6): 2488-97.

Kumar, R., D. Harnden and H. F. DeLuca. 1976. Metabolism of 1,25-dihydroxyvitamin D_3: evidence for side-chain oxidation. Biochemistry 15(11): 2420-3.

Laing, C. J. and N. E. Cooke. 2005. Chapter 8: Vitamin D binding protein. In *Vitamin D, 2nd Edition*, edited by D. Feldman, J. W. Pike and F. H. Glorieux. Burlington, MA: Elsevier Academic Press.

Leerbeck, E. and H. Sondergaard. 1980. The total content of vitamin D in human milk and cow's milk. British Journal of Nutrition 44(1): 7-12.

Lensmeyer, G. L., D. A. Wiebe, N. Binkley and M. K. Drezner. 2006. HPLC method for 25-hydroxyvitamin D measurement: comparison with contemporary assays. Clinical Chemistry 52(6): 1120-6.

LeVan, L. W., H. K. Schnoes and H. F. DeLuca. 1981. Isolation and identification of 25-hydroxyvitamin D_2 25-glucuronide: a biliary metabolite of vitamin D_2 in the chick. Biochemistry 20(1): 222-6.

Li, P., C. Li, X. Zhao, X. Zhang, S. V. Nicosia and W. Bai. 2004. p27(Kip1) stabilization and G(1) arrest by 1,25-dihydroxyvitamin D(3) in ovarian cancer cells mediated through down-regulation of cyclin E/cyclin-dependent kinase 2 and Skp1-Cullin-F-box protein/Skp2 ubiquitin ligase. Journal of Biological Chemistry 279(24): 25260-7.

Liel, Y., J. Edwards, J. Shary, K. M. Spicer, L. Gordon and N. H. Bell. 1988. The effects of race and body habitus on bone mineral density of the radius, hip, and spine in premenopausal women. Journal of Clinical Endocrinology and Metabolism 66(6): 1247-50.

Lips, P. 2006. Vitamin D physiology. Progress in Biophysics and Molecular Biology 92(1): 4-8.

Liu, P. T., S. Stenger, H. Li, L. Wenzel, B. H. Tan, S. R. Krutzik, M. T. Ochoa, J. Schauber, K. Wu, C. Meinken, D. L. Kamen, M. Wagner, R. Bals, A. Steinmeyer, U. Zugel, R. L. Gallo, D. Eisenberg, M. Hewison, B. W. Hollis, J. S. Adams, B. R. Bloom and R. L. Modlin. 2006. Toll-like receptor triggering of a vitamin D-mediated human antimicrobial response. Science 311(5768): 1770-3.

Liu, S., A. Gupta and L. D. Quarles. 2007. Emerging role of fibroblast growth factor 23 in a bone-kidney axis regulating systemic phosphate homeostasis and extracellular matrix mineralization. Current Opinion in Nephrology and Hypertension 16(4): 329-35.

Liu, N., L. Nguyen, R. F. Chun, V. Lagishetty, S. Ren, S. Wu, B. Hollis, H. F. DeLuca, J. S. Adams and M. Hewison. 2008. Altered endocrine and autocrine metabolism of vitamin D in a mouse model of gastrointestinal inflammation. Endocrinology 149(10): 4799-808.

Lohnes, D. and G. Jones. 1992. Further metabolism of 1α,25-dihydroxyvitamin D3 in target cells. Proceedings of the First International Congress on Vitamins and Biofactors in Life Science. Journal Nutritional Science and Vitaminology (Special Issue) 75-78.

Looker, A. C. 2005. Body fat and vitamin D status in black versus white women. Journal of Clinical Endocrinology and Metabolism 90(2): 635-40.

Looker, A. C. 2007. Do body fat and exercise modulate vitamin D status? Nutrition Reviews 65(8 Pt 2): S124-6.

Looker, A. C., C. M. Pfeiffer, D. A. Lacher, R. L. Schleicher, M. F. Picciano and E. A. Yetley. 2008. Serum 25-hydroxyvitamin D status of the US population: 1988-1994 compared with 2000-2004. American Journal of Clinical Nutrition 88(6): 1519-27.

Lubin, D., E. H. Jensen and H. P. Gies. 1998. Global surface ultraviolet radiation climatology from TOMS and ERBE data. Journal of Geophysical Research 103(D20): 26061-91.

Lucas, J. A., M. J. Bolland, A. B. Grey, R. W. Ames, B. H. Mason, A. M. Horne, G. D. Gamble and I. R. Reid. 2005. Determinants of vitamin D status in older women living in a subtropical climate. Osteoporosis International 16(12): 1641-8.

Ma, J. F., L. Nonn, M. J. Campbell, M. Hewison, D. Feldman and D. M. Peehl. 2004. Mechanisms of decreased vitamin D 1alpha-hydroxylase activity in prostate cancer cells. Molecular and Cellular Endocrinology 221(1-2): 67-74.

MacLaughlin, J. and M. F. Holick. 1985. Aging decreases the capacity of human skin to produce vitamin D_3. Journal of Clinical Investigation 76(4): 1536-8.

Mahdy, T., S. Atia, M. Farid and A. Adulatif. 2008. Effect of Roux-en Y gastric bypass on bone metabolism in patients with morbid obesity: Mansoura experiences. Obesity Surgery 18(12): 1526-31.

Makin, H. L. J., G. Jones, M. Kaufman and M. J. Calverley. 2010. Chapter 11: Analysis of vitamins D, their metabolites and analogs. In *Steroid Analysis*, edited by H. L. J. Makin and D. B. Gower. New York: Springer.

Mantell, D. J., P. E. Owens, N. J. Bundred, E. B. Mawer and A. E. Canfield. 2000. 1 Alpha,25-dihydroxyvitamin D(3) inhibits angiogenesis in vitro and in vivo. Circulation Research 87(3): 214-20.

Martinez, M. E., M. T. Del Campo, M. J. Sanchez-Cabezudo, G. Balaguer, A. Rodriguez-Carmona and R. Selgas. 1995. Effect of oral calcidiol treatment on its serum levels and peritoneal losses. Peritoneal Dialysis International 15(1): 65-70.

Masuda, S., V. Byford, A. Arabian, Y. Sakai, M. B. Demay, R. St-Arnaud and G. Jones. 2005. Altered pharmacokinetics of 1alpha,25-dihydroxyvitamin D_3 and 25-hydroxyvitamin D_3 in the blood and tissues of the 25-hydroxyvitamin D-24-hydroxylase (Cyp24a1) null mouse. Endocrinology 146(2): 825-34.

Masuda, S. and G. Jones. 2006. Promise of vitamin D analogues in the treatment of hyperproliferative conditions. Molecular Cancer Therapeutics 5(4): 797-808.

Matsuoka, L. Y., J. Wortsman, J. G. Haddad and B. W. Hollis. 1989. In vivo threshold for cutaneous synthesis of vitamin D_3. Journal of Laboratory and Clinical Medicine 114(3): 301-5.

McDuffie, J. R., K. A. Calis, S. L. Booth, G. I. Uwaifo and J. A. Yanovski. 2002. Effects of orlistat on fat-soluble vitamins in obese adolescents. Pharmacotherapy 22(7): 814-22.

Misra, M., D. Pacaud, A. Petryk, P. F. Collett-Solberg and M. Kappy. 2008. Vitamin D deficiency in children and its management: review of current knowledge and recommendations. Pediatrics 122(2): 398-417.

Moreno, J., A. V. Krishnan, S. Swami, L. Nonn, D. M. Peehl and D. Feldman. 2005. Regulation of prostaglandin metabolism by calcitriol attenuates growth stimulation in prostate cancer cells. Cancer Research 65(17): 7917-25.

Morris, J. F. and M. Peacock. 1976. Assay of plasma 25-hydroxy vitamin D. Clinica Chimica Acta 72(3): 383-91.

Mulligan, G. B. and A. Licata. 2010. Taking vitamin D with the largest meal improves absorption and results in higher serum levels of 25-hydroxyvitamin D. Journal of Bone and Mineral Research 25(4): 928-30.

Murphy, S. C., L. J. Whited, L. C. Rosenberry, B. H. Hammond, D. K. Bandler and K. J. Boor. 2001. Fluid milk vitamin fortification compliance in New York State. Journal of Dairy Science 84(12): 2813-20.

Olds, W. J., A. R. McKinley, M. R. Moore and M. G. Kimlin. 2008. In vitro model of vitamin D3 (cholecalciferol) synthesis by UV radiation: dose–response relationships. Journal of Photochemistry and Photobiology. B, Biology 93(2): 88-93.

Park, E. A. 1940. The therapy of rickets. JAMA 94: 370-9.

Penna, G., S. Amuchastegui, N. Giarratana, K. C. Daniel, M. Vulcano, S. Sozzani and L. Adorini. 2007. 1,25-Dihydroxyvitamin D_3 selectively modulates tolerogenic properties in myeloid but not plasmacytoid dendritic cells. Journal of Immunology 178(1): 145-53.

Phinney, K. W. 2009. Methods development and standard reference materials for 25(OH) D. Presented at the Committee to Review Dietary Reference Intakes for Vitamin D and Calcium Information-gathering Workshop, August 4, 2009. Washington, DC.

Picciano, M. F., J. T. Dwyer, K. L. Radimer, D. H. Wilson, K. D. Fisher, P. R. Thomas, E. A. Yetley, A. J. Moshfegh, P. S. Levy, S. J. Nielsen and B. M. Marriott. 2007. Dietary supplement use among infants, children, and adolescents in the United States, 1999-2002. Archives of Pediatrics and Adolescent Medicine 161(10): 978-85.

Pike, J. W., N. K. Shevde, B. W. Hollis, N. E. Cooke and L. A. Zella. 2008. Vitamin D—binding protein influences total circulating levels of 1,25-dihydroxyvitamin D-3 but does not directly modulate the bioactive levels of the hormone in vivo. Endocrinology 149(7): 3656-67.

Quarles, L. D. 2008. Endocrine functions of bone in mineral metabolism regulation. Journal of Clinical Investigation 118(12): 3820-8.

Radimer, K., B. Bindewald, J. Hughes, B. Ervin, C. Swanson and M. F. Picciano. 2004. Dietary supplement use by US adults: data from the National Health and Nutrition Examination Survey, 1999-2000. American Journal of Epidemiology 160(4): 339-49.

Rapuri, P. B., H. K. Kinyamu, J. C. Gallagher and V. Haynatzka. 2002. Seasonal changes in calciotropic hormones, bone markers, and bone mineral density in elderly women. Journal of Clinical Endocrinology and Metabolism 87(5): 2024-32.

Rapuri, P. B., J. C. Gallagher and G. Haynatzki. 2004. Effect of vitamins D_2 and D_3 supplement use on serum 25OHD concentration in elderly women in summer and winter. Calcified Tissue International 74(2): 150-6.

Reeve, L. E., R. W. Chesney and H. F. DeLuca. 1982. Vitamin D of human milk: identification of biologically active forms. American Journal of Clinical Nutrition 36(1): 122-6.

Reichel, H., H. P. Koeffler and A. W. Norman. 1989. The role of the vitamin D endocrine system in health and disease. New England Journal of Medicine 320(15): 980-91.

Reinehr, T., G. de Sousa, U. Alexy, M. Kersting and W. Andler. 2007. Vitamin D status and parathyroid hormone in obese children before and after weight loss. European Journal of Endocrinology/European Federation of Endocrine Societies 157(2): 225-32.

Reinhardt, T. A., C. F. Ramberg and R. L. Horst. 1989. Comparison of receptor binding, biological activity, and in vivo tracer kinetics for 1,25-dihydroxyvitamin D_3, 1,25-dihydroxyvitamin D_2, and its 24 epimer. Archives of Biochemistry and Biophysics 273(1): 64-71.

Riedt, C. S., M. Cifuentes, T. Stahl, H. A. Chowdhury, Y. Schlussel and S. A. Shapses. 2005. Overweight postmenopausal women lose bone with moderate weight reduction and 1 g/ day calcium intake. Journal of Bone and Mineral Research 20(3): 455-63.

Riedt, C. S., R. E. Brolin, R. M. Sherrell, M. P. Field and S. A. Shapses. 2006. True fractional calcium absorption is decreased after Roux-en-Y gastric bypass surgery. Obesity (Silver Spring) 14(11): 1940-8.

Roborgh, J. R. and T. de Man. 1959. The hypercalcemic activity of dihydrotachysterol-2 and dihydrotachysterol-3 and of the vitamins D_2 and D_3: comparative experiments on rats. Biochemical Pharmacology 2: 1-6.

Roborgh, J. R. and T. de Man. 1960. The hypercalcemic activity of dihydrotachysterol-2 and dihydrotachysterol-3 and of the vitamins D_2 and D_3 after intravenous injection of the aqueous preparations. 2. Comparative experiments on rats. Biochemical Pharmacology 3: 277-82.

Rosenstreich, S. J., C. Rich and W. Volwiler. 1971. Deposition in and release of vitamin D_3 from body fat: evidence for a storage site in the rat. Journal of Clinical Investigation 50(3): 679-87.

Roth, H. J., H. Schmidt-Gayk, H. Weber and C. Niederau. 2008. Accuracy and clinical implications of seven 25-hydroxyvitamin D methods compared with liquid chromatography-tandem mass spectrometry as a reference. Annals of Clinical Biochemistry 45(Pt 2): 153-9.

Sawada, N., T. Sakaki, M. Ohta and K. Inouye. 2000. Metabolism of vitamin D(3) by human CYP27A1. Biochemical and Biophysical Research Communications 273(3): 977-84.

Silver, J., T. Naveh-Many, H. Mayer, H. J. Schmelzer and M. M. Popovtzer. 1986. Regulation by vitamin D metabolites of parathyroid hormone gene transcription in vivo in the rat. Journal of Clinical Investigation 78(5): 1296-301.

Singh, R. J., R. L. Taylor, G. S. Reddy and S. K. Grebe. 2006. C-3 epimers can account for a significant proportion of total circulating 25-hydroxyvitamin D in infants, complicating accurate measurement and interpretation of vitamin D status. Journal of Clinical Endocrinology and Metabolism 91(8): 3055-61.

Siu-Caldera, M. L., H. Sekimoto, S. Peleg, C. Nguyen, A. M. Kissmeyer, L. Binderup, A. Weiskopf, P. Vouros, M. R. Uskokovic and G. S. Reddy. 1999. Enhanced biological activity of 1alpha,25-dihydroxy-20-epi-vitamin D_3, the C-20 epimer of 1alpha,25-dihydroxyvitamin D_3, is in part due to its metabolism into stable intermediary metabolites with significant biological activity. Journal of Steroid Biochemistry and Molecular Biology 71(3-4): 111-21.

Sjoden, G., C. Smith, U. Lindgren and H. F. DeLuca. 1985. 1 alpha-hydroxyvitamin D_2 is less toxic than 1 alpha-hydroxyvitamin D_3 in the rat. Proceedings of the Society for Experimental Biology and Medicine 178(3): 432-6.

Slatopolsky, E., C. Weerts, J. Thielan, R. Horst, H. Harter and K. J. Martin. 1984. Marked suppression of secondary hyperparathyroidism by intravenous administration of 1,25-dihydroxycholecalciferol in uremic patients. Journal of Clinical Investigation 74(6): 2136-43.

Smith, S. M., K. K. Gardner, J. Locke and S. R. Zwart. 2009. Vitamin D supplementation during Antarctic winter. American Journal of Clinical Nutrition 89(4): 1092-8.

Snellman, G., H. Melhus, R. Gedeborg, S. Olofsson, A. Wolk, N. L. Pedersen and K. Michaelsson. 2009. Seasonal genetic influence on serum 25-hydroxyvitamin D levels: a twin study. PLoS ONE [Electronic Resource] 4(11): e7747.

Sneve, M., Y. Figenschau and R. Jorde. 2008. Supplementation with cholecalciferol does not result in weight reduction in overweight and obese subjects. European Journal of Endocrinology/European Federation of Endocrine Societies 159(6): 675-84.

Specker, B. L., B. Valanis, V. Hertzberg, N. Edwards and R. C. Tsang. 1985. Sunshine exposure and serum 25-hydroxyvitamin D concentrations in exclusively breast-fed infants. Journal of Pediatrics 107(3): 372-6.

Springbett, P., S. Buglass and A. R. Young. 2010. Photoprotection and vitamin D status. Journal of Photochemistry and Photobiology B: Biology 101(2):160-8.

Stamp, T. C., J. G. Haddad, Jr., A. N. Exton-Smith, A. Reuben and C. A. Twigg. 1976. Assay of vitamin D and its metabolites. Annals of Clinical Biochemistry 13(6): 571-7.

Stamp, T. C., J. G. Haddad and C. A. Twigg. 1977. Comparison of oral 25-hydroxycholecalciferol, vitamin D, and ultraviolet light as determinants of circulating 25-hydroxyvitamin D. Lancet 1(8026): 1341-3.

Steenbock, H. and A. Black. 1924. Fat-soluble vitamins. Journal of Biological Chemistry 61(2): 405-22.

Strushkevich, N., S. A. Usanov, A. N. Plotnikov, G. Jones and H. W. Park. 2008. Structural analysis of CYP2R1 in complex with vitamin D_3. Journal of Molecular Biology 380(1): 95-106.

Stubbs, J. R., A. Idiculla, J. Slusser, R. Menard and L. D. Quarles. 2010. Cholecalciferol supplementation alters calcitriol-responsive monocyte proteins and decreases inflammatory cytokines in ESRD. Journal of the American Society of Nephrology 21(2): 353-61.

Suda, T., H. F. DeLuca, H. K. Schnoes and J. W. Blunt. 1969. The isolation and identification of 25-hydroxyergocalciferol. Biochemistry 8(9): 3515-20.

Suda, T., N. Takahashi and E. Abe. 1992. Role of vitamin D in bone resorption. Journal of Cellular Biochemistry 49(1): 53-8.

Sundaram, S., M. Chaudhry, D. Reardon, M. Gupta and D. A. Gewirtz. 2000. The vitamin D_3 analog EB 1089 enhances the antiproliferative and apoptotic effects of adriamycin in MCF-7 breast tumor cells. Breast Cancer Research and Treatment 63(1): 1-10.

Sutton, R. A., N. L. Wong and J. H. Dirks. 1976. Effects of parathyroid hormone on sodium and calcium transport in the dog nephron. Clinical Science and Molecular Medicine 51(4): 345-51.

Talwar, S. A., J. F. Aloia, S. Pollack and J. K. Yeh. 2007. Dose response to vitamin D supplementation among postmenopausal African American women. American Journal of Clinical Nutrition 86(6): 1657-62.

Tanaka, Y. and H. F. DeLuca. 1983. Stimulation of 1,25-dihydroxyvitamin D_3 production by 1,25-dihydroxyvitamin D_3 in the hypocalcaemic rat. Biochemical Journal 214(3): 893-7.

Tanner, J. T., J. Smith, P. Defibaugh, G. Angyal, M. Villalobos, M. P. Bueno, E. T. McGarrahan, H. M. Wehr, J. F. Muniz, B. W. Hollis et al. 1988. Survey of vitamin content of fortified milk. Journal—Association of Official Analytical Chemists 71(3): 607-10.

Thompson, G. R., B. Lewis and C. C. Booth. 1966. Absorption of vitamin D3-3H in control subjects and patients with intestinal malabsorption. Journal of Clinical Investigation 45(1): 94-102.

Thompson, P. D., P. W. Jurutka, G. K. Whitfield, S. M. Myskowski, K. R. Eichhorst, C. E. Dominguez, C. A. Haussler and M. R. Haussler. 2002. Liganded VDR induces CYP3A4 in small intestinal and colon cancer cells via DR3 and ER6 vitamin D responsive elements. Biochemical and Biophysical Research Communications 299(5): 730-8.

Tjellesen, L., A. Gotfredsen and C. Christiansen. 1985. Different actions of vitamin D_2 and D_3 on bone metabolism in patients treated with phenobarbitone/phenytoin. Calcified Tissue International 37(3): 218-22.

Trang, H. M., D. E. Cole, L. A. Rubin, A. Pierratos, S. Siu and R. Vieth. 1998. Evidence that vitamin D3 increases serum 25-hydroxyvitamin D more efficiently than does vitamin D_2. American Journal of Clinical Nutrition 68(4): 854-8.

Trump, D. L., K. K. Deeb and C. S. Johnson. 2010. Vitamin D: considerations in the continued development as an agent for cancer prevention and therapy. Cancer Journal 16(1): 1-9.

Turner, M., P. E. Barre, A. Benjamin, D. Goltzman and M. Gascon-Barre. 1988. Does the maternal kidney contribute to the increased circulating 1,25-dihydroxyvitamin D concentrations during pregnancy? Mineral and Electrolyte Metabolism 14(4): 246-52.

Tzotzas, T., F. G. Papadopoulou, K. Tziomalos, S. Karras, K. Gastaris, P. Perros and G. E. Krassas. 2010. Rising serum 25-hydroxy-vitamin D levels after weight loss in obese women correlate with improvement in insulin resistance. Journal of Clinical Endocrinology and Metabolism 95(9): 4251-7.

Urushino, N., K. Yasuda, S. Ikushiro, M. Kamakura, M. Ohta and T. Sakaki. 2009. Metabolism of 1alpha,25-dihydroxyvitamin D_2 by human CYP24A1. Biochemical and Biophysical Research Communications 384(2): 144-8.

Valderas, J. P., S. Velasco, S. Solari, Y. Liberona, P. Viviani, A. Maiz, A. Escalona and G. Gonzalez. 2009. Increase of bone resorption and the parathyroid hormone in postmenopausal women in the long-term after Roux-en-Y gastric bypass. Obesity Surgery 19(8): 1132-8.

van der Mei, I. A., A. L. Ponsonby, O. Engelsen, J. A. Pasco, J. J. McGrath, D. W. Eyles, L. Blizzard, T. Dwyer, R. Lucas and G. Jones. 2007. The high prevalence of vitamin D insufficiency across Australian populations is only partly explained by season and latitude. Environmental Health Perspectives 115(8): 1132-9.

van Dijk, C. E., M. R. de Boer, L. L. Koppes, J. C. Roos, P. Lips and J. W. Twisk. 2009. Positive association between the course of vitamin D intake and bone mineral density at 36 years in men. Bone 44(3): 437-41.

Vieth, R. 1990. The mechanisms of vitamin D toxicity. Bone and Mineral 11(3): 267-72.

Vieth, R. 2004. Why the optimal requirement for vitamin D_3 is probably much higher than what is officially recommended for adults. Journal of Steroid Biochemistry and Molecular Biology 89-90(1-5): 575-9.

Wang, L., J. N. Flanagan, L. W. Whitlatch, D. P. Jamieson, M. F. Holick and T. C. Chen. 2004. Regulation of 25-hydroxyvitamin D-1alpha-hydroxylase by epidermal growth factor in prostate cells. Journal of Steroid Biochemistry and Molecular Biology 89-90(1-5): 127-30.

Wang, T. J., F. Zhang, J. B. Richards, B. Kestenbaum, J. B. van Meurs, D. Berry, D. P. Kiel, E. A. Streeten, C. Ohlsson, D. L. Koller, L. Peltonen, J. D. Cooper, P. F. O'Reilly, D. K. Houston, N. L. Glazer, L. Vandenput, M. Peacock, J. Shi, F. Rivadeneira, M. I. McCarthy, P. Anneli, I. H. de Boer, M. Mangino, B. Kato, D. J. Smyth, S. L. Booth, P. F. Jacques, G. L. Burke, M. Goodarzi, C. L. Cheung, M. Wolf, K. Rice, D. Goltzman, N. Hidiroglou, M. Ladouceur, N. J. Wareham, L. J. Hocking, D. Hart, N. K. Arden, C. Cooper, S. Malik, W. D. Fraser, A. L. Hartikainen, G. Zhai, H. M. Macdonald, N. G. Forouhi, R. J. Loos, D. M. Reid, A. Hakim, E. Dennison, Y. Liu, C. Power, H. E. Stevens, L. Jaana, R. S. Vasan, N. Soranzo, J. Bojunga, B. M. Psaty, M. Lorentzon, T. Foroud, T. B. Harris, A. Hofman, J. O. Jansson, J. A. Cauley, A. G. Uiterlinden, Q. Gibson, M. R. Jarvelin, D. Karasik, D. S. Siscovick, M. J. Econs, S. B. Kritchevsky, J. C. Florez, J. A. Todd, J. Dupuis, E. Hypponen and T. D. Spector. 2010. Common genetic determinants of vitamin D insufficiency: a genome-wide association study. Lancet 376(9736): 180-8.

Ward, L. M., I. Gaboury, M. Ladhani and S. Zlotkin. 2007. Vitamin D-deficiency rickets among children in Canada. Canadian Medical Association Journal 177(2): 161-6.

Wastney, M. E., J. Ng, D. Smith, B. R. Martin, M. Peacock and C. M. Weaver. 1996. Differences in calcium kinetics between adolescent girls and young women. American Journal of Physiology 271(1 Pt 2): R208-16.

Webb, A. R., L. Kline and M. F. Holick. 1988. Influence of season and latitude on the cutaneous synthesis of vitamin D_3: exposure to winter sunlight in Boston and Edmonton will not promote vitamin D_3 synthesis in human skin. Journal of Clinical Endocrinology and Metabolism 67(2): 373-8.

Webb, A. R., B. R. DeCosta and M. F. Holick. 1989. Sunlight regulates the cutaneous production of vitamin D_3 by causing its photodegradation. Journal of Clinical Endocrinology and Metabolism 68(5): 882-7.

Weber, F. 1981. Absorption mechanisms for fat-soluble vitamins and the effect of other food constituents. Progress in Clinical and Biological Research 77: 119-35.

Weber, F. 1983. Absorption of fat-soluble vitamins. International Journal for Vitamin and Nutrition Research (Suppl 25): 55-65.

Weber, K., M. Goldberg, M. Stangassinger and R. G. Erben. 2001. 1Alpha-hydroxyvitamin D_2 is less toxic but not bone selective relative to 1alpha-hydroxyvitamin D_3 in ovariectomized rats. Journal of Bone and Mineral Research 16(4): 639-51.

Willnow, T. and A. Nykjaer. 2005. Chapter 10: Endocytic pathways for 25-(OH) vitamin D_3. In *Vitamin D, 2nd Edition*, edited by D. Feldman, J. W. Pike and F. Glorieux. Burlington, MA: Elsevier.

Wortsman, J., L. Y. Matsuoka, T. C. Chen, Z. Lu and M. F. Holick. 2000. Decreased bioavailability of vitamin D in obesity. American Journal of Clinical Nutrition 72(3): 690-3.

Xie, S. P., S. Y. James and K. W. Colston. 1997. Vitamin D derivatives inhibit the mitogenic effects of IGF-I on MCF-7 human breast cancer cells. Journal of Endocrinology 154(3): 495-504.

Xu, Y., T. Hashizume, M. C. Shuhart, C. L. Davis, W. L. Nelson, T. Sakaki, T. F. Kalhorn, P. B. Watkins, E. G. Schuetz and K. E. Thummel. 2006. Intestinal and hepatic CYP3A4 catalyze hydroxylation of 1alpha,25-dihydroxyvitamin D(3): implications for drug-induced osteomalacia. Molecular Pharmacology 69(1): 56-65.

Yamamoto, M., Y. Kawanobe, H. Takahashi, E. Shimazawa, S. Kimura and E. Ogata. 1984. Vitamin D deficiency and renal calcium transport in the rat. Journal of Clinical Investigation 74(2): 507-13.

Yanagisawa, J., Y. Yanagi, Y. Masuhiro, M. Suzawa, M. Watanabe, K. Kashiwagi, T. Toriyabe, M. Kawabata, K. Miyazono and S. Kato. 1999. Convergence of transforming growth factor-beta and vitamin D signaling pathways on SMAD transcriptional coactivators. Science 283(5406): 1317-21.

Yasuda, H., K. Higashio and T. Suda. 2005. Vitamin D and osteoclastogenesis. In *Vitamin D, Volume 1*, edited by D. Feldman, J. W. Pike and F. H. Glorieux. San Diego, CA: Elsevier Academic Press. Pp. 665-85.

Yetley, E. A. 2008. Assessing the vitamin D status of the US population. American Journal of Clinical Nutrition 88(2): 558S-64S.

Yetley, E. A., D. Brule, M. C. Cheney, C. D. Davis, K. A. Esslinger, P. W. Fischer, K. E. Friedl, L. S. Greene-Finestone, P. M. Guenther, D. M. Klurfeld, M. R. L'Abbe, K. Y. McMurry, P. E. Starke-Reed and P. R. Trumbo. 2009. Dietary reference intakes for vitamin D: justification for a review of the 1997 values. American Journal of Clinical Nutrition 89(3): 719-27.

Zinser, G. M. and J. Welsh. 2004. Accelerated mammary gland development during pregnancy and delayed postlactational involution in vitamin D_3 receptor null mice. Molecular Endocrinology 18(9): 2208-23.

Zittermann, A., S. Frisch, H. K. Berthold, C. Gotting, J. Kuhn, K. Kleesiek, P. Stehle, H. Koertke and R. Koerfer. 2009. Vitamin D supplementation enhances the beneficial effects of weight loss on cardiovascular disease risk markers. American Journal of Clinical Nutrition 89(5): 1321-7.

4

Review of Potential Indicators of Adequacy and Selection of Indicators: Calcium and Vitamin D

APPROACH

The first step in the decision-making process associated with the development of Dietary Reference Intakes (DRIs) is the identification of potentially useful measures—indicators—that reflect a health outcome associated with the intake of the nutrient. As described in Chapter 1, this is classically referred to as hazard identification, the first step of risk assessment. The available data are examined to determine their relevance and validity as well as strengths and limitations for elucidating a relationship between the health outcome of interest (including chronic disease risk) and the intake of the nutrient.

In considering reference values for calcium and vitamin D, there are challenges in organizing a data review to examine these nutrients independently, because they act in concert and are often administered together in experimental studies. To the extent possible, the independent effects of these nutrients were explored and taken into account; when this was not possible or not appropriate, the combined effect was considered. This chapter reviews evidence for calcium and vitamin D jointly to avoid redundancy. Evidence related to potential indicators for adverse effects of excess intake of calcium and vitamin D is reviewed separately in Chapter 6.

Identification of Potential Indicators for Calcium and Vitamin D

The array of potential health outcomes to be considered for these two nutrients was identified using five sources:

1. Agency for Healthcare Research and Quality (AHRQ) evidence report issued in 2007 (Cranney et al., 2007), hereafter referred to in this chapter as AHRQ-Ottawa without a reference citation; and

2. AHRQ evidence report issued in 2009 (Chung et al., 2009), hereafter referred to in this chapter as AHRQ-Tufts without a reference citation;

3. The Institute of Medicine (IOM) report *Dietary Reference Intakes for Calcium, Phosphorus, Magnesium, Vitamin D, and Fluoride* (IOM, 1997);

4. Literature searches conducted by the committee;

5. Publicly available input from stakeholders either through written submissions to the committee or as presented during the information gathering workshop.

As outlined in Chapter 1, the ARHQ analyses are highly relevant to DRI development. Evidence-based systematic reviews have been identified as a useful tool for the purposes of dietary reference value development (Russell et al., 2009), and the work of this committee was enhanced by the availability of these two high-quality evidence reports from AHRQ. The approach used, questions asked, data search criteria, and the detailed results from the AHRQ-Ottawa and AHRQ-Tufts can be found in Appendixes C and D.

In sum, the focus of AHRQ-Ottawa was on the:

- Association of specific circulating 25-hydroxyvitamin D (25OHD) concentrations with bone health outcomes in children, women of reproductive age, postmenopausal women, and elderly men;
- Effect of vitamin D dietary intake (fortified foods and/or supplements) and sun exposure on serum 25OHD levels;
- Effect of vitamin D on bone mineral density (BMD) and fracture or fall risk; and
- Identification of potential harms associated with vitamin D exposures above current reference intakes.

The AHRQ-Tufts evidence report analyzed data related to calcium and vitamin D with respect to a broader spectrum of health outcomes. AHRQ-Tufts also served to update and expand AHRQ-Ottawa. Specifically, AHRQ-Tufts focused on the:

- Relationship between vitamin D and growth, cardiovascular disease (CVD), body weight, cancer, immunological outcomes, bone health, all-cause mortality, hypertension/blood pressure, and BMD and bone mineral content (BMC); and

- Relationship between calcium and growth, CVD, body weight, and cancer.

Neither AHRQ report reviewed calcium alone as a factor in bone health.

A key component of systematic reviews of scientific literature is a specification of the quality of the available data. The AHRQ grading system is summarized in Box 4-1. In the case of the systematic analysis carried out by AHRQ-Ottawa, the Jadad scale (Jadad et al., 1996) was used for quality assessments of randomized controlled trials (RCTs). The Jadad scale is a validated scale designed to assess the methods used to generate random assignments and double blinding. The scale also scores whether there is a description of dropouts and withdrawals by intervention group. Jadad scores range from 1 to 5, and a total score of 3 and above indicates studies of higher quality. Further, to assess the quality of the observational studies, a grading system adapted from R. P. Harris et al. (2001) was used. In the case of the AHRQ-Tufts analysis, a three-category grading system ("A," "B," or "C") was adapted from the AHRQ Methods Reference Guide for Effectiveness and Comparative Effectiveness Reviews (AHRQ, 2007). This system defines a generic grading system that is applicable to each type of study design including interventional and observational studies; it is summarized in Box 4-1.

The committee's literature search identified relevant evidence outside the scope of, or not included in, the two AHRQ reports as well as newer data available after the cutoff date of the AHRQ-Tufts analysis in 2009. The nature of the literature search is outlined in Appendix E. The literature base that was included in the 1997 report of the IOM committee tasked with DRI development for calcium and vitamin D (IOM, 1997) was also considered. Additionally, information gathered as part of a public workshop and several open committee sessions (see Appendix J) and a white paper requested by the committee (Towler, 2009) were taken into account.

Through use of the five data sources listed above, health outcomes of potential interest were identified. They are listed alphabetically in Table 4-1 and are grouped by general outcome. In addition, there is the possibility of intermediate variables that are not validated biomarkers of effect for health outcomes, but which may have the potential to be useful in the development of DRIs. Two such variables were considered: serum 25OHD concentrations and levels of parathyroid hormone (PTH).

Review of Data

General Principles

Within the scientific and clinical literature, there is a general hierarchy of study design. The lowest form of evidence is the idea or opinion,

BOX 4-1
AHRQ Critical Appraisal and Grading of Evidence

Grading system used by AHRQ-Ottawa:

Basic Jadad score is assessed based on the answer to five questions listed below. Questions that are answered with a "yes" gain 1 point; questions answered with a "no" receive 0 points; the maximum score is 5. A score of 0 to 2 points is considered "low" quality, and a score of 3 to 5 points is considered "high" quality.

1. Was the study described as random?
2. Was the randomization scheme described and appropriate?
3. Was the study described as double-blind?
4. Was the method of double-blinding appropriate? (Were both the patient and the assessor appropriately blinded?)
5. Was there a description of dropouts and withdrawals?

Grading system used by AHRQ-Tufts (based on criteria below):

A = highest quality
   Studies have the least bias and results are considered valid. These studies adhere mostly to the commonly held concepts of high quality, including the following: a formal study design; clear description of the population, setting, interventions, and comparison groups; appropriate measurement of outcomes; appropriate statistical and analytical methods and reporting; no reporting errors; less than 20 percent dropout; clear reporting of dropouts; and no obvious bias. Studies must provide valid estimation of nutrient exposure from dietary assessments and/or biomarkers with reasonable ranges of measurement errors and justifications for approaches to control for confounding in their design and analyses.

B = medium quality
   Studies are susceptible to some bias, but not sufficient to invalidate the results. They do not meet all the criteria in category "A"; they have some deficiencies, but none likely to cause major bias. The study may be missing information, making it difficult to assess limitations and potential problems.

C = low quality
   Studies have significant bias that may invalidate the results. These studies have serious errors in design, analysis, or reporting; there are large amounts of missing information or discrepancies in reporting.

SOURCES: Jadad et al., 1996; Cranney et al., 2007; Chung et al., 2009.

TABLE 4-1 Alphabetical Listing of Potential Indicators of Health Outcomes for Nutrient Adequacy

Indicator	AHRQ (Ottawa and Tufts)
Cancer/neoplasms	
• All cancers	✓
• Breast cancer	✓
• Colorectal cancer/colon polyps	✓
• Prostate cancer	✓
Cardiovascular diseases and hypertension	✓
Diabetes (type 2) and metabolic syndrome (obesity)	✓
Falls	✓
Immune response	✓
• Asthma	—[a]
• Autoimmune disease	✓
○ Diabetes (type 1)	✓
○ Inflammatory bowel and Crohn's disease	✓
○ Multiple sclerosis	✓
○ Rheumatoid arthritis	✓
○ Systemic lupus erythematosus	—[a]
• Infectious diseases	✓
○ Tuberculosis	—[a]
○ Influenza/upper respiratory infections	—[a]
Neuropsychological functioning	—[b]
• Autism	—[b]
• Cognitive function	—[b]
• Depression	—[b]
Physical performance[c]	✓
Preeclampsia, pregnancy-induced hypertension, and other non-skeletal reproductive outcomes	✓
Skeletal health (commonly bone health)	
• Serum 25OHD, as intermediate	✓
• Parathyroid hormone, as intermediate	✓
• Calcium absorption	✓
• Calcium balance	✓
• Bone mineral content/bone mineral density	✓
• Fracture risk	✓
• Rickets/osteomalacia	✓

[a]Specific condition not reviewed as a health outcome in AHRQ.
[b]Outcome category not considered in AHRQ.
[c]In the discussions within this chapter, physical performance is considered together with falls to avoid redundancy.

followed, in ascending order, by case reports, case series, case–control studies, cohort studies, and, finally, the highest form of evidence, the randomized, controlled, double-blind trial (Croswell and Kramer, 2009). Only the RCT can show a causal relationship between an intervention and an outcome. Observational evidence can show only associative links, not causality. The highest level of observational evidence is the cohort study—a large, population-based, prospective investigation to compare an exposed group with an unexposed group. However, the cohort study does not reach the level of evidence of an RCT, because the intervention is not a random or chance event; rather it is the choice of the investigator (Croswell and Kramer, 2009). Nested case–control studies are a type of cohort study and were considered at that level of evidence; in some literature, populations from RCTs were evaluated as a cohort (adjusting for treatment assignment or limiting the analysis to the control group) and thus are at the same level of evidence as other observational research.

A summary of the strengths and weaknesses of the various types of observational studies and RCT studies is shown in Table 4-2. Flaws, biases, and confounding effects are an inevitable aspect of any study design, and the strength of a study therefore depends on the ability of the investigator to control such methodological obstacles. In addition, even well-designed studies can be weakened by complications such as loss to follow-up, missing outcomes, subject non-compliance, and a biased selection process (Baker and Kramer, 2008).

The Process

In addition to its consideration of the AHRQ analyses, the committee conducted searches of several online bibliographical databases, including Medline, Science Direct, and WorldCat/First Search. Evidence searches were carried out to identify relevant RCTs in support of a causal relationship between vitamin D and/or calcium and the health outcome under consideration, and these were weighted as the strongest type of evidence for development of a DRI. The second tier of evidence considered was observational to support associative relationships between vitamin D and/or calcium and a health outcome. Further examination was carried out to determine the quality of the observational evidence and whether the results were in agreement with RCT outcomes for a specific indicator. Potential confounders were also taken into account. Figure 4-1 shows the committee's ranking of evidence by the strength of the study design. In the figure, RCTs prevail over observational and ecological studies as the strongest evidential support and were therefore necessary for a health outcome indicator to be further considered for DRI development. When the totality of evidence, including causal evidence, was supported by concordance

TABLE 4-2 Comparison of the Strengths and Weaknesses of Observational Study Designs and Randomized Controlled Trials for Use in DRI Development

Study Type/ Definition	Strengths	Weaknesses	Quality Ranking For DRI Development
Ecological *An observational study in which the units of analysis are populations or groups of people, rather than individuals*	• Provides an exploratory overview or indication for a potential association with outcome of interest	• Outcome measures are not predictable at the individual level	Low
Cross–sectional *An observational study in which a statistically significant sample of a population is used to estimate the relationship between an outcome of interest and population variables as they exist at one particular time*	• Allows for study of either a whole population or a representative sample • Provides estimates of prevalence of all factors measured • Facilitates greater generalizability	• Possible selection bias • Susceptible to mis-classification • Poor design for uncommon diseases or conditions • Simultaneous data collection obscures the order of effects	Low moderate
Case–control *An observational epidemiological study of persons with the outcome variable of interest and a suitable control group of persons without the variable of interest*	• Good design for uncommon diseases or conditions • Time and resource efficient	• Does not provide an estimate of incidence or prevalence of the disease, unless data about the population size are available • Possible selection bias • Susceptible to mis-classification • Simultaneous data collection obscures the order of effects	Moderate

continued

TABLE 4-2 Continued

Study Type/ Definition	Strengths	Weaknesses	Quality Ranking For DRI Development
Cohort *A method of epidemiological study in which subsets of a defined population can be identified as exposed to a factor hypothesized to influence the probability of occurrence of an outcome*	• Good design for common diseases or conditions • Relative timing of exposure and disease is less confusing than with other observational study designs	• Can be expensive and time-consuming • Possible selection bias from loss to follow-up • Statistically inefficient	High moderate
Randomized controlled trial *An experimental study design in which exposure is randomly assigned and in which the frequency of the outcome of interest is compared between one or more groups receiving an experimental treatment and a group receiving a placebo or the current standard of care*	• More similar to experimental study design than to observational design • Provides strongest evidence for causality • Fulfills the basic assumption of statistical hypothesis tests	• Expensive and time-consuming • Subjects may not be representative of all who might receive treatment	High

SOURCE: Gordis (2009).

between RCTs and high-quality observational evidence and had strong biological plausibility, the committee gave further consideration to a potential indicator for development of a DRI. When observational evidence failed to support the findings of RCTs, the indicator's validity for consideration was reevaluated, and a decision to give further consideration was made on the balance of the totality of evidence.

For each potential indicator discussed in this chapter, the review of evidence included consideration of the analytical approach, study population, and research protocol design and the overall quality of the evidence for each study reviewed. The introductory statement for each indicator includes ecological studies. Observations made from such studies require caution in their interpretation because the outcome measures are not known at the individual level, and inferring individual characteristics or

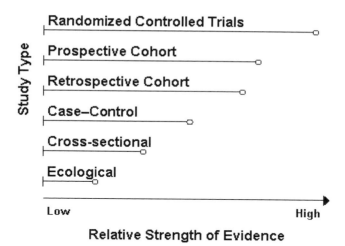

FIGURE 4-1 Ranking study designs: Ranking is shown in descending order of quality from top to bottom; the length of bars is arbitrary and indicates the relative strength of a study design.

relationships from group-level measures would be fallacious. Ecological studies, however, can contribute important information in more than an exploratory manner. Where it was relevant or needed in the absence of human studies, evidence for biological plausibility was included in the review as gleaned from experimental animal and mechanistic studies. The observational evidence reviewed included cross–sectional, case–control, and cohort (prospective and retrospective) studies. As pointed out previously, the strongest evidence among observational studies is from the cohort study. This study design offers an advantage over the case–control design in that it allows for observation of the incidence of a health outcome or the rate at which the health outcome develops in association with vitamin D or calcium intake or status in the population under study. In case–control studies, cases are included without identifying the entire "exposed" and "unexposed" populations from which they were derived, thus inferences drawn about a health outcome related to vitamin D or calcium intake or status are less reliable using this type of design.

As a tool to aid in the review process, the committee developed evidence "maps" for each indicator to provide an overarching view of the balance of relevant evidence from ecological and biological plausibility studies, observational studies, systematic reviews, and RCTs (including trials where the indicator was a primary outcome as well as other evidence from trials where the indicator was a secondary or non-pre-specified outcome). These served largely as an organizing tool and are included in Appendix

F. The organizational construct of the maps did not allow distinctions between studies relative to the quality of the study design; however, this was considered by the committee in the overall evaluation of data.

The nature of the data surrounding each potential indicator is described below, beginning with a brief statement about the condition under consideration, followed by a summary of the evidence for ecological and biological plausibility studies, observational studies, systematic reviews from the two AHRQ reports, and additional evidence not covered in the AHRQ reviews. Each indicator is then evaluated in a summary discussion of the utility of the evidence for DRI development.

REVIEW OF POTENTIAL INDICATORS

Owing to the importance of a variety of acute and chronic diseases as public health concerns and the accumulating data focused on the hypothesis that vitamin D and/or calcium may have an impact on disease risk, it was crucial that this committee consider a wide spectrum of indicators for DRI development. After reviewing the available data, including recent systematic reviews from AHRQ and other literature, the committee chose to focus on areas where the research database is most compelling and the indicator is of public health concern within the context of DRI development. The following discussions review the roles of vitamin D and calcium in the reduction of risk for the health indicators identified in Table 4-1.

The entirety of evidence for each indicator that was reviewed by the committee cannot be presented in detail here, and the following discussions are a summary of relevant evidence. In drawing its conclusions about an indicator, the committee evaluated the strengths and weaknesses of the studies considered for each indicator, including an examination of the methods used for measuring an indicator, its relevance to total intake and functional or physiological outcomes, and the strength of the study design. This approach is summarized in Box 4-2.

Cancer/Neoplasms

As the second leading cause of death in the United States, cancer is a major public health concern. Cancer encompasses a wide range of malignancies with many variations in etiology and pathogenesis. Thus, the committee considered not only total cancer, but also specific malignancies in which vitamin D and/or calcium have been examined for an interaction thought to play a role.

Cancer is a disease in which genetically damaged cells within a tissue experience uncontrolled growth and invasion with subsequent spread to other host organs. The metastatic spread leads to dysfunction of vital organs causing significant morbidity and culminating in death. An expanding

---

BOX 4-2
Evaluation of Evidence for DRI Development

In its review of evidence, the committee used a qualitative approach to determine its confidence in interpreting positive or negative relationships between vitamin D and/or calcium and indicators of disease outcomes for DRI development. In analyzing and weighing the data, the committee considered the following factors:

- Preliminary evidence in support of a relationship between vitamin D and/or calcium and a disease outcome is not always complete or well substantiated.
- Evidence for the effect of vitamin D and/or calcium on disease outcomes is heterogeneous and may not provide strong support for a consistent and predictable outcome.
- Clinical trials have the greatest influence in moderating confidence in a relationship between vitamin D and/or calcium and a disease outcome.

The committee's findings and conclusions were derived from its weighing of the totality of evidence and its ranking of evidence based on examination of study methods, relevance to dietary intake, effect of vitamin D and/or calcium on disease outcome, and overall strength of the study design.

---

array of experimental studies examining cells in culture and rodent models of cancer are providing evidence that vitamin D may have an impact on carcinogenesis at several organ sites (Deeb et al., 2007; Welsh, 2007; Davis, 2008). In parallel, epidemiological investigations of diverse approaches are examining the role of vitamin D in human cancer (WCRF/AICR, 2007; Yetley et al., 2009). In contrast, very few randomized and controlled prospective intervention trials with vitamin D targeting cancer as the primary outcome have been undertaken, leaving major gaps in understanding of causal relationships. Although more challenging to study in vitro, studies of dietary calcium in rodent models have also suggested a potential role in cancer risk; there are, as discussed below, experimental and clinical studies providing evidence in support of calcium as a modulator of carcinogenesis, particularly in the colon and rectal mucosa.

All Cancers

Cancer represents hundreds of different histopathologically distinct types of malignancy derived from virtually all organs and tissues. Investigations into the cellular defects contributing to the carcinogenic process indicate that cancers, regardless of tissue origin, share in a specific set of defective biological processes (Hanahan and Weinberg, 2000) that enhance cell proliferation, survival, invasion, and metastasis. Although cancer studies initially suggested the possibility of a tissue-specific gene expression signature unique to a cancer type, it is now appreciated that multiple different mutational patterns contribute to the heterogeneity in biology and response to intervention among humans with cancer.

Biological plausibility   Serum 25OHD levels are determined by both dietary intake and endogenous synthesis in the skin upon exposure to ultraviolet B (UVB) light. UVB exposure is often used as an indirect estimate of endogenous production of vitamin D in ecological studies of cancer incidence patterns. Several investigators associated lower UVB exposure with higher cancer mortality beginning decades ago (Apperley, 1941) and continuing with improved methods of estimating exposure (Boscoe and Schymura, 2006), as reviewed by IARC (2008). However, a large literature suggests that increasing latitude cannot be equated with decreasing vitamin D status, and cancer risk factors (exposure to UVB or other forms of ionizing radiation) vary with latitude. Importantly, an opposite gradient is well established for skin cancers, with a greater risk among populations residing in areas of high sun exposure (IARC, 1992). In general, ecological studies based upon estimated UVB exposure, vitamin D status, and cancer risk have many potential biases due to methodological considerations making causal biological inferences, particularly at the level of the individual, impossible.

Systematic reviews and meta-analyses   Assessment of total cancer risk has been the subject of systematic reviews, including IARC (2008), WCRF/AICR (2007), and AHRQ-Tufts. Several studies, including those reviewed in AHRQ-Tufts, were examined by the committee in detail. Three intervention trials that examined total cancer as an outcome were identified from these reviews; these trials were originally designed to assess fracture risk, and none included total cancer as a pre-specified primary outcome (see Table 4-3). In both the Trivedi et al. (2003) and Lappe et al. (2007) osteoporosis trials cancer risk was determined from a secondary analysis of safety data that relied upon subjects notifying the investigators of the new diagnosis. Neither trial indicated a significant reduction in cancer incidence with vitamin D supplementation, whether given alone (Trivedi et al., 2003) or in combination with calcium and compared with calcium supplementation alone (Lappe et al., 2007). In the Lappe et al. (2007) trial, however, logistic regression analysis showed a significant reduction in risk for all cancers in the vitamin D plus calcium treatment group when

TABLE 4-3 Vitamin D, Calcium,[a] and Total Cancer: Results of RCTs Reviewed in AHRQ-Tufts[b]

Reference; Location (Latitude)	Population Description	Background Calcium and Serum 25OHD	Outcome	Intervention, Daily Dose	n Event/N Total	Outcomes: Metric (Comparison); Result; 95% CI
Lappe et al., 2007 Nebraska, United States (41°N)	Postmenopausal women Mentally and physically fit Mean age 67 years	25OHD: 71.8 nmol/L	Incident cancer (all causes)	Vit D$_3$ 1,000 IU + Ca (citrate 1,400 mg or carbonate 1,500 mg)	13/446	RR (Vit D + Ca vs. Ca) 0.76
				Ca (citrate 1,400 mg or carbonate 1,500 mg)	17/445	0.38–1.55
			Incident cancer (restricted to patients who were free of cancer at 1-year intervention)	Vit D$_3$ 1,000 IU + Ca (citrate 1,400 mg or carbonate 1,500 mg)	8/403	RR (Vit D + Ca vs. Ca) 0.55
				Ca (citrate 1,400 mg or carbonate 1,500 mg)	15/416	0.24–1.28
Trivedi et al., 2003 Oxford, UK (52°N)	General population Mean age 75 (65–85) years	25OHD: 53.4 nmol/L Calcium intake: 742 mg/day (at 4 years; no difference by treatment allocation)	Incident cancer (all causes)	Vit D$_3$ ~ 833 IU (100,000 IU every 4 months)	188/1,345	HR (Vit D vs. placebo) 1.09
				Placebo	173/1,341	0.86–1.36
			Total cancer mortality	Vit D$_3$ ~ 833 IU (100,000 IU every 4 months)	63/1,345	HR (Vit D vs. placebo) 0.86
				Placebo	72/1,341	0.61–1.2

NOTE: CI = confidence interval; HR = hazard ratio; IU = International Units; RR = relative risk; UK = United Kingdom; Vit = vitamin.
[a]Calcium is included in Lappe et al. (2007) only.
[b]This table has been truncated for the purposes of this chapter, but it can be found in its entirety in Appendix D.
SOURCE: Modified from Chung et al. (2009).

compared with the placebo group. Notably, the investigators could not exclude that cancers had been present at baseline or that cancers remained unnoticed at the end of the study. Moreover, the analysis of the multitude of outcomes in safety data raises the possibility of chance results that seem to be statistically significant but are the result of multiple comparisons being made within one data set.

Observational evidence in AHRQ-Tufts included a large 12-year prospective study of a cohort from the Third National Health and Nutrition Examination Survey (NHANES III) that examined associations between serum 25OHD levels and total cancer mortality as well as specific cancer mortalities. Serum 25OHD levels were found to be associated with gender, educational level, and race/ethnicity, but not with season/latitude. No interaction was detected, however, between serum 25OHD level and total cancer mortality (Freedman et al., 2007). In one frequently cited study included in the AHRQ-Tufts review, Giovannucci et al. (2006) prospectively examined a large cohort from the Health Professionals Follow-up Study (HPFS) for 14 years for multiple determinants of vitamin D, including diet, supplements, skin pigmentation, adiposity, and geography, and their associations with cancer mortality. This study found that each incremental increase in serum 25OHD level of 25 nmol/L was associated with a 17 percent reduction in total cancer incidence and a 29 percent reduction in total cancer mortality. Each of the determinants considered was found to influence plasma 25OHD levels among older men. These results should be viewed with caution, however, because of heterogeneity in serum 25OHD levels that is not accounted for by the variables used in the study, which included intakes based on self-administered semiquantitative food frequency questionnaires and self-reported weight and physical activity levels.

Taken together, the studies reviewed by AHRQ-Tufts, IARC (2008), and WCRF/AICR (2007) as a whole are not supportive of a role for vitamin D, with or without calcium in reducing risk for cancer.

Additional evidence from randomized controlled trials In addition to the trials identified in AHRQ-Tufts, a secondary analysis of data from the Women's Health Initiative (WHI) trial examined the effect of combined supplementation of vitamin D and calcium (400 International Units [IU] of vitamin D and 1,000 mg of elemental calcium) on various health outcomes including cancer mortality (Lacroix et al., 2009). The results, with an average of 7 years of follow-up, indicated a non-significant trend toward reduction in risk for cancer mortality among postmenopausal women.

Observational studies One additional large cohort study, not included in the AHRQ reviews, was identified that examined serum 25OHD levels and risk for cancer mortality. This study examined cancer mortality among patients referred for coronary disease after a median of 7.75 years and found a significant correlation between low serum 25OHD level defined as less than 25.5 nmol/L, and increased cancer mortality. No associations were detected, however, between calcitriol level and cancer mortality (Pilz et al., 2008). In total, the observational studies reviewed suggest that the association between 25OHD level and risk of death from all cancers is generally weak when considered over a broad range of serum 25OHD levels because of variability in outcomes between the studies reviewed. However, there may be a stronger association between low serum 25OHD levels and cancer risk. The evidence reviewed was not strong enough to conclude that associations between cancer mortality were dependent on latitude, or race/ethnicity.

The role of calcium in cancer risk was examined in one large prospective cohort study over 7 years of follow-up (Park et al., 2009). Calcium intake was found not to be related to total cancer risk in men, but a non-linear reduction in total cancer incidence in women was reported. A decreased cancer risk was found for calcium intakes up to approximately 1,300 mg/day, although no additional risk reduction was observed for higher intakes. Taken together, the heterogeneity among outcomes exhibited in these studies and the discrepancy in outcomes between observational and randomized trial evidence do not support a relationship between vitamin D or calcium and total cancer risk.

Concluding statement   The totality of the available evidence from RCTs and observational association studies for a relationship between vitamin D and/or calcium and the risk for either incidence of or mortality from all cancers does not support the use of cancer mortality as an indicator for DRI development. The interpretation of the evidence reviewed is limited by the small number of studies identified and lack of consistency in associations between vitamin D intake or serum 25OHD levels and all cancer mortality. Interpretation is further complicated by the absence of large-scale RCTs examining total cancer risk as a pre-specified primary outcome. Given the lack of consistent evidence on associations between vitamin D intake or serum 25OHD level and total cancer, and the paucity of evidence on cancer as a primary outcome of vitamin D or calcium intervention in randomized trials, as well as inconsistency between findings in the available research for an effect of vitamin D or calcium supplementation or status on reducing risk for cancer, the committee could not draw a conclusion about the utility of the evidence for this indicator to support DRI development.

Breast Cancer

Risk for breast cancer is largely defined by reproductive endocrinology, with increased risk for those with early age of menarche, late menopause, no pregnancy, later age of first pregnancy, shorter duration of lactation, the use of postmenopausal hormonal supplementation (Fentiman, 2002; Velie et al., 2005; Narod, 2006; Parsa and Parsa, 2009; Dietel, 2010). Dietary-related factors have been extensively reviewed with alcoholic drinks, adult attained height, and adult weight gain likely contributing to risk and with physical activity showing some benefit (WCRF/AICR, 2007). These characteristics must be considered when evaluating other putative breast cancer risk factors.

Biological plausibility   The influence of the active form of vitamin D (calcitriol) on breast cancer cells in vitro is well characterized and includes anti-cancer effects such as cell cycle inhibition, reduced proliferation, enhanced sensitivity to apoptosis, and induction of differentiation markers (Welsh, 2004), which are likely mediated by the vitamin D receptor (VDR) (Matthews et al., 2010). A shortcoming in applying results from cell culture studies to risk for disease, however, is that the dose of calcitriol necessary to achieve tumor inhibition in vivo is frequently associated with hypercalcemic toxicity (Welsh, 2004; Matthews et al., 2010). Novel genomic approaches have begun to elucidate the gene expression signature of vitamin D in breast cancer cells and the mammary glands of mice (Matthews et al., 2010). Many of the genes identified show a consensus vitamin D response element (VDRE) in their promoter elements, indicating that they are specific targets of the vitamin D receptor (VDR[1]) complex (Swami et al., 2003; Matthews et al., 2010). Since the discovery of polymorphisms in the *Vdr* gene, a search for associations of mutations with breast cancer has been undertaken, but with indeterminate results (Bertone-Johnson, 2009; McKay et al., 2009). An inverse association has been postulated between mammographic density, a putative breast cancer risk factor, and serum 25OHD levels in premenopausal women (Berube et al., 2004; Brisson et al., 2007). The role of dietary calcium intake and in breast cancer risk, however, is less well studied, and the potential biological mechanisms of action are not understood.

Systematic reviews and meta-analyses   AHRQ-Tufts did not find any qualified systematic reviews that evaluated associations between vitamin D and calcium intake or serum 25OHD levels and risk for breast cancer. Three observational studies of sufficient methodological quality were identified that examined the relationship between 25OHD levels and breast cancer risk. A prospective cohort study described above for total cancer mortality reported that women whose 25OHD levels were in a higher stratification, were at significantly lower risk for breast cancer. There were, however,

---

[1]In this report, the term VDR is used to refer to the protein. The term *Vdr* is used to refer to the gene, whether in animals or humans.

only eight women in the higher stratification and a linear trend analysis was not significant (Freedman et al., 2007). A nested case–control study using data from the Nurses' Health Study (NHS) (Bertone-Johnson et al., 2005) found no significant relationship between higher plasma 25OHD concentrations and decreased risk for breast cancer overall, except when the population was restricted to women over 60 years of age. Another nested case–control cohort study of postmenopausal women participating in the Prostate, Lung, Colorectal, and Ovarian (PLCO) Cancer Screening Trial also found no evidence supporting the hypothesis that higher plasma 25OHD concentrations were associated with reduced risk of breast cancer in this cohort (Freedman et al., 2008).

Analysis of the results of RCTs reviewed in AHRQ-Tufts found no significant effect of supplementation with both vitamin D and calcium on breast cancer incidence and no association between the intervention and risk for death from breast cancer. Subjects with lower baseline 25OHD levels were found to be at increased risk for breast cancer; however, the association was not significant after adjusting for body mass index and physical activity (Chlebowski et al., 2008).

A meta-analysis of evidence from observational studies carried out by IARC (2008) evaluated associations between serum vitamin D levels and cancer. The analyses for breast cancer risk indicated no significant or con-sistent associations. A literature review and all-inclusive meta-analysis of published studies of heterogeneous quality individually examined the im-pact of estimated vitamin D intake, circulating 25OHD levels, and calcium intake on breast cancer risk (Chen et al., 2010). Their analysis suggests an inverse relationship between risk and level of vitamin D intake, serum $25OHD_3$ level, and calcium intake.

Additional evidence from randomized controlled trials   WHI was used as a data source in an 8-year follow-up study for risk of benign proliferative breast disease, a putative premalignant condition associated with increased risk of subsequent cancer (Rohan et al., 2009). This study identified an association between risk for breast cancer and baseline age but found no effect of supplemental calcium and vitamin D intervention on reducing risk for breast cancer.

Observational studies   Several case–control and cohort studies conducted subsequent to the systematic reviews were identified that examined associa-tions between dietary and supplemental intake of vitamin D and calcium and risk for breast cancer, and these have shown mixed results. Rossi et al. (2009), a large case–control study in Italy, found an inverse association between vitamin D intake and risk for breast cancer at intakes of 188 IU/ day or greater, suggesting a threshold effect; however, when risk was calculated in the upper three deciles compared with the lower seven deciles the significant difference was attenuated. A population-based case–control study of women ages 25 to 74 years in Canada compared vitamin D and calcium intake from food alone or from food and supplements. When intake above 400 IU of vitamin D per day was compared with no intake, a reduced risk was found. Calcium supplement intake alone, however, did not correlate with reduced risk, although a significant inverse trend was identified (Anderson et al., 2010). Two studies were identified that examined associations between dairy intake and risk of breast cancer. Shin et al. (2002) analyzed data from the NHS 1980 cohort for dairy intake and incident breast cancer. Over 16 years of follow-up, a significant inverse association was found for premenopausal women consuming low-fat dairy products and breast cancer risk. No association was found for calcium and vitamin D intake and postmenopausal breast cancer risk. Supplemental calcium intake had no linear association and supplemental vitamin D intake a weak but non-significant association with breast cancer risk in both premenopausal and postmenopausal women. Using a similar study design, McCullough et al. (2005), in an analysis of participants from the Cancer Prevention Study II Nutrition Cohort, found that two or more daily servings of dairy products were inversely associated with breast cancer risk; however, no association was found for either calcium or vitamin D supplementation. Women with dietary calcium intakes above 1,250 mg/day had lower breast cancer risk than women with intakes at or below 500 mg/day. Altogether, these observational studies were of lower quality and thus not considered as strong support for an association between vitamin D and risk for breast cancer, and they were not well supported by randomized trial evidence.

Concluding statement In summary, although experimental studies are suggestive of a role for vitamin D in breast biology, a review of the available evidence from both RCTs and observational studies of associations between vitamin D and calcium and risk of breast cancer shows a lack of consistency between study outcomes and insufficiently strong evidence to support DRI development. Both retrospective and prospective studies do not show consistent associations between estimated vitamin D intake or 25OHD status and breast cancer risk. A paucity of RCTs of vitamin D, calcium, or both with breast cancer as a primary outcome further limited the strength of the evidence.

Colorectal Cancer/Colon Polyps

Foods, nutrients, and physical activity all interact in a complex array of mechanisms to influence colorectal cancer risk. There is convincing evidence that physical activity protects against colorectal cancer, whereas red and processed meat, body fatness, and alcohol may increase the risk (WCRF/AICR, 2007). The committee's review of studies on vitamin D and calcium and risk for colorectal cancers and possible protective benefits identified for calcium and vitamin D was inconclusive.

Biological plausibility   A major role of the active form of vitamin D is to enhance calcium absorption by the intestine, and the molecular and cell biology has been well defined (Song and Fleet, 2007; Xue and Fleet, 2009). The VDR and the vitamin D converting enzyme, 1α-hydroxylase, are both expressed in the colon and rectum (Cross et al., 1997; Holt et al., 2002). Vitamin D has been reported to act on colonic epithelial and cancer cells to regulate growth factor and inhibitor expression and signaling pathways, including modulation of the cell cycle, sensitivity to apoptosis, and enhancement of cellular differentiation (Harris and Go, 2004; Yang et al., 2007). Many rodent models of colon carcinogenesis suggest that there is an increased risk for colon cancer associated with vitamin D deficiency; and a decreased risk associated with supplementation (Harris and Go, 2004; Yang et al., 2008; Newmark et al., 2009). However, few studies were identified that examined vitamin D over a range of dose levels. A recent review of findings from the *Vdr*-null mouse model indicates an increase in hyperplasia of the distal colonic epithelium and greater deoxyribonucleic acid (DNA) damage in vitamin D–deficient compared with wild-type mice (Bouillon et al., 2008). The independent role of calcium in modulating colon cancer risk is also under investigation. Although intracellular calcium plays a key role in cell biology and influences growth control processes that may be related to carcinogenesis, serum calcium is tightly regulated over a wide range of intakes. Thus, the potential mechanisms by which serum calcium levels could mediate risk for colon cancer may be through indirect effectors in metabolic pathways involved in tumorigenesis.

Systematic reviews and meta-analyses
   Colorectal cancer   The AHRQ-Tufts systematic review considered evidence for associations between 25OHD levels and risk for colorectal cancer mortality or incidence. One RCT found no significant difference between colorectal mortality or incidence and supplementation with vitamin D in an elderly population. One cohort study was identified that found an inverse association between high serum 25OHD levels and risk for colorectal cancer mortality, and two nested case–control studies in women found an inverse trend between serum 25OHD level and colorectal cancer incidence. Two nested case–control studies in men and three in both men and women found no significant associations between serum 25OHD level and risk of colorectal cancer.
   The IARC (2008) meta-analysis found a significant protective effect for

serum 25OHD level against risk for colorectal cancer that correlated with each 2.5 nmol/L increase, although there was significant between-study heterogeneity. The results did not significantly differ by gender, mean population age, or cancer subsite (colon or rectum). The review noted that, based on multiple studies of circulating 25OHD and colorectal cancer risk, individuals in the high quartile or quintile of 25OHD level had about half the risk of colorectal cancer as did those in the lowest group. In another systematic review of studies examining associations between serum 25OHD levels and colorectal cancer, Bischoff-Ferrari et al. (2006a) concluded that the protective effect of 25OHD for decreased risk of colorectal cancers began at 75 nmol/L, and optimal levels were between 90 and 100 nmol/L. In contrast to these findings, the AHRQ-Ottawa systematic review reported that the studies reviewed were too inconsistent to permit conclusions to be drawn about specific serum 25OHD levels that conferred a decrease in risk.

Colorectal adenomas/polyps   The AHRQ-Tufts systematic review considered evidence for associations between 25OHD levels and risk for colorectal adenomas. Colorectal adenomas or polyps are precursor lesions for colon cancer, and a number of investigations focused on the influence of vitamin D or calcium on the incidence of these surrogate markers for human colon carcinogenesis. A meta-analysis by Wei et al. (2008) of seven studies suggested that at the upper quintiles of circulating 25OHD levels there was a significant decrease in risk for colorectal adenoma. In parallel, these authors conducted a meta-analysis of vitamin D intake and colorectal adenoma risk in seven cohort and five case–control studies and found a marginally significant (11 percent) decreased risk among persons with high compared with low vitamin D intakes. The cut-points for the highest category of vitamin D intake varied between studies, with about one-third of the studies reporting cut-points of approximately 600 IU/day, one-third reporting cut-points between 250 and 600 IU/day, and one-third reporting cut-points of below 250 IU/day.

Stronger evidence has accumulated for a role of dietary calcium. The AHRQ-Tufts analysis identified four good quality cohort studies that evaluated the association between calcium intake and risk for colorectal adenoma. Two of these studies recruited men and women with a history of previous colorectal adenoma. One study found a significant inverse association between total calcium intake and colorectal adenoma recurrence after an average of 3.1 years of follow-up (highest [> 1,279 mg/day] vs. lowest [< 778 mg/day]) intake, whereas another found no significant association. Among two studies of healthy women without a history of colorectal adenoma one found a significant inverse association between total calcium intake and colorectal adenoma (highest vs. lowest intake, whereas the other found a borderline significant trend (highest [median, 1,451 mg/day] vs. lowest [median, 584 mg/day] intake. A Cochrane systematic review identified two randomized trials that found that calcium supplementation reduced the incidence of recurrent colorectal adenoma (Weingarten et al., 2008). Overall, the evidence is suggestive that vitamin D and probably calcium may reduce the risk of this intermediate endpoint for colorectal cancer, but the available data are not sufficient to allow a definitive assessment of the effects of vitamin D, calcium, and their interactions on risk for new or recurrent colorectal adenomas.

Additional evidence from randomized controlled trials   The committee did not identify any additional relevant RCTs assessing vitamin D or calcium intake and risk for colorectal cancer or adenomas.

Observational studies   The European Prospective Investigation into Cancer and Nutrition (EPIC) study has recently reported data on more than 1,200 colorectal cancer cases and an equal number of controls (Jenab et al., 2010). In this report, serum concentrations lower than the pre-defined mid-level concentrations of 25OHD (50 to 75 nmol/L) were associated with higher colorectal cancer risk. Jenab et al. (2010) also reported that higher 25OHD concentrations of 75 to less than 100 nmol/L and 100 nmol/L and higher were associated with a decreased risk. No other relevant observational studies were identified outside the AHRQ reviews. Although this evidence was largely in agreement with the IARC (2008) findings and Bischoff-Ferrari et al. (2006a), the committee did not consider it convincing enough to outweigh the conclusions from both AHRQ reviews.

Concluding statement   Taken in aggregate, epidemiological studies examining associations between vitamin D status and colorectal cancer incidence generally support an inverse association, although the shape of the dose–response relationship curve over a wide range of vitamin D intake remains very speculative. The biological plausibility is supported by data from cell culture and rodents, with additional support from surrogate biomarker studies in humans. There remains a paucity of prospective randomized intervention studies, and those available have not shown a significant relationship at this time. Thus, the data are insufficient for the committee to utilize colon cancer as an outcome for establishment of vitamin D DRIs. The data for an effect of dietary calcium on colorectal cancer risk are also highly suggestive of a protective effect, but there are not sufficient data available on dose–response relationships to utilize colorectal cancer as a health outcome for DRI development.

Prostate Cancer

Prostate cancer risk is strongly associated with aging and is clearly dependent upon prolonged exposure to testosterone. Unlike breast cancer in women, however, where specific reproductive events define risk, further characterization of the relationship has been challenging. Specific dietary and nutritional hypotheses, including a role for vitamin D and calcium, have been proposed but evidence supporting these relationships is not conclusive.

Biological plausibility   Studies in vitro document that prostate cancer and prostate epithelial cells in culture respond to calcitriol with anti-proliferative effects and that calcitriol stimulates cell differentiation (Washington and Weigel, 2010). Evidence indicates that these effects, as for epithelial cells of other tissue origins, are mediated by the VDR expressed on prostate cells (Kivineva et al., 1998; Thorne and Campbell, 2008). Gene expression array studies provide evidence that calcitriol induces a pattern of gene expression that inhibits growth factor signaling and cell cycle progression, promotes differentiation, and is anti-inflammatory and anti-angiogenic (Krishnan et al., 2004; Peehl et al., 2004; Kovalenko et al., 2010). The role of dietary calcium intake in prostate cancer risk is less well studied, with inconsistent results, and the potential biological mechanisms of action are highly speculative.

Systematic reviews and meta-analyses   The AHRQ-Tufts systematic review found no qualified systematic reviews assessing associations between serum 25OHD levels and incidence of prostate cancer. Among observational studies reviewed, 8 of 12 nested case–control studies found no association between baseline serum 25OHD levels and risk for prostate cancer, and only 1 (C-rated) (Ahonen et al., 2000) reported a significant association between baseline serum 25OHD levels below 30 nmol/L and higher risk of prostate cancer, compared to those with levels greater than 55 nmol/L. Further, the effect appeared to be stronger for men younger than age 52 at entry into the study. A meta-analysis by Huncharek et al. (2008) of 45 observational studies on dairy and milk intake and risk of prostate cancer showed no significant association between dietary intake of vitamin D and prostate cancer risk.

Additional evidence from randomized controlled trials   No relevant RCTs that were not reviewed by AHRQ were identified for vitamin D or calcium intervention and risk for prostate cancer.

Observational studies   Three observational studies not included in either AHRQ-Ottawa or AHRQ-Tufts were identified as potentially relevant to prostate cancer as a health indicator for vitamin D and calcium. Schwartz and Hulka (1990) suggested that vitamin D deficiency was a causative factor in prostate cancer based upon the observation that the prevalence of vitamin D deficiency increases with age and is greater in those with dark-pigmented skin types and northern European populations, coupled with the observation that mortality rates for prostate cancer appear to be inversely related to sun exposure. However, a more recent case–control analysis of data from the Alpha-Tocopherol, Beta-Carotene Cancer Prevention (ATBC) Study, which examined male smokers, found no association; including any age-related associations to support a relationship between serum 25OHD levels and incidence of prostate cancer (Faupel-Badger et al., 2007). A potential procarcinogenic effect of higher dietary calcium was suggested by the HPFS (Giovannucci et al., 1998), which reported that calcium intake from the diet or from diet and supplements was independently associated with risk of locally advanced or metastatic prostate cancer especially when intakes exceeded 2,000 mg per day. The potential role for calcium as a risk factor for prostate cancer is discussed in detail in Chapter 6.

Because of the complexity of assessing vitamin D exposure over time relative to prostate cancer risk, high-quality evidence from observational studies was limited. The results of the HPFS, the only large, prospective cohort study identified for calcium, are not supported by evidence from available RCTs. Therefore, the evidence from human studies is insufficient to permit the committee to draw conclusions about a role for vitamin D and/or calcium in reducing prostate cancer risk.

Concluding statement   Overall experimental data indicating that cultured prostate epithelial and prostate cancer cells respond to vitamin D via the VDR suggest a role for vitamin D in prostate cancer. However, associational studies of vitamin D status and risk of prostate cancer have provided mixed results, and randomized controlled clinical trials of substantial quality examining incidence or mortality have not been reported. Thus, there are insufficient data to permit the committee to draw a conclusion about the utility of the evidence for this indicator to support DRI development.

Cardiovascular Diseases and Hypertension

CVD broadly describes a range of diseases affecting the heart and blood vessels. Diseases that fall under the umbrella of CVD comprise coronary artery disease, myocardial infarction, stroke/cerebrovascular disease, peripheral artery disease, atherosclerosis, hypertension, arrhythmias, heart failure, and other vascular disorders. CVD is a public health concern because it is associated with an enormous burden of illness, disability, and mortality. CVD and hypertension were considered as potential indicators based on proposed hypotheses that vitamin D alone or in combination with calcium may help to prevent CVD or hypertension. Calcium has also been implicated independently as a nutrient related to reducing risk for development of CVD. Limited data were available for this indicator in the 1997 DRI report (IOM, 1997); however, additional experimental animal and observational studies for both vitamin D and calcium and CVD have been published in the interim.

Biological Plausibility

Vitamin D has been linked to decreased risk for CVD. Ecological studies suggest that there is higher cardiovascular mortality during the winter and in regions with less average exposure to UVB radiation from sunlight (Zittermann et al., 2005). Various biological mechanisms have been proposed in support of this hypothesis. Experimental animal studies failed to demonstrate an effect of vitamin D on risk for hypertension (Li et al., 2004) and increased thrombogenicity (Aihara et al., 2004). In rodents, administration of calcitriol or its analogues enhances vascular reactivity (Hatton et al., 1994). In support of the hypothesis that biological activation of vitamin D is relevant to cardiovascular function, the *Vdr*-null mouse has been used to model CVD.

High dietary calcium intake may help to reduce CVD risk through its roles in decreasing intestinal absorption of lipids and increasing lipid excretion, lowering blood cholesterol levels, and promoting calcium influx into cells.

Systematic Reviews and Meta-Analyses

The AHRQ-Tufts report identified one RCT and four relevant observational studies for vitamin D and cardiovascular outcomes. The RCT (Trivedi et al., 2003) found no statistically significant difference in incidence of cardiovascular events and deaths for subjects treated with 100,000 IU of vitamin D every 4 months over 5 years of follow-up. Among the observational studies reviewed, the Framingham Offspring Study found a significant association between low serum 25OHD levels and incident CVD (T. J. Wang et al., 2008). However, a closer look at the individuals with the highest serum 25OHD levels suggests that there was no additional reduction in risk at levels greater than 75 nmol/L and that the dose–response relationship may be U-shaped above 75 nmol/L. In the HPFS, Giovannucci et al. (2008), using a nested case–control design, found a significant association between low (< 37.5 nmol/L) serum 25OHD levels and incident myocardial infarction. A study using data from NHANES III, however, found no significant association between serum 25OHD levels and cardiovascular mortality overall, although individuals with the lowest 25OHD levels experienced a significant increase in total mortality compared with those with the highest levels. Echoing the findings for incident CVD in the Framingham Offspring Study, a closer examination of the highest 25OHD levels suggested a U-shaped dose–response relationship, with increased total mortality at both the lowest and highest 25OHD levels in this cohort (Melamed et al., 2008). The fourth observational study reported in AHRQ-Tufts (Marniemi et al., 2005) also failed to find an association between serum 25OHD levels and total CVD incidence, although it did find that vitamin D intake predicted a decreased risk for stroke. With the exception of one case–control study, the overall findings from the observational studies reviewed reaffirm a lack of significant association between 25OHD level and CVD risk and that higher 25OHD levels may incur an increased risk for CVD. From this, AHRQ-Tufts concluded that the evidence was insufficient to support a relationship between vitamin D or calcium and risk for CVD.

A recent meta-analysis of randomized trials using calcium supplements (without vitamin D) suggested that calcium supplementation was associated with an increase in the risk of myocardial infarction (Bolland et al., 2010a). However, another recent meta-analysis that included CVD as a secondary outcome found a slightly reduced, but not significant, risk for CVD with vitamin D supplementation, no association with calcium supplementation, and no association with a combination of vitamin D plus calcium supplementation (Wang et al., 2010).

Additional Evidence from Randomized Controlled Trials

No new RCTs were identified that examined CVD as a pre-specified primary outcome although several trials analyzed CVD as a secondary treatment outcome, and the findings of secondary outcome studies were not supportive of a reduction in CVD risk for either vitamin D or calcium. Among the additional RCTs reviewed outside the AHRQ reviews examining CVD as a secondary outcome (Hsia et al., 2007 [400 IU vitamin D_3/1,000 mg calcium]; Major et al., 2007 [400 IU vitamin D/1,200 mg calcium]; Margolis et al., 2008 [400 IU vitamin D_3/1,000 mg calcium]; Prince et al., 2008 [1,000 IU vitamin D_2/1,000 mg calcium]; Manson et al., 2010 [400 IU vitamin D_3/1,000 mg calcium]), none found a significant treatment-related effect of vitamin D on risk of CVD (see Evidence Map in Appendix F). In a 5-year study of calcium intake and risk for CVD in New Zealand, Bolland et al. (2008) found that women taking 1,000 mg of elemental calcium had a significantly higher risk (compared to placebo) for myocardial infarction and a composite CVD endpoint of myocardial infarction, stroke, and sudden death. However, when unreported events identified from a national database were added to the analysis, the increased cardiovascular risks in the calcium group were no longer statistically significant. A bone density trial, also conducted in New Zealand, assessing self-reported composite vascular events among men was also not significant for an interaction between 1,000 mg of calcium daily and CVD outcomes (Reid et al., 2008). The results of these trials are in agreement with the null findings of the AHRQ-Tufts review described above. The additional clinical trials reviewed did not show a statistically significant causal relationship between either vitamin D or calcium and decreased cardiovascular risk, and reductions in risk that were noted in some trials were not well supported by data analyses. Therefore, the totality of the evidence does not support an interaction between either vitamin or calcium and risk for CVD. Adverse cardiovascular effects associated with excess calcium intake were also noted, and these are discussed further in Chapter 6.

Observational Studies

In addition to the clinical trials reviewed, including those from AHRQ, several observational studies were identified that examined a role for vitamin D and/or calcium in reducing CVD risk. Two large, prospective cohort studies were identified. In one study of individuals at high risk of CVD, among coronary angiography patients followed for more than 7 years, those with the lowest serum 25OHD levels had significantly higher total mortality and cardiovascular mortality compared with those with the highest levels (Dobnig et al., 2008). Melamed et al. (2008) assessed 25OHD levels and prevalence of peripheral artery disease using data from NHANES 2001 to 2004. This study found a graded association between levels of 25OHD up to 29.1 nmol/L and levels of 29.2 nmol/L and above. In a trend analysis, a statistically significant difference was found between the lower 25OHD levels compared with the higher levels.

A number of small cohort studies were identified that evaluated serum 25OHD or calcitriol levels in patients at risk for various CVD indicators compared with control subjects who were free of CVD indicators. Watson et al. (1997) assessed calcitriol levels in subjects at high risk for developing coronary heart disease compared with asymptomatic individuals and found a significant inverse association between calcitriol and amount of vascular calcification in both groups, although the difference was greater in the at-risk group. Poole et al. (2006) compared serum 25OHD levels in a small group of patients admitted for a first stroke with those of healthy controls and found that serum 25OHD levels were significantly lower among stroke patients. Zittermann et al. (2003) compared both 25OHD and calcitriol levels against serum levels of biomarkers indicative of congestive heart failure in a small group of patients admitted for treatment and in free-living controls. The study found a significant difference in biomarker levels between treated patients compared with controls for both 25OHD and calcitriol levels.

One small case–control study was identified that determined the relationship between serum 25OHD levels and risk for myocardial infarction in at-risk patients compared with normal controls. In this study, Scragg et al. (1990) found that serum 25OHD levels were significantly lower in myocardial infarction cases than in controls and that the difference was greater (but not significantly so) during the winter.

Although these studies together provide evidence for lower serum 25OHD levels in individuals with CVD, whether the low serum 25OHD levels are sufficient to predict risk for CVD has not been clearly established. Additional evidence indicates that low serum 25OHD levels are associated with risk factors for CVD—specifically, increased carotid arterial thickness (Targher et al., 2006)—and apparent CVD in patients with type 2 diabetes (Cigolini et al., 2006; Chonchol et al., 2008). Additionally, some studies suggest a positive association between vitamin D intake and CVD risk factors associated with other chronic conditions, including hypertension (Krause et al., 1998; Pfeifer et al., 2001; Forman et al., 2007; L. Wang et al., 2008; Wang et al., 2010), impaired glucose tolerance or type 2 diabetes (Liu et al., 2005; Pittas et al., 2006, 2007a; Mattila et al., 2007), and inflammation (Timms et al., 2002; Schleithoff et al., 2006; Shea et al., 2008).

Risk of incident hypertension in relation to dietary vitamin D intake has been evaluated in three large prospective study cohorts; NHS 1, NHS 2, and the HPFS for 8 years and longer. Women in NHS 1 and NHS 2 (a younger cohort) showed no association between vitamin D intake and risk for incident hypertension. Likewise, among men from the HPFS no association was found between vitamin D intake and risk for incident hypertension. Al-Delaimy et al. (2003) also found no association between calcium intake, vitamin D intake, or total dairy intake and risk for total ischemic heart disease in men enrolled in the HPFS. Similarly, no association was found when the cohort was analyzed for calcium supplement intake, although an inverse association was identified between calcium intake among supplement users compared with nonusers and fatal ischemic heart disease only.

In contrast to the intake studies, in a prospective study, Forman et al. (2007) found inverse associations between incidence of hypertension and measured serum 25OHD levels in a larger cohort in the HPFS and in women from a larger cohort in NHS.

In summary, three of four large, prospective cohort studies reviewed found associations between serum 25OHD levels and risk for CVD. Among the many smaller observational studies of lower quality that were identified, most did not find a significant positive association between vitamin D and calcium intake and risk for CVD. Taken together, this observational evidence was strong enough to support a relationship between serum 25OHD levels and incident disease, but not a conclusion that higher serum 25OHD levels were associated with a lower risk for CVD. Additionally, the review of randomized trial evidence does not support a causal relationship between vitamin D intake and risk for CVD.

Concluding Statement

Review of the available evidence, from both RCTs and observational studies on associations between vitamin D and calcium intake and risk for CVD shows that although observational evidence supports a relationship between serum 25OHD levels and the presence of CVD, it does not show a relationship with risk for developing CVD, and evidence was not found for a causal relationship between vitamin D intake and development of disease. Given the lack of statistically significant evidence supporting associations between vitamin D intake or serum 25OHD level and risk for CVD and the lack of evidence on CVD as a primary outcome of treatment in RCTs with vitamin D and/or calcium, the committee could not draw an inference about the efficacy of this indicator to support DRI development.

Diabetes and Metabolic Syndrome

Type 2 diabetes is a blood glucose disorder characterized by insulin resistance and relative insulin deficiency. Metabolic changes that accompany chronic elevated blood glucose levels frequently lead to functional impairment in many organ systems, particularly the cardiovascular system, which contributes to substantially increased risk of morbidity and mortality.

Metabolic syndrome is a condition characterized by a constellation of metabolic risk factors, including abdominal obesity, atherogenic dyslipidemias, elevated blood pressure, insulin resistance, prothrombotic state, and proinflammatory state (e.g., elevated C-reactive protein).

Individuals with metabolic syndrome are at increased risk of coronary heart disease, stroke, peripheral vascular disease, and type 2 diabetes. Adiposity is a component of both type 2 diabetes and metabolic syndrome, which may have an impact on vitamin D status. Since the release of the 1997 DRIs (IOM, 1997), a number of studies have been published on relationships between vitamin D with or without calcium and type 2 diabetes and metabolic syndrome. The committee recognized that obesity can be a confounder to vitamin D analysis. However, as it is a component of the health outcome and because of the prevalence of both obesity and metabolic syndrome in the general population, this indicator was considered as a candidate for DRI development.

Biological Plausibility

Vitamin D was first implicated as a modulator of pancreatic endocrine function and insulin synthesis and secretion in studies using rodent models more than three decades ago (Norman et al., 1980; Clark et al., 1981; Chertow et al., 1983). Since then, the role of calcitriol in the synthesis and secretion of insulin and regulation of calcium trafficking in β-islet cells as well as its effects on insulin action have been established in both rodent models and in vitro cell culture models (Frankel et al., 1985; Cade and Norman, 1986; Faure et al., 1991; Sergeev and Rhoten, 1995; Billaudel et al., 1998; Bourlon et al., 1999). These findings stimulated observational and intervention studies examining the role of vitamin D and calcium in type 2 diabetes and metabolic syndrome in humans.

Systematic Reviews and Meta-Analyses

Neither AHRQ-Ottawa nor AHRQ-Tufts included type 2 diabetes or metabolic syndrome in its systematic review, although AHRQ-Tufts did include body weight as a health outcome and found no effect of vitamin D or calcium on changes in body weight. A systematic review and meta-analysis by Pittas et al. (2007b) included a large body of observational evidence and six intervention studies (four small short-term and two long-term studies) of vitamin D supplementation, one study using combined vitamin D and calcium supplementation and five studies using calcium alone or dairy supplementation. The results from these trials were largely negative; among the short-duration vitamin D trials, three studies reported no effect, and one reported enhanced insulin secretion but no improvement in glucose tolerance following vitamin D supplementation. In one study included in the review, however, the relationship was statistically significant only when non-Hispanic blacks were excluded from the meta-analysis.

Overall, the evidence reviewed from the intervention studies did not support a role for vitamin D alone, although vitamin D in combination with calcium supplementation may have a role in preventing type 2 diabetes in populations already at risk. The observational evidence in the review included cross–sectional and case–control studies in which serum vitamin D and calcium levels were determined from individuals in a population with established glucose intolerance. Similar confounding and a lack of adjustment for confounders limited the cohort studies. Thus, the one meta-analysis that included both observational and intervention studies could not be considered as supportive for a relationship between either vitamin D or calcium and the health outcomes of diabetes or metabolic syndrome.

Additional Evidence from Randomized Controlled Trials

Two randomized trials were identified that evaluated the effect of vitamin D supplementation with or without supplemental calcium on markers of glucose tolerance as a primary outcome and four additional trials were identified that evaluated glucose metabolism as a secondary outcome. A trial in New Zealand that examined the effect of supplementation with 4,000 IU of vitamin D_3 per day for 6 months on insulin resistance in non-diabetic overweight South Asian women found a significant improvement in insulin sensitivity compared with those in the placebo group after 6 months (von Hurst et al., 2010). Among women who had low serum 25OHD levels at the beginning of the study, those who achieved a serum 25OHD level above 80 nmol/L at 6 months had significant improvement in insulin sensitivity. In contrast, sub-analysis of data from the Randomised Evaluation of Calcium and/Or vitamin D (RECORD) trial examining the association between incidence of self-reported development of type 2 diabetes or initiation of treatment for type 2 diabetes and supplementation with 800 IU of vitamin D_3 and 1,000 mg of calcium in an elderly population found no association (Avenell et al., 2009a). Zittermann et al. (2009), in a weight loss trial evaluating the effect of supplemental vitamin D on markers of CVD in overweight adults as a primary outcome, found no significant difference for an effect on glucose metabolism. Jorde et al. (2010), in a 1-year trial in Norway with overweight or obese subjects, found no change in measures of blood glucose in vitamin D–supplemented subjects compared with control subjects, but they did identify an unexpected and significant increase in systolic blood pressure in the supplemented group compared with controls. Without further analysis, however, it is not possible to determine whether the increase in blood pressure was related to 25OHD levels in blood. A trial in India evaluated the effect of short-term vitamin D supplementation on homeostasis model assessment and oral glucose insulin sensitivity in healthy, centrally obese men (Nagpal et al., 2009). In an intention-to-treat analysis, the difference was not significant. Overall, higher waist-to-hip ratios and lower baseline serum 25OHD levels were significant predictors of improvement in oral glucose insulin sensitivity. A posthoc analysis of a trial testing the effects of long-term supplementation with 700 IU of vitamin D and 500 mg of calcium daily on health, including associations between combined supplementation and changes in fasting glucose levels, found that subjects with impaired fasting glucose who followed the supplementation regimen for 3 years had a significantly lower rise in fasting glucose levels and less insulin resistance compared with placebo controls (Pittas et al., 2007a). Although the findings of this study are in agreement with a previous secondary analysis of data from the NHS cohort (see below: Pittas et al., 2006), the study is limited by the small number of outcomes measured compared with the total cohort; thus, an unintended bias cannot be ruled out. In addition, the study was designed for skeletal outcomes as the primary analysis. When the totality of the evidence was considered, the negative findings from the clinical trials for an effect of vitamin D or calcium on risk for type 2 diabetes together with the lack of significant evidence from either the AHRQ reviews or the meta-analysis by Pittas et al. (2007b) compelled the committee to conclude that there was not sufficient evidence to establish a causal relationship.

Observational Studies

Low serum 25OHD levels have been implicated in metabolic syndrome, abdominal obesity, and hyperglycemia.

In a prospective cohort analysis of data from NHS, women were followed for 20 years to examine associations between vitamin D and calcium intake and risk for type 2 diabetes (Pittas et al., 2006). A significant inverse association was found between total vitamin D intake and calcium intake and risk for type 2 diabetes. A separate analysis of the association between risk for type 2 diabetes and dairy food consumption found that women who consumed three or more dairy servings per day were at lower risk compared with those who consumed less than one dairy serving per day. These findings suggest that risk for type 2 diabetes is associated with vitamin D or dairy food intake. A small cohort study in obese and overweight individuals found that in addition to a significant inverse association between serum 25OHD level and weight and waist circumference there was a weak inverse relationship with hemoglobin A1c. However, no association between serum 25OHD level and any other indicators of type 2 diabetes or metabolic syndrome were observed (McGill et al., 2008).

In other observational evidence reviewed, a cross–sectional survey of Polynesian and white adult populations in New Zealand found a significantly lower serum 25OHD level in subjects with newly diagnosed diabetes and impaired glucose tolerance compared with controls. In addition, among the control groups, the native New Zealand populations (Maori and Pacific Islanders) were found to have significantly lower serum 25OHD levels compared with Europeans. The authors speculated that the low serum 25OHD level in the native populations explained, in part, the higher prevalence of diabetes in those groups (Scragg et al., 1995). Isaia et al. (2001), in a cross–sectional study in Italy, found that postmenopausal women diagnosed with type 2 diabetes had significantly higher body mass indexes (BMIs), lower activity scores, higher prevalence of serum 25OHD levels below 12.5 nmol/L, and lower dietary calcium intake compared with controls. In summary, these observational studies fail to provide conclusive support of a relationship between vitamin D intake and risk for either type 2 diabetes or metabolic syndrome because of the lack of consistency among studies, the paucity of high-quality large cohort studies, and the lack of strength for an association between vitamin D status and incidence of type 2 diabetes or metabolic syndrome.

Concluding Statement

The available evidence from observational studies of the associations between vitamin D and calcium and risk for type 2 diabetes or metabolic syndrome and secondary analyses from RCTs on markers of glucose tolerance proved insufficiently strong to support DRI development. The association studies linking lower serum 25OHD levels to increased risk for type 2 diabetes may be confounded by overweight and obesity, which not only predispose individuals to type 2 diabetes, but also cause lower serum 25OHD levels as a result of sequestration in fat and possibly other mechanisms. Although both retrospective and prospective studies tend to support an inverse association between serum 25OHD levels and type 2 diabetes, these studies are limited by the study design and cannot show a causal relationship. Evidence from RCTs on the effect of vitamin D supplements on incident diabetes or markers of glucose homeostasis is variable, and few RCTs showing significant results were identified. Taken together, the evidence in support of a role for vitamin D as a modulator of pancreatic endocrine function and insulin synthesis and secretion is not conclusive and therefore is not sufficient to support glucose tolerance as an indicator for DRI development.

Falls and Physical Performance

The committee considered falls and physical performance as independent indicators. However, because of the integration of these indicators in the literature reviewed by the committee, the evidence for both indicators is examined together in this section.

The risk of falling is a major concern among the elderly, because falls can lead to fracture and long-term disability or death in this population. Vitamin D is necessary for normal development and growth of muscle fibers, and vitamin D deficiency may adversely affect muscle strength. Muscle weakness and pain (myopathy) are characteristics of rickets and osteomalacia and contribute to poor physical performance (Prineas et al., 1965; Skaria et al., 1975; Yoshikawa et al., 1979). Thus vitamin D-deficiency muscle weakness and the implications of poor muscle tone suggest a relationship between serum 25OHD level and risk for falling and/or poor physical performance in susceptible populations.

Biological Plausibility

Experimental evidence suggests that vitamin D exerts its effect on muscle tissue via the VDR, but it may also use other pathways. In vitro and in vivo experiments provide evidence to support calcitriol regulation of calcium uptake by muscle, which, in turn, controls muscle contraction and relaxation, synthesis of muscle cytoskeletal proteins involved in muscle contraction, and muscle cell proliferation and differentiation (reviewed in Ceglia, 2008). Because intracellular calcium levels control the contraction and relaxation of muscle, thus affecting muscle function, it is possible that calcium intake may also affect risk for falls and poor physical performance (reviewed in Ceglia, 2008). However, the topic is not considered in more detail here because of the lack of observational and RCT data on the relationship between calcium intake and physical performance.

Systematic Reviews and Meta-Analyses

The AHRQ-Ottawa systematic review identified a total of 14 RCTs in addition to five prospective cohort studies and one case–control study that examined vitamin D and risk for falls in postmenopausal women and elderly men. The evidence between the RCTs and observational studies was discordant. Overall the review reported that the evidence for an association between low serum 25OHD levels and risk of falls and measures of physical performance among postmenopausal women and elderly men was inconsistent and rated the evidence as "fair." The AHRQ-Tufts systematic review identified three additional RCTs (Bunout et al., 2006; Burleigh et al., 2007; Lyons et al., 2007), but these studies did not find a significant effect of vitamin D supplementation on reducing risk of falls or poor performance in the elderly and were given a "C" rating. No additional observational evidence was found for this indicator in the AHRQ-Tufts review.

A meta-analysis reported in AHRQ-Tufts, which included the AHRQ-Ottawa RCTs, highlighted the inconsistency of findings from RCTs on the effect of vitamin D treatment on reduction in risk or prevention of falls. A smaller meta-analysis by Bischoff-Ferrari et al. (2004a) examined RCTs in elderly populations for evidence of a reduction in risk for falls with "vitamin D"; however, only three studies used vitamin D, and the other two studies used calcitriol/1α-hydroxycholecalciferol. Some of the studies identified in this meta-analysis were also included in the AHRQ-Tuft analysis. In contrast to the AHRQ-Tufts analysis, Bischoff-Ferrari et al. (2004a) found, from pooled results, a significant reduction in risk of falling among subjects treated with vitamin D compared with those treated with calcium or placebo. This disparity in findings is best explained by the small numbers in the Bischoff-Ferrari et al. (2004a) analysis and the fact that none of the vitamin D studies pooled by Bischoff-Ferrari et al. (2004a) was individually significant.

A meta-analysis published in 2009 by Bischoff-Ferrari et al. (2009a) examined fall prevention based on supplemental intake and serum 25OHD concentrations. From this analysis of the eight RCTs ($n = 2,426$ subjects) that met the inclusion criteria, the authors concluded that supplemental vitamin D intake (700 to 1,000 IU/day) reduced the risk of falling among older subjects by 19 percent and that serum 25OHD concentrations less than 60 nmol/L may not reduce the risk of falling. This meta-analysis as conducted has major limitations.

First, the stated inclusion/exclusion criteria and their application are problematic. As stated by the authors, to be included in the primary analysis, the trial design had to be double-blinded and the assessment of falls had to be a primary or secondary endpoint defined at the onset of the trial. The study had to include a definition of falls and how they were assessed, and falls had to be assessed for the entire trial period. Studies using patients with Parkinson's disease, organ transplant recipients, or stroke patients were excluded as were trials using intramuscular injection of vitamin D. Of concern is the fact that some studies that met the inclusion/exclusion criteria were omitted, and at least one study that failed to meet the criteria was included. The Broe et al. (2007) study, did not have a secondary analysis that pre-specified falls as an outcome, was never powered to examine the incidence of falls; with the wide confidence interval due to small sample size the results are questionable. This study influenced the analysis considerably; other than the work of Pfeifer et al. (2009), it was the single largest contributor to the effect. The work of Law et al. (2006) was excluded because it was a cluster randomization design instead of individual randomization; however, such a design does not appear to violate the authors' stated criteria. It was also excluded because the dose of oral vitamin D (50,000 IU) was given every 3 months; however, the serum 25OHD increased from 45 to 75 nmol/L, indicating an adequate therapeutic level. Had the Law et al. (2006) study been included, in which 44 percent of the vitamin D–treated group and 43 percent of the control group were fallers (not significantly different), the overall results would have been negative.

Second and more importantly, Figure 3 as reported in Bischoff-Ferrari et al. (2009a) is inappropriately presented. The figure is intended to demonstrate fall prevention with dose of vitamin D and achieved serum 25OHD concentrations. Specifically, the figure is a meta-regression analysis of the relative risk (RR) against vitamin D dose or serum 25OHD concentration. However, the meta-regression appears to be incorrectly carried out, or the authors used assumptions that were not specified in the methods section of their publication. In their analysis, the dependent variable appearing in the graph is RR (linear scale of 0 to 2.5); however, log(RR) is typically used in this type of meta-regression, which is a weighted linear regression with each study being the unit of analysis. Even when RR is to be reported, a meta-regression of log(RR) against the predictor variable should be carried out and then retransformed back to the RR scale, in which case the line will be curvilinear instead of straight. Carrying out a meta-regression analysis using untransformed RR in the linear scale assumes an exponential relationship of the dose with effect. Moreover, the predictor variable (x-axis) is equally spaced for data points, but the data points are not equally spaced according to the vitamin D doses (or serum 25OHD concentrations). In the top panel of Figure 3 in Bischoff-Ferrari et al. (2009a), the dose intervals between the data points range from 0 IU (two 400 IU studies; two 800 IU studies) to 100 IU (between 600 IU and 700 IU) to 200 IU (between 200 IU and 400 IU, 400 IU and 600 IU, 800 IU and 1,000 IU). Two data points were also composed of multiple trials "collapsed" into a single data point for two levels (800 IU of vitamin D_3; 1,000 IU of vitamin D_2) of the predictor variables. This introduces considerable uncertainty as to the appropriateness of the location of the regression line. If the measurement intervals had been appropriately and evenly spaced, it is very likely that the conclusion of the analysis would have been that no significant relationship was demonstrated.

The importance of the limitations of this study becomes clear when the data are reanalyzed in the appropriate statistical manner. As shown in Figures 4-2 and 4-3, no dose–response relationship between vitamin D intake and risk of falls is evident. For this analysis, which used the STATA program, analyses were repeated by fitting a random effects meta-regression with the log(RR) of sustaining at least one fall as the response variable and the daily dose of vitamin D supplementation or the mean achieved 25OHD serum concentration in the vitamin D supplementation arm as the predictor variable (both predictor variables are continuous variables). Specifically, the results do not show a significant dose–response relationship between the risk of sustaining at least one fall and the daily dose of vitamin D supplementation or achieved 25OHD serum concentration (beta coefficient = −0.0005 ± 0.0003 and = −0.0087 ± 0.0056 standard error [SE], respectively; relative risk reduction = 0.95 for risk of falls per 100 IU/day and increased in dose of vitamin D, $p = 0.13$; relative risk reduction = 0.92 for risk of falls for every 10 nmol/L increase in 25OHD level, $p = 0.17$). Both analyses had significant heterogeneity across studies ($I^2 = 47$ percent, $p = 0.05$; $I^2 = 54$ percent, $p = 0.03$, respectively). Further, a non-linear dose–response relationship was explored by adding a quadratic term of the predictor variable to the model. The result suggests that a U-shaped curve

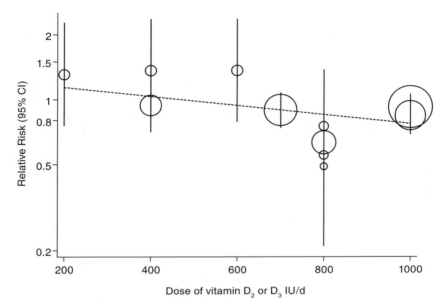

FIGURE 4-2 Relative risk of falls and vitamin D supplementation doses: Correct meta-regressions with continuous predictors showing non-significance.
NOTE: Relative risk reduction is 0.95 (95% confidence interval [CI] 0.89 to 1.02; $p = 0.13$) per 100 IU/day difference (increase) in dose.

better describes the relationship between the risk of sustaining at least one fall and the achieved serum 25OHD concentrations.

Additional Evidence from Randomized Controlled Trials

As discussed above, among RCTs that tested for effects of vitamin D with and without calcium on reduction in risk for falls, no consistent outcome was found. As described above, the data related to falls are questionable, and among muscle performance studies one included 12 subjects who were post-stroke patients and a second included 16 subjects for whom the study was only 8 weeks in length.

Two recent studies published after the AHRQ-Tufts analysis was completed have failed to show efficacy in reducing falls. A randomized but not placebo-controlled trial examined the effect of either 800 or 2,000 IU of vitamin D per day combined with enhanced or standard physiotherapy on the rate of falls and hospital re-admission following hip fracture in free-living adults with a mean age of 84 years (Bischoff-Ferrari et al., 2010). Neither of the two dosages of vitamin D_3 reduced the rate of falls or improved

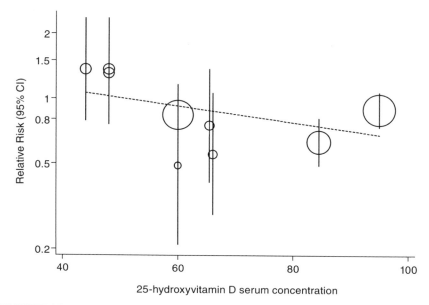

FIGURE 4-3 Relative risk of falls and mean achieved serum 25OHD concentrations: Correct meta-regressions with continuous predictors showing non-significance.
NOTE: Relative risk reduction is 0.92 (95% confidence interval [CI] 0.80 to 1.05; $p =$ 0.17) per 10 nmol/L difference (increase) in mean achieved 25OHD concentration.

strength or function compared with physiotherapy. Another study (Sanders et al., 2010) that examined the incidence of falls and fractures in elderly women treated with 500,000 IU of vitamin D_3 annually for 3 years found a significant increase in falls and fractures in the treatment group compared with the placebo group. Notably, the increased incidence of falls was significant in the treatment group by 3 months following administration of the supplemental vitamin D. Further, as described in Chapter 6, the authors of this study concluded that levels of 65 nmol/L were not consistent with reduced rates of fall or fractures.

When this committee considered the totality of evidence for causality pertinent to the relationship between vitamin D and incidence of or risk for falls, it became clear that the greater part of the causal evidence indicated no significant reduction in fall risk related to vitamin D intake or achieved level in blood. Table 4-4 illustrates the range of clinical trial data assessing changes in fall incidence or risk for falls with varying levels of vitamin D treatment that were taken into account. Of the 18 studies considered, including several studies identified in Bischoff-Ferrari et al. (2009a), only 4 (Pfeifer et al., 2000; Harwood et al., 2004; Flicker et al.,

162

TABLE 4-4 Outcome Measures for Falls: Summary of Evidence from Randomized Trials with Vitamin D and Calcium

Reference; Study Duration; Outcome	N	Vitamin D Dose	Calcium Dose	Serum 25OHD level (nmol/L) Baseline	Serum 25OHD level (nmol/L) Achieved	Falls	Fallers	RR/OR (95% CI) / (p-value)
Studies using oral doses								
Bischoff et al., 2003[a] 12 weeks follow-up (primary analysis)	122	Placebo 800 IU/d	1,200 mg/d 1,200 mg/d	29.0 (23.0–25.0) 30.8 (23.0–55.0)	28.0 (24.5–41.5) 65.5 (49.8–82.8)	✓	✓	0.68 (0.30–1.54) 0.70 (0.30–1.50)
Bischoff-Ferrari et al., 2006b 3-year trial (secondary outcome of primary analysis)	Women: 246 Men: 199	Women: Placebo 700 IU/d Men: Placebo 700 IU/d	Women: Placebo 500 mg/d Men: Placebo 500 mg/d	Women: 63.0 (± 30.3) 70.0 (± 33.0) Men: 83.0 (± 33.5) 82.0 (± 37.5)	Women: 68.0 (± 32.5) 104.0 (± 41.8) Men: 76.5 (± 27.3) 110.0 (± 34.0)		Women: ✓ Men: ✓	Women: 0.44 (0.21–0.90) Men: 0.84 (0.42–1.66)
Bischoff-Ferrari et al., 2010 12-month trial (primary outcome)	173	800 IU/d 2,000 IU/d	500 mg/d 500 mg/d	30.8 (± 19.3) 33.0 (± 20.3)	88.5 (± 25.3) 111.8 (± 26.0)	✓		28 (−4.0–68.0)
Broe et al., 2007 5-month study period (secondary analysis)	124	Placebo 200 IU/d 400 IU/d 600 IU/d 800 IU/d	None None None None None	53.0 (± 28.5) 44.5 (± 23.0) 51.8 (± 29.0) 41.3 (± 18.5) 53.5 (± 23.0)		✓		1.10 (0.49–2.50) 1.05 (0.48–2.28) 1.21 (0.55–2.61) **0.28 (0.10–0.75)**[b]
Burleigh et al., 2007[a] 30 days (primary outcome)	203	Placebo 800 IU/d	1,200 mg/d 1,200 mg/d	24.7 (± 10.0) 21.7 (± 7.1)		✓	✓	0.82 (0.59–1.16)

Study	N	Intervention	Calcium					Result
Chapuy et al., 2002 2-year trial (secondary analysis)	583	Placebo	none	22.8 (±17.3)	15.0		✓	1.08 (0.75–1.55) treatment groups combined
		800 IU/d or Ca combined	1,200 mg/d	22.5 (±16.5)	80.0			
		800 IU/d + Ca given separately	1,200 mg/d	21.3 (±13.3)	75.0			
Flicker et al., 2005 2-year follow-up (primary outcome)	540	Placebo	600 mg/d	42.5		✓	✓	0.73 (0.57–0.95)[b]
		10,000 IU/wk later 1,000IU/d	600 mg/d	40.0				0.82 (0.59–1.12)
Graafmans et al., 1996 28-week follow-up (primary outcome)		Placebo	none			✓	✓	1.00 (0.60–1.80)
		400 IU/d	none	65.0				1.00 (0.60–1.50)
Grant et al., 2005[c] 24- to 62-month follow-up (secondary analysis)	5,292	Placebo	none	38.0	45.4	✓	✓	Subjects on Vit D vs no vit D
		Calcium	1,000 mg/d		42.0			
		800 IU/d	none		62.5			
		800 IU/d + Ca	1,000 mg/d		62.0			0.97 (0.84–1.12)
Larsen et al., 2005 42-month trial (primary outcome)	2,426	No intervention	none				✓	Women:
		400 IU/d	1,000 mg/d	35.0				0.89 (0.79–1.03) Men: 1.07 (0.90–1.27)

continued

TABLE 4-4 Continued

Reference; Study Duration; Outcome	N	Vitamin D Dose	Calcium Dose	Serum 25OHD level (nmol/L)		Falls	Fallers	RR/OR (95% CI) / (p-value)
				Baseline	Achieved			
Law et al., 2006 10-month trial (primary outcome)	3,717	No pills 1,100 IU/d	none none	47.0 (35.0–102.0)	74.0 (52.0–110.0)	✓	✓	1.09 (0.95–1.25) 1.36 (0.80–2.34)
Pfeifer et al., 2009 12-month trial; follow-up at 20 months (primary outcome)	242	Placebo 800 IU/d	1,000 mg/d 1,000 mg/d	54.0 (± 18.0) 55.0 (± 18.0)	57.0 (± 20.0) 84.0 (± 18.0)	✓	✓	**0.61 (0.34–0.76)**[b] **0.40 (p < 0.001)**
Pfeifer et al., 2000 8-week trial (primary outcome)	137	Placebo 800 IU/d	1,200 mg/d 1,200 mg/d	24.6 (± 12.1) 25.7 (± 13.6)	42.9 (± 20.1) 66.2 (± 27.0)	✓	✓	**0.55 (0.29–1.06)**[d]
Prince et al., 2008 1-year trial (primary outcome)	302	Placebo 1,000 IU/d	1,000 mg/d 1,000 mg/d	44.3 (± 12.8) 42.3 (± 12.5)	44.3 60.0		✓	0.66 (0.41–1.06)
Trivedi et al., 2003[c] 5-year trial (secondary analysis)	2,686	Placebo 100,000 IU 3 doses/y	none none		53.4 (±21.1) 74.3 (± 20.7)		✓	Women: 1.03 (0.72–1.48) Men: 0.87 (0.68–1.12)
Studies using injected doses								
Dhesi et al., 2004[a] 6-month trial (secondary outcome)	123	Placebo 600,000 IU IM injection once	none none	25.0 (23.8–26.3) 26.8 (25.5–28.0)	31.5 (28.5–34.5) 43.8 (41.3–46.3)	✓	✓	0.24 (p = 0.28) 11 (p = 0.52)

Study	N	Intervention	Calcium	Value	Value			RR/OR (95% CI)
Harwood et al., 2004[c] 1-year trial (secondary analysis)	150	No treatment 300,000 IU IM once 300,000 IU IM once 800 IU/d	0 mg/d 0 mg/d 1,000 mg/d 1,000 mg/d	30.0 (12.0–64.0) 28.0 (10.0–67.0) 30.0 (12.0–85.0) 30.0 (12.0–64.0)	27.0 40.0 44.0 50.0		✓	0.48 (0.3–0.9)
Latham et al., 2003 6-month follow-up (secondary outcome)	122	Placebo 300,000 IU once	none none	47.5 40.0	47.5 62.5	✓		1.12 (0.79–1.59)
Sanders et al., 2010 3-year trial (primary outcome)	2,256	Placebo 500,000 IU/y	none none	45.0 (40.0–57.5) 53.0 (40.0–65.0)	Median 55.0–75.0	✓	✓	1.15 (1.02–1.30) 0.74 (*p* = 0.03)
Smith et al., 2007 3-year trial (secondary analysis)	9,440	Placebo 300,000 IU IM injection/y	none none	56.5 56.5	56.5 68.5	✓		0.98 (0.94–1.04)

NOTE: CI = confidence interval; IM = intramuscular; IU = International Units; OR = odds ratio; RR = relative risk; y = year.
[a]Included in AHRQ-Ottawa (Cranney et al., 2007) and/or AHRQ-Tufts (Chung et al., 2009).
[b]**Bolding** indicates significant difference and is presented for assessment of causality.
[c]Discussed in the "Skeletal Health" section below.
[d]Data provided in Bischoff-Ferrari et al. (2009a).

2005; Broe et al., 2007) found a significant effect of vitamin D on fall incidence. The only two significant studies for fallers are Pfeifer et al. (2000, 2009), although Pfeifer et al. (2000) was a 2-month study and administered calcium with the vitamin D placebo.

Observational Studies

Observational studies have long suggested an association between a higher serum 25OHD level and a lower risk of falls in elderly persons; however, when analyzed as a whole in the AHRQ reviews, there was no consistency between study findings. Snijder et al. (2006), a study of elderly subjects participating in the Longitudinal Aging Study Amsterdam, a prospective cohort study, was not included in the AHRQ reviews. This study found that a low serum 25OHD level (< 25 nmol/L) was independently associated with an increased risk of falling for subjects who experienced two or more falls compared with those who did not fall or fell once; however the study outcome does not affect the discordant findings among observational studies identified in the AHRQ reviews.

Most observational studies of associations between serum 25OHD levels and physical performance have been cross–sectional, which limits causal inference. A cross–sectional study of 4,100 older adults from NHANES III found higher serum 25OHD concentrations associated with better lower-extremity function (Bischoff-Ferrari et al., 2004b). Much of the improvement occurred at concentrations ranging from 22.5 nmol/L to approximately 40 nmol/L, but some improvement was also seen from 40 to 94 nmol/L (the top of the reference range). Results were similar in men and women, three racial/ethnic groups (whites, African Americans, and Mexican Americans), active and inactive persons, and those with high and low calcium intakes. A study of Dutch adults 65 years of age and older found that serum 25OHD concentrations below 20 nmol/L were significantly associated with poorer physical performance at baseline and a greater decline in physical performance over a 3-year period (Wicherts et al., 2007). Another cross–sectional study of healthy post-menopausal women found that serum 25OHD level was significantly associated with physical fitness indexes, including balance, handgrip strength, androidal fat mass, and lean mass (Stewart et al., 2009). Finally, a cross–sectional study of 60 men and women with heart failure (mean age of 77 years) found a significant association between serum 25OHD level and 6-minute walk distance and frailty status (Boxer et al., 2008). Taken together, however, this evidence is weakened by the cross–sectional study design, does not provide strong support for an association between serum 25OHD level and physical performance, and does not contradict the findings of the AHRQ reviews.

Concluding Statement

A problem in a number of the RCTs is that falls rather than fallers are analyzed; consequently, individuals who fell more than once were also counted more than once in the primary outcome analysis. The studies generally did not have the statistical power to detect a significant difference in the number of fallers but relied on repeat fallers to achieve the desired number of total falls. Moreover, the meta-analyses described above combined data from the few trials in which fallers were counted with data from trials in which falls were the outcome. By comparison, the U.S. Food and Drug Administration (FDA) mandated primary outcomes in osteoporosis and cardiovascular trials are the number of individuals with fractures or cardiovascular events rather than the number of events. It remains uncertain whether a reduction in the number of falls can be used to infer that the number of fallers would be significantly reduced.

The committee's review of the available evidence, including the results from RCTs and observational associations between vitamin D with or without calcium and risk for falls and poor physical performance, indicates a lack of sufficiently strong evidence to support DRI development. A limited review of observational data outside of the AHRQ reviews found some support for an association between 25OHD levels and physical performance. However, high-quality observational evidence from large cohort studies was lacking. Additionally, although the cross–sectional studies were more supportive of an association between high serum 25OHD levels and reduced risk for falls, evidence from RCTs in particular showed outcomes that varied in significance and thus did not support the observational findings or a causal relationship. The evidence was also not consistently supportive for a role for vitamin D combined with calcium in reduction of risk for falls.

Overall, data from RCTs suggest that vitamin D dosages of at least 800 IU/day, either alone or in combination with calcium, may confer benefits for physical performance measures. Although high doses of vitamin D (i.e., ≥ 800 IU/day) appear to provide greater benefit for physical performance than low doses (i.e., 400 IU/day), evidence is insufficient to define the shape of the dose–response curve for higher levels of intake. Thus, the outcome of physical performance is appropriate for identifying Estimated Average Requirements (EARs) of vitamin D, with or without calcium, in adults above the age of 50, but cannot be used to define the shape of the dose–response curve at higher levels of intake.

Immune Responses

Vitamin D has been reported to modulate immune functioning in cell culture and animal models. Vitamin D, specifically its active form, calcitriol, is a regulator of both adaptive and innate immune responses. However, its role is complex and not fully understood. Many factors influence the specific effect of vitamin D on immune function including its target cells; the nature of the immune challenge and response (either autoimmune or anti-infective); the status and availability of calcium, depending on the tissue or cell type; the physiological, differentiated or activated stage of the tissue or cell type; and the expression and polymorphisms of the genes for the *Vdr* and 1α-hydroxylase.

Asthma

Asthma is a chronic lung disease that manifests as inflammation in bronchial tissue. The disease is characterized by recurrent periods of wheezing, chest tightness, shortness of breath, and coughing and may be accompanied by comorbidities, such as eczema or atopic dermatitis. Diet has long been linked to asthma and allergic disease. Dietary sodium and magnesium intakes were implicated as risk factors for asthma in the 1980s and 1990s (Burney, 1987; Britton et al., 1994a, b). Dietary lipids have also been hypothesized to contribute to increased prevalence of asthma (Black and Sharpe, 1997). More recently, vitamin D has been linked to asthma incidence in the developing fetus and in young children (Litonjua and Weiss, 2007).

Biological plausibility   Genetic studies mapping the *Vdr* gene in animal models of asthma suggest that *Vdr* polymorphism is linked with expression of asthma. In humans, Poon et al. (2004) compared *Vdr* genetic variants between members of a family-based cohort (223 families of 1,139 individuals) with and without asthma. Their analysis found significant associations between six polymorphisms in the *Vdr* gene and clinical diagnosis of asthma. Wjst (2005) conducted genotyping on 951 individuals from pedigrees that had at least two asthmatic children to determine whether transmission of *Vdr* polymorphism was associated with asthma in the children. Preferential transmission of candidate polymorphisms in asthmatic children could not be confirmed; however, the authors did hypothesize the possibility of transmitting a protective effect to unaffected offspring based on their finding of a low probability of an unaffected phenotype in an affected cohort.

Systematic reviews and meta-analyses   No systematic reviews or meta-analyses were identified for this indicator.

Additional evidence from randomized controlled trials   No RCTs were identified for this indicator.

Observational studies   A few studies were identified that examined a genetic linkage between vitamin D and risk for asthma or related conditions, and these were discussed above. Additional observational studies examined the relationship between perinatal serum 25OHD levels and risk of asthma in offspring. Devereux et al. (2007) examined associations between vitamin D intake during pregnancy and risk for childhood wheezing in a large prospective cohort study; a significant inverse association was found between maternal intake of vitamin D from diet and supplements and symptoms of wheezing at 2 and 5 years of age, although there was no significant association with diagnosed asthma at 5 years of age. In another study, Camargo et al. (2007) assessed the relationship between maternal dietary intake of vitamin D during pregnancy and risk of wheezing in children in Project Viva, a large prospective cohort study examining prenatal factors and pregnancy and child health outcomes. Overall, higher maternal intake of vitamin D during pregnancy was significantly associated with a lower risk for recurrent wheezing in the offspring at 3 years of age when compared with the lowest maternal vitamin D intake. Other associated symptoms of respiratory infection and eczema, however, were not significantly associated with maternal vitamin D intake. Similarly, Hypponen et al. (2004) found in a large prospective cohort study in Finland, that the prevalence of atopy and allergic rhinitis in subjects at age 31 years was higher among those who received regular vitamin D supplementation as infants than among those who did not; however, this study relied on retrospective recall of supplementation by the mother.

These large prospective cohort studies support an association between maternal or infant vitamin D intake and risk related to symptoms of asthma, particularly wheezing, but not with diagnosed disease. Several other observational studies have examined associations between 25OHD level in blood and risk for asthma. Gale et al. (2008), in a small prospective cohort study, found a five times increased risk for asthma at 9 years among children whose mothers' serum 25OHD level was below 27.5 nmol/L, compared with those whose mothers had levels above 75 nmol/L. The small size of the cohort that was followed to 9 years of age (178 subjects) was a limitation to the reported finding. In contrast, a larger analysis of NHANES data found no association between serum 25OHD level and sensitization to allergens (Wjst and Hypponen, 2007). The study did identify an increased prevalence of allergic rhinitis across levels of 25OHD, although unrecognized confounding may account for the association.

In a cross–sectional study examining associations between vitamin D status and markers of allergic or asthmatic response, Brehm et al. (2009) found that serum vitamin D levels below 75 nmol/L were identified in 28 percent of children and that inflammatory markers (immunoglobulin E

[IgE] and eosinophil count) were significantly and inversely associated with vitamin D status. These lower quality observational studies largely support the associations with symptoms of asthma identified in the larger cohort studies but do not support an association between 25OHD level in blood and diagnosed asthma.

Although genetic studies support a possible biological mechanism for a functional role of vitamin D in development of asthma there are no RCTs to demonstrate a causal role.

Autoimmune Diseases

Autoimmune diseases such as multiple sclerosis (MS), rheumatoid arthritis (RA), inflammatory bowel disease (IBD), and lupus are characterized by abnormal T cell response to self, resulting in inflammatory reactions in peripheral tissues. Models of autoimmune diseases support a role for vitamin D in regulating the T helper 1 (Th1) immune response, an integral component of immune tolerance with regard to recognition of self (reviewed in Cantorna and Mahon, 2005; Szodoray et al., 2008). Recent genomic analyses for polymorphisms in the *Vdr* gene suggest that single nucleotide polymorphisms identified in individuals with type 1 diabetes could negatively modulate calcitriol synthesis and thereby play a detrimental role in autoimmune response and subsequent manifestation of the disease (Israni et al., 2009).

Diabetes (type 1) Type 1 diabetes is a chronic disease resulting from loss of β-cell function in the pancreas. The disease is characterized by diminished or absent insulin production and loss of control of blood glucose. Emerging evidence for an association between low vitamin D status and increased risk for type 1 diabetes comes from experimental animal, ecological, and observational studies; however, no intervention trials using supplemental vitamin D (not analogues) were identified to provide causal support for a relationship.

Biological plausibility Experimental animal, ecological, and observational evidence support a relationship between vitamin D status and risk for type 1 diabetes, although treatment protocols and dosages vary. Ecological evidence has suggested a link between type 1 diabetes risk and limited erythemal UVB exposure in Newfoundland (Sloka et al., 2009, 2010). Mohr et al. (2008) plotted incidence rates for type 1 diabetes by latitude in an ecologic study comparing geographical distribution, estimated UVB exposure and disease incidence and, using a polynomial analysis to best fit the data points, determined that the incidence of type 1 diabetes was greater at higher latitudes.

In nonobese diabetic (NOD) mice, which are genetically predisposed to develop insulitis and type 1 diabetes, disease developed earlier when the mice were fed vitamin D–deficient diet and reared in the absence of UV light (Giulietti et al., 2004). However, type 1 diabetes was not prevented when NOD mice were treated with a supraphysiological dose of vitamin D, beginning from conception and continuing to 10 weeks of age (Hawa et al., 2004). Additionally, in a study in which NOD mice were cross bred with mice null for the *Vdr* gene, the rate of disease presentation did not differ from that in mice carrying only the NOD mutation, even though immune abnormalities were aggravated by the absence of the VDR (Gysemans, 2008). These results indicate that severe vitamin D and UV deficiency can increase the risk of type I diabetes in a genetically predisposed animal, yet neither vitamin D nor the absence of the *Vdr* gene affects the onset of type 1 diabetes.

Systematic reviews and meta-analyses   Neither AHRQ-Ottawa nor AHRQ-Tufts included type 1 diabetes as a health outcome in its systematic reviews. Another recent systematic review and meta-analysis of five observational, four case–control and one cohort study (no RCTs were found) assessed whether vitamin D supplementation of infants reduced risk for type 1 diabetes later in life (Zipitis and Akobeng, 2008). The meta-analysis of data from the four case–control studies revealed a significant 29 percent reduction in risk for type 1 diabetes among vitamin D–supplemented infants compared with controls, which was further supported by the cohort study. The authors also cited evidence for a dose–response effect based on studies indicating reduced likelihood for developing diabetes among subjects who received regular vitamin D supplements, whereas subjects who developed rickets early in life were more likely to develop diabetes. A limitation of this meta-analysis is that two of the studies included had study designs that relied on delayed retrospective recalls by the mothers of vitamin D–supplemented infants. Additionally, no other meta-analyses were identified that either support or refute the findings of Zipitis and Akobeng (2008).

Additional evidence from randomized controlled trials   No RCTs were identified for this indicator.

Observational studies   No additional observational evidence that was not included in the systematic reviews and meta-analysis was identified for consideration.

Inflammatory bowel and Crohn's disease   IBD is a group of conditions of chronic inflammation that usually involve the distal portion of the ileum. In Crohn's disease, inflammation spreads to the colon and upper gastrointestinal tract and causes local abscesses, scarring, and bowel obstruction; the condition is also characterized by diarrhea, cramping, and loss of appetite and weight. Vitamin D status has been linked to IBD in association studies of sun exposure and in genetic studies through down-regulation of the Th1-mediated immune response.

Biological plausibility   Ecological studies have linked vitamin D, particularly 25OHD levels, to a number of autoimmune diseases. A connection between seasonal vitamin D status and risk for Crohn's disease was proposed by Peyrin-Biroulet et al. (2009), based largely on ecological evidence for an association between low 25OHD levels in blood and other autoimmune diseases. The effect of seasonal variation on serum 25OHD levels in patients with Crohn's disease, compared to matched controls found that mean serum 25OHD was lower in Crohn's patients despite having vitamin D intake from foods and supplements and sunlight exposure similar to those of matched controls (McCarthy et al., 2005). Genetic evidence in humans and in animal models provides some support for a biological association between polymorphisms in the *Vdr* and susceptibility to IBD and Crohn's disease. In a human study, a linkage analysis, used to identify the *TaqI* polymorphism in the *Vdr* gene, suggested that the variant may be a candidate for conferring susceptibility to IBD (Simmons et al., 2000). Animal model studies in both vitamin D–deficient and *Vdr* null mice suggested that the risk of developing IBD is increased in several respects: spontaneous occurrences are increased, the disease is more severe, and the disease is more easily provoked in response to agents that induce IBD or bacterial infections transferred from an affected animal (reviewed in Bouillon et al., 2008).

Systematic reviews and meta-analyses   The AHRQ-Tufts systematic review found no RCTs for immune function clinical outcomes and no evidence for IBD or Crohn's disease. Thus, the evidence was insufficient for further analysis in the systematic review. No meta-analyses were identified for this indicator.

Additional evidence from randomized controlled trials   No RCTs were identified for this indicator.

Observational studies   Two observational studies were identified that evaluated 25OHD levels in patients with Crohn's disease and/or IBD. A cross–sectional assessment of serum 25OHD levels in children and young adults with IBD living in Boston found that prevalence of low 25OHD status (≤ 38 nmol/L) averaged 34.6 percent overall, with higher prevalence in winter compared with summer (Pappa et al., 2006). A small population-based cohort of patients with Crohn's disease and ulcerative colitis in Scandinavia found a prevalence of 25OHD levels below 30 nmol/L in 27 percent of those with Crohn's disease and 15 percent of those with ulcerative colitis. In addition, patients with Crohn's disease had lower mean serum 25OHD levels compared with those with ulcerative colitis or the reference population (Jahnsen et al., 2002). The study design and poor controls characteristic of these observational studies diminish the reliability of their findings. Another confounding problem is that vitamin D is absorbed with fat in the terminal ileum, and this is the area that is most inflamed in Crohn's disease (and can become inflamed in ulcerative colitis). Consequently, low 25OHD levels can be expected to occur as a consequence of the inflammatory condition. The question not answered by these studies is whether low 25OHD levels can predispose individuals to the conditions.

Multiple sclerosis   MS is a chronic disease of the central nervous system that manifests as numbness in the limbs or, in more severe cases, paralysis or loss of vision. The progress, severity, and specific symptoms of MS are unpredictable and vary among individuals. The disease is an autoimmune response directed against myelin. Damaged myelin forms scar tissue (sclerosis), which impairs nerve impulse conduction, producing the variety of symptoms associated with the disease.

Biological plausibility   Similar to findings with other autoimmune-related diseases, low solar exposure, latitude, and polymorphisms in the *Vdr* gene have been implicated in susceptibility to MS (Partridge et al., 2004; Dwyer et al., 2008; Sloka et al., 2008; Dickinson et al., 2009). However, whether a lack of sun exposure is causally related to MS cannot be shown. Findings from animal models are not consistent. In a mouse model, vitamin D deficiency accelerated development of autoimmune encephalomyelitis (the murine model of MS in humans), whereas treatment with calcitriol reduced it (Cantorna et al., 1996). In contrast, a subsequent study, using a mouse model null for the *Vdr* gene, found that the *Vdr* null mice were protected from development of the disease compared with wild-type mice (Meehan and DeLuca, 2002). A recent genetic study in humans evaluating associations between specific *Vdr* gene polymorphisms (*Apal* and *Taq1*) and serum 25OHD levels in healthy adults compared with those with MS, found no relationship between mutations in *Apal* and *Taq1* and incidence of MS (Smolders et al., 2009). Taken together, neither ecological studies nor genetic studies in animal models and humans show consistency in finding a significant relationship between serum 25OHD level and presence of MS.

Systematic reviews and meta-analyses   The AHRQ-Tufts systematic review found no RCTs for immune function clinical outcomes and no evidence for MS related to vitamin D. In a recent review paper of observational studies on the effects of vitamin D on incidence and severity of MS, Smolders et al. (2008) concluded that there was no strong direct evidence supporting the ability of vitamin D to modulate MS or influence risk for the disease. Their review included observational evidence in humans linking low serum 25OHD levels with incidence of MS in white American adolescents; associations between lower circulating levels of 25OHD after onset of MS;

associations between skin pigmentation and lower disability scores in females; congruence of geographical distribution of MS with geographical distribution of low vitamin D levels; associations between seasonal variation in birth and in disease severity with the seasonal variation of low vitamin D levels; associations between remission and pregnancy (when calcitriol levels increase); and variations in risk associated with polymorphisms in the *Vdr* gene. In addition to the lack of positive evidence, the authors raised concerns about the safety of calcitriol treatment for MS because of the dose-dependent risk for hypercalcemia identified with calcitriol treatment in animal models. No meta-analyses were identified for this indicator.

Additional evidence from randomized controlled trials   No RCTs were identified for this indicator.

Observational studies   Observational studies in humans have also failed to show a consistent association between serum 25OHD levels and MS. A small longitudinal study of 23 MS patients and 23 controls found no differences in circulating 25OHD levels, no difference in seasonal variation, and comparable rates of vitamin D deficiency or insufficiency based on serum 25OHD levels between MS patients and controls (Soilu-Hanninen et al., 2008). Interestingly, in this study, serum 25OHD levels were significantly lower during relapse episodes, whereas serum levels of intact PTH were significantly higher than in remission periods in MS patients. A prospective nested case–control study in military personnel reported that, for white subjects, serum 25OHD levels were inversely related to the risk of MS and that effect was even greater when serum 25OHD levels were low in individuals under 20 years of age (Munger et al., 2006). Overall, serum 25OHD levels were lower in black and Hispanic compared to white subjects and 25OHD levels were more frequently in the range of 25 to 40 nmol/L in MS patients compared to controls. These findings, however, were unrelated to risk for MS (Munger et al., 2006). In a small population-based case–control study of individuals living at latitudes of 41 to 43°S (similar to New York City and Boston), van der Mei et al. (2007) found that serum 25OHD levels below 25 nmol/L were moderately associated with MS, compared with levels above 40 nmol/L. With more consistent serum 25OHD levels and less seasonal variability, there was an association with less disability.

Taken together, these observational studies show widely variable outcomes for associations between serum 25OHD levels and MS and such associations are not supported by meta-analyses. In addition, the lack of causal evidence further diminishes the likelihood for a relationship between vitamin D and MS.

Rheumatoid arthritis   RA is a chronic disease characterized by systemic inflammation that may affect many tissues and organs, but particularly the joints. In RA inflammatory synovitis of the joints can progress to destruction of the articular cartilage and ankylosis. RA can also produce diffuse inflammation in the lungs, pericardium, pleura, and sclera, as well as nodular lesions under the skin. This progressive disease can result in chronic pain, loss of function, and eventual disability.

Biological plausibility In experimental studies, Tetlow and Wooley (1999) found that the VDR was strongly expressed in cells associated with rheumatoid lesions, including macrophages, synovial fibroblasts, and chondrocytes, but weakly or not at all in normal articular cartilage tissue, suggesting an up-regulation of VDR-mediated activity in tissues affected by RA. Smith et al. (1999) found that cultured human synovial fibroblasts, but not human articular chondrocytes, when treated with the inflammatory cytokine, interleukin 1 (IL-1), followed by calcitriol, indicated inhibition of expression of the matrix metalloproteinases associated with RA. In a mouse model of RA, treatment with calcitriol decreased arthritis symptoms induced by injection with bovine collagen and halted the progression of arthritis after arthritic lesions were apparent (Cantorna et al., 1998). Together, this evidence is suggestive of an immunomodulatory role for vitamin D in expression of arthritic changes in some, but not all, cell types associated with RA.

Systematic reviews and meta-analyses The AHRQ systematic reviews found no RCTs for immune function clinical outcomes related to RA and no evidence that RA was related to vitamin D. No meta-analyses were identified for this indicator.

Additional evidence from randomized controlled trials No RCTs were identified for an effect of vitamin D and/or calcium on risk for RA.

Observational studies A number of studies have been conducted to determine whether serum 25OHD level and incidence of RA are associated. In a prospective cohort study, a small subset of subjects from the Iowa Women's Health Study were followed to determine if dietary vitamin D intake (primary outcome) and/or calcium intake (secondary outcome) were associated with incident RA (Merlino et al., 2004). No significant associations were found for dietary (not supplemented) vitamin D intake and risk for RA, although the association was significant for daily supplemental intakes of 400 IU or more compared with less than 400 IU. No association was found between calcium intake and risk for incident RA. A cross–sectional analysis of women with RA living in Brazil, found a significant correlation between higher mean serum calcium level and normal BMD compared with calcium levels in women with osteopenia, although no significant difference was found between calcium and vitamin D intake and BMD (Sarkis et al., 2009).

With no large prospective cohort studies and no clinical trials to support a relationship between vitamin D and/or calcium and RA, along with a paucity of other observational evidence, the committee could not conclude that either vitamin D or calcium is related to risk for RA.

Systemic lupus erythematosus Systemic lupus erythematosus (SLE) is a chronic generalized connective tissue disorder characterized by skin eruptions, arthralgia, arthritis, leukopenia, anemia, visceral lesions, neurological manifestations, and lymphadenopathy. It has been proposed that vitamin D plays a role in maintenance of immune homeostasis, and recent studies have linked SLE to vitamin D deficiency although a causal relationship has not been established.

Biological plausibility Mouse models of SLE have been reported to produce high levels of IgG2a immune cells that are implicated in the pathogenesis of lupus (Slack et al., 1984). However, owing to the complexity of the disease, experimental animal studies have not shown consistent outcomes on questions regarding the role for vitamin D in preventing or alleviating manifestations of the disease. Administration of calcitriol in a murine SLE model using a treatment protocol of daily dosing with a low-calcium diet for 4 weeks followed by dosing every other day for 18 weeks resulted in attenuation of symptoms of SLE, including reduced dermatological lesions. All SLE mice in the study developed proteinuria by 20 weeks; however, among those treated with vitamin D, lower urinary protein/creatinine ratios indicated reduced levels of proteinuria (Lemire et al., 1992). In contrast to these findings, when Vaisberg et al. (2000) injected SLE-prone mice with vitamin D_3, they found a worsening of the histopathological effects of SLE in the kidney. Upon examining serum levels of calcitriol and 25OHD in SLE patients compared with unaffected controls, Muller et al. (1995) found lower levels of calcitriol but not 25OHD, but were unable to speculate on a cause for the difference. In humans, vitamin D has been proposed to modulate maturation and induction of interferon alpha-(IFN-α)–mediated monocyte differentiation into dendritic cells that are activated in SLE. The findings of Ben-Zvi et al. (2010) suggest that such a role is likely via vitamin D–mediated inhibition of over-expression of IFN-regulated genes in cultured monocytes from both normal and SLE patients following exposure to an activation factor. Altogether, however, there is a lack of consistency in study outcomes between animal models and human experimental studies, and thus findings are not supportive of a biological role for vitamin D in SLE.

Systematic reviews and meta-analyses The AHRQ systematic reviews found no RCTs for immune function clinical outcomes related to SLE and no evidence for a relationship between SLE and vitamin D. No meta-analyses were identified for this indicator.

Additional evidence from randomized controlled trials No RCTs were identified that examined a role for vitamin D or calcium in reducing risk for or manifestations of symptoms of SLE.

Observational studies Epidemiological evidence to support an association between vitamin D status and incidence of SLE shows variability in the levels of 25OHD associated with SLE. Kamen et al. (2006), in a small subset of a larger population-based cohort, found that 22 out of 123 SLE patients across race, age, and gender groups had 25OHD levels below 25 nmol/L and that African Americans had levels significantly lower than whites (40 nmol/L compared with 78 nmol/L [p = 0.04]). In a small pilot study of 50 subjects (25 per group), Huisman et al. (2001) found that 50 percent of female SLE patients had 25OHD levels below 50 nmol/L. The associations between vitamin D status and incidence of SLE identified in these studies are not borne out by evidence from a prospective cohort study of dietary factors and risk for developing SLE. An analysis of a small subset of women participating in NHS over a period of 22 years found no association between vitamin D (or calcium) intake assessed with a food frequency questionnaire and risk for developing SLE or RA (Costenbader et al., 2008). In a cross–sectional survey, Ruiz-Irastorza et al. (2008) found that 75 percent of patients with SLE had serum 25OHD levels below 75 nmol/L and 15 percent had levels below 25 nmol/L, and 25OHD levels in blood in patients with SLE were not responsive to calcium and vitamin D treatment. Thus, it is not clear whether therapeutic treatment would have any effect on disease manifestation. The few relevant studies identified for review, and the lack of uniformly significant findings between studies, which may be a result of the small study populations (< 200 participants), are not sufficient to permit the committee to draw a conclusion about an association between SLE and vitamin D intake or 25OHD levels in blood.

Infectious Diseases

Tuberculosis   Pulmonary tuberculosis (TB) is a granulomatous infection in which hypercalcemia occurs in a subset of patients (Sharma et al., 1972; Abbasi et al., 1979; Need and Phillips, 1979). The increased production of immune and inflammatory cells in patients with TB correlates with increased serum levels of calcitriol (Adams et al., 1989) and with calcitriol in pleural fluid (Cadranel et al., 1994). Treatment of alveolar macrophages with IFN-γ appears to stimulate synthesis of calcitriol (Koeffler et al., 1985; Reichel et al., 1987). Although vitamin D has been used as a therapeutic agent in the management of TB (Martineau et al., 2007a), treatment of individuals with active TB with supplemental vitamin D exacerbates or reveals hypercalcemia (Sharma, 1981).

Biological plausibility   Vitamin D may be an important factor in innate immunity in the upper respiratory tract (reviewed in Bartley, 2010). Although calcitriol does not have direct anti-bacterial activity, it induces anti-tubercular actions in cultured monocytes and macrophages (Chan et al., 1994). Recent evidence, stemming from the molecular cloning of 1α-hydroxylase (Monkawa et al., 2000), supports macrophages as the source of 1α-hydroxylase that converts 25OHD to calcitriol and stimulates the mobilization of calcium seen in inflammatory diseases (Inui et al., 2001; Yokomura et al., 2003; Karakelides et al., 2006). Animal models provide additional evidence that calcitriol levels increase in tubercular infection. Rhodes et al. (2003) identified a transient increase in calcitriol levels following infection of cattle with bovine mycobacterium, but only among animals that went on to develop TB. This increase in activated vitamin D that accompanied infection suggests a role for vitamin D in the host immune reactivity to TB infection. In a mouse model, calcitriol increased production of nitric oxide, an endogenously produced anti-infective compound, suggesting a bactericidal mechanism for vitamin D in TB-infected animals (Waters et al., 2004). Other more recent studies have identified the peripheral cellular conversion of 25OHD to calcitriol as a mechanism for rapid local induction of anti-microbial peptides as a direct mechanism for killing TB and staphylococcal bacteria (Liu et al., 2006; Schauber et al., 2006). Immune responses to increased 25OHD levels may vary among individuals as a result of the genetic expression of *Vdr* polymorphisms. For example, Selvaraj et al. (2008) found that allelic variations in the Cdx-2 polymorphism were associated with either resistance or susceptibility to TB bacteria; however, more research is needed to better understand the genetic relationship between *Vdr* polymorphisms and TB susceptibility.

Systematic reviews and meta-analyses The AHRQ reviews did not identify relevant evidence for TB as an outcome. Nnoaham and Clarke (2008) systematically reviewed and meta-analyzed the relationship between low serum 25OHD levels and TB among diverse community- and hospital-based population groups in both developed and developing countries. The meta-analysis was restricted to studies that compared serum 25OHD levels in TB patients not on a treatment regimen with healthy matched controls. Seven observational studies were included in the meta-analysis, which found a 70 percent probability that a person without TB would have a higher serum 25OHD level than a person with TB. Whether this association predicts low serum 25OHD as a risk factor for active TB cannot be concluded from the analysis; however, the findings would increase the strength of similar findings from other high-quality observational studies or from a larger meta-analysis.

Additional evidence from randomized controlled trials Even though treatment of individuals with active TB with supplemental vitamin D can lead to hypercalcemia, vitamin D has been used as a therapeutic agent in the management of the disease. A small double-blind RCT of 131 individuals who had come into close contact with patients with TB (or TB contacts) in the United Kingdom (UK) measured the ability of a single oral dose of 100,000 IU of vitamin D to inhibit growth of recombinant mycobacteria, an indicator of TB exposure, grown in vitro and detected using the Barger-Lux (BCG-*lux*) assay, from the study subjects (Martineau et al., 2007b). Compared with placebo, subjects who received the vitamin D treatment showed a significant increase in serum 25OHD levels for 6 weeks without hypercalcemia, as well as inhibition of in vitro growth of mycobacteria. Another small intervention trial examined the effect of UVB exposure on TB in recent Asian immigrants to the UK who have a higher TB prevalence than indigenous populations (Yesudian et al., 2008). Anti-microbial activity, expressed as response to the BCG-*lux* assay, varied between the subjects, showing a small transient decrease but no significant change following UVB exposure. Another RCT testing the effect of vitamin D supplementation on the clinical course of patients with TB also found no significant change in clinical outcome or reduction in mortality in patients treated with 100,000 IU of vitamin D three times over 8 months (Wejse et al., 2009). Only one of the two studies reviewed showed a significant effect of vitamin D treatment on 25OHD levels in TB patients, and none of the clinical trials showed a significant effect of vitamin D on clinical outcome. Thus, evidence from RCTs does not support a reduction in TB infections with vitamin D treatment.

Observational studies   Because TB is rare in industrialized countries, particularly the United States, most observational studies are on populations from developing countries that have immigrated to developed countries. Gibney et al. (2008), in a retrospective analysis of hospitalized patients, found that low serum 25OHD levels in patients born in sub-Saharan African countries who immigrated to Australia were predictive of any form of TB infection as well as current and past infection. Another analysis of a small study of patients reporting to a TB clinic prior to treatment (Sita-Lumsden et al., 2007) found a statistically significant difference in serum 25OHD levels between TB patients and their contacts and the greatest difference among those patients with the lowest 25OHD levels. Although there was no difference in dietary intake of vitamin D between TB patients and their contacts, the TB patients did demonstrate a stronger correlation between dietary intake and measures of vitamin D in serum. Sun exposure did not differ between patients and their contacts. Strachan et al. (1995), in a case–control study of Asian immigrants to the UK who had a diagnosis of active TB, found a trend of increasing risk of TB correlated with a decreasing frequency of consumption of meat or fish and an 8.5-fold increased risk for TB among lactovegetarians compared with daily meat or fish eaters. Many observational studies of an effect of vitamin D on susceptibility to TB are confounded by endogenous production of calcitriol in infected individuals (Adams et al., 1989; Cadranel et al., 1994) and thus must be cautiously interpreted. Nevertheless, the few small studies identified support the findings of the meta-analysis from Nnoaham and Clarke (2008) for higher serum 25OHD levels in TB patients; however, these studies did not uniformly find significant associations between vitamin D intake and risk for TB.

Influenza and upper respiratory infections   Influenza is an acute contagious viral infection characterized by inflammation of the respiratory tract, fever, chills, and muscular pain. Upper respiratory infections are most commonly viral infections characterized by inflammation of the respiratory tract. Vitamin D has been hypothesized to act through the immune system to prevent influenza infections.

Biological plausibility   Environmental observations of seasonal variation in serum 25OHD levels and occurrence of influenza have been proposed as an indicator to show a correlation between vitamin D and risk for influenza (Cannell et al., 2006; Hayes, 2009). In an animal study (Underdahl and Young, 1956), mice deficient in vitamins A, D, and E and inoculated with influenza had the same intensity of influenza infection as those mice replete in vitamins A, D, and E, showing no effect of vitamin D status on reducing influenza infection. This finding contrasts with earlier work by Young et al. (1949), which suggested that vitamin D could reduce the susceptibility of mice to influenza.

Systematic reviews and meta-analyses   The AHRQ studies did not identify any relevant studies for influenza as a health outcome. There were no meta-analyses identified for this indicator.

Additional evidence from randomized controlled trials   Available data from RCTs do not provide strong support for a role for vitamin D in reducing susceptibility to influenza infection. A small RCT testing the effect of 1,200 IU of vitamin D supplementation per day for 4 months found that for influenza A as the primary outcome, occurrence between days 1 and 30 was not significantly different between the vitamin D group and placebo, but between days 31 and 60, influenza A occurred significantly less often in the vitamin D than in the placebo group; between day 61 and the end of the study, the occurrence of influenza A was not significantly different between the vitamin D and placebo groups (Urashima et al., 2010). Analysis of other related secondary outcomes showed no significant difference for influenza B, influenza-like illness (negative in rapid influenza diagnostic tests), non-specific fever, gastroenteritis, pneumonia, hospital admission, or absence from school. Overall, the absolute reduction in influenza A cases was offset by a similar increase in the number of influenza B cases. These may be chance findings, however, as a result of confounding by the loss of subjects. In another 3-month prospective double-blind RCT (Li-Ng et al., 2009), even though 73 percent of subjects supplemented with 2,000 IU of vitamin D_3 daily achieved a serum 25OHD level above 75 nmol/L, no benefit of supplementation was seen for either prevention of self-reported upper respiratory infections or a decrease in their severity. This evidence from RCTs in both children and adults shows no causal role for vitamin D in either reducing or preventing influenza.

Observational studies   Only one study of 16 patients was identified in which plasma 25OHD levels were measured in children undergoing tympanosotomy tube placement. The study showed that 50 percent of the children had 25OHD levels less than 50 nmol/L and 31 percent had levels between 52.5 and 72.5 nmol/L (Linday et al., 2008). The authors concluded from this finding that there was a possible relationship between vitamin D and susceptibility to bacterial infection and influenza. This small observational study is not adequate to support a relationship between vitamin D and one outcome related to influenza infection and no additional evidence was found to verify any causal or associative relationship between vitamin D and influenza.

Concluding Statement

The committee's review of the results of large cohort studies showed support for a positive association between vitamin D intake and reduction in symptoms associated with asthma but not with diagnosed disease. Other observational evidence of lower quality was found to largely support an association between risk for asthma and 25OHD level in blood, but associations have not been shown for diagnosed asthma. The lack of causal evidence and the lack of observational data demonstrating a relationship between vitamin D and diagnosed asthma led the committee to conclude that development of a DRI for this indicator is not supported by the totality of the evidence reviewed.

Emerging observational evidence in humans and experimental studies in animals inversely links vitamin D measures to risk of autoimmune disorders such as type 1 diabetes, MS, and IBD as well as infectious diseases such as TB (Maruotti and Cantatore, 2010). However, even though animal models indicate plausibility for a mechanistic role for vitamin D in autoimmune or anti-microbial function, results from RCTs as well as from observational associations between vitamin D and calcium and risk for either autoimmune or infectious diseases show a lack of consistency. Although both retrospective and prospective studies tend to support an inverse association between serum 25OHD levels and autoimmune and infectious diseases, these studies are limited in their interpretation owing to confounding effects that require further verification. The evidence available from RCTs is of limited utility because of the small size of the trials, inconsistency in measured outcomes, and lack of dose–response data. Overall, the evidence was not consistently supportive of a causal role for vitamin D combined with calcium or for vitamin D alone in reducing risk for developing autoimmune or infectious diseases. In the absence of verifiable dose–response data from RCTs a conclusion about asthma, autoimmune, or infectious diseases as indicators for DRI development cannot be reached.

Neuropsychological Functioning

Emerging evidence is suggestive of a role for vitamin D in neuropsychological functioning, including a range of diseases from autism to Alzheimer's.

Autism

Autism is a neurodevelopmental disorder of unknown etiology that manifests as repetitive behaviors, social withdrawal, and communication deficits. A number of factors are implicated in development of the disorder, including genetic (Abrahams and Geschwind, 2008) and environmental (Deth et al., 2008) factors.

Biological plausibility Although mechanistic studies using animal models tend to support an association between vitamin D intake during pregnancy and subsequent development of autism, these studies are limited in their interpretation and extrapolation to humans. There are some animal models suggesting a mechanism whereby vitamin D may influence the development of autism (reviewed in McGrath et al., 2004). These experiments demonstrate that pre-natal deprivation of vitamin D_3 results in gross abnormalities in fetal rat brains at birth. Feron et al. (2005) subsequently reported that vitamin D deprivation and associated disruptions in brain development seen in rat pups at birth persisted into adulthood.

In humans, *Vdr* gene polymorphisms have been proposed as a possible link to psychiatric diseases, including autism. Yan et al. (2005) analyzed the coding sequences and splice junctions of 100 patients with schizophrenia and, in a pilot study within the same population, 24 patients with autism. The frequency of the sequence variants identified, however, was not significantly different from that of sequence variants found in control subjects.

Systematic reviews and meta-analyses The AHRQ reviews did not identify evidence to support autism as a relevant health outcome for vitamin D. No meta-analyses were identified for this indicator.

Additional evidence from randomized controlled trials No RCTs were identified for this indicator.

Observational studies No large, prospective cohort studies were identified that examined associations between either vitamin D intake or 25OHD levels in blood and risk for autism. Three lower-quality observational studies were identified for further consideration: one retrospective chart review, one small cohort from a developing country, and one cross–sectional study. A recent study in Sweden that retrospectively reviewed serum 25OHD levels from medical records of out-patients receiving psychiatric care, including autism, suggested a high prevalence of vitamin D insufficiency in psychiatric outpatients (Humble et al., 2010). Although the study did not include matched controls, comparisons made with previously published samples from healthy Swedish populations suggested that the prevalence of vitamin D insufficiency was greater in the population receiving psychiatric care. The study, however, did not take into account dietary intake of vitamin D. Fernell and Gillberg (2010) tested the association between serum 25OHD levels and prevalence of autism in an analysis of a small cohort of mothers of children with autism from Somalia and Sweden, but they found no statistically significant differences in serum 25OHD levels between either group of mothers and controls.

Herndon et al. (2009), in a cross–sectional study, examined associations between vitamin D and calcium in dairy foods and autism. This study found that children with autism spectrum disorders consumed less calcium and fewer servings of dairy foods compared with children with typical development. Interpretation of this evidence for an association between vitamin D measures and risk for autism, however, is confounded by other potential factors that could influence vitamin D measures.

Concluding statement   Owing to the lack of causal evidence from RCTs and a paucity of evidence, as well as a lack of data from large, prospective cohort studies and inconsistent findings for an association between vitamin D and incidence of autism from largely cross–sectional observational studies, autism was not considered further as an indicator for DRI development.

Cognitive Function

     Loss of cognitive function in the form of dementia is frequently associated with aging. Between the ages of 60 and 85, the prevalence of dementia in the general population increases from 1 to 40 percent (Bolla et al., 2000). Dementia is classified into four major subtypes: Alzheimer's disease, Lewy body dementia, frontotemporal dementia, and vascular dementia (Bolla et al., 2000; Grossman et al., 2006). Vitamin D has been hypothesized to confer neuroprotective effects and reduce the risk for developing dementia (Buell and Dawson-Hughes, 2008; McCann and Ames, 2008).

Biological plausibility   Vitamin D has been proposed to prevent cognitive decline, and plausible biological mechanisms support this hypothesis. Vitamin D may protect against cognitive decline by promoting vascular health through anti-inflammatory or other pathways, but may also have direct neuroprotective effects (Buell and Dawson-Hughes, 2008; McCann and Ames, 2008). Rodent models show morphological and biochemical effects of vitamin D on brain tissue. Early experiments on rat brain revealed that vitamin D-deficiency reduced vitamin D–dependent enzyme activity in the cerebral context, including non-sodium-mediated glucose transport, that was restored when rats were treated with calcitriol (Stio et al., 1993). Subsequent work in mouse models demonstrated that developmental vitamin D deficiency had a negative effect on brain development, as manifested by changes in brain size and shape and ventricular size and reduced nerve growth factor expression (McGrath et al., 2004; Feron et al., 2005), as well as effects on brain function and exploratory behavior (Harms et al., 2008). When adult offspring of dams deprived of vitamin D during pregnancy underwent learning tests, they displayed impaired learning at 30 weeks of age but not at 60 weeks (de Abreu et al., 2010).

VDR and 1α-hydroxylase are found throughout the brain. Vitamin D affects gene and protein expression in brain tissue, including expression of neurotropins and glial cell–derived neurotrophic factor (Naveilhan et al., 1996; Sanchez et al., 2002). A battery of 40 different tests in *Vdr*-null mice showed them to have normal cognitive function but abnormal muscle and motor behavior, although the abnormal neuromuscular function may be due to hypocalcemia rather than a direct effect of loss of the VDR (reviewed in Bouillon et al., 2008). In neurological tissue, vitamin D modulates certain calcium-binding proteins, including calbindin-D28K, parvalbumin, and calretinin, which are important for brain function (de Viragh et al., 1989; Alexianu et al., 1998). In addition, calcitriol down-regulates the expression of calcium channel currents in rat hippocampal cells (Brewer et al., 2006), stimulates neurogenesis in human neuroblastoma cells (Moore et al., 1996; Taniura et al., 2006), and may affect other pathways (Garcion et al., 1997; Baas et al., 2000; Brown et al., 2003; Obradovic et al., 2006). Vitamin D restriction results in unfavorable structural and biochemical changes in the brain (Ko et al., 2004; Feron et al., 2005). However, experiments in rats rendered vitamin D deficient by dietary and UV radiation restriction and in *Vdr* null mice have not consistently shown learning impairments, although the data are sparse (Becker et al., 2005; Minasyan et al., 2007). Calcium independently of or in concert with vitamin D is involved in many physiological processes related to neural functioning, and disturbed calcium homeostasis is also characteristic of neurodegenerative disorders (Canzoniero and Snider, 2005; Mattson, 2007; Toescu and Verkhratsky, 2007).

Systematic reviews and meta-analyses   The AHRQ reviews did not identify sufficient evidence to support cognition (or cognitive decline) as a relevant health outcome for vitamin D. No meta-analyses were identified for this indicator.

Additional evidence from randomized controlled trials   In the WHI trial, a subset of participants completed a cognitive test battery, but results of analyses examining the vitamin D intervention's effect on cognitive function are not yet available.

Observational studies   Numerous observational studies that examined associations between vitamin D, serum 25OHD level, or calcium and cognitive function were identified as potentially relevant to DRI development. The greatest number of studies, however, were cross–sectional. No large prospective cohort studies were identified for review, although two analyses of data from large population-based annual surveys and several small cohort studies were included.

Low serum 25OHD levels have been associated with decreased cognitive function in various population groups. A cross–sectional analysis of 752 women 75 years of age and older in the Epidémiologie de l'Ostéoporose (EPIDOS) study found that participants with vitamin D deficiency (serum 25OHD level < 25 nmol/L) had twice the odds of cognitive impairment as other participants (Annweiler et al., 2010). In a population-based cross–sectional study, Lee et al. (2009) examined associations between serum 25OHD level and cognitive function and mood among adult men in a European population. In a spline regression model, significant associations were found between slower information processing and serum 25OHD levels below 35 nmol/L in men ages 40 years and older. In contrast to these findings, a more recent cross–sectional study found that among 1,604 men up to 65 years of age in the Osteoporotic Fractures in Men (MrOS) Study, there were no associations between serum 25OHD level and cognitive impairment, even after adjusting for age, race/ethnicity, education, and other potential confounders (Slinin et al., 2010). This study also examined vitamin D measures as a predictor of subsequent cognitive decline over a mean of 4.6 years of follow-up and found only a borderline significant trend across the first three quartiles of serum 25OHD levels, ($\leq$ 49.75 nmol/L, 50.0 to < 62.75 nmol/L, and 62.75 to < 74.5 nmol/L, respectively), compared with the fourth quartile ($\geq$ 74.5 nmol/L); serum 25OHD level did not predict decline on a timed test of executive function.

In a cross–sectional study of 318 older individuals (mean age 74 years) receiving home health care services, those who received a neurological exam and cranial magnetic resonance imaging (MRI), a lower serum 25OHD level (< 50 nmol/L) was associated with at least twice the odds for all-cause dementia, Alzheimer's disease, and stroke, as well as increased white-matter hyperintensity volume and prevalence of large-vessel infarcts (Buell et al., 2010). Among three age groups (adolescent, adult, and elderly) examined from NHANES III, no association was found between high serum 25OHD levels and learning or memory, and only the elderly population group was found to have an inverse association between 25OHD level and performance on a task of learning and memory. Within the elderly population group, those in the highest quintile for serum 25OHD level were also the most impaired; thus, the results fail to confirm the hypothesis that serum 25OHD level enhances performance in learning and memory (McGrath et al., 2007).

There are few observational studies on calcium and cognitive function. In a cross–sectional study on Korean adults 60 years of age and older, a positive association was found between calcium intake and score on the Mini-Mental State Examination for Koreans (MMSE-K) in women but not in men after adjustment for age (Lee et al., 2001). In contrast, another study in Portuguese adults more than 65 years of age found no association between calcium intake and MMSE score after 8.5 months of follow-up (Velho et al., 2008). Using a cross–sectional analysis, Wilkins et al. (2009) found, as expected, lower serum 25OHD levels among the African American population compared with the white population, and poorer cognitive performance among African Americans with the lowest 25OHD levels compared with those with higher levels. Similarly, in a cross–sectional analysis in a British population of adults ages 65 years or older with serum 25OHD levels reported in quartiles, Llewellyn et al. (2009) found a greater risk for impaired cognitive performance among persons in the lowest (8 to 30 nmol/L) compared with the highest quartile (66 to 170 nmol/L). Even though the committee identified a large number of observational studies that evaluated associations between vitamin D and calcium and cognitive function, these were predominantly lower quality cross–sectional studies or small cohort studies, and their results were mixed. No causal evidence was found to support experimental evidence for biological plausibility and the relatively weak observational evidence. The committee took into account the generally lower quality of the study designs in its interpretation of the findings and in drawing conclusions about outcomes associated with this indicator.

Depression

Depression is a disease with characteristic signs and symptoms that interfere with the ability to work, sleep, eat, and enjoy once-pleasurable activities. These signs and symptoms include loss of interest in activities; a persistently sad or anxious mood; feelings of hopelessness, pessimism, guilt, worthlessness, or helplessness; social withdrawal; fatigue; sleep disturbances; difficulty in concentrating or making decisions; unusual restlessness or irritability; persistent physical problems that do not respond to treatment; and thoughts of death or suicide or suicide attempts. Depressive disorders include major depressive disorder, dysthymic disorder, psychotic depression, postpartum depression, and seasonal affective disorder, with major depressive disorder and dysthymic disorder being the most common.[2] Whether there is a functional relationship between measures of serum vitamin D or intake and mood or depression has not been determined.

Biological plausibility   Seasonal affective disorder occurs more often at northern latitudes, and the etiology is presumed to be due, at least in part, to lack of sunlight exposure. In turn, lack of sunlight exposure causes low serum 25OHD levels unless the diet is adequate in vitamin D. Investigators have pursued the hypothesis that the low serum 25OHD levels are a cause of seasonal affective disorder, although it must be considered that the lack of sunlight may independently cause both seasonal affective disorder and low serum 25OHD levels without a direct link between them.

Systematic reviews and meta-analyses   The AHRQ reviews did not identify sufficient evidence to support depression as a relevant health outcome for vitamin D. No meta-analyses were identified for this indicator.

Additional evidence from randomized controlled trials   One RCT was identified that evaluated effects of vitamin D supplementation on depressive symptoms. Jorde et al. (2008) gave either 20,000 or 40,000 IU of vitamin D_3 or a placebo treatment weekly for 1 year to men and women ages 21 to 70 years, living in Norway. Symptoms of depression were evaluated using the Beck Depression Inventory (BDI), and serum 25OHD level and BMI were measured. Participants whose serum 25OHD levels were below 40 nmol/L had significantly higher BDI scores, indicating a higher incidence of depressive disorder, compared with those whose serum 25OHD levels were 40 nmol/L and above after 1 year. Both treatment groups indicated significant improvement in BDI score compared with placebo.

Results of other randomized trials testing the effects of vitamin D on a subtype of depression that occurs during the winter months have been mixed. Three small, short-term trials examining effects of treatment with vitamin D for seasonal affective disorder reported that vitamin D improves mood (Lansdowne and Provost, 1998; Gloth et al., 1999; Vieth et al., 2004), but a larger, longer-term trial found no effect (Thys-Jacobs et al., 1998). Vieth et al. (2004) treated adults with serum 25OHD concentrations below 61 nmol/L with the equivalent of either 4,000 or 600 IU of vitamin D per day for 3 months over two consecutive winters and found evidence of a significant difference in measures of improved well-being at the higher compared with the lower dose. Lansdowne and Provost (1998) assigned healthy adults to 5 days of treatment with either 400 or 800 IU of vitamin

---

[2]Available online at http://www.nimh.nih.gov/health/publications/depression/what-are-the-different-forms-of-depression.shtml (accessed April 5, 2010).

D or placebo and found that both vitamin D doses increased positive affect and decreased negative affect compared with placebo. Gloth et al. (1999) assigned 15 people to either 100,000 IU of vitamin D or broad-spectrum light therapy for 1 month and found an increase in serum 25OHD level was significantly associated with improvement in depressive symptoms. However, Harris and Dawson-Hughes (1993) randomized 250 middle-aged and older women to treatment with 400 IU of vitamin D per day of vitamin D plus 377 mg of calcium per day or to calcium alone for 1 year and found no treatment-related changes in seasonal mood as assessed by the Profile of Mood States (POMS) questionnaire.

Observational studies   Among four cross–sectional studies on small population groups ($n < 50$) that evaluated associations between serum 25OHD level and evidence for clinical diagnosis of depression in women (Michelson et al., 1996; Herran et al., 2000; Eskandari et al., 2007) or men and women (Schneider et al., 2000), only Eskandari et al. (2007) found a significant association between serum 25OHD level and diagnosis of depression and Michelson et al. (1996) found a significant association with calcitriol level. Another large population-based cross–sectional study among middle-aged and elderly Chinese also found, after controlling for confounders and geographic location, no significant associations between serum 25OHD level (grouped by tertile) and symptoms of clinical depression (Pan et al., 2009). In contrast to the cross–sectional studies, Hoogendijk et al. (2008) found, in a cohort study in the Netherlands, a significantly lower mean serum 25OHD level (47.5 nmol/L) among individuals with both major and minor depression compared with a mean level of 55 nmol/L among those who did not have depression.

Concluding Statement

Although some observational studies support an association between low measures of vitamin D exposure and risk for cognitive impairment or changes in mood, results have been inconsistent, and the majority of studies were cross–sectional in study design, including possible selection bias or other confounding factors that diminish the quality ranking of the studies. In addition, few or no clinical trials were identified to support biological plausibility. As a result of the many shortcomings in study design and quality of observational evidence and the paucity of high-quality evidence from RCTs identified by the committee, the findings for neuropsychological indicators are inconclusive. The committee's review of the available evidence for either associations or a causal relationship between vitamin D and calcium and risk for cognitive disorders shows a lack of sufficient evidence to support DRI development.

Preeclampsia, Pregnancy-Induced Hypertension, and Other Non-Skeletal Reproductive Outcomes

Preeclampsia is a serious condition in which hypertension and proteinuria arise in pregnancy. It can affect both the mother and the unborn child. Pregnancy-induced hypertension is a transient hypertension without proteinuria that occurs during pregnancy. Pregnancy is a type of immunological challenge, and women with some autoimmune diseases, particularly type 1 diabetes and RA, are at increased risk for developing preeclampsia (Evers et al., 2004; Wolfberg et al., 2004). Clinical observations have noted that urinary calcium excretion is low in women with preeclampsia, whereas it is elevated in women during normal pregnancy. Calcium intake has been examined relative to reducing the risk of preeclampsia.

Biological Plausibility: Preeclampsia and Pregnancy-Induced Hypertension

Vitamin D metabolism may be altered under conditions of preeclampsia (August et al., 1992), when calcitriol level is low and hypocalciuria is present, but it is unclear whether these are causes or consequences of preeclampsia. The placenta and deciduas both express 1α-hydroxylase and activate 25OHD in vitro. Calcitriol regulates immunomodulatory cytokine production in cultured decidual cells (Evans et al., 2006) and placental trophoblasts (Diaz et al., 2009). However, the specific role of vitamin D in vivo is less clear. Its actions in vitro may provide some clues as to its physiological relevance, but these hypotheses need to be examined rigorously in future studies.

As mentioned above, it has long been observed that urinary excretion of calcium is increased during pregnancy, and hypercalciuria may result. In contrast, women with preeclampsia often have hypocalciuria. This observation has prompted a number of investigations to test whether low calcium intake predisposes a pregnant woman to both hypocalciuria and preeclampsia, although a biological mechanism to explain how low calcium intake would cause the preeclampsia has not been clearly elucidated.

Systematic Reviews and Meta-Analyses: Preeclampsia and Pregnancy-Induced Hypertension

The AHRQ-Tufts analysis identified a single nested case–control study (rated B for methodological quality) that evaluated the association between serum 25OHD concentration and the risk of preeclampsia (Bodnar et al., 2007). The researchers found a significant association between preeclampsia and serum 25OHD concentrations when the serum values were less than 37.5 nmol/L early in pregnancy.

A 2007 systematic review of evidence incorporated 12 RCTs (15,528 women) to examine the relationship between calcium supplementation and preeclampsia prevention (Hofmeyr et al., 2007). Calcium supplementation reduced overall hypertension in 11 of the studies reviewed and incidence of preeclampsia in 12 of them. There was also a significant effect for calcium among women at high risk, which was greatest among those with lower baseline calcium intakes.

Additional Evidence from Randomized Controlled Trials:
Preeclampsia and Pregnancy-Induced Hypertension

Additional RCTs not included in the review from Hofmeyr et al. (2007), although of lower-quality study design, also reported similar results suggesting that there may be no effect from daily calcium supplementation when dietary calcium intake is already adequate (Hofmeyr et al., 2006 [1,000 mg/day]; Villar et al., 2006 [2,000 mg/day]; Hiller et al., 2007 [1,800 mg/day]; Kumar et al., 2009 [500 mg/day]).

A prospective non-randomized clinical trial of the effect of vitamin D (0.5 mg/day) and calcium (312 mg/day) supplementation in women at risk for preeclampsia found that the incidence of preeclampsia was 10.9 percent lower in treated women than in controls (Ito et al., 1994). However, women who had the highest level of angiotensin II, a marker for preeclampsia, also had the lowest incidence of preeclampsia; thus, the role of calcium and vitamin D supplementation in preventing of preeclampsia is not clear from this trial (Ito et al., 1994). A small randomized trial of pregnant women in India supplemented with 600,000 IU of vitamin D in the seventh and eighth months of pregnancy compared with controls found no significant difference in incidence of preeclampsia, although a significant reduction in systolic blood pressure of 8 mmHg was seen in the vitamin D–supplemented group (Marya et al., 1987). The relationship of this small decrease in blood pressure to pregnancy-induced hypertension is unclear.

Observational Studies: Preeclampsia and Pregnancy-Induced Hypertension

Findings from observational studies have shown mixed results. In addition to the nested case–control study reviewed in AHRQ-Tufts, the committee identified one large prospective cohort study, a large retrospective cohort study, and two small case–control studies examining vitamin D intake or serum 25OHD level and risk for preeclampsia, as well as one small case–control study of serum calcitriol level and pregnancy-induced hypertension (Lalau et al., 1993). In the large prospective study, Haugen et al. (2009) examined associations between risk for preeclampsia and intake of vitamin D from diet and supplements. This study found that women who developed preeclampsia did not have a lower intake of vitamin D from foods compared with women without preeclampsia, but they did have a significantly lower intake of vitamin D from supplements, although the dose of the supplement was not correlated with prevalence of preeclampsia. Risk for preeclampsia was reduced by 31 percent in women who achieved a total vitamin D intake from food plus supplements between 300 and 400 IU/day, and the minimum combined intake of vitamin D needed for a protective effect was 200 IU/day. Hypponen et al. (2007) retrospectively examined the use of vitamin D supplements in infants of women with previously diagnosed preeclampsia in the Northern Finland Birth Cohort of 1966. The female children of mothers who had preeclampsia had a greater prevalence of preeclampsia in their own pregnancies, but vitamin D supplementation was significantly associated with a lower subsequent risk of developing preeclampsia. In contrast to these findings, two case–control studies, one in the United States (Seely et al., 1992) and one in Denmark (Frolich et al., 1992), found no significant difference in serum 25OHD levels between women with preeclampsia and those without, even though serum calcium levels were significantly lower in the women with pregnancy-induced hypertension or preeclampsia, respectively. In a small case–control study, women with pregnancy-induced hypertension had lower total and free serum calcitriol levels than did normotensive women during pregnancy (Lalau et al., 1993), but serum 25OHD levels and vitamin D intake were not measured.

Concluding Statement: Preeclampsia and Pregnancy-Induced Hypertension

Overall, two observational studies identified associations between supplementary vitamin D and incidence of preeclampsia, but data on associations between serum 25OHD level and preeclampsia were not conclusive. Similarly, only one observational study reported an association of pregnancy-induced hypertension with lower serum total and free calcitriol levels (Lalau et al., 1993), and no placebo-controlled RCTs were identified that examined a causal relationship between vitamin D and preeclampsia or pregnancy-induced hypertension.

Calcium supplementation has not been shown to have an effect on the incidence of preeclampsia in normal women meeting calcium requirements, but it may be of benefit in cases of low calcium intake. Associations between serum 25OHD level (as well as calcitriol level) and the onset of preeclampsia have not been well studied and a mechanism of action is unclear. Thus, because of the lack of a causal relationship and the inconsistent results in the observational studies for both vitamin D and calcium the committee concluded that neither preeclampsia nor pregnancy-induced hypertension can be considered as an indicator for DRI development.

Other Non-Skeletal Reproductive Outcomes

Neither AHRQ-Ottawa nor AHRQ-Tufts addressed maternal non-skeletal outcomes beyond preeclampsia and pregnancy-induced hypertension. However, other non-skeletal outcomes may include maternal events such as cesarean section, obstructed labor, and vaginosis. Regarding fetal outcomes, so-called developmental programming of health outcomes in the offspring may focus on immune-related outcomes such as type 1 diabetes and atopic eczema, which has been included above in autoimmune response, as well as measures of BMD and skeletal development, discussed below in the Skeletal Health section. Infant birthweight is also of interest.

One observational study has reported an increased risk of approximately 65 percent and 26 percent of bacterial vaginosis in women with serum 25OHD levels below 20 nmol/L and below 50 nmol/L, respectively, compared with those with serum 25OHD levels of 75 nmol/L (Bodnar et al., 2009). Two observational studies reported conflicting results for the association of serum 25OHD levels with maternal delivery (cesarean/obstructed), with one finding an inverse association (Merewood et al., 2009) and the other finding no relationship with serum 25OHD levels. Overall, insufficient evidence makes maternal Cesarean delivery/obstructed labor uninformative for DRI development.

Regarding infant birthweight, AHRQ-Tufts discussed two RCTs (Mallet et al., 1986 and Maxwell et al., 1981; quality graded B and C, respectively) and reported no effect of supplemental vitamin D during pregnancy on offspring's birthweight or length, and also one RCT (Marya et al., 1988; quality graded C) that reported an increased birthweight in vitamin D–supplemented pregnant women with low dietary intakes of vitamin D. One additional RCT published after the AHRQ-Tufts report (Yu et al., 2009) also reported no effect of vitamin D on infant birthweight.

Brooke et al. (1980) reported on an RCT that involved 126 women treated with either a dose of vitamin D or a placebo during pregnancy. The intended dose for the treated group was 1,000 IU/day, but it appears that a higher dose was administered (10,000 IU/day) as the achieved cord level of 25OHD was 138 nmol/L for the treated group versus 10 nmol/L. In any case, no change in birthweight was evidenced. In a smaller study of 40 pregnant women, Delvin et al. (1986) showed no effect on birthweight comparing 1,000 IU/day versus a placebo.

Several observational studies have also examined this relationship, again with conflicting results. In a nested case–control study, a U-shaped relationship was found only in white women, with an increased probability (2.4 to 3.9) of small-for-gestational-age measures in those women in the lowest (21 to 58 nmol/L) and the highest (90.7 to 245.0 nmol/L) quartiles of serum 25OHD levels (Bodnar et al., 2010). In the same study, despite lower serum 25OHD levels in black women, no relationship was found between small-for-gestational-age measures and maternal serum 25OHD levels. In a prospective cohort observational study, mean birthweight was lowest in infants born to women with 25OHD levels below 30 nmol/L, intermediate in those born to women with 25OHD levels 30 to 50 nmol/L, and highest in those born to women with 25OHD levels above 50 nmol/L (Leffelaar et al., 2010). Birthweight was 60 g lower for the infants of women who consumed less than 200 IU of vitamin D per day during pregnancy compared to those who consumed 200 IU of vitamin D or more per day, and there was a significant linear trend for increased birthweight from lowest to highest quintile of intake (Scholl and Chen, 2009). Morley et al. (2006) enrolled 475 women in a study that compared maternal serum 25OHD levels during pregnancy to offspring birth size. No relationship was reported. Other observational studies reported no effect of vitamin D on birthweight (Brunvand et al., 1998; Gale et al., 2008; Farrant et al., 2009). The relationship, however, has not been tested in a sufficiently powered clinical trial. Corrections for differences in gestational length and other potentially confounding factors are not usually possible with associational studies. The available evidence for non-skeletal outcomes is limited and presently conflicting among both RCTs and observational studies, precluding the ability to find these data useful at this time for DRI development.

Skeletal Health

Skeletal health, referred to commonly as bone health, is manifested by desirable growth and maintenance of skeletal tissue, including bones and teeth. The use of bone health outcomes as reflective of calcium and vitamin D requirements is long-standing. Bone health served as an indicator for determining the calcium and vitamin D DRIs in 1997, when nutrient reference values for these nutrients were last reviewed (IOM, 1997). Since that time, additional studies have added to the scientific understanding of the relationships between calcium and vitamin D and bone health and are reflected to a large extent in AHRQ-Ottawa and AHRQ-Tufts, completed in 2007 and 2009, respectively.

Bone health is a concern throughout the life span. Initially, it comprises skeletal development during the times of gestational development and growth in infancy, childhood, and adolescence; this is followed by bone maintenance in adulthood. Menopause and aging result in bone loss. Various measures and health conditions are relevant to considerations of bone health; these include BMC/BMD, calcium balance, rickets/osteomalacia, and fracture risk. The latter is particularly germane to older adults. Further, while not health outcomes, measures of serum 25OHD concentrations and of circulating PTH levels have been incorporated into studies as intermediates related to bone health. Finally, although physical performance and the incidence of falls are defined by some as a component of bone health, these measures are reviewed separately in this report.

Compared with other potential indicators, this health outcome is characterized by a sizable number of RCTs as well as numerous observational studies from large cohorts. However, many of the studies evaluated calcium and vitamin D in combination, and there are relatively few studies that have evaluated the effects of calcium alone without vitamin D supplementation or vice versa. Given the nature of the available data and the need to integrate information to develop a set of measures reflective of bone health as a potential indicator for developing DRIs, this section is organized differently from those for other potential indicators. The understandings that link calcium and vitamin D to bone health and provide the basis for biological plausibility for an effect on bone health have been described in Chapters 2 and 3 and are therefore not repeated here. The many observational studies are briefly summarized.

Given the depth and breadth of the available AHRQ systematic analyses for the topic of bone health, the AHRQ analyses are considered in a single section. The two AHRQ analyses systematically reviewed, first, the published literature on the relationship between bone health and vitamin D (often in combination with calcium) (AHRQ-Ottawa) and, second, the relationship between bone health and vitamin D alone or vitamin D in combination with calcium (AHRQ-Tufts). Neither of the two AHRQ analyses considered calcium alone in relation to bone health. These two analyses have been described at the beginning of this chapter, and specific information about the studies included in AHRQ can be found in Appendixes C and D. Relevant information has been summarized and included in the tables presented below.

AHRQ included only minimal information about reproductive outcomes, and therefore the literature related to skeletal health during pregnancy and lactation is highlighted. AHRQ also included only minimal information about PTH level, a measure some investigators relate to bone health, so PTH level as a potential measure for bone health is examined separately.

The final component of this section integrates the available data on the basis of bone accretion, bone maintenance, and bone health. The preliminary step of specifying the utility of serum 25OHD level as a marker as well as the relationship between calcium absorption and serum 25OHD level provides the opening discussions for the integration section.

Summary of Observational Studies

The observational studies surrounding bone health are myriad. However, as is the case with the evidence hierarchy, the basis for the relationship between the two nutrients and bone health is more appropriately explored by examining evidence from controlled interventions, although data from observational studies can lend support and offer confirmatory input. Observational data regarding calcium intake and bone health are mixed regarding the finding that a range of increasing calcium intakes above deficiency levels are associated with improved bone mass and reduced fracture risk. These studies are confounded by an array of variables that have an impact on measures of bone density.

Regarding serum 25OHD concentrations and bone health, the AHRQ-Ottawa analysis concluded that observational studies suggested a correlation between higher serum 25OHD concentrations and increased BMC for older children and adolescents. For postmenopausal women and elderly men, observational studies reviewed in AHRQ-Ottawa provided *fair evidence* to support an association between serum 25OHD level and BMD or changes in BMD at the femoral neck. This analysis noted that the observational data overall were discordant with the results from available RCTs. Newer observational studies for the most part are consistent with older observational studies with respect to a relationship between low serum 25OHD levels and outcomes such as bone loss, fractures, or osteomalacia (Cauley et al., 2008; Looker and Mussolino, 2008; van Schoor et al., 2008; Ensrud et al., 2009; Bolland et al., 2010b; Cauley et al., 2010; Melhus et al., 2010). However, there are confounders related to such studies, including age, calcium intake, and social situation.

Bone mineral content/bone mineral density: Serum 25OHD   AHRQ conducted its analyses for serum 25OHD concentrations on the basis of certain age and gender groups, as presented below.

Infants   Overall, AHRQ-Ottawa, for which some studies included combinations of calcium and vitamin D, has reported that there is inconsistent evidence for an association between serum 25OHD concentrations and BMC measures in infants. Of the two RCTs examining BMC (Greer et al., 1982; Zeghoud et al., 1997), one demonstrated no significant benefit of higher serum 25OHD concentrations on radial bone mass, whereas the other showed a transient increase of BMC compared with the unsupplemented group at 12 weeks, but not at 26 weeks. Based on case–control studies (Okonofua et al., 1986; Bougle et al., 1998; Namgung et al., 1998; Park et al., 1998), greater whole-body BMC was related to higher serum 25OHD levels. Data are summarized in Table 4-5. AHRQ-Tufts found no additional RCTs for infants published in the period since the completion of the AHRQ-Ottawa review.

Children and adolescents   For children and adolescents, there was fair evidence from AHRQ-Ottawa of an association between serum 25OHD levels and baseline BMD and change in BMD or BMD indexes. However, the results from the RCTs (Ala-Houhala et al., 1988; El-Hajj Fuleihan et al.,

TABLE 4-5 Serum 25OHD Levels and Bone Health Outcomes for Infants: Summary from AHRQ-Ottawa Analyses[a]

Reference; Country; Jadad Score for RCTs[b]	Population Description	Intervention/ Duration	Bone Health Outcomes	Results
RCTs				
Greer et al., 1982 United States Jadad = 3	Healthy full-term infants; exclusively breast-fed $n = 18$ 66% female 17 Caucasian 1 Asian-Indian	IG1: 400 IU vit D_2/d CG: placebo 12 wk (double-blind) At 6 mo, unblinded to mother, and placebo group began to receive 400 IU vit D_2/d Followed to 1 y	Distal L radius BMC (SPA) Measured at 3, 6, 12, 26, 40, and 52 wks	Serum 25OHD, mean (nmol/L) Baseline: no significant difference between groups 12 wk: IG1: 95* (graph) CG: 50 26 wk: IG1: 81.8 CG: 32.3 BMC, mean (SEM) (mg/cm) 12 wk: IG1 79 (3); CG 64 (3); $p < 0.003$ 26 wk: IG1 70 (6); CG 75 (5); NS 52 wk: IG1 108 (20); CG 120 (19) (CG receiving vit D for 6 mo)

continued

Greer and Marshall, 1989 United States Jadad = 4	Healthy full-term infants born to mothers willing to breastfeed for 6 mo $n = 46$ (+ 12 controls) 46% female All infants had Caucasian mothers (fathers included 1 black, 1 American Indian)	IG1: 400 IU vit D_2/d CG: placebo 6 mo, starting at birth	Distal L radius BMC (SPA) Measured at 1.5, 3.0, and 6.0 mo	Total serum 25OHD, mean (SD) (nmol/L) At birth: IG1: 59.7 (11.8) CG: 58.8 (19.1) 6 mo: IG1: 92.4 (29.7) CG: 58.8 (24.9), $p < 0.01$ BMC, mean (SD) (mg/cm) No significant difference between groups at 1.5 and 3.0 mo. At 6.0 mo, CG was significantly greater than IG1: IG1 89.5 (12.5) vs. CG 101.0 (17.9), $p < 0.05$ However, change in mean BMC from 1.5 to 6.0 mo was not different between groups

198

TABLE 4-5 Continued

Reference; Country; Jadad Score for RCTs[b]	Population Description	Intervention/ Duration	Bone Health Outcomes	Results
Zeghoud et al., 1997 France Jadad = 1	Healthy neonates and their mothers $n = 80$ European	IG1: 500 IU vit D_2/d IG2: 1,000 IU vit D_2/d Starting at 3–6 d after birth All infants fed formula with mean (SD) 426 (46) IU vit D_3/L	iPTH (RIA) Measured at 3–6 d, 1 mo, 3 mo	Serum 25OHD, mean (SD) Baseline total sample: 29.5 (13.8) nmol/L; range 10–80 nmol/L 51/80 (63.7%) ≤ 30 nmol/L iPTH was significantly higher in neonates with 25OHD < 16 nmol/L than in those born with 25OHD > 30 nmol/L: mean (SD) 70 (30) pmol/L Mean baseline 25OHD by group** Group 1 ($n = 14$): 25OHD ≤ 30 nmol/L and iPTH > 60 ng/L: 17.9 (7.8) Group 2 ($n = 36$): 25OHD ≤ 30 nmol/L and iPTH < 60 ng/L: 22.7 (6.5) Group 3 ($n = 29$): 25OHD > 30 nmol/L and iPTH < 60 ng/mL: 43.7 (10.6) At 1 mo, all 3 groups (pooled vit D doses): mean serum 25OHD was significantly increased, and there was no significant difference between groups Group 1: 53.1 (12.0) nmol/L Group 2: 59.8 (17.7) nmol/L Group 3: 59.2 (11.4) nmol/L At 3 mo, mean 25OHD for total sample (pooled doses) was 69.0 nmol/L; highest value 92.5 nmol/L IG1 (500 IU D_2/d): For group 1, at 1 mo (45.5 nmol/L) and 3 mo (56.1 nmol/L), serum 25OHD values were significantly lower than in the other 2 groups receiving same dose and lower than in all groups receiving 1,000 IU/d IG2 (1,000 IU vit D_2/d): Change in serum 25OHD (3 mo) was not significantly different between the 3 groups

Case–control studies

Study	Population		Outcome	Results
Okonofua et al., 1986 UK	Healthy full-term infants $n = 21$ 47.6% Caucasian 52.4% Asian	NA	Fractures during birth	Serum 25OHD, mean (SD) (nmol/L): Lower in Asian vs. white full-term infants ($p < 0.01$) White: 15 (5) (range 9–39) Asian: 6 (4) (range < 5–20) Maternal 25OHD in white mothers was 30 (11) nmol/L and in Asian mothers was 15 (10) nmol/L; serum PTH was higher in Asian mothers 25OHD levels in mothers were significantly higher than neonatal levels; the two were correlated ($r = 0.60$) Fractures during birth: 0
Bougle et al., 1998 France	Healthy full-term infants $n = 82$ (also 44 preterm) Asian	NA	LS BMD and BMC (DXA)	Full-term infants: Serum 25OHD, mean (SD) nmol/L (range) 75 (52.5) (10.0–292.5) 25OHD negatively related to BMD ($r = -1.7$, $p = 0.02$) and to BMC ($r = -0.04$, $p = 0.02$) in a simple regression analysis, but not related to BMC or BMD in a multiple regression analysis

continued

TABLE 4-5 Continued

Reference; Country; Jadad Score for RCTs[b]	Population Description	Intervention/ Duration	Bone Health Outcomes	Results
Namgung et al., 1998 Korea	Healthy full-term infants $n = 71$ (37 born in summer and 34 in winter) Summer 59% female Winter 38% female Korean	NA	Whole-body BMC measured before 3 d of age (DXA)	Serum 25OHD, mean (SD) (nmol/L): Winter-born infants had lower 25OHD than summer-born infants ($p < 0.001$) Winter born: 26.8 (19.0) Summer born: 75.0 (24.0) % of infants with levels < 27.5 nmol/L Winter born: 97% Summer born: 47% Winter-born infants had 8% lower whole-body BMC than summer-born infants ($p = 0.0002$) BMC LSM (SD) (g/cm): Winter born: 86.7 (7.7) Summer born: 93.9 (7.8) Whole-body BMC correlated positively with serum 25OHD ($r = 0.243$, $p = 0.047$) Maternal 25OHD was lower in winter than in summer: 24 (13) vs. 43 (18), $p < 0.001$

Park et al., 1998 Korea	Healthy full-term infants born in winter (some exclusively breast-fed [n = 18] or formula-fed with 400 IU vit D [n = 17]); n = 35; Breast-fed 28% female; Formula-fed 47% female; Korean	LS BMC and BMD (DXA)	NA	Serum 25OHD, mean (SD) (nmol/L): Mean was lower in breast-fed vs. formula-fed infants, $p = 0.001$
				Breast-fed: 39.9 (28.2)
				Formula-fed: 72.5 (22.2)
				% with 25OHD < 28 nmol/L
				Breast-fed: 8/18 (44%)
				Formula-fed: 1/17 (6%), $p = 0.01$
				LS BMD no difference between breast-fed (n = 14/18) and formula-fed infants (n = 14/17) (data NR)
				LS BMC, mean (SD) (g/cm)
				No difference between groups
				Breast-fed: 0.62 (0.2)
				Formula-fed: 0.65 (0.2)
				25OHD did not correlate with BMC ($r = 0.173$, $p = 0.39$, n = 28)

NOTE: *SEM provided in graph but not estimable; **1/80 infants did not clearly fit into any category and had findings suggestive of transient congenital hypoparathyroidism; BMC = bone mineral content; BMD = bone mineral density; CG = control group; d = day; DXA = dual-energy X-ray absorptiometry; IG = intervention group; iPTH = intact parathyroid hormone; IU = International Units; L = Left; LS = lumbar spine; LSM = least squares mean; mo = month(s); NA = not applicable; NR = not reported; NS = not significant; RCT = randomized controlled trial; RIA = radioimmunoassay; SD = standard deviation; SEM = standard error of the mean; SPA = single-photon absorptiometry; UK = United Kingdom; vit = vitamin; wk = week(s); y = year(s).

*a*This table has been truncated for the purposes of this chapter, but it can be found in its entirety in Appendix C.

*b*Jadad score is based on a scale of 1 to 5. See Box 4-1 for details on the scoring system.

SOURCE: Modified from Cranney et al. (2007).

2006) did not confirm a consistent benefit on BMD or BMC across skeletal sites and age groups. Some studies included combinations of calcium and vitamin D.

There were seven studies in older children and adolescents (two RCTs, three cohort studies, one case–control study, and one before-and-after study) that evaluated the relationship between serum 25OHD concentrations and BMC or BMD (see Table 4-6). In older children, there was one RCT, one prospective cohort study, and one before-and-after study. The RCT (Ala-Houhala et al., 1988) did not find an association between serum 25OHD concentrations and distal radial BMC. Two of three non-RCT studies found a positive association between baseline serum 25OHD concentrations and BMC or BMD. The effect of bone size and muscle mass on these outcomes in relation to baseline serum 25OHD concentrations was not reported.

One RCT with children and adolescent girls (El-Hajj Fuleihan et al., 2006) demonstrated a significant relationship between baseline serum 25OHD concentrations and baseline BMD of the lumbar spine, femoral neck, and radius. However, only high dose supplementation with 14,000 IU of vitamin D_3 per week increased BMC of the total hip.

AHRQ-Tufts identified two RCTs available after the AHRQ-Ottawa analysis, both rated C, that compared the effect of vitamin D supplementation alone on BMC in healthy girls between 10 and 17 years of age (El-Hajj Fuleihan et al., 2006; Andersen et al., 2008). Both RCTs were rated C because the results were not adjusted for important potential confounders, such as height, bone area, lean mass, sun exposure, and pubertal status. One RCT (Andersen et al., 2008) analyzed 26 healthy girls, who were Pakistani immigrants primarily living in the Copenhagen area of Denmark (latitude 55°N). Girls were randomly assigned to receive either a daily dose of 400 or 800 IU of vitamin D_3 or placebo for 1 year. The mean baseline dietary calcium intake was 510 mg/day, and the serum 25OHD concentration was 11 nmol/L. At the end of the study, there were no significant differences in whole-body BMC changes between groups receiving the two doses of vitamin D_3 (400 or 800 IU/day) and the placebo group. A second RCT (El-Hajj Fuleihan et al., 2006) analyzed 168 healthy girls living in the Greater Beirut area, Lebanon (latitude 33°N). Girls were randomly assigned to receive either weekly oral vitamin D doses of 1,400 IU (equivalent to 200 IU/day) or 14,000 IU (equivalent to 2,000 IU/day) or placebo for 1 year. The mean baseline dietary calcium intake was 677 mg/day, and the 25OHD concentration was 35 nmol/L. At the end of the study, there were no significant differences in whole-body BMC changes between either the low-dose vitamin D group (200 IU/day) or the high-dose vitamin D group (2,000 IU/day) and the placebo group. The same findings were seen when analyses were restricted to either premenarcheal or postmenarcheal girls.

TABLE 4-6 Serum 25OHD Levels and Bone Health Outcomes for Older Children and Adolescents: Summary from AHRQ-Ottawa Analyses[a]

Reference; Country; Jadad Score for RCTs[b]	Population Description	Intervention/ Duration	Bone Health Outcomes	Results
RCTs				
Ala-Houhala et al., 1988 Finland Jadad = 1	Children, 8–10 y old n = 60 IG1: 62% female CG: 48% female Caucasian	IG1: 400 IU vit D_2 5–7×/wk CG: placebo 13 mo	Distal radius BMC (SPA)	Serum 25OHD, mean (SD) (nmol/L) Baseline (winter): IG1: 49.3 (19.0) vs. CG: 46.0 (15.5) Mid-study (autumn): IG1: 78.0 (24.3) vs. CG 59.0 (17.8) End-of-study (winter): IG1: 71.3 (23.4) vs. CG 43.3 (19.5), $p < 0.01$ No difference between groups in distal radius BMC at 13 mo

continued

TABLE 4-6 Continued

Reference; Country; Jadad Score for RCTs[b]	Population Description	Intervention/ Duration	Bone Health Outcomes	Results
El-Hajj Fuleihan et al., 2006 Lebanon Jadad = 4	Children and adolescent girls (premenarcheal and postmenarcheal), 10–17 y n = 179 Middle Eastern	IG1: 1,400 IU vit D/wk IG2: 14,000 IU vit D/wk CG: placebo 1 y	BMD and BMC LS, forearm, total body (DXA)	25OHD, mean (SD) (nmol/L) baseline: IG1: 35.0 (22.5) IG2: 35.0 (20.0) CG: 35.0 (17.5) 1 y: IG1: 42.5 (15.0) IG2: 95.0 (77.5) CG: 40.0 (20.0) Covariates: percentage change in bone area, percentage change in lean mass Significant association between baseline serum 25OHD and: LS BMD ($r = 0.16$, $p = 0.033$) Femoral neck ($r = 0.17$, $p = 0.028$) Radius BMD levels ($r = 0.24$, $p = 0.002$) Radius BMC levels ($r = 0.16$, $p = 0.033$) Largest increases in bone mass in IG2 (high dose) subjects with lowest 25OHD levels at baseline

continued

Prospective cohort studies

Guillemant et al., 1999 France	Healthy adolescent boys from a jockey training center; age range 13 y 5 mo to 16 y 1 mo $n = 175$ Caucasian	NA	iPTH (immunoradiometric assay, Nichols)	25OHD, mean (SD) (nmol/L) Post-summer 58.5 (10.0) Post-winter 20.6 (6.0), $p = 0.0001$ At serum 25OHD > 83 nmol/L, iPTH plateau occurred at 2.48 pmol/L
Javaid et al., 2006 UK	Children with known maternal 25OHD status in third trimester; 9 y old $n = 198$ Caucasian	NA	Total body and LS BMC and areal BMD, calculated volumetric BMD (DXA Lunar DPX-L)	Maternal serum 25OHD in late pregnancy: 18% had serum 25OHD levels < 27.5 nmol/L and 31% had levels 27.5–50.0 nmol/L Mothers with lower 25OHD during pregnancy had children with reduced total body ($r = 0.21$, $p = 0.0088$) and lumbar spine BMC ($r = 0.17$, $p = 0.03$). Adjustment for height did not weaken the relationship between total body BMC and 25OHD; volumetric LS BMD was not associated with maternal 25OHD. Adjusted for age of child

TABLE 4-6 Continued

Reference; Country; Jadad Score for RCTs[b]	Population Description	Intervention/ Duration	Bone Health Outcomes	Results
Lehtonen-Veromaa et al., 2002 Finland	Healthy adolescent girls; 12.9 (1.7) y, range 9–15 y n = 191 Caucasian	NA	LS BMD and BMAD FN BMD and BMAD (DXA)	25OHD, mean (SD) (nmol/L) Baseline: 34.0 (13.2) (winter) 1 y: 33.2 (11.1) 3 y: 40.6 (15.8) Baseline 25OHD correlated with Δ LS BMD ($r = 0.35$, $p < 0.001$) and Δ FN BMD ($r = 0.32$, $p < 0.001$) Baseline 25OHD correlated with Δ LS BMAD (0.35, $p < 0.001$) and Δ FN BMAD (0.24, $p < 0.002$) Adjusted for: baseline reproductive year, bone mineral values, increases in height and weight, mean intake of calcium, and mean amount of physical activity Significant correlation between baseline 25OHD and Δ 3-y adjusted LS or FN BMD and BMAD Difference in mean 3-y Δ LS BMD between group with baseline 25OHD < 20 nmol/L and group with baseline 25OHD ≥ 37.5 was 4%

continued

Case–control studies

Marwaha et al., 2005	Healthy school children	NA	BMD (distal forearm and calcaneum) using DXA	Serum 25OHD, mean (SD) (nmol/L): 29.5 (18.0) LSES: 26 (1); USES: 34 (1)
India	(from LSES and USES); age range 10–18 y			25OHD < 22.5 nmol/L: 35.7%; LSES 42.3% vs. USES 27%, *p* < 0.01
	n = 5,137 (3,089 LSES; 2,048 USES)			Prevalence of clinical vit D deficiency (defined by genu varum or genu valgum): LSES 11.6% vs. USES 9.7%, *p* = 0.07
				Forearm mean BMD significantly higher (*p* < 0.01) in USES group compared with LSES
	LSES 65.1% female USES 52.7% female			BMD adjusted for height and weight
				Serum calcium not significantly different between groups, but dietary calcium intake lower in LSES group
	Indian			No significant correlation between BMD and serum 25OHD in either group

TABLE 4-6 Continued

Reference; Country; Jadad Score for RCTs[b]	Population Description	Intervention/ Duration	Bone Health Outcomes	Results
Before-and-after studies				
Rajakumar et al., 2005 United States	Healthy 6–10 y olds Tanner stage I/II (81% I) Skin type III/IV (81% IV); mean age 8.9 (1.2) y (range 6–10 y) Vit D dietary intake: mean (SD) 277 (146) IU/d 16/41 (39%) dietary intake < 200 IU/d n = 42 34% female African American	400 IU vit D/d (isoform not specified) 1 mo	iPTH (Immulite iPTH chemiluminescent assay)	Serum 25OHD, mean (SD) (nmol/L) Baseline: 60.0 (26.3) 49% < 50 71% < 75 Group 1 = 25OHD < 50 nmol/L at baseline: 38.5 (8.0) Group 2 = 25OHD > 50 nmol/L at baseline: 80.3 (20.5) 1 mo (total group): 68.8 (18.8) Group 1: 57.5 (16.0) Group 2: 79.5 (14.5) Increase in serum 25OHD was observed only in group 1 7/39 (18%) of group 1 continued to have a level < 50 nmol/L after 1 mo of supplementation Negative correlation of 25OHD with body weight ($r = -0.378$, $p = 0.015$) at baseline No significant differences at baseline or 1 mo in markers of bone turnover, $1,25(OH)_2D$ or PTH between groups with 25OHD < 50 nmol/L or > 50 nmol/L at baseline

NOTE: BMAD = bone mineral apparent density; BMC = bone mineral content; BMD = bone mineral density; CG = control group; DXA = dual-energy X-ray absorptiometry; FN = femoral neck; IG = intervention group; iPTH = intact parathyroid hormone; IU = International Units; LS = lumbar spine; LSES = lower socioeconomic status; mo = month(s); NA = not applicable; PTH = parathyroid hormone; RCT = randomized controlled trial; SD = standard deviation; SPA = single-photon absorptiometry; UK = United Kingdom; USES = upper socioeconomic status; vit = vitamin; wk = week(s); y = year(s).

[a]This table has been truncated for the purposes of this chapter, but it can be found in its entirety in Appendix C.

[b]Jadad score is based on a scale of 1 to 5. See Box 4-1 for details on the scoring system.

SOURCE: Modified from Cranney et al. (2007).

Postmenopausal women and elderly men   Overall, regarding serum 25OHD and bone density measures, AHRQ-Ottawa, which included some studies that combined calcium and vitamin D, reported discordance between the results from RCTs and the majority of observational studies; the authors attributed this as likely due to the impact of confounders relative to observational data as a general matter. Nineteen studies (see Table 4-7) evaluated the association between serum 25OHD levels and BMD. Of these, six studies were RCTs. One RCT (Ooms et al., 1995b) reported an association between serum 25OHD concentrations and BMD or bone loss, whereas the other five RCTs (Dawson-Hughes et al., 1995; Storm et al., 1998; Schaafsma et al., 2002; Cooper et al., 2003; Aloia et al., 2005) and three cohort studies did not. Four cohort studies found a significant association between 25OHD concentrations and bone loss, which was most evident at the hip sites, but the evidence for an association between 25OHD concentrations and lumbar spine BMD was weak. Six case–control studies suggested an association between 25OHD concentrations and BMD, and the association was most consistent at the femoral neck. A forest plot showing the effect of vitamin D plus calcium supplementation (versus placebo) for femoral neck BMD at 1 year is shown in Figure 4-4. Overall, significant increases at the femoral neck were observed with a combined estimate as reported in Table 4-7 of 1.37 percent (95% confidence interval [CI]: 0.24–2.50) from three trials after 1 year.

Based on the results from the observational studies, there is fair evidence to support an association between serum 25OHD levels and BMD or changes in BMD at the femoral neck. Specific circulating concentrations of 25OHD below which bone loss at the hip was increased ranged from 30 to 80 nmol/L.

AHRQ-Tufts identified two more recent RCTs, one that combined calcium with vitamin D and one that did not. The first, an A-quality RCT (Zhu et al., 2008a), compared the effect of vitamin D_2 supplementation on hip BMC in 256 elderly women between 70 and 90 years of age. All elderly women in this trial had normal physical functioning. They were randomly assigned to receive either vitamin D_2 (1,000 IU/day) plus calcium (1,200 mg/day) supplement or calcium (1,200 mg/day) supplement alone for 1 year. The mean baseline dietary calcium intake was 1,097 mg/day, and the mean serum 25OHD concentration was 44.3 nmol/L. Total hip BMD increased significantly in both groups, with no difference between the vitamin D_2 plus calcium and calcium alone groups (hip BMD change: vitamin D, +0.5 percent; control, +0.2 percent).

The second, a B-quality RCT (Andersen et al., 2008), analyzed 89 healthy adult women and 83 healthy adult men separately. The participants were Pakistani immigrants living in the Copenhagen area of Denmark (latitude 55°N). Women and men were randomly assigned to receive either a daily dose of 400 or 800 IU vitamin D_3 or placebo for 1 year. For women,

TABLE 4-7 Serum 25OHD Levels and BMC/BMD in Postmenopausal Women and Older Men: Summary from AHRQ-Ottawa Analyses[a]

Reference; Country; Jadad Score for RCTs[b]	Population Description	Intervention/ Duration	Bone Health Outcomes	Results
RCTs				
Aloia et al., 2005 United States Jadad = 5	PM women; IG1: 59.9 (6.2) y CG: 61.2 (6.3) y *n* = 208 100% African American	IG: 800 IU vit D$_3$ for 2 y, then 2,000 IU for 1 y + 1,200–1,500 mg CaCG: 1,200–1,500 mg Ca 3 y	BMD: LS, total hip, total body, mid radius (DXA)	No association between serum 25OHD and Δ BMD Analyses examining those with low baseline 25OHD or high PTH showed no influence of 25OHD on Δ BMD
Cooper et al., 2003 Australia Jadad = 4	PM women not on HRT; IG1: 56.5 (4.2) y, CG: 56.1 (4.7) y *n* = 187 Caucasian	IG1: 10,000 IU vit D$_2$/wk + 1,000 mg Ca/d CG: 1,000 mg Ca/d 2 y	BMD: LS, FN, Ward's triangle, Tr, proximal forearm (DXA)	No significant correlation between baseline 25OHD concentration and Δ BMD at any site or between Δ 25OHD and Δ BMD at any site
Dawson-Hughes et al., 1995 United States Jadad = 3	Healthy, ambulatory PM women; IG1: 63.0 y CG: 64.0 y *n* = 247 Caucasian	IG1: 700 IU vit D$_3$ + 500 mg Ca citrate malate CG: 100 IU vit D$_3$ + 500 mg Ca daily 2 y	BMD: LS, FN, and total body (DXA)	25OHD concentrations during either season did not correlate with Δ BMD at any site

Ooms et al., 1995b Netherlands Jadad = 4	Elderly women; IG1: 80.1 (5.6) y CG: 80.6 (5.5) y n = 348	IG1: 400 IU vit D_3/d CG: placebo 2 y	BMD: FN, Tr, and distal radius (DXA)	Effect of vitamin D supplementation was independent of baseline 25OHD as well as 25OHD corrected for season
Schaafsma et al., 2002 Netherlands Jadad = 4	Healthy, PM women 50–70 y n = 85 Caucasian	IG1: eggshell powder + 200 IU vit D_3 IG2: Ca carbonate + 200 IU vit D_3 CG: placebo 12 mo	BMD: LS, hip (DXA)	No significant correlation between 25OHD and BMD
Storm et al., 1998 Netherlands Jadad = 4	PM women without OP n = 60 Caucasian	IG1: 4 glasses of fortified milk (325 IU vit D/quart) daily IG2: Ca carbonate daily CG: placebo 2 y	BMD: Tr, FN, LS (DXA)	Serum 25OHD was not a significant determinant of FN BMD at baseline, during winter ($p = 0.23$), or over the entire study period
Prospective cohort studies				
Bischoff-Ferrari et al., 2005 United States	Individuals with knee OA: 74.4 (11.1) y n = 228 64% female	1–2 y	BMD: FN (DXA Lunar DPX-L)	Significant positive association between 25OHD and BMD independent of age, gender, BMI, knee pain, physical activity, and disease severity Significant trend between being in a higher serum 25OHD group and having higher BMD ($p < 0.04$)

continued

TABLE 4-7 Continued

Reference; Country; Jadad Score for RCTs[b]	Population Description	Intervention/ Duration	Bone Health Outcomes	Results
del Puente et al., 2002 Italy	Active, noninstitutionalized females (menopausal and premenopausal); 58 (9) y n = 139 Caucasian	2 y	BMD: LS and FN (DXA)	25OHD independent predictor of BMD change at FN and LS (FN Δ BMD [β = 0.26 (0.13), p = 0.04] and LS Δ BMD [β = 0.07 (0.03), p = 0.04]) In stepwise analysis discrimination models, only FN significant (partial R^2 = 0.26, p = 0.04)
Dennison et al., 1999 UK	Healthy adults age 60–75 y n = 316 45% female	4 y	BMD: LS and proximal femur (DXA)	No association between baseline 25OHD and BMD at LS and proximal hip (β = 0.002 spine, 0.001 hip) and no association between 25OHD and bone loss after adjustment for adiposity
Gerdhem et al., 2005 Sweden	Ambulatory independently living women; 75 (75–75.9) y n = 1,044	3 y	BMD: FN and LS (DXA)	No association between baseline 25OHD and BMD
Melin et al., 2001 Sweden	Healthy, independent elderly individuals; 83.7 y n = 64 81% female Caucasian	1 y	BMD: FN (DXA)	FN BMD associated with serum 25OHD after summer (r = 0.38, p = 0.003) and winter (r = 0.37, p = 0.003) After adjusting for BMI, 25OHD remained a significant determinant after winter (adjusted R^2 = 0.14, p = 0.005)

Rosen et al., 1994 United States	Healthy independently living elderly women; 77 (2) y $n = 18$	2 y	BMD: LS and FN (DXA)	Δ 25OHD between summer and winter was associated with LS BMD in 2nd y ($r = 0.59$, $p = 0.04$), but not FN BMD
Stone et al., 1998 United States	Healthy elderly females > 65 y, random sample, subcohort of individuals not on HRT from Study of Osteoporotic Fractures $n = 261$ Caucasian	42–71 mo	BMD: total hip (DXA), calcaneal (SPA)	Significant association between lower 25OHD levels and total hip BMD loss Lower 25OHD levels associated with increased loss at total hip after adjusting for estradiol, testosterone, SHBG, season, and use of supplements 25OHD not associated with calcaneal BMD after adjusting for age and weight
Case–control studies				
Al-oanzi et al., 2006 UK	Men with idiopathic OP Cases: 59.6 (13.6) y Controls: 62.4 (10.4) y $n = 56$ (+ 114 controls) Caucasian	NA	BMD diagnosis of OP based on T-score FN and LS	No significant difference between plasma 25OHD in cases and controls, but mean free plasma 25OHD was about 33% lower in men with OP vs. controls ($p < 0.0001$)

continued

TABLE 4-7 Continued

Reference; Country; Jadad Score for RCTs[b]	Population Description	Intervention/ Duration	Bone Health Outcomes	Results
Boonen et al., 1999 Belgium	PM women (hip fracture patients and controls) n = 100 Cases: 74.2 (7.8) y Controls: 75.8 (5.6) y	NA	BMD: FN and Tr (DXA) Fractures	Mean 25OHD$_3$ was lower in cases vs. controls ($p < 0.001$) Vit D deficiency (< 30 nmol/L): 64% of cases vs. 8% controls within the same 4-mo sampling period (no relation between 25OHD and month of sample collection) FN and Tr BMD were significantly lower in cases than in controls. No significant relation found between the 25OHD$_3$–PTH axis and BMD in cases and controls. In multiple regression of pooled data, models using 25OHD$_3$ and PTH were highly predictive of FN BMD ($R^2 = 32\%$, $p < 0.001$).
Landin-Wilhelmsen et al., 1999 Sweden	PM patients with OP and age-matched controls from outpatient clinic n = 128 (+ 227 age-matched controls) Cases: 59 (6) y Controls: 59 (5) y	NA	BMD and BMC: LS, total body, and FN (DXA) Fractures	25OHD significantly lower in OP patients vs. controls ($p < 0.05$) OP patients had lower body weight and BMI vs. controls ($p < 0.001$)

| Villareal et al., 1991 United States (Midwest) | Ambulatory, independently living PM women, women with low (< 38 nmol/L) 25OHD and controls

$n = 98$

Cases: 64 y
Controls: 63 y

Caucasian | NA | BMD: (LS, T12-L3), QCT | Women with low 25OHD levels had a reduced LS BMD. In the low 25OHD group, LS BMD correlated with 25OHD ($r = 0.41$, $p < 0.01$).

In multivariate analysis, iPTH was the major determinant of a decrease in LS BMD |
| Thiebaud et al., 1997 Switzerland | Hip fracture patients, hospital controls, and community controls

$n = 179$ (+ 180 controls)

Cases: 81.0 y (women) and 77.7 y (men); hospital controls: 80.9 y (women) and 76.9 y (men); community controls: 71.7 y (women) and 71.3 y (men) | NA | BMD: FN, total hip, and Tr (DXA)

Fractures | Women and men with hip fractures significantly lower 25OHD levels vs. controls

Fracture patients had lower hip BMD vs. controls ($p < 0.001$)

Significant biochemical markers in the multivariate logistic regression model of the risk for hip fracture were serum albumin and PTH

In women FN, Tr BMD weakly correlated with 25OHD, and the only significant association was at the Tr ($r = 0.13$, $p < 0.05$) |

continued

216

TABLE 4-7 Continued

Reference; Country; Jadad Score for RCTs[b]	Population Description	Intervention/ Duration	Bone Health Outcomes	Results
Yan et al., 2003 China 42°N and UK 52°N	Older individuals (60–83 y) n = 352 Chinese: 50% female British: 50% female 64% Chinese (Asian), 36% British (Caucasian)	NA	BMC: FN (DXA)	Significantly higher 25OHD levels in British subjects Weak association ($r = 0.054$, $p = 0.05$) between 25OHD and FN BMC in British subjects after adjusting for size, but not in Chinese subjects

NOTE: BMC = bone mineral content; BMD = bone mineral density; BMI = body mass index; CG = control group; DXA = dual-energy X-ray absorptiometry; FN = femoral neck; HRT = hormone replacement therapy; IG = intervention group; iPTH = intact parathyroid hormone; IU = International Units; LS = lumbar spine; mo = month(s); NA = not applicable; OA = osteoarthritis; OP = osteoporosis; PM = postmenopausal; PTH = parathyroid hormone; QCT = quantitative computed tomography; RCT = randomized controlled trial; SHBG = sex hormone binding globulin; SPA = single-photon absorptiometry; Tr = trochanter; UK = United Kingdom; vit = vitamin; wk = week(s); y = year(s).

[a]This table has been truncated for the purposes of this chapter, but it can be found in its entirety in Appendix C.

[b]Jadad score is based on a scale of 1 to 5. See Box 4-1 for details on the scoring system.

SOURCE: Modified from Cranney et al. (2007).

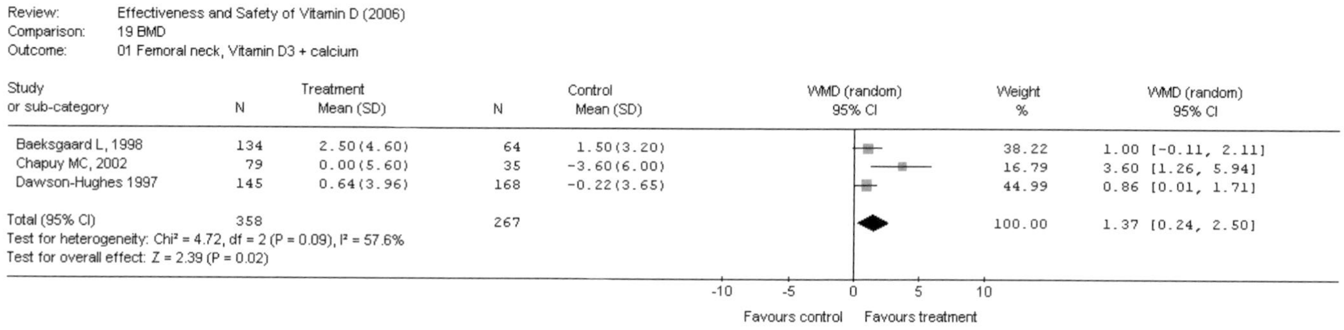

FIGURE 4-4 Forest plot: Effect of vitamin D_3 + calcium vs. placebo on femoral neck BMD at 1 year.
SOURCE: Cranney et al. (2007).

the mean baseline dietary calcium intake was 495 mg/day, and the mean serum 25OHD concentration was 12 nmol/L. For men, the mean baseline dietary calcium intake was 548 mg/day, and the mean serum 25OHD concentration was 21 nmol/L. At the end of the study, in both women and men, there were no significant differences in lumbar spine BMD changes between the groups receiving the two doses of vitamin D_3 (400 or 800 IU/day) and the placebo group.

Pregnant or lactating women   Overall, from AHRQ-Ottawa, there was insufficient evidence on the association between 25OHD concentration and change in bone density during pregnancy. Four studies (no RCTs, three cohort studies, one before-and-after study) assessed vitamin D nutriture at various time points in pregnancy, with vitamin D deficiency being observed in 0 to 50 percent of subjects, but only one cohort study ($n = 115$) rated

---

BOX 4-3
AHRQ Findings by Life Stage for Serum
25OHD Measures and BMC/BMD*

0–6 months: Inconsistent evidence for an association between a specific serum 25OHD concentration and the bone health outcome BMC in infants.

7 months–2 years: Fair evidence of an association between 25OHD concentrations and baseline BMD and change in BMD or BMC indexes from the studies in older children and adolescents.

3–8 years: Fair evidence of an association between 25OHD concentrations and baseline BMD and change in BMD or BMC indexes from the studies in older children and adolescents.

9–18 years: Fair evidence of an association between 25OHD concentrations and baseline BMD and change in BMD or BMC indexes from the studies in older children and adolescents. Two new RCTs identified by AHRQ-Tufts enrolled only girls in this life stage. The results showed no significant differences in whole-body BMC changes between groups receiving either lower doses of vitamin D (200 or 400 IU/day) or higher doses of vitamin D (800 or 2,000 IU/day) and the placebo group.

19–50 years: Discordance between the results from RCTs and the majority of observational studies in postmenopausal women and elderly men. Based on results of the observational studies, there is fair evidence to support an association between serum 25OHD concentration and BMD or changes in BMD at the femoral neck. One new RCT identified by AHRQ-Tufts enrolled primarily men and women in this life stage. The

as good quality included maternal BMD as an outcome, and there was no relationship between vitamin D status and postpartum changes in BMD. Information on the four studies can be found in Appendix C. AHRQ-Tufts found no new RCTs.

Summary   Evidence regarding serum 25OHD concentrations and BMC/BMD measures varied by life stage. The findings from the AHRQ analyses are summarized by DRI-relevant life stage group in Box 4-3 below.

Bone mineral content/bone mineral density: Vitamin D supplementation with or without calcium   AHRQ addressed data primarily for menopausal women. One RCT for girls was also identified. Overall, AHRQ-Ottawa concluded that there is good evidence that vitamin D_3 plus calcium supplementation resulted in small increases in BMD of the spine, total body,

---

results showed that there were no significant differences in lumbar spine BMD changes between the groups receiving two doses of vitamin D_3 (400 or 800 IU/day) and the placebo group.

51–70 years: Discordance between the results from RCTs and the majority of observational studies in postmenopausal women and elderly men. Based on results of the observational studies, there is fair evidence to support an association between serum 25OHD concentration and BMD or changes in BMD at the femoral neck. One new RCT identified by AHRQ-Tufts enrolled some men in this life stage. The results showed that there were no significant differences in lumbar spine BMD changes between the groups receiving two doses of vitamin D_3 (400 or 800 IU/day) and the placebo group.

≥71 years: Discordance between the results from RCTs and the majority of observational studies in postmenopausal women and elderly men. Based on results of the observational studies, there is fair evidence to support an association between serum 25OHD and BMD or changes in BMD at the femoral neck. One new RCT identified by AHRQ-Tufts enrolled only elderly women in this life stage. The results showed that vitamin D_2 supplementation (1,000 IU/day) had no additional effect on hip BMD compared with calcium supplementation alone.

Pregnant or lactating women: Insufficient evidence for an association between a specific serum 25OHD concentration and the bone health outcome BMC.

---

*Evidence from AHRQ-Ottawa; information from AHRQ-Tufts as noted.
SOURCE: Modified from Chung et al. (2009).

femoral neck and total hip. Based on included trials, it was less certain whether vitamin D_3 supplementation alone has a significant effect on BMD.

Seventeen RCTs evaluated the effect of supplemental vitamin D_2 or vitamin D_3 on BMD, predominantly in populations of late menopausal women (see Table 4-8). Only one small RCT included premenopausal women, and two trials included older men (> 60 years). Most trials were 2 to 3 years in duration and used vitamin D doses of up to 800 IU daily. Most trials used vitamin D_3 and also included 500 mg of calcium as a co-intervention.

Meta-analysis results of 17 RCTs comparing vitamin D_3 plus calcium with placebo (AHRQ-Tufts) were consistent with a small effect on lumbar spine, femoral neck, and total body BMD. The WHI trial found a significant benefit of supplementation with 400 IU of vitamin D_3 plus 1,000 mg of calcium on total hip BMD. However, when the effect of supplementation with vitamin D_3 plus calcium versus supplementation with calcium alone was assessed by AHRQ-Tufts, no significant increase in BMD was observed with either intervention, suggesting that vitamin D_3 may be of less benefit in calcium-replete postmenopausal women. It is noted, however, that the dose administered was 400 IU/day, which is a lower level than has been used commonly, although the authors of the report did measure background intakes of vitamin D for participants, which, when added to the 400 IU dose results in an average intake of approximately 750 IU/day. Vitamin D_3 alone versus placebo did not result in a significant increase in BMD in postmenopausal women, except in one trial that noted an increase in femoral neck BMD. Only a few trials reported the impact of baseline serum 25OHD concentrations on BMD; in all of these trials, baseline 25OHD concentration was not associated with increased BMD.

AHRQ-Tufts identified four RCTs that were made available after the completion of AHRQ-Ottawa, one of which focused on children (see Table 4-9). Two of the three new RCTs for women and elderly men indicated a significant increase in hip or total BMD in postmenopausal women, comparing vitamin D_3 or vitamin D_2 (300 or 1,000 IU/day, respectively) plus calcium (1,200 mg/day) with placebo. The RCT that focused on healthy girls, ages 10 to 12 years (Cheng et al., 2005) compared the effect of vitamin D_3 (200 IU/day) plus calcium (1,000 mg/day) supplementation on bone indexes with placebo. The mean background dietary calcium intake was 670 mg/day. The intention-to-treat analyses suggested that after 2 years of supplementation, there was no significant difference in the BMC changes between girls who received vitamin D plus calcium supplement or placebo. The methodological quality of this study was rated C, as a result of being underpowered and having low compliance rate. The findings from AHRQ are summarized by DRI-relevant life stage groups in Box 4-4.

TABLE 4-8 Effect of Vitamin D_2 or Vitamin D_3 on BMD by Site in Individual Trials (for Women of Reproductive Age, Postmenopausal Women, and Older Men): Summary from AHRQ-Ottawa Analyses[a]

Reference	Duration; Sample Size (n/Total N)	Vitamin D Dose (IU/day); Mean Dietary Vitamin D Intake (Tx/Control)	Lumbar Spine BMD % change (SD) Tx	Control (e.g., placebo, calcium, or lower dose of vit D)	Femoral Neck BMD % change (SD) Tx	Control	Total Body BMD % change (SD) Tx	Control
Aloia et al., 2005	3 years 208	800 D_3 for 2 y, then 2,000 D_3 for 1 y + calcium 184 IU/d	0.25 (1.82)	0.30 (1.82)	NR	NR	-0.35 (1.60)	-0.30 (1.50)
Baeksgaard et al., 1998	2 years 240	560 D_3 + 1,000 mg calcium 158/140 IU/d	1.6	-0.2	1	0.4	NR	NR
Chapuy et al., 1992	1.5 years 56 (56/3270)	800 D_3 + 1,200 mg calcium NR	NR	NR	2.90 (6.40)	1.80 (9.40)	NR	NR
Chapuy et al., 2002	2 years 114 (114/583)	800 D_3 + 1,200 mg calcium 40/42 IU/d	NR	NR	-1.20 (7.40)	-4.50 (7.10)	NR	NR
Cooper et al., 2003	2 years 276 (187/187)	10,000 D_2/wk + 1,000 mg calcium NR	0.21 (4.89)	1.66 (5.27)	0.87 (4.95)	3.32 (5.10)	NR	NR

continued

TABLE 4-8 Continued

Reference	Duration; Sample Size (n/Total N)	Vitamin D Dose (IU/day); Mean Dietary Vitamin D Intake (Tx/Control)	Lumbar Spine BMD % change (SD)		Femoral Neck BMD % change (SD)		Total Body BMD % change (SD)	
			Tx	Control (e.g., placebo, calcium, or lower dose of vit D)	Tx	Control	Tx	Control
Dawson-Hughes et al., 1991	1 year 261 (220–246/276)	400 D_3 + 377 mg calcium; During treatment, 106/87 IU/d, August–November	0.85 (2.41)	0.15 (2.62)	NR	NR	0.03 (1.35)	−0.08 (1.25)
Dawson-Hughes et al., 1995	2 years 215 (215–246/261)	700 D_3 + 500 mg calcium; 120/107 IU/d	−0.31 (2.87)	−0.11 (3.15)	−1.06 (3.76)	−2.54 (4.07)	−0.20 (1.66)	−0.35 (1.56)
Dawson-Hughes et al., 1997b	3 years 389	700 D_3 + 500 mg calcium; Women: 174/184 IU/d; Men: 202/197 IU/d	2.12 (4.06)	1.22 (4.25)	0.50 (4.80)	−0.70 (5.03)	0.06 (1.83)	−1.09 (1.71)
Grados et al., 2003a; Companions: Grados et al., 2003b; Brazier et al., 2005	1 year 192 (67–72/192)	800 D_3 + 1,000 mg calcium; 84.9/83.9 IU/d	2.98*	−0.21*	1.19*	−0.83*	0.99*	0.11*

Study	Duration	N	Intervention/Dose						
Harwood et al., 2004	1 year	150 (40/150)	800 D$_3$ + 1,000 mg calcium 300,000 D$_2$ single injection 300,000 D$_2$ single injection + 1,000 mg calcium NR	−1.6	8.2	−1.9	−0.9	NR	NR
Hunter et al., 2000	2 years	128 Comparison of 64 pairs of twins	800 D$_3$ 135/134 IU/d	0.00 (5.62)	0.00 (5.56)	—	—	—	—
Jackson et al., 2006	7 years	2,431 of total sample	400 D$_3$ + 1,000 mg calcium Total vit D intake diet and supplements: 365/368 IU	Graph	Graph	Graph	Graph	Graph	Graph
Jensen et al., 2002	3 years	68/83	400 D$_3$ + 1,450 mg calcium NR	1.20 (4.32)	0.73 (4.08)	NR	NR	−1.10 (1.78)	−1.78 (1.56)
Komulainen et al., 1998	5 years	206/425	300 D$_3$ + 500 mg calcium NR	−4.6 (5.08)	−4.5 (4.90)	−4.3 (5.03)	−4.3 (4.9)	NR	NR

continued

TABLE 4-8 Continued

Reference	Duration; Sample Size (n/Total N)	Vitamin D Dose (IU/day); Mean Dietary Vitamin D Intake (Tx/Control)	Lumbar Spine BMD % change (SD)		Femoral Neck BMD % change (SD)		Total Body BMD % change (SD)	
			Tx	Control (e.g., placebo, calcium, or lower dose of vit D)	Tx	Control	Tx	Control
Meier et al., 2004	2 years 55 (43/55)	500 D$_3$ + 500 mg calcium NR	0.8	NR	0.1	NR	NR	NR
Ooms et al., 1995b	2 years 348	400 D$_3$ NR	NR	NR	1.47 (6.13) left femoral neck	−0.21 (6.12)	NR	NR
Patel et al., 2001	2 years 70	800 D$_3$ NR	NA crossover trial					

NOTE: * Median % change; Dawson-Hughes et al. (1997b) included 176/389 men (45% of participants) and Meier et al. (2004) included 19/55 men (35% of participants). All other studies included women only. BMD = bone mineral density; IU = International Units; NA = not applicable; NR = not reported; SD = standard deviation; Tx = treatment; vit = vitamin; wk = week(s).

^{a}This table has been truncated for the purposes of this chapter, but it can be found in its entirety in Appendix C.
SOURCE: Modified from Cranney et al. (2007).

TABLE 4-9 Combined Vitamin D and Calcium and Bone Mineral Density/Bone Mineral Content: Characteristics of RCTs Published after AHRQ-Ottawa Report: Summary from AHRQ-Tufts Analyses[a]

Reference; Location (Latitude)	Population Description	Background Calcium Intake and Vitamin D Data	Comparisons	Compliance	Comments
Cheng et al., 2005 Jyvaskyla, Finland (62°24′N)	Health status: Healthy Mean age (range), y: 11.2 (10–12) Male (%): 0	Diet vit D: 100 IU/d Ca: 670 mg/d	200 IU vit D_3/d + 1,000 mg Ca carbonate/d vs. placebo	65% completed intervention with > 50% compliance	
Bolton-Smith et al., 2007 UK (54°N)	Health status: Healthy (assumed postmenopausal) Mean age (range), y: 68 (≥ 60) Male (%): 0	25OHD: 59.4 nmol/L Ca: 1,548 mg/d	400 IU vit D_3/d + 100 mg elemental Ca/d vs. placebo	Good supplement adherence based on pill count (median, 99; IQE 97.3–99.8%)	Noncompliant women were excluded
Zhu et al., 2008b Western Australia	Health status: nd (assumed postmenopausal) Mean age (SD), y: 74.8 (2.6) Male (%): 0	25OHD: 68 nmol/L Ca: 1,010 mg/d	1,000 IU vit D_2/d + 1,200 mg Ca citrate/d vs. placebo	No differences in adherence among groups (81–89% by tablet counting)	
Moschonis and Manios, 2006 Greece (31°N)	Health status: Postmenopausal Mean age (range), y: 61 (55–65) Male (%): 0	Diet vit D: 23.6 IU/d Ca 680.0 mg/d	300 IU vit D_3/d + 1,200 mg Ca/d (from low-fat dairy products) vs. control (usual diet)	Dairy group 93% (assessed via information obtained at the biweekly sessions)	Control group had no intervention (or usual diet), so compliance issue not applicable

NOTE: IU = International Units; nd = not determined; SD = standard deviation; UK = United Kingdom; vit = vitamin; y = year(s).
[a]This table has been truncated for the purposes of this chapter, but it can be found in its entirety in Appendix D.
SOURCE: Chung et al. (2009).

BOX 4-4
AHRQ Findings by Life Stage for Vitamin D
and Calcium and BMC/BMD*

0–6 months: No data

7 months–2 years: No data

3–8 years: No data

9–18 years: One RCT showed that, compared with placebo, there was no significant effect of vitamin D_3 (200 IU/day) plus calcium (1,000 mg/day) on BMC changes in healthy girls between 10 and 12 years of age.

19–50 years: No data

51–70 years: No new data were identified in AHRQ-Tufts

≥ 71 years: No new data were identified in AHRQ-Tufts

Postmenopause: Findings from the AHRQ-Ottawa report showed that vitamin D_3 (≤ 800 IU/day) plus calcium (~500 mg/day) supplementation resulted in small increases in BMD of the spine, total body, femoral neck, and total hip in predominantly populations of late-menopausal women. Two of the three new RCTs showed a significant increase in hip or total BMD in postmenopausal women, comparing vitamin D_3 or vitamin D_2 (300 or 1,000 IU/day, respectively) plus calcium (1,200 mg/day) with placebo.

Pregnant and lactating women: No new data were identified in AHRQ-Tufts

---

*Evidence from AHRQ-Ottawa; information from AHRQ-Tufts as noted.
SOURCE: Modified from Chung et al. (2009).

Fractures and BMD in postmenopausal women and older men: Serum 25OHD   The association between risk of fractures and vitamin D in combination with calcium, as well as vitamin D alone, was addressed by AHRQ. Neither analysis focused on fracture risk and calcium intake alone.

AHRQ-Ottawa, which included some studies that combined calcium and vitamin D, identified observational studies (ranging from poor to fair quality) that reported on the association between serum 25OHD concentrations and fractures. The studies are identified in Table 4-10. The analysis concludes that there is inconsistent evidence to support an association between serum 25OHD concentration and an increased risk of fracture. Five studies of good quality evaluated the association between serum 25OHD concentration and risk of falls (see discussion in section above on Falls and

TABLE 4-10 Serum 25OHD Levels and Fractures in Postmenopausal Women and Older Men: Summary from AHRQ-Ottawa Analyses[a]

Reference; Country	Population Description	Duration (or Matching Variables)	Bone Health Outcomes	Covariates; Summary of Results
Prospective cohort studies				
Cummings et al., 1998 United States	Subset of a cohort of ambulatory community-dwelling women ≥ 65 years of age (nested case–control study); 72.6 y (subset) n = 9,704 Caucasian	5.9 y	Hip fractures	Adjusted for age, weight, and calcaneal BMD (SPA)
			Vertebral fractures	There were no statistically significant unadjusted or adjusted (age, weight, season, use of vit D supplements) associations between serum 25OHD or PTH and the risk of hip or vertebral fracture
			BMD calcaneus (SPA)	For women in the lowest quintile of serum 25OHD levels, there was no increased risk for hip or vertebral fracture
				Women in the lowest quintile of serum 1,25(OH)$_2$D had a significant increase in hip fracture risk (RR 2.1, 95% CI 1.2–3.5), but not vertebral fracture risk
Gerdhem et al., 2005 Sweden	Ambulatory independently living women, 75 y (range 75–75.9 y) n = 1,044	3 y	Fractures (low energy)	119/986 (12%) had a total of 159 low-energy fractures (29 hip, 28 wrist, 12 proximal humerus, 43 vertebral, and 47 other)
				9/43 (21%) with 25OHD < 50 nmol/L had one or more fractures vs. 110/943 (12%) with 25OHD > 50 nmol/L: HR 2.04 (95% CI 1.04–4.04)
				Fracture association was independent of season, although a seasonal difference was noted in mean level of 25OHD (September 101 nmol/L vs. February 89.8 nmol/L)

continued

TABLE 4-10 Continued

Reference; Country	Population Description	Duration (or Matching Variables)	Bone Health Outcomes	Covariates; Summary of Results
Woo et al., 1990 Hong Kong	Elderly ≥ 60 y living independently in sheltered housing n = 470 60% females Asian (Chinese)	30 mo	Fractures	Adjusted for age, gender, drinking, smoking, and BMI Subjects with lower serum 25OHD (males < 79 nmol/L and females < 66 nmol/L) had a nonsignificant increase in adjusted RR for fracture
Case–control studies				
Bakhtiyarova et al., 2006 Russian Federation	Hip fracture cases (spontaneous or low trauma) and controls admitted to ophthalmology department Cases: 68.8 (9.5) y Controls: 70.2 (8.3) y n = 64 (+ 97 controls) Cases: 69% female Controls: 55% female Caucasian	NR	Hip fractures	Median serum 25OHD levels significantly lower in hip fracture cases vs. controls (graph only) Hip fracture patients more likely to have serum 25OHD < 25 nmol/L than controls (65% vs. 47%, p = 0.006)

Reference, Location	Population	Matching/Adjustment	Outcome	Results
Boonen et al., 1997 Belgium	Elderly women with hip fractures and community-dwelling controls; $n = 117$ (+ 117 controls); Caucasian	Age, PM status, gender, ethnicity	Hip fractures; BMD (FN and Tr) (DXA)	Serum 25OHD significantly lower in cases vs. controls ($p = 0.001$); Hip BMD (FN and Tr) significantly lower in cases vs. controls ($p < 0.001$)
Boonen et al., 1999 Belgium	PM women (osteoporotic hip fracture patients and independently living controls); Cases: 79.2 y; Controls: 77.7 y; $n = 50$ (+ 50 controls)	Age, gender, PM status, sampled at the same time of year	Fractures; BMD (FN and Tr) (DXA)	Adjusted for age; Mean 25OHD$_3$ was significantly lower in cases vs. controls; 25OHD < 30 nmol/L: 64% of cases vs. 8% controls within the same 4-mo sampling period (no relation between 25OHD and month of sample collection); FN and Tr BMD were significantly lower in cases than in controls
Cooper et al., 1989 UK	Hip fractures and healthy controls; Cases: 77.4 (8.6) y; Controls: 73.3 (10.5) (inpatients) and 66.9 (11.8) y (outpatients); $n = 41$ (+ 40 controls)	Age (cases and one of the two control groups similar), gender	Hip fractures	Age and albumin; Mean 25OHD was significantly lower in cases vs. controls ($p < 0.01$). When age and albumin were used as covariates in the analysis, there was no residual difference in serum 25OHD levels. More hip fracture cases (49%) had 25OHD levels < 25 nmol/L vs. 15% of inpatient and 10% of outpatient controls

continued

TABLE 4-10 Continued

Reference; Country	Population Description	Duration (or Matching Variables)	Bone Health Outcomes	Covariates; Summary of Results
Diamond et al., 1998 Australia	Men with hip fracture and healthy controls Cases: 79.6 y Controls: 78.7 y and 77 y n = 41 (+ 82 controls)	Age, gender	Hip fractures	Age, body weight, comorbidity score, smoking history, alcohol intake, serum calcium, albumin, 25OHD, and free testosterone Men with hip fractures had significantly lower 25OHD levels vs. controls ($p = 0.007$) 25OHD < 50 nmol/L: 63% of fracture patients vs. 25% of combined controls, OR 3.9 (95% CI 1.74–8.78) Multiple regression analysis showed that serum 25OHD level < 50 nmol/L was strongest predictor of hip fracture ($r = 0.34$ [0.19], $p = 0.013$) Age was the best determinant of a serum 25OHD level < 50 nmol/L, $p = 0.028$
Erem et al., 2002 Turkey	Women with hip fractures and healthy PM women, all independent community-dwellers Cases: 76.7 (6.5) y Controls: 75.4 (6.3) y n = 21 (+ 20 controls) Far Eastern	Age, gender, PM status	Hip fractures	NR Nonsignificant difference in 25OHD levels in hip fracture patients vs. controls 25OHD levels in all groups < 37.5 nmol/L

Study	Sample	Covariates	Outcomes	Results
Landin-Wilhelmsen et al., 1999 Sweden	PM women with OP, controls from outpatient clinic Osteoporotic women: 59 (6) y Controls: 59 (5) y n = 128 (+ 227 controls)	Age, gender, PM status	Fractures BMD and BMC: LS, TB, and FN (DXA)	NR 25OHD significantly lower in osteoporotic women vs. controls (p < 0.05); PTH significantly higher in osteoporotic women vs. controls (p < 0.001) Fracture history in 56% of osteoporotic women vs. 4% of controls (p < 0.001) Osteoporotic women had lower body weight and BMI vs. controls (p < 0.001)
Lau et al., 1989 Hong Kong	Hip fracture patients in hospital and community-living controls Age range: 49–93 y (cases), 60–90 y (controls) n = 200 (+ 427 controls) Asian	Ethnicity	Hip fractures	NR 25OHD levels were significantly lower in cases vs. controls (p < 0.01) Hip fracture patients with low 25OHD (male < 36.5 nmol/L, female < 34.3 nmol/L, defined by lower limit of 95% CI for controls) were less mobile than those with normal 25OHD; 33% with low 25OHD could walk outdoors without an aid vs. 61% of those with a normal 25OHD level
LeBoff et al., 1999 United States	Community-dwelling women [30 with hip fracture and OP (group 1); 68 women admitted for elective joint replacement with (17) or without (51) OP (group 2)] Group 1: 77.9 y Group 2: OP 69.9 y; non-OP 64.4 y n = 98	Gender, PM status, setting, surgical procedure OP in group 1 and subset of group 2	Hip fractures BMD: LS, FN, Tr, TB (DXA)	Adjusted for age and estrogen replacement therapy Women with hip fracture and OP had significantly lower 25OHD vs. women with OP admitted for surgery (p = 0.01) and vs. women without OP admitted for surgery (p = 0.02) % of women with 25OHD < 30 nmol/L: Significantly more in group 1 (50%) vs. OP or non-OP group 2 (graph only ~ 5% for OP and 10% for non-OP) (p < 0.002) Mean BMD (LS, FN, Tr) was significantly less in women with acute hip fracture/OP vs. elective surgery non-OP controls

continued

TABLE 4-10 Continued

Reference; Country	Population Description	Duration (or Matching Variables)	Bone Health Outcomes	Covariates; Summary of Results
Lips et al., 1983, 1987 Netherlands	Consecutive patients with FN fracture and 74 healthy community controls Cases: 75.9 (11) y Controls: 75.6 (4.2) $n = 125$ (+ 74 controls) Cases: 67% female Controls: 73% female	Age	Hip fractures	Adjusted for age and sex Serum 25OHD levels lower in cases vs. controls ($p < 0.001$)
Lund et al., 1975 Denmark	67 consecutive cases of proximal femur fractures Controls: middle-aged (30–59 y, $n = 27$) and elderly healthy individuals (60–95 y, $n = 67$) at same time of year	Age	Proximal femur fractures	There was no statistically significant difference in serum 25OHD levels vs. either controls
Punnonen et al., 1986 Finland	Cases of hip fracture and controls (from gynecological clinic) Cases: 77.1 (8.6) y Controls: 73.8 (8.4) y $n = 40$ (+ 25 controls)	Age, gender, setting	Hip fractures (FN)	NR 25OHD levels were significantly lower in cases vs. controls ($p < 0.01$)

	Age, setting (for cases and one control group)	Fractures	
Thiebaud et al., 1997 Switzerland	179 hip fracture patients; 180 hospital controls; 55 community controls	Cases: women 81.0 y; men 77.7 y Hospital controls: women 80.9 y, men 76.9 y Community controls: women 71.7 y, men 71.3 y Cases: 76% female Hospital controls: 75% female Community controls: 85% female	BMD: FN, TH, Tr (DXA)	Adjusted for age, sex, and creatinine Women and men with hip fractures had significantly lower 25OHD levels vs. controls. Fracture patients had lower hip (TH, FN) BMD vs. either control group ($p < 0.001$). In multivariate logistic regression of the risk for hip fracture, serum albumin and PTH were significant. In women, BMD was weakly correlated with 25OHD, and the only significant association was at the Tr ($r = 0.13$, $p < 0.05$).

NOTE: Total 25OHD or either isoform of 25OHD (isoform not specified); BMC = bone mineral content; BMD = bone mineral density; BMI = body mass index; CI = confidence interval; DXA = dual-energy X-ray absorptiometry; FN = femoral neck; HR = hazard ratio; mo = month(s); LS = lumbar spine; NR = not reported; OP = osteoporosis; OR = odds ratio; PM = postmenopausal; PTH = parathyroid hormone; RR = relative risk; SPA = single-photon absorptiometry; TB = total body; TH = total hip; Tr = trochanter; vit = vitamin; y = year(s).

*a*This table has been truncated for the purposes of this chapter, but it can be found in its entirety in Appendix C.

SOURCE: Modified from Cranney et al. (2007).

Physical Performance). Nineteen studies assessed the association between serum 25OHD concentrations and BMD, and there is fair evidence from observational studies for an association between serum 25OHD concentrations and changes in hip BMD sites. Some studies identified specific serum concentrations of 25OHD below which falls, fractures, or bone loss increased; these values ranged from approximately 40 to 80 nmol/L.

The findings from AHRQ are summarized by DRI-relevant life stage groups in Box 4-5.

Fractures in postmenopausal women and older men: Vitamin D supplementation with or without calcium[3]   Overall, AHRQ-Ottawa concluded that supplementation with vitamin D (most studies used vitamin D_3) plus calcium is effective in reducing fractures in institutionalized older populations. AHRQ-Tufts did not identify new RCTs examining the combined effect of vitamin D plus calcium supplementation on fractures in postmenopausal women and older men.

As reported by AHRQ-Ottawa, 15 RCTs evaluated the effect of vitamin D_2 or vitamin D_3 (with or without calcium supplementation) on fractures in postmenopausal women and older men (Table 4-11). The majority of the trials used vitamin D_3 preparations (300 to 800 IU/day). Ten trials were of higher quality, although high losses to follow-up and inadequate reporting of allocation concealment were limitations of a number of trials. Vertebral fractures were not included as an outcome in most trials. Vitamin D_3 (700 to 800 IU/day) combined with calcium supplements (500 to 1,200 mg/day) significantly reduced non-vertebral and hip fractures although the benefit was predominantly in older subjects living in institutionalized settings (hip fractures: odds ratio [OR] = 0.69; 95% CI 0.53–0.90). The benefit of vitamin D and calcium on fractures in community-dwelling individuals was inconsistent across trials.

Specifically, AHRQ-Ottawa conducted a meta-analysis of 13 of the RCTs (omitting Anderson et al. [2004], which is an abstract only, and Larsen et al. [2004], which included no placebo control). Included in the 13 RCTs was the report from Jackson et al. (2006), which reflected data from the WHI trials based on 36,282 subjects. Reproduced in Figures 4-5 through 4-7 are the relevant forest plots for the outcomes related to total fractures from studies that used either oral vitamin D_3 or vitamin D_2 plus or minus calcium versus calcium or placebo, total fractures for studies that used vitamin D_3 plus calcium versus placebo, and hip fractures (by setting)

---

[3]As an aside, it was noted that one RCT of premenopausal women, ages 17 to 35 years, showed that 800 IU/day of vitamin D in combination with 2,000 mg/day of calcium supplementation can reduce the risk of stress fracture from military training compared with placebo (Lappe et al., 2008).

BOX 4-5
AHRQ Findings by Life Stage for 25OHD and Fractures*

0–6 months: Not reviewed

7 months–2 years: Not reviewed

3–8 years: Not reviewed

9–18 years: Not reviewed

19–50 years: No data

51–70 years: The AHRQ-Ottawa report concluded that the associations between serum 25OHD concentrations and risk of fractures are inconsistent. No new data were identified in the AHRQ-Tufts report.

≥ 71 years: Findings from three new RCTs did not show significant effects of either vitamin D_2 or vitamin D_3 supplementation (daily doses ranged from 400 to 822 IU) in reducing the risk of total fractures among men and women in this life stage.

Postmenopause: The AHRQ-Ottawa report concluded that the associations between serum 25OHD concentrations and risk of fractures are inconsistent. No new data were identified in the AHRQ-Tufts report.

Pregnant and lactating women: Not reviewed

---

*Evidence from AHRQ-Ottawa; information from AHRQ-Tufts as noted.
SOURCE: Modified from Chung et al. (2009).

---

for studies that used vitamin D_3 plus or minus calcium versus placebo. As highlighted above, the benefit in community-dwelling individuals was inconsistent, but benefit was evidenced for institutionalized individuals.

As reported by AHRQ-Tufts, findings from three RCTs that postdated AHRQ-Ottawa (Bunout et al., 2006; Burleigh et al., 2007; Lyons et al., 2007) did not show significant effects of either vitamin D_2 or vitamin D_3 supplementation (daily doses of 400 to 822 IU) in reducing the risk of total fractures (Table 4-12). The findings from AHRQ are summarized by DRI-relevant life stage groups in Box 4-6.

Rickets in children Rickets was explored by AHRQ-Ottawa relative to serum 25OHD measures only. Overall, there was fair evidence for an association between low serum 25OHD concentrations and confirmed rickets, regardless of the types of assays used to measure serum 25OHD concentrations. There is inconsistent evidence to determine whether there is a

TABLE 4-11 Odds Ratio (95% Confidence Interval) for Total Fractures from Individual RCTs of Vitamin D: Summary from AHRQ-Ottawa Analyses[a]

Reference; Jadad Score for RCTs[b]	Duration (y)	Sample Size (n)	Vitamin D (IU/day) Follow-up	Mean Baseline 25OHD for IG (nmol/L)	End of trial 25OHD for IG (nmol/L)	OR (95% CI)
Chapuy et al., 2002 Jadad = 3	2	583	800 D$_3$ + 1,200 mg Ca	22	75 (graph)	0.79 (0.54–1.17)
Chapuy et al., 1992 Jadad = 2	1.5	3,270	800 D$_3$ + 1,200 mg Ca	40	105	0.72 (0.58–0.90)
Lips et al., 1996 Jadad = 5	4	2,578	400 D$_3$	27	62	1.12 (0.86–1.44)
Dawson-Hughes et al., 1997b Jadad = 4	3	389	700 D$_3$ + 500 mg Ca	82.7 M, 67.5 F	112	0.42 (0.20–0.88)
Law et al., 2006 Jadad = 2	1	3,717	1,100 D$_2$	59	77	1.4 (0.9–2.0)
Pfeifer et al., 2000 Jadad = 3	1	148	800 D$_3$ + 1,200 mg Ca	25.6	66.1	0.48 (0.12–1.99)
Komulainen et al., 1998 Jadad = 3	5	232	300 D$_3$ + 500 mg Ca	28.6	37.5	0.71 (0.31–1.61)
Grant et al., 2005 Jadad = 5	5	5,292	800 D$_3$ with or without 1,000 mg Ca	39	62.2	1.02 (0.84–1.22)
Flicker et al., 2005 Jadad = 4	2	625	1,100 D$_2$ + 1,000 mg Ca	NR	NR	0.69 (0.4–1.18)

TABLE 4-11 Continued

Reference; Jadad Score for RCTs[b]	Duration (y)	Sample Size (n)	Vitamin D (IU/day) Follow-up	Mean Baseline 25OHD for IG (nmol/L)	End of trial 25OHD for IG (nmol/L)	OR (95% CI)
Jackson et al., 2006 Jadad = 4	7	36,282	400 D$_3$ + 1,000 mg Ca	46	NR	0.97 (0.91–1.03)
Porthouse et al., 2005 Jadad = 3	2	3,314	800 D$_3$ + 1,000 mg Ca	—	—	0.96 (0.65–1.46) Unequal 1.09 (0.60–1.96) Equal
Trivedi et al., 2003 Jadad = 3	5	2,686	100,000 D$_3$ 4 mo	NR	74.3	0.78 (0.60–1.00)
Harwood et al., 2004 Jadad = 3	1	150	800 D$_3$ + 1,000 mg Ca	28–30	40–50	0.58 (0.13–2.64)

NOTE: CI = confidence interval; F = female; IG = intervention group; IU = International Units; OR = odds ratio; M = male; mo = month(s); NR = not reported; y = year(s).

[a]This table has been truncated for the purposes of this chapter, but it can be found in its entirety in Appendix C.

[b]Jadad score is based on a scale of 1 to 5. See Box 4-1 for details on the scoring system.
SOURCE: Modified from Cranney et al. (2007).

threshold concentration of serum 25OHD above which rickets does not occur.

Six studies (one RCT, three before-and-after studies, and two case–control studies) reported mean or median serum 25OHD concentrations below 30 nmol/L in children with rickets, whereas the other studies reported that the mean or median serum 25OHD concentrations were above 30 nmol/L (and up to 50 nmol/L). In seven of eight case–control studies, serum 25OHD concentrations were lower in children with rickets compared with controls. Information on the 13 studies is shown in Table 4-13.

AHRQ-Tufts identified no new RCTs concerning rickets since the completion of AHRQ-Ottawa.

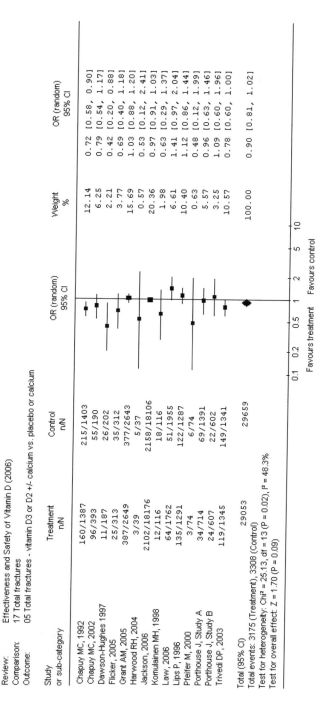

Review:	Effectiveness and Safety of Vitamin D (2006)
Comparison:	17 Total fractures
Outcome:	05 Total fractures - vitamin D3 or D2 +/- calcium vs. placebo or calcium

Study or sub-category	Treatment n/N	Control n/N	OR (random) 95% CI	Weight %	OR (random) 95% CI
Chapuy MC, 1992	160/1387	215/1403		12.14	0.72 [0.58, 0.90]
Chapuy MC, 2002	96/393	55/190		6.25	0.79 [0.54, 1.17]
Dawson-Hughes 1997	11/187	26/202		2.21	0.42 [0.20, 0.88]
Flicker, 2005	25/313	35/312		3.77	0.69 [0.40, 1.18]
Grant AM, 2005	387/2649	377/2643		15.69	1.03 [0.88, 1.20]
Harwood RH, 2004	3/39	5/37		0.57	0.53 [0.12, 2.41]
Jackson, 2006	2102/18176	2158/18106		20.36	0.97 [0.91, 1.03]
Komulainen MH, 1998	12/116	18/116		1.98	0.63 [0.29, 1.37]
Law, 2006	64/1762	51/1955		6.61	1.41 [0.97, 2.04]
Lips P, 1996	135/1291	122/1287		10.40	1.12 [0.86, 1.44]
Pfeifer M, 2000	3/74	6/74		0.63	0.48 [0.12, 1.99]
Porthouse J, Study A	34/714	69/1391		5.57	0.96 [0.63, 1.46]
Porthouse J, Study B	24/607	22/602		3.25	1.09 [0.60, 1.96]
Trivedi DP, 2003	119/1345	149/1341		10.57	0.78 [0.60, 1.00]
Total (95% CI)	29053	29659		100.00	0.90 [0.81, 1.02]

Total events: 3175 (Treatment), 3308 (Control)
Test for heterogeneity: Chi² = 25.13, df = 13 (P = 0.02), I² = 48.3%
Test for overall effect: Z = 1.70 (P = 0.09)

0.1   0.2   0.5   1   2   5   10
Favours treatment   Favours control

FIGURE 4-5 Forest plot comparing risk of total fractures with vitamin D_2 or vitamin D_3 with or without calcium vs. placebo or calcium.

SOURCE: Cranney et al. (2007).

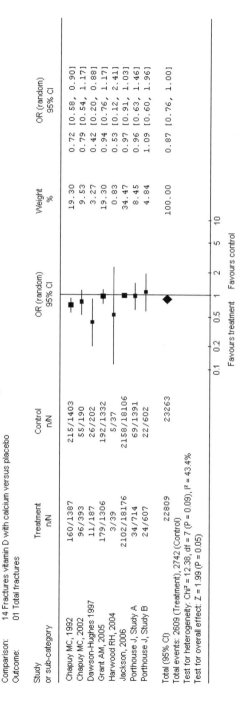

FIGURE 4-6 Forest plot comparing the risk of total fractures with vitamin D_3 combined with calcium vs. placebo.
SOURCE: Cranney et al. (2007).

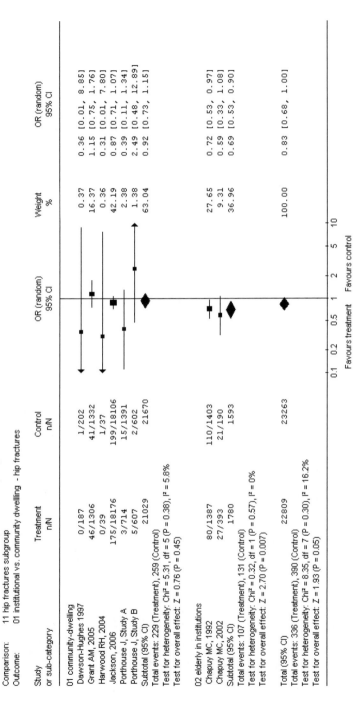

FIGURE 4-7 Forest plot comparing risk of hip fractures with vitamin D_3 with or without calcium vs. placebo by setting.
SOURCE: Cranney et al. (2007).

TABLE 4-12 Vitamin D and Bone Health: Characteristics of RCTs Published after AHRQ-Ottawa[a]

Reference; Location (Latitude)	Population Description		Background Calcium Intake and Vitamin D Data	Comparisons	Compliance
Lyons et al., 2007 South Wales, UK (52°N)	Health status	Living in care facilities including some elderly with mobility, cognitive, visual, hearing, or communication impairments	nd	100,000 IU vit D_2 4× monthly vs. placebo	80% (percentage of occasions observed to take tablets)
	Mean age (range), y	84 (62–107)			
	Male (%)	23.7			
Burleigh et al., 2007 Scotland (55°57′N)	Health status	Inpatient with high levels of comorbidity, mortality, and polypharmacy	25OHD: 22 nmol/L	800 IU vit D_3/d + 1,200 mg Ca carbonate/d vs. 1,200 mg Ca carbonate/d	Ca group = 87%, vit D + Ca group = 89% (total study drug taken/total study drug prescribed, as recorded in drug prescription charts)
	Mean age (SD), y	83 (7.6)			
	Male (%)	40			
Bunout et al., 2006 Chile (32°S)	Health status	Healthy	25OHD: ≤ 40 nmol/L	800 mg Ca/d vs. 800 mg Ca/d + 400 IU vit D/d (with and without exercise training)	92% (tablet counting)
	Mean age (SD), y	76 (4)			
	Male (%)	11.6			

NOTE: IU = International Units; nd = not determined; SD = standard deviation; UK = United Kingdom; vit = vitamin; y = year(s)

[a]This table has been truncated for the purposes of this chapter, but it can be found in its entirety in Appendix D.

SOURCE: Modified from Chung et al. (2009).

BOX 4-6
AHRQ Findings by Life Stage for Vitamin D and
Calcium for Clinical Outcomes of Bone Health*

0–6 months: Not reviewed

7 months–2 years: Not reviewed

3–8 years: Not reviewed

9–18 years: Not reviewed

19–50 years: The AHRQ-Ottawa report concluded that supplementation with vitamin D (most studies used vitamin D_3) plus calcium is effective in reducing the risk of fractures in institutionalized populations. One RCT of female Navy recruits ages 17 to 35 years showed that vitamin D (800 IU/day) in combination with calcium (2,000 mg/day) supplementation can reduce the risk of stress fractures from military training compared with placebo.

51–70 years: No new data were identified in the AHRQ-Tufts report

≥ 71 years: No new data were identified in the AHRQ-Tufts report

Pregnant and lactating women: No data

---

*Evidence from AHRQ-Ottawa; information from AHRQ-Tufts as noted.
SOURCE: Modified from Chung et al. (2009).

Pregnancy, Fetal Development, and Lactation

Pregnancy and lactation constitute specific, unique life stages that are of current interest regarding calcium and vitamin D functions and nutritional requirements. The body of evidence concerning skeletal health as it relates to the calcium and vitamin D nutriture of pregnancy, lactation, and fetal development is integrated below so as to provide context for the selection of indicators for DRI development.

Pregnancy: Calcium   The developing fetus requires calcium, especially during the third trimester when the skeleton is undergoing mineralization. Direct measurements of the calcium content of the newborn skeleton have indicated that 25 to 30 g of calcium is transferred to the fetus by the end of gestation (Givens and Macy, 1933; Trotter and Hixon, 1974). Maternal intestinal calcium absorption doubles beginning early in pregnancy even though little calcium is transferred to the embryo at this stage (Heaney

continued

TABLE 4-13 Serum 25OHD Levels in Infants and Young Children with Established Rickets: Summary from AHRQ-Ottawa[a]

Reference; Country	Population Description	Intervention; Duration	Bone Health Outcomes	Results
RCTs				
Cesur et al., 2003 Turkey	Infants with nutritional rickets 10.7 (6.1) mo (range 3–36 mo) 36% female *n* = 56	IG1: 150,000 IU vit D IG2: 300,000 IU vit D IG3: 600,000 IU vit D (single dose) 2 mo	Rickets	25OHD$_3$, mean (SD) (nmol/L): Stage I: 15.8 (6.4) Stage II: 15.4 (4.8) Stage III: 14.7 (3.9) Ca, mean (SD) (mmol/L): All patients 1.9 (0.33)
Before-and-after studies				
Bhimma et al., 1995 South Africa	Children with rickets: vit D deficiency rickets (25OHD < 25 nmol/L); Ca deficiency rickets; phosphopenic rickets; healing/healed rickets Age range 1–12 y Vit D deficiency rickets 56% female *n* = 23	5,000–10,000 IU vit D$_3$/d (plus 500–1,000 mg Ca/d) 12 mo	Rickets	25OHD, mean (SD) (nmol/L): Vit D–deficient rickets: 9.3 (8.8) Ca-deficient rickets: 45.5 (10.0) Ca, mean (SD) (mmol/L): Vit D–deficient rickets: 2.09 (0.27) Ca-deficient rickets: 2.16 (0.28)

TABLE 4-13 Continued

Reference; Country	Population Description	Intervention; Duration	Bone Health Outcomes	Results
Elzouki et al., 1989 Libya	Children < 2 y admitted for treatment of rickets $n = 22$ 37.5% female African black	1–3 h/d of sunshine followed by single IM injection of 600,000 IU vit D_2 Follow-up median 17 d	Rickets	25OHD: At diagnosis, 50% of patients had 25OHD > 20 nmol/L Range 4–65 nmol/L (graph) Ca: ND
Garabedian et al., 1983 France/Belgium	Infants and children with rickets and controls Infants and young children: range 4–26 mo Older children: range 4–12 y $n = 20$ (+ 60 controls) 80% immigrants from North Africa, Black Africa, Turkey, Portugal, Pakistan	IG1: 2,000 IU vit D_2/d IG2: 400 IU vit D_3/kg (single dose) 6 mo	Rickets	25OHD mean (SD) (nmol/L): All patients: 11.5 (8.0) Ca, mean (SD) (mmol/L): All patients: 1.8 (0.27)
Markestad et al., 1984 Norway	Children with rickets 11 (64.7%) immigrants from Pakistan, Cape Verde Islands, Turkey, Morocco, Sri Lanka, and West Africa; 6 (35.3%) Norwegians	1,700–4,000 IU vit D_2/d (reduced to 500–1,000 IU in 3 children at 2–4 wk) 10 wk	Rickets	25OHD median (range) (nmol/L): $n = 9$ diagnosed in summer: 21.0 (4.1–30.6) $n = 8$ diagnosed in winter: 12.1 (3.8–19.4) Ca: ND

244

Case–control studies

Study	Population	Treatment	Condition	Results
Arnaud et al., 1976 Canada/Midwest United States	Children with mild, moderate, and severe rickets and controls; 2 mo–3.5 y $n = 9$ (+ 9 controls) Rickets: 22% female Canadian (First Nations, West Indian black, Portuguese) and American (mid-northwestern United States)	5,000 IU vit D/d 4 wk	Rickets	25OHD, mean (SD) (range) (nmol/L): Mild rickets: 45.0 (7.5) (range 40.0–52.5) Moderate rickets: 30 (5) Severe rickets: 20 (NR) Controls: 90 (30) Ca, mean (SD) (mmol/L): ND for mild, moderate, severe subgroups Stage II rickets: 2.4 (0.15) Age-matched controls: 2.53 (0.1)
Balasubramanian et al., 2003 India	Children and adolescents with rickets/osteomalacia and controls Children: Rickets: median 33 mo (range 11–120 mo) Controls: median 27 mo (range 6–84 mo) Adolescents: Rickets: median 198 mo (range 168–240 mo) Controls: median 156 mo (range 120–228 mo) $n = 40$ (+ 53 controls) Rickets: 54.1% female Controls: 47% female Hindu/Muslim	Cases: 6,000 IU vit D/d or single dose of 600,000 IU 3 mo	Rickets	25OHD, mean (SD) (nmol/L): Children: Rickets: 50.0 (38.9) Controls: 61.3 (35.9), NS Adolescents: Rickets: 12.6 (7.1) all but one < LLN Controls: 46.0 (45.4), $p < 0.001$ Ca, mean (SD) (mmol/L): Children: Rickets: 2.2 (0.3) Controls: 2.4 (0.3), NS Adolescents: Rickets: 2.1 (0.2) Controls: 2.3 (0.2), $p = 0.008$

continued

TABLE 4-13 Continued

Reference; Country	Population Description	Intervention; Duration	Bone Health Outcomes	Results
Dawodu et al., 2005 United Arab Emirates	Children with rickets and historical controls Rickets: 13.5 mo Controls: 13.0 mo $n = 38$ (+ 50 controls) Rickets: 50% female Controls: 40% female Arab	NA	iPTH (rickets group only)	25OHD, median (IQR) (nmol/L): Rickets: 8.0 (3.8–15.3) Controls: 43.8 (25–64.3), $p = 0.001$ PTH showed a trend toward negative correlation with 25OHD (data NR) Ca, median (IQR) (mmol/L): Rickets: 2.22 (1.88–2.35) Controls: 2.4 (2.25–2.5), $p = 0.001$
Graff et al., 2004 Nigeria	Children with rickets and controls (unrelated) Rickets: 46 (22) mo Controls: 47 (22) mo $n = 15$ (+ 15 controls) 60% female Rickets: 7 Muslim and 8 Christian Controls: 4 Muslim and 11 Christian	Cases: 1,000 mg Ca/d (no vit D supplement) Treatment duration: 6 mo Follow-up: 12 mo	Rickets	25OHD, mean (SD) (nmol/L): Significantly lower in children with rickets Rickets: 37.5 (13.5) Controls: 72.5 (11.5), $p < 0.001$ Ca, mean (SD) (mmol/L): Rickets: 2.13 (0.2) Controls: 2.4 (0.1), $p < 0.001$

continued

Majid Molla et al., 2000 Kuwait	Children with rickets and controls Rickets: 14.5 (5.2) mo (range 9 mo–8 y) Controls: 15.2 (6.3) mo $n = 103$ (+ 102 controls) 96.1% from mothers with hijab use	NA	Rickets	25OHD, mean (SD) (nmol/L): Significantly lower in children with rickets Rickets: 26.5 (15.5) Controls: 83.5 (74.75), $p < 0.0001$ Ca, mean (SD) (mmol/L): Rickets: 2.24 (0.28) Controls: 2.45 (0.15), $p < 0.0001$
Oginni et al., 1996 Nigeria	Children with active rickets and healthy controls Children with rickets age range: 1–5 y $n = 26$ (+ 90 controls) Rickets: 50% female Controls: 61% female Nigerian	NA	Rickets	25OHD, mean (SD) (range) (nmol/L): Significantly lower in rickets group Rickets: 36 (28), range 7–147 Controls: 69 (22), range 32–140, $p < 0.0002$ Ca (albumin-corrected), mean (SD) (mmol/L): Rickets: 2.06 (0.23) Controls: 2.35 (0.14), $p < 0.001$
Thacher et al., 2000 Nigeria	Active rickets and controls Rickets: median (25th and 75th percentile) age: 46 (34–63) mo Controls: 42 (25–70) mo $n = 123$ (+ 123 controls) 49.6% female Christian/Islam: Rickets: 82/41 Controls: 57/66	NA	Rickets	25OHD median (25th and 75th percentile) (nmol/L): Rickets: 32 (22, 40); < 30: 37% Controls: 50 (42, 62), $p < 0.0001$ Ca, mean (SD) (mmol/L): Rickets: 1.93 (0.22) Controls: 2.24 (0.15), $p < 0.0001$

TABLE 4-13 Continued

Reference; Country	Population Description	Intervention; Duration	Bone Health Outcomes	Results
Thacher, 1997 Nigeria	Children with active rickets (median duration of 14 mo) and healthy controls with normal weight Rickets: 3.16 (1.53) y Controls 3.14 (1.51) y n = 37 (+ 37 controls) 47% female All Nigerian	NA	Rickets	25(OH)D Rickets: levels > LLN in 16/28 (57%); 2/28 (7%) had values < 12.5 nmol/L Controls: ND Ca, mean (SD) (mmol/L): Rickets: 2.09 (0.30) Controls: 2.08 (0.31), NS 55% of rickets and 51% of controls were hypocalcemic (< 2.1)

NOTE: h = hours; IG = intervention group; IM = intramuscular; iPTH = intact parathyroid hormone; IQR = interquartile range; IU = International Units; LLN = lower limit of normal reference range; mo = month(s); NA = not applicable; ND = not determined; NR = not reported; NS = not significant; PTH = parathyroid hormone; SD = standard deviation; vit = vitamin; wk = week(s); y = year(s).

*a*This table has been truncated for the purposes of this chapter, but it can be found in its entirety in Appendix C.

SOURCE: Modified from Cranney et al. (2007).

and Skillman, 1971). The increased intestinal calcium absorption causes a net positive calcium balance in the mother early in pregnancy (Heaney and Skillman, 1971). However, in the third trimester, the rapid maternal-fetal calcium transfer results in a maternal calcium balance that is zero or perhaps slightly negative by the end of pregnancy.

There is controversy about the mobilization of calcium from maternal bone during pregnancy and its contribution to fetal calcium needs. A possible loss of BMC has been seen longitudinally using the modern technique of dual-energy X-ray absorptiometry (DXA), but measurements were done 1 to 18 months prior to pregnancy and 1 to 6 weeks postpartum (i.e., not during pregnancy) making it uncertain whether the measured calcium loss had truly occurred during pregnancy (Kovacs and Kronenberg, 1997; Kovacs and Fuleihan Gel, 2006). Further, the effect of pregnancy on bone mineral content may depend on the site examined, with decreases reported for trabecular bone (Black et al., 2000; Naylor et al., 2000; More et al., 2001; Kaur et al., 2003; Ulrich et al., 2003; Akesson et al., 2004; Pearson et al., 2004), but not cortical bone (Naylor et al., 2000; Pearson et al., 2004). Two studies (Kaur et al., 2003; Olausson et al., 2008) used contemporaneous non-pregnant and non-lactating age-matched controls to compare, to the extent feasible, the effects of pregnancy and age on BMD. Kaur et al. (2003) found no significant difference in BMD before and after pregnancy. Olausson et al. (2008) found a significant 1 to 4 percent decrease in whole-body, spine, and total hip BMC before and 2 weeks after pregnancy, whereas controls had an increase in whole-body BMC and a smaller (0.5 to 1 percent) decrease in BMD at the spine and hip. These skeletal changes were unrelated to calcium intake in either group. Collectively, the evidence tends to suggest that mineral mobilization is variable during pregnancy and may contribute, to some extent, to fetal calcium needs.

Relatively few studies have examined the effect of calcium supplementation on either fetal or maternal outcomes. In a placebo-controlled double-blind randomized trial conducted in the United States, Koo et al. (1999) demonstrated that calcium supplementation during pregnancy may benefit the offspring's bone health, but only in those infants whose mothers had very low calcium intake (600 mg/day), based on a post-hoc subgroup analysis. In contrast to this possible benefit to the offspring, calcium supplementation during pregnancy of Gambian women with low calcium intakes resulted surprisingly in greater decreases in BMC and BMD and related biochemical evidence, consistent with higher bone mineral mobilization during lactation (Jarjou et al., 2010).

Maternal serum calcium levels fall during pregnancy (Pedersen et al., 1984) as a consequence of plasma volume expansion and reduced albumin concentration; lower calcium levels do not imply calcium deficiency. The ionized calcium (i.e., the physiologically important fraction of calcium) and the albumin-corrected serum calcium levels do not change during pregnancy (Seely et al., 1997). Pregnant women consuming "moderate" calcium (800 to 1,000 mg/day) (Gertner et al., 1986; Allen et al., 1991) to "high" calcium (1,950 mg/day) (Cross et al., 1995) are often hypercalciuric as a result of increased intestinal calcium absorption (i.e., absorptive hypercalciuria); as such, pregnancy itself is a risk factor for kidney stones. Urinary calcium excretion increases as early as the 12th week of gestation and averages 300 ± 61 mg/24 hours in the third trimester with hypercalciuric levels not uncommon (Pedersen et al., 1984; Gertner et al., 1986; Allen et al., 1991; Cross et al., 1995; Seely et al., 1997). While urinary calcium excretion goes up in normal pregnancy, it decreases in women who are developing preeclampsia. The risk of preeclampsia can be reduced with supplemental calcium when the dietary calcium intake is very low; however, there appears to be no effect when dietary calcium intake is adequate (Hofmeyr et al., 2006; Villar et al., 2006; Hiller et al., 2007; Kumar et al., 2009).

In the adolescent, whose skeleton is still growing, pregnancy could theoretically reduce peak bone mass and increase the long-term risk of osteoporosis. Most cross–sectional studies that have compared the BMD in teens early postpartum with that in never-pregnant teens have suggested that there is no reason to be concerned about BMD or bone mass after adolescent pregnancy (Kovacs and Kronenberg, 1997). A few smaller observational studies have reported that lower adolescent age at first pregnancy is associated with lower BMD in the adult (Sowers et al., 1985, 1992; Fox et al., 1993). In contrast, an analysis of NHANES III data on BMD by DXA for 819 women ages 20 to 25 years found that women pregnant as adolescents had the same BMD as women pregnant as adults and as nulliparous women (Chantry et al., 2004). This study's population is diverse and representative of the general U.S. population and thus reassures that teen pregnancy does not reduce BMD in most women. An additional study (O'Brien et al., 2003) found that fractional calcium absorption doubles during adolescent pregnancy (as it does in adults) and during the first 2 months postpartum. Mean BMD of previously pregnant—but not lactating—adolescents was above the expected BMD for age in this study, also suggesting that no loss of BMD had occurred during pregnancy. These data indicate that adolescent women meet the calcium demands of pregnancy by increasing intestinal calcium absorption while preserving maternal bone mass.

Pregnancy: Vitamin D

Maternal outcomes Total calcitriol levels double early in pregnancy and remain at this increased level until delivery (Bikle et al., 1984; Cross et al., 1995; Ardawi et al., 1997; O'Brien et al., 2006; Papapetrou, 2010).

This is related to a concomitant increase in plasma vitamin D binding protein (DBP) (Bikle et al., 1984; Ardawi et al., 1997). Free calcitriol levels do not increase until the third trimester (Bikle et al., 1984; Specker, 2004; Kovacs, 2008). The main source of calcitriol is from the maternal renal 1α-hydroxylase, with little contribution from the placenta even though it expresses 1α-hydroxylase, based on the case report of a pregnant anephric woman whose low levels of calcitriol increased less than 15 percent by the beginning of the third trimester (Turner et al., 1988). Despite the increased synthesis of calcitriol during pregnancy and the passage of 25OHD across the placenta to the fetus, maternal serum 25OHD levels are relatively unaffected by pregnancy (Hillman et al., 1978; Brooke et al., 1980; Cross et al., 1995; Ardawi et al., 1997; Morley et al., 2006; Papapetrou, 2010), although one report noted a significant decline by the third trimester in Saudi women (Ardawi et al., 1997). Even when baseline serum 25OHD level was in the severely deficient range (mean 20.1 ± 1.9 nmol/L), the serum levels did not change significantly by the end of pregnancy (Brooke et al., 1980).

The increase in maternal intestinal calcium absorption has been positively associated with the increase in maternal serum calcitriol levels in observational studies in humans (Cross et al., 1995; Ritchie et al., 1998). Certain results from studies in animal models are relevant to understanding the changes in vitamin D physiology that occur during human pregnancy. Intestinal calcium absorption is markedly up-regulated in pregnant vitamin D–deficient rats and in mice lacking the VDR (*Vdr*-null mice) to the same high rate achieved in pregnant vitamin D–replete rats and wild-type mice, respectively (Halloran and DeLuca, 1980a; Brommage et al., 1990; Fudge and Kovacs, 2010). This suggests that factors other than vitamin D (e.g., estrogen, placental lactogen, and prolactin) stimulate intestinal calcium absorption during pregnancy.

Very few clinical trials of vitamin D supplementation during pregnancy have been conducted. The work of Wagner et al. (2010a, b), reported currently in abstract form, has focused on high doses of vitamin D (4,000 versus 2,000 and 400 IU/day) in intervention trials in which the focus was on non-skeletal outcomes. A final report from these studies is expected soon. To date, the available intervention studies have shown little effect of vitamin D supplementation on maternal, fetal, or neonatal outcomes, although it would be expected that higher serum 25OHD levels in the newborn should protect against neonatal hypocalcemia (Specker, 2004; Kovacs, 2008). In a study of Asian women with initially low 25OHD levels (mean of 20 nmol/L) at baseline, daily supplementation with 1,000 IU of vitamin D per day did not affect cord blood calcium level or the newborns' crown–heel length, forearm length, triceps skinfold thickness, or head circumference, but it did reduce the fontanelle area by 32.7 percent (Brooke et al.,

1980). The achieved serum 25OHD level in the vitamin D–supplemented group was 168 nmol/L compared with 10 nmol/L in the control group, raising the question as to whether the actual supplemented dose was considerably higher than the intended dose of 1,000 IU/day. In another trial, 1,000 IU of vitamin D per day was administered during the last trimester of pregnancy, compared with controls with no supplementation (Mallet et al., 1986). Supplementation resulted in higher maternal and cord blood 25OHD levels but had no effect on maternal, cord blood, or neonatal calcium levels or anthropometric parameters in the infants. In a study of vitamin D–deficient Asian women given a single dose of 800,000 IU of vitamin D in the third trimester, cord blood calcium level increased slightly, but there was no other benefit compared with women who received either no supplement or a daily dose of 1,200 IU of vitamin D (Marya et al., 1981, 1988). One small randomized but not blinded intervention trial found that maternal supplementation with 800 IU of vitamin D per day increased both maternal serum and cord blood 25OHD levels significantly, but did not affect gestational age at delivery, compared with unsupplemented controls (Yu et al., 2009). Observational studies have reported an uneventful clinical course of pregnancy in women with abnormalities of the VDR (vitamin D–dependent rickets type I [VDDR I] or VDDR II) when normo-calcemia is maintained (Malloy et al., 1997; St-Arnaud et al., 1997).

Fetal outcomes   Animal models (e.g., mice, rats, guinea pigs, and sheep) have contributed to elucidating aspects of the physiology of fetal vitamin D nutriture that cannot be studied during human pregnancy. Studies in genetically altered animal models have provided information about the requirements for vitamin D and VDR signaling during pregnancy. For this reason, reference to such studies is included extensively in this component of the literature review.

There is evidence that 25OHD crosses the placenta relatively freely based on animal studies (Haddad et al., 1971; Noff and Edelstein, 1978) and studies of human perfused placenta (Ron et al., 1984). In contrast, calcitriol transfers across the human perfused placenta (Ron et al., 1984), but not the rat placenta (Noff and Edelstein, 1978). Overall, however, the net transfer from the human mother to fetus appears to be low. By term, cord blood 25OHD levels are typically 75 to 90 percent of maternal 25OHD levels (Seino et al., 1982; Kovacs, 2008), whereas cord blood calcitriol levels are low compared to maternal levels. As already highlighted in previous discussions regarding calcium, fetal serum calcium, ionized calcium, and phosphorus levels are raised above the maternal values, whereas PTH and calcitriol levels are lower. The higher calcium and phosphorus levels in the fetus suppress the 1α-hydroxylase in the placenta and fetal kidneys, and likely explain the low circulating calcitriol levels in normal fetuses.

Despite widespread expression of the VDR in the early embryo and later in many different fetal tissues, evidence suggests that vitamin D, calcitriol, and VDR are not required for skeletal development or mineralization prior to birth, as demonstrated in experimental animal studies and human observations.

Experimental animal studies have examined vitamin D deficiency as well as the genetic absence of the VDR (*Vdr*-null mice). In *Vdr*-null fetuses, the rate of placental calcium transfer rates and the expression of the calcium transient receptor potential cation channel, vanilloid family member 6 (TRPV6), increase compared with normal littermates (Kovacs, 2005). Further, in multiple animal models fetuses and neonates have been shown to have normal calcium homeostasis—i.e., normal blood calcium, phosphorus, PTH, and skeletal mineral content—under conditions of severe vitamin D deficiency as shown in: rats (Halloran and DeLuca, 1979, 1980b, 1981; Halloran et al., 1979; Miller et al., 1983); pigs with a null mutation of the 1α-hydroxylase (Lachenmaier-Currle and Harmeyer, 1989); 1α-hydroxylase-null mice (Dardenne et al., 2001; Panda et al., 2001); and *Vdr*-null mice (Li et al., 1997, 1998; Kovacs et al., 2005; Fudge and Kovacs, 2010). In contrast to the fetus, the mothers in these models exhibit severe hypocalcemia, hypophosphatemia, and osteomalacia.

Further, serum calcium levels and skeletal mineral content remain normal for the first 2 to 3 weeks after birth in vitamin D–deficient rats and *Vdr*-null mice (Kovacs et al., 2005). After weaning, the deficient and *Vdr*-null animals develop progressive hypocalcemia, hypophosphatemia, and histomorphometric evidence of rickets, not seen in normal or heterozygous littermates. This situation parallels the maturation of calcium absorption in the intestine, which changes from a non-saturable, passive process in the newborn to an active, saturable, calcitriol-dependent process in the rat (Ghishan et al., 1980, 1984; Halloran and DeLuca, 1980c). It is also consistent with observational evidence from human studies, as discussed below. It should be noted that the guinea pig stands in contrast to other animal models. Vitamin D deficiency in pregnant guinea pigs reduces fetal whole-body BMC, but not BMD (Rummens et al., 2002; Finch et al., 2010). It also appears to reduce guinea pig weight at birth (Rummens et al., 2002; Finch et al., 2010).

The information gleaned from these studies highlights the importance of calcitriol in the regulation of intestinal calcium absorption and the facilitation of skeletal mineralization in the weaned young, adolescent, and adult, but not in the fetus or early neonate. Collectively, the physiological data from several different animal models indicate that fetal calcium homeostasis and skeletal development/mineralization are regulated independently of vitamin D, calcitriol and its receptor. Heterozygous and null fetuses of *Vdr*-null mothers were, however, smaller and weighed less despite maintaining normal blood calcium levels and normal mineral content for their proportionately smaller skeletons (Kovacs et al., 2005).

Evidence from humans is mixed on whether the movement of calcium into the fetal body requires calcitriol (Specker, 2004). Both RCTs and observational evidence suggest that calcium transfer and fetal skeletal outcomes are not affected by vitamin D deficiency (Kovacs, 2008). Brooke et al. (1980) reported on an RCT of 126 women in which babies born of placebo-treated mothers had a mean serum 25OHD level of 10 nmol/L and there were no radiographic signs of rickets. Delvin et al. (1986), reporting on an RCT, found that maternal vitamin D supplementation had no effect on cord blood calcium level but resulted in higher 25OHD levels in both the maternal and cord blood. An observational study found no relationship between maternal 25OHD level and whole-body BMC and BMD and a positive relationship of gestational age and birth weight (Akcakus et al., 2006). Another observational study (Congdon et al., 1983) reported that maternal vitamin D supplementation did not affect neonatal BMC for offspring from Asian women with very low serum 25OHD levels.

In human babies lacking the 1α-hydroxylase (VDDR I) or lacking the VDR (VDDR II or hereditary vitamin D–resistant rickets) normal skeletons and blood calcium at birth have been reported (Silver et al., 1985; Takeda et al., 1997; Teotia and Teotia, 1997; Kitanaka et al., 1998; Bouillon et al., 2006). Regarding rickets, observational studies of babies born of severely vitamin D–deficient mothers generally show normal skeletal mineral content with no radiological evidence of rickets at birth (Maxwell and Miles, 1925), followed by the development of hypocalcemia or rickets only in postnatal weeks to months (Pereira and Zucker, 1986; Campbell and Fleischman, 1988; Specker, 1994; Beck-Nielsen et al., 2009). Although some isolated reports have indicated the presence of congenital rickets at birth, the diagnosis was actually made within the first or second week (Begum et al., 1968; Ford et al., 1973; Moncrieff and Fadahunsi, 1974; Sann et al., 1976; Park et al., 1987; Teotia et al., 1995). Radiographic findings have reported rickets present at day 15 but not day 2 (Sann et al., 1976). In many cases, the cause was not isolated vitamin D deficiency, but malnutrition, malabsorption (e.g., celiac disease, pancreatic insufficiency), or very low maternal intakes of both calcium and vitamin D (Begum et al., 1968; Teotia et al., 1995; Innes et al., 2002). In a study in China, neonatal rickets was not found, even though 57 percent of the infants had low cord blood 25OHD levels (Specker et al., 1992).

Overall, data are not consistent regarding skeletal development, in that several observational studies have found an adverse effect of low maternal vitamin D on fetal skeletal outcomes. An ecological study reported a positive association of imputed UVB exposure during the last trimester with some neonatal bone outcomes (Sayers and Tobias, 2009). Another study in Korean infants born in winter reported seasonal low neonatal total BMC and maternal 25OHD levels (Namgung et al., 1998). Lower levels of maternal and neonatal serum 25OHD were found for infants with craniotabes (softening of the skull bones along suture lines) compared with those without (Reif et al., 1988). Another study reported only a small non-significant reduced knee–heel length at birth in neonates whose mothers had a serum 25OHD level below 28 nmol/L (Morley et al., 2006). Recently, Mahon et al. (2010) identified an inverse relationship of femur metaphyseal cross–sectional area and splaying index with maternal 25OHD levels at 34 weeks, using high-resolution three-dimensional ultrasound at the 19th and 34th weeks of gestation. Viljakainen et al. (2010), based on a study of 124 mothers and their infants, reported impaired fetal neonatal tibia BMC and cross–sectional area, but not BMD, when maternal 25OHD levels were below the median of 42.6 nmol/L. It is noted that Mahon et al. (2010) concluded that the higher cross–sectional area was evidence of prenatal rachitic deformity, while Viljakainen et al. (2010) considered the higher cross–sectional area to predict higher bone mass in childhood. It is unclear whether the investigators in these various studies examined multiple skeletal measurements in multiple long bones, and these differences may explain some of the differences in the reports.

Regarding so-called developmental programming, recent associational studies have suggested possible adverse programming (including skeletal and selected immunological outcomes) in offspring of mothers with low maternal serum 25OHD levels (Arden et al., 2002; Cooper et al., 2005; Javaid et al., 2006; Miyake et al., 2009; Nwaru et al., 2010) as well as high maternal serum 25OHD levels (Gale et al., 2008). However, a recent observational study reported no association of maternal 25OHD levels with autoimmunity or type 1 diabetes (Marjamaki et al., 2010). Skeletal parameters at birth and nine months were normal but BMC determined later in childhood were reported to be higher in offspring of women with higher serum 25OHD levels during pregnancy compared with those with the lowest serum 25OHD levels (Javaid et al., 2006). The interpretation of these associational studies may be confounded by factors that are associated with maternal serum 25OHD level during pregnancy and affect fetal growth, such as increased maternal weight, lower socioeconomic status, and poorer nutrition. These factors may also be conferred on the offspring during childhood development, complicating the ability to establish a causal relationship.

Overall, the human and experimental animal data indicate that the development and mineralization of the fetal skeleton, as well as fetal blood calcium and phosphorus levels, are generally normal despite extremes of severe vitamin D deficiency, absence of calcitriol, and absence of the VDR. In contrast, the data confirm that vitamin D deficiency that is present at birth and left uncorrected will more readily lead to neonatal hypocalcemia and the postnatal development of rickets.

Lactation: Calcium   Key physiological changes in the female adolescent or adult occur to meet the calcium demands of lactation that are higher than those in pregnancy, but the adaptations differ from those that occur during pregnancy (Kovacs and Kronenberg, 1997, 2008; Kalkwarf, 1999; Prentice, 2003). Maternal bone resorption is markedly up-regulated (Specker et al., 1994; Kalkwarf et al., 1997), and it appears that most of the calcium present in milk derives from the maternal skeleton. This bone resorption is driven by low estradiol and high plasma PTH-related protein (PTHrP) levels (and possibly other factors), which act through osteoblasts to up-regulate osteoclast number and activity. Maternal BMD can decline 10 to 45 percent during 2 to 6 months of exclusive breastfeeding, but it normally returns to baseline over the succeeding 6 to 12 months post-weaning (Kalkwarf, 1999).

The effect of dietary intake of calcium on the skeletal resorption that occurs during lactation has been examined through randomized trials and in observational studies comparing North American and Gambian women. The consistent finding is that calcium intakes ranging from very low (< 500 mg/day) to supplemented well above normal (1.0 to 2.5 g/day) have no effect on the degree of skeletal demineralization that occurs during lactation, but calcium supplementation does increase urinary calcium excretion (Cross et al., 1995; Fairweather-Tait et al., 1995; Prentice et al., 1995; Kalkwarf et al., 1997; Laskey et al., 1998; Polatti et al., 1999).

The effect of calcium intake on skeletal recovery after weaning has not been rigorously studied. In one RCT that enrolled 95 lactating women prior to weaning, use of a 1 g/day calcium supplement resulted in a 5.9 percent increase in lumbar spine BMD compared with a 4.4 percent increase in women who took a placebo, as well as a 2.5 percent increase in non-lactating women compared with a 1.6 percent increase in women who took a placebo (Kalkwarf et al., 1997). These studies suggest that a higher calcium intake during post-weaning recovery might be beneficial for ensuring restoration of skeletal mineral content; conversely, a low calcium intake during post-weaning might be expected to impair skeletal recovery. However, skeletal recovery was complete in Gambian women with habitually very low calcium intakes. Moreover, the large associational studies mentioned above found no effect (and some found a protective effect) of a history of lactation or the number of months that a mother recalled breastfeeding her child on BMD, osteoporosis, or fracture risk later in life (Sowers, 1996; Kovacs and Kronenberg, 1997). Thus, in the long term, a history of lactation does not increase the risk of low BMD or osteoporosis.

The efficiency of intestinal calcium absorption, which is up-regulated during pregnancy, decreases to the non-pregnant level in the puerperium, and remains at that level during lactation (Kent et al., 1991; Specker et al., 1994; O'Brien et al., 2006), then increases slightly during post-weaning compared with the level in non-pregnant or lactating women (Kalkwarf et al., 1996). Urinary calcium excretion also decreases (Allen et al., 1991; O'Brien et al., 2006) and may reach the lower end of the normal range, especially in women with low calcium intakes (Specker et al., 1994). This effect presumably is due to the influence of PTHrP, which stimulates renal calcium reabsorption.

Breast milk calcium content is homeostatically regulated and unaffected by maternal calcium intake. The evidence includes randomized trials in which supplemental calcium from 1 g/day (Kalkwarf et al., 1997) to 1.5 g/day in Gambian women whose habitual calcium intake was low (Jarjou et al., 2006) showed no effect on breast milk calcium content. These results are consistent with the notion that the calcium content of milk derives from resorption of the maternal skeleton and local regulation within mammary tissue. At least one study has confirmed that the breast milk output predicts the decline in maternal BMD during lactation, whereas calcium intake, breast milk calcium concentration, and VDR genotype have no effect (Laskey et al., 1998).

In lactating women, the albumin-corrected serum calcium as well as the ionized calcium levels are normal or slightly increased (Hillman et al., 1981; Specker et al., 1991). The mean ionized calcium level of exclusively lactating women is higher than that of normal controls (Dobnig et al., 1995; Kovacs and Chik, 1995). Also, mothers nursing twins have significantly higher total calcium levels compared with mothers nursing singletons (Greer et al., 1984).

These physiological responses appear to be similar for lactating adolescents. In fact, the largest and most reassuring data set from NHANES III (described previously), which obtained BMD using the DXA method in 819 women ages 20 to 25 years (Chantry et al., 2004) indicates that young women who had breast-fed as adolescents have higher BMD than those who had not breast-fed, even after controlling for obstetrical variables. This indicates that the normal loss of BMD during lactation and recovery afterward occur in adolescent women and may even lead to a higher BMD post-weaning.

Lactation: Vitamin D   Breast milk is not normally a significant source of vitamin D for the infant. Because vitamin D (calciferol) is usually present in the circulation only for short intervals after meals, typically very little passes into breast milk. As discussed below, preliminary data may suggest that levels of vitamin D and 25OHD in breast milk can be increased by high levels of vitamin D supplementation. Neither 25OHD nor calcitriol passes readily into breast milk.

With respect to the effects of vitamin D supplementation on serum levels of 25OHD in the infant, several studies have examined supplementation of infants with 300 or 400 IU of vitamin D per day, which raised levels above 75 nmol/L (Hollis and Wagner, 2004; Basile et al., 2006; Wagner et al., 2006); however, administering supplements of 300 to 2,000 IU/day to the lactating mother did not increase serum levels of the infant (Greer et al., 1982; Rothberg et al., 1982; Ala-Houhala, 1985; Ala-Houhala et al., 1988; Greer and Marshall, 1989; Hollis and Wagner, 2004). However, very high doses of vitamin D (4,000 to 6,400 IU/day) given to the mother have been reported to raise infant serum 25OHD levels (Hollis and Wagner, 2004; Wagner et al., 2006). As described by the authors, the work was a pilot study and involved 19 subjects. Specifically, when 4,000 IU of vitamin D per day was given to the mothers, the mean serum 25OHD level of the infants exceeded 75 nmol/L; with a dose of 6,400 IU/day, the serum 25OHD level of all infants exceeded this value. However, the functional impact of raising infants' serum 25OHD levels above 75 nmol/L by increasing maternal dietary intake to such high levels is not clear, and the small sample size of this pilot study ($n = 19$) precluded conclusions about safety. One RCT found no benefit in raising infants' serum 25OHD level above 50 nmol/L relative to measures of weight, length, and skeletal mineral content (Chan et al., 1982). Other work with the administration of high dosages of vitamin D to the mother has not specifically reported any functional health outcome to the breast-fed infant other than increased serum 25OHD levels; the breast milk calcium content is unaffected (Hollis and Wagner, 2004; Wagner et al., 2006). The administration of 400 IU/day to the infant remains the American Academy of Pediatrics' recommendation (Wagner and Greer, 2008).

Serum 25OHD levels do not appear to change significantly during lactation compared with non-lactating states, although this has been assessed in only two small studies (Kent et al., 1990; Sowers et al., 1998). Because 25OHD does not pass readily into milk, it is not lost to the mother via this route. One study (Cross et al., 1995) reported an increase in maternal serum 25OHD level post-weaning, and although calcitriol levels increased in two studies (Cross et al., 1995; Kalkwarf et al., 1997), they did not in another (Specker et al., 1991). Studies have generally shown that providing vitamin D to lactating mothers increased their serum 25OHD levels, but otherwise had no significant effect on maternal outcome parameters (Cancela et al., 1986; Okonofua et al., 1987; Takeuchi et al., 1989; Kent et al., 1990; Alfaham et al., 1995; Sowers et al., 1998) and in clinical trials (Rothberg et al., 1982; Ala-Houhala, 1985; Ala-Houhala et al., 1988; Kalkwarf et al., 1996; Hollis and Wagner, 2004; Basile et al., 2006; Wagner et al., 2006; Saadi et al., 2007).

An observational study in Gambian women consuming a low-calcium diet reported no relationship between maternal 25OHD levels and breast milk calcium (Prentice et al., 1997). However, many studies measured no outcome other than the achieved serum 25OHD level in mothers and neonates and were not powered to examine outcomes such as hypocalcemia or clinical rickets (Rothberg et al., 1982; Ala-Houhala, 1985; Hollis and Wagner, 2004; Basile et al., 2006; Wagner et al., 2006).

Maternal skeleton recovers BMC after lactation ceases, but no RCTs have tested whether vitamin D sufficiency affects the speed and net recovery of maternal skeletal mineral content after weaning. An observational study in Saudi women found no relationship of serum 25OHD level with BMD at the lumbar spine, femoral neck, Ward's triangle, or trochanter, as well as no difference in BMD at these sites in women with or without severe hypovitaminosis D (Ghannam et al., 1999). None of the intervention studies that examined the use of vitamin D supplementation during lactation enrolled sufficient adolescent women to permit conclusions to be drawn about the effect of the intervention.

As noted above, animal models are of interest; in the case of vitamin D, rodent models have predominated. Unlike the situation in humans, calcitriol levels in lactating rodents remain elevated, but increase further in response to a low-calcium diet or larger litter size (Lobaugh et al., 1990, 1992). This may indicate a compensatory mechanism that increases intestinal calcium absorption even further when extra demands are placed on the mother during lactation. However, studies in vitamin D–deficient rats and *Vdr*-null mice have indicated that sufficiency of vitamin D, or responsiveness to calcitriol is not required for lactation. Vitamin D–deficient rats and *Vdr*-null mice lactated normally and resorbed the expected proportion of bone (Halloran and DeLuca, 1980b; Miller et al., 1982; Fudge and Kovacs, 2010), although one study in vitamin D–deficient rats found that more skeletal mineral content was lost than normal (Marie et al., 1986). Intestinal calcium absorption was twice the control level in lactating vitamin D–deficient rats, confirming that vitamin D is not required for the intestinal adaptation to take place (Halloran and DeLuca, 1980a; Boass et al., 1981).

In rodents, the skeleton is substantially resorbed during lactation, and this is followed in the post-lactation period by an interval of up-regulated bone formation, which effectively restores BMD to a normal level within 10 to 14 days. Two studies of vitamin D–deficient rats reported at least partial recovery of skeletal mineral content after lactation, with the final value exceeding the pre-pregnancy value in one study (Halloran and DeLuca, 1980b; Miller et al., 1982). Likewise, in *Vdr*-null mice, BMC after weaning also exceeded the pre-pregnancy level (Fudge et al., 2006). Thus, these animal studies suggest that calcitriol may not be required for the skeleton to recover its normal mineral content after lactation is completed.

In both *Vdr*-null and 1α-hydroxylase-null mice, the provision of a high-calcium, high-phosphorus, lactose-enriched diet, initiated in the neonates prior to weaning, prevented the development of rickets in the adult (Li et al., 1998; Amling et al., 1999; Van Cromphaut et al., 2001; Hoenderop et al., 2002; Dardenne et al., 2003; Rowling et al., 2007). Similar outcomes have been reported for children with VDDR-I or VDDRI-II in which rickets is mitigated with high levels of oral calcium or intermittent intravenous infusions of calcium (Balsan et al., 1986; Hochberg et al., 1992; Kitanaka et al., 1998). These results indicate that the main role of calcitriol is to stimulate active intestinal calcium absorption rather than to directly affect skeletal development. Moreover, it suggests that the role of calcitriol can be bypassed if the calcium content of the experimental diet is suitably manipulated.

Other Measures of Interest Related to Bone Health: PTH

PTH is potentially of interest as an indicator of bone health because vitamin D intake can lower serum PTH levels (Malabanan et al., 1998) and because elevated serum PTH levels have been recognized as a risk factor for osteoporosis (Hodsman et al., 2002). The role of PTH in the calcium–vitamin D homeostatic system is highlighted in Chapter 2. A critical question is what levels of PTH are harmful to bone, as only a small amount of PTH is needed to maintain a normal level of serum 25OHD.

Measures that have been explored are the levels of serum 25OHD at which PTH levels rise as well as the level of serum 25OHD at which PTH levels no longer decline (Aloia et al., 2006a; Durazo-Arvizu et al., 2010). However, because serum PTH levels increase with age, it is not clear what level of PTH should be regarded as normal (Dawson-Hughes et al., 1997a; Vieth et al., 2003) or whether the relationship is meaningful for all age groups (Abrams et al., 2005). These studies have led some to suggest that a serum 25OHD level of 75 nmol/L is consistent with the PTH plateau point (Malabanan et al., 1998) and hence demarcates sufficiency and insufficiency for vitamin D. However, a review of the literature does not show widespread agreement on a plateau consistent with a serum 25OHD level of 75 nmol/L. In most cases, serum PTH level reaches a plateau at different levels of serum 25OHD varying between 37.5 and 125.0 nmol/L. Box 4-7 summarizes the study outcomes.

Race/ethnicity may be a factor in determining the relationship between serum 25OHD and PTH levels, although the measures used have focused on calcitriol rather than serum 25OHD concentrations. African American and dark-skinned populations have lower serum 25OHD and calcitriol levels compared with white populations (Bell, 1995, 1997). A study of more than 500 healthy women ages 20 to 80 years found that PTH

BOX 4-7
Studies Demonstrating PTH Plateaus at Various Serum 25OHD Levels

Serum 25OHD < 30 nmol/L:
- Ooms et al. (1995a)

Serum 25OHD < 50 nmol/L:
- Malabanan et al. (1998)
- Levis et al. (2005)
- Steingrimsdottir et al. (2005)
- Aloia et al. (2006a)

Serum 25OHD < 75 nmol/L:
- Vieth et al. (2003)
- Holick et al. (2005)
- Durazo-Arvizu et al. (2010)

Serum 25OHD ~ 88 nmol/L:
- Kinyamu et al. (1998)

Serum 25OHD 100–125 nmol/L:
- Krall et al. (1989)
- Dawson-Hughes et al. (1997a)

No plateau:
- Bates et al. (2003)
- Benjamin et al. (2009)

No relationship:
- Rucker et al. (2002)

---

and calcitriol levels were higher in black than in white women and that the black women had lower bone turnover rates compared with white women (Aloia et al., 1996b). Some evidence, however, suggests that PTH levels are similar in both populations (Benjamin et al., 2009).

As reviewed by Prentice et al. (2008), an inverse relationship between PTH and serum 25OHD concentrations has been reported in many cross–sectional and intervention studies in elderly people (Krall et al., 1989; Ooms et al., 1995a; Chapuy et al., 1997; Bates et al., 2003), post menopausal women (Krall et al., 1989; Lappe et al., 2006), and young persons (Guillemant et al., 1999). Some studies suggest that the plasma PTH concentration reaches a plateau as the 25OHD concentration increases

(Chapuy et al., 1997; Lappe et al., 2006), whereas others describe an exponential inverse relationship (linear when the data are expressed in logarithms) throughout the physiological range of 25OHD concentrations (Bates et al., 2003; Vieth et al., 2003). The reasons for these discrepancies are unclear, but they could reflect differences among the populations studied and statistical methods used (Prentice, 2008).

Further, the plasma PTH concentration varies widely within and among individuals at any given concentration of 25OHD (Chapuy et al., 1997; Bates et al., 2003), because the plasma PTH concentration depends upon many factors other than vitamin D, such as stage of life, ethnic background, intakes of dietary calcium (Steingrimsdottir et al., 2005) and phosphorus, time of day, kidney function (Ooms et al., 1995a), physical activity level, and drug use (Slovik et al., 1981; van der Wiel et al., 1991; Vieth et al., 2003; Fraser et al., 2004; Patel et al., 2007; Prentice, 2008). In addition, the choice of assay method is important because an assay could detect both PTH fragments and intact molecules (van der Wiel et al., 1991).

Most of the studies supporting the use of serum PTH level as either a biomarker of exposure or a biomarker of biological effect have been conducted among older white persons living in Europe and the United States. However, the available studies in other age groups and in people from different geographic locations and ethnic backgrounds do not provide evidence that PTH measures can be universally applied relative to information about vitamin D intakes and effects. Studies in Africa and China, for example, have reported that plasma PTH measures are elevated in populations with low calcium intake, even when vitamin D nutriture is good, and the inverse correlations between plasma PTH measures and bone health outcomes such as BMD and fracture risk observed in Western countries are not found (Yan et al., 2003; Aspray et al., 2005). Also, PTH measures increase during puberty (Abrams et al., 2005; Tylavsky et al., 2005), a period of skeletal growth. Therefore, although the potential for PTH as a useful indicator of bone health is acknowledged, it is not a useful indicator for DRI development at this point in time.

Integration of Evidence for the Potential Indicator of Bone Health

To be useful for judging bone health outcomes as potential indicators for DRI development, the available evidence must be considered in the context of its relevance to bone accretion, bone maintenance, and bone loss. The committee therefore arranged the data consistent with these physiological states. Although the AHRQ analyses were useful overall for this purpose, the committee recognized that there were useful studies published after the completion of the AHRQ-Tufts as well as several relevant studies that did not meet the inclusion criteria stipulated by the

AHRQ analyses. These are included and identified in the discussions below. The following sections integrate data on bone accretion, maintenance, and loss and refer to the DRI life stage groups as appropriate. Initially, the utility of serum 25OHD level for the purposes of DRI development is discussed, as is the relationship between calcium absorption and serum 25OHD concentrations.

Utility of serum 25OHD level for examining bone health outcomes   Although serum 25OHD is indicative of vitamin D exposure (see Chapter 3), the seemingly logical next step of using serum 25OHD level to explore the levels at which vitamin D effects a health outcome requires caution. There are a number of studies of good quality that report serum 25OHD concentrations in relation to health outcomes such as fracture incidence—and which have been described in the AHRQ analyses—but such associations are not necessarily causal or predictive, and not all of the variables associated with serum 25OHD levels are reported. In short, these associations are not yet an adequate basis for validating serum 25OHD concentrations as a "biomarker of effect" (see Chapter 1) for either an intermediate health endpoint (e.g., blood pressure) or disease (e.g., rickets or osteoporosis).

Others have also concluded that the usefulness of serum 25OHD level as an indicator of functional outcomes has not been demonstrated in many cases, with the possible exception of elderly people (Brannon et al., 2008). Further, Brannon et al. (2008) pointed out that the value of the measure appears to be most useful at the extremes of the range for detecting deficiency and toxicity, but may be less useful in the middle range and subject to confounders. Additionally, it has not been ruled out that vitamin D may act to produce health outcomes in a manner that is separate from circulating 25OHD levels and thereby function in a pathway different from that known for 25OHD. Currently there is no evidence confirming pathways not involving 25OHD, although their existence is plausible.

Nonetheless, serum 25OHD concentration is a useful measure for several reasons, not the least of which is that 25OHD has a long half-life in the circulation and its concentration is not under tight homeostatic control. It generally demonstrates a direct relationship with "exposure" or "supply" (i.e., dietary intake and cutaneous synthesis), although, as discussed in Chapter 3, the relationship is known to vary with factors ranging from body adiposity to aging and is also known to be curvilinear, with decreased response as intakes increase. Despite these caveats, serum 25OHD concentration is a useful biomarker of the supply of vitamin D available to target tissues in most situations (Prentice et al., 2008). It therefore is relevant as a stand-in for overall vitamin D nutriture, although distinguishing between concentrations due to intake and those due to sun exposure is not possible for most studies.

The utility of serum 25OHD level as a biomarker of effect is less certain. Prentice et al. (2008) pointed out that the adequacy of the vitamin D supply in meeting functional requirements depends upon many factors, including the uptake of 25OHD by target cells, the rate of conversion of calcitriol and its delivery to target tissues, the expression and affinity of the VDR in target tissues, the responsiveness of cells to the activated VDR, and the efficiency of induced metabolic pathways.

Nonetheless, despite these uncertainties, serum 25OHD levels can be regarded as a useful tool in considering vitamin D requirements; in fact, such measures are virtually the only tool available at this time. As pointed out by AHRQ-Tufts, when a non-validated intermediate outcome must be considered, the implicit assumption is that it would have the properties of a validated surrogate outcome, and this assumption should be made explicit and the uncertainties identified. This is a reasonable approach and allows the appropriate inclusion of consideration of serum 25OHD concentrations for the purposes of specifying the potential indicator of bone health.

Relationship between calcium absorption and serum 25OHD level   Ensuring desirable rates of calcium uptake from the intestinal lumen into the body—calcium absorption—is an important aspect of bone health. Because vitamin D is instrumental in calcium absorption, the relationship between vitamin D and calcium absorption is relevant to an indicator for bone health. The literature in this area focuses on fractional calcium absorption (i.e., fraction of a given dose of calcium that is absorbed) and its association with serum 25OHD level.

Although calcitriol has been shown to stimulate intestinal calcium absorption directly and calcitriol levels correlate with absorption, the understanding of the current relationship between 25OHD level and calcium absorption requires examination. Widely quoted as evidence of the threshold for maximal calcium absorption at serum 25OHD levels above 75 nmol/L is an analysis of results from three separate studies (Barger-Lux and Heaney, 2002; Bischoff et al., 2003; Heaney et al., 2003) as put forward by Heaney (2005). Less widely understood is the nature of the evidence from each of these studies and, thus, the limitations of this graphic analysis. In only one of these studies (Barger-Lux and Heaney, 2002) was calcium absorption directly measured using a single calcium isotope method; the difference between the lower (approximately 75 nmol/L) and higher (approximately 125 nmol/L) serum 25OHD levels was non-significant. Although the single-isotope method is considered less accurate than the dual-isotope method for measuring calcium absorption, this method is viewed as appropriate. The two values from the Barger-Lux and Heaney

(2002) study are the most reliable of the values in this analysis. Two additional values taken from Heaney et al. (2003) in this graphic analysis (at approximately 50 and 85 nmol/L) are not direct measures of calcium absorption, but instead are indirect pharmacokinetic measures based on the plasma calcium response to a 500 mg oral calcium load (Heaney et al., 2003). Thus, the committee found these values limited in their usefulness in this analysis. The remaining 25OHD level of a calcium absorption of 0.15 at serum 25OHD 29 nmol/L was taken from Bischoff et al. (2003). It does not represent either a direct or indirect measurement of calcium absorption, but was derived from measured urinary calcium excretion using subjects that did not reduce serum PTH while on calcium supplements (Heaney, 2005; personal communication, R. P. Heaney, Creighton University, Omaha, NE, August 25, 2009). This approach is not generally acceptable, and the committee could not consider the value to be valid. In conclusion, the portion of this analysis showing a rise in calcium absorption with an increase in 25OHD level from approximately 28 nmol/L to 80 or 90 nmol/L is unreliable, because the two values showing this rise either are not based on directly measured calcium absorption or are based on an unreliable method for estimating calcium absorption as discussed by Aloia et al. (2010) and as described below. The remaining two values, although reliable, are insufficient to determine the relationship of 25OHD level to calcium absorption, if any exists.

The gold standard for assessing fractional calcium absorption is to administer two calcium isotopes (one orally, one intravenously) under conditions in which blood and/or urine can be collected and assayed for both isotopes. Alternatively, calcium absorption can be assessed using a single isotope test, although results may be less precise. As discussed below, the data from studies published after the Heaney (2005) paper either do not show increased calcium absorption with higher levels of 25OHD or show only a very slight increase in calcium absorption as serum 25OHD level rises.

With respect to children, Abrams et al. (2009) performed dual-label calcium absorption studies in 251 children ranging from 4.9 to 16.7 years of age and found no effect of higher serum 25OHD level on fractional calcium absorption. In fact, children with 25OHD levels of 28 to 50 nmol/L had higher fractional calcium absorption than did children with 25OHD levels of 50 to 80 or greater than 80 nmol/L. Data from a 2008 study in girls (Weaver et al., 2008) indicated that serum 25OHD level did not predict net calcium absorption and retention. A study conducted in Nigeria (Thacher et al., 2009) demonstrated that in children with rickets, increases in serum 25OHD level did not coincide with increased fractional calcium absorption.

With respect to adults, there are a number of single-isotope studies of interest. Need et al. (2008) studied fractional calcium absorption in 319 men (66 ± 10 years) with serum 25OHD levels less than 40 nmol/L. Fractional calcium absorption was 0.36 in men with the lowest quartile serum 25OHD levels (< 10 nmol/L) and rose significantly to 0.56 in the second quartile (11 to 20 nmol/L). No further change in fractional calcium absorption occurred with 25OHD levels of 21 to 30 or 31 to 40 nmol/L (Need et al., 2008). Kinyamu et al. (1998) performed a cross–sectional study of 376 healthy women (71 ± 4 years) and compared calcium absorption in those who took vitamin D supplements with that in non-supplemented women. Serum 25OHD level was significantly higher in women who took vitamin D (87.9 ± 28.2 nmol/L vs. 73.6 ± 23.0 nmol/L), whereas fractional calcium absorption did not differ between the two groups (Kinyamu et al., 1998). In addition, Devine et al. (2002) used a single isotope of calcium in a study of 120 older women and plotted a linear relationship between intestinal calcium absorption and serum 25OHD level. Intestinal calcium absorption rose from 35 percent at a mean serum 25OHD level of 15 nmol/L to 50 percent at 150 nmol/L. However, there were few data points at any serum 25OHD level, and an alternative fit to the data suggested an increase to 50 nmol/L and a plateau thereafter.

Hansen et al. (2008) studied 18 postmenopausal women before and after 15 days of supplementation with 50,000 IU of vitamin D_2 daily. Serum 25OHD level rose markedly from 55 ± 10 nmol/L to 160 ± 53 nmol/L (p < 0.001), while fractional calcium absorption changed only modestly from 24 ± 7 percent at baseline to 27 ± 6 percent after vitamin D repletion (p < 0.04), indicating that the large rise in serum 25OHD levels was statistically significant, as was the small rise in intestinal calcium absorption. The 3 percent absolute increase in fractional calcium absorption was considered by the authors to be a minor increment given the large increase in serum 25OHD level (Hansen et al., 2008).

In a randomized controlled study, postmenopausal women with a mean baseline serum 25OHD level of 44 nmol/L receiving 1,000 mg of calcium citrate daily were randomized to daily placebo or 1,000 IU of vitamin D_2 (Zhu et al., 2008a). Using a single-isotope method, this research group found a 36 nmol/L rise in serum 25OHD level and no increase in calcium absorption. This outcome is consistent with findings from their longer-term study (over 5 years), also demonstrating no rise in absorption (Zhu et al., 2008a). In both placebo and vitamin D groups, the calcium absorption decreased compared with baseline, most likely as a result of greater calcium intake (1 g calcium supplementation in both treatment arms). Also, Francis et al. (1996) found that 500 to 1,000 IU of vitamin D_2 did not increase calcium absorption in elderly women. In a randomized double-blind controlled pilot trial in women (mean age = 57 years; dual-isotope method) with a baseline serum 25OHD level of 52 nmol/L, it was found that 400 IU of vitamin D per day raised serum 25OHD level (by 14 nmol/L) and did not significantly increase calcium absorption compared with placebo.[4]

In a recent study, Aloia et al. (2010) performed a single-isotope assay of intestinal calcium absorption in 492 white and black women ages 20 to 80 years. They tested whether serum 25OHD or calcitriol level predicted the rate of intestinal calcium absorption in a multivariate model that included age, menopausal status, calcium intake, and other factors. The serum 25OHD levels ranged from 30 to 150 nmol/L, and were 51.62 ± 33.67 nmol/L overall or 32.87 ± 21.20 nmol/L in blacks and 67.73 ± 34.11 nmol/L in whites. Whereas calcitriol level was an important predictor of intestinal calcium absorption in the final model, 25OHD level had no effect. The authors concluded that serum 25OHD level is not an indicator of intestinal calcium absorption efficiency by itself, but 25OHD does interact at low levels with calcitriol to predict calcium absorption.

Overall, the data are mixed, but most studies show no increase in intestinal calcium absorption across a broad range of serum 25OHD levels. The single-isotope study by Need et al. (2008) indicates no increase in fractional calcium absorption above 20 nmol/L. The single-isotope studies by Heaney et al. (2003), Kinyamu et al. (1998), and Aloia et al. (2010) indicate no change in fractional calcium absorption across higher ranges of 25OHD levels—specifically, from 60 to 154 nmol/L in Heaney et al. (2003), from 50 to 116 nmol/L in Kinyamu et al. (1998), and from 30 to 150 nmol/L in Aloia et al. (2010). Others (Francis et al., 1996; Patel et al., 2001; Zhu et al., 2008a, b) demonstrate no effect on absorption of increasing the serum 25OHD concentrations by 14 to 36 nmol/L, whereas the Hansen et al. (2008) study indicates a 3 percent increase in absorption after raising the serum 25OHD level from 55 to 160 nmol/L in the short-term (15 days).

The data currently suggest that fractional calcium absorption reaches a maximum between 30 and 50 nmol/L in both children and adults. A value of 50 nmol/L allows for some uncertainty in the data and a buffer against seasonal and dietary variations in calciferol intake that, in turn, cause fluctuations in serum 25OHD levels.

Bone accretion   Bone accretion resulting in bone growth and skeletal development occurs during the younger life stages. Measures of the amount of calcium needed to achieve normal bone accretion as well as the levels of vitamin D that support accretion are, therefore, relevant considerations. The topics of pregnancy and lactation among adolescent girls, who are still accruing bone tissue, are discussed in other sections below jointly with pregnancy and lactation among women.

---

[4]Personal communication, S. Shapses, Rutgers University, New Brunswick, NJ, April 10, 2010.

Calcium retention levels   Total body calcium at birth in healthy, full-term infants is approximately 30 g (Givens and Macy, 1933; Widdowson et al., 1951). Based on bone mineral accretion derived as a function of change in body weight, total body calcium increases to approximately 80 g by 1 year of age (Leitch and Aitken, 1959). This suggests an average accretion rate of approximately 140 mg calcium per day during the first year of life. This greatly exceeds the earlier accretion rate estimates, derived from cadaveric sources, of approximately 30 to 35 mg/day and 50 to 55 mg/day for infants through 4 months of age and 4 through 12 months of age, respectively (Fomon and Nelson, 1993; Koo and Tsang, 1997). Yet another mean accretion rate of approximately 80 mg/day during the first year of life has been derived using metacarpal morphometry data (Garn, 1972; Weaver, 1994). Resolution of these different values for usual accretion rate is not currently possible, but assessment of these data and the balance data suggests that a mean accretion rate of about 100 mg/day overall during the first year of life may serve as a reasonable approximation for primarily breast-fed infants (Abrams, 2010).

Information about bone accretion in young children is limited given the impracticalities associated with studies of young subjects. Lynch et al. (2007), using an isotope-based method, evaluated the relationship between calcium intake and balance in healthy children 1 to 4 years of age. They reported mean calcium retention of 161 mg/day with a mean calcium intake of 551 mg/day, reflecting a positive calcium balance. Linear and non-linear modeling indicated that calcium intakes of 470 mg/day yielded a calcium retention of 140 mg/day, consistent with the growth needs of this population (Lynch et al., 2007).

For slightly older children in the 7- to 8-year age range, the work by Abrams et al. (1999) has also demonstrated that the average calcium accretion rate is 140 mg/day[5] calcium. A small increase is seen in late pre-puberty (Leitch and Aitken, 1959; Ellis et al., 1996), yielding a bone calcium accretion rate ranging from 140 to 160 mg/day across this age group, within which a small percentage will be pre-pubertal. Based on modeling, a curvilinear dose–response relationship between calcium intake and retention was made evident as shown in Figure 4-8.

A recent publication from Wu et al. (2010) that focused on Chinese American boys and girls 11 to 15 years of age reported calcium retention to be 1,100 mg/day in boys and 970 mg/day in girls, but these estimates were based on intakes to achieve maximal calcium retention as opposed to average calcium retention, the value needed to determine an EAR. A recent study of white children in Canada (Vatanparast et al., 2010) has provided bone calcium accretion levels for children and adolescents between the

---

[5]The 140 mg/day value is a modeled value as described in the study (Abrams et al., 1999).

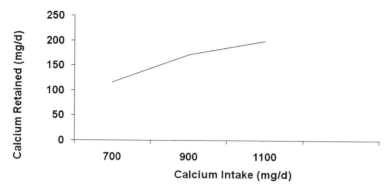

FIGURE 4-8 Dose–response relationship between calcium intake and retention.
SOURCES: Abrams et al. (1999); Ames et al. (1999).

ages of 9 and 18 years as shown in Table 4-14. The differences between girls and boys and between the 9- to 13-year and the 14- to 18-year age groups are small, but statistically significant. The data provide a basis for estimating intake levels needed for this age group relative to bone accretion.

Although it would be expected that bone maintenance is characteristic of young adults overall, there is some evidence of a small accretion of bone mass for persons in their 20s. The magnitude of this reported accretion varies. Specifically, Recker et al. (1992) followed 156 college-age women for 5 years and reported an increase of 12.4 percent per decade (about 1.24 percent per year) in whole-body BMC, but there were smaller increases in clinically relevant sites such as the forearm (4.8 percent per decade or 0.48 percent per year) and the lumbar spine (5.9 percent per decade or 0.59 percent per year). Further, the rate of increase declined each year for this group. The variance was also large in this study, which may be due to the method selected to assess BMC. Barger-Lux et al. (2005) more recently reported an accretion rate of 0.28 percent per year for women in the 20-

TABLE 4-14 Mean Bone Calcium Accretion for Three Age Groupings of Girls and Boys

Age (years)	Mean Bone Calcium Accretion (mg/day)	
	Girls	Boys
9–13	151	141
14–18	92	210
9–18	121	175

SOURCE: Vatanparast et al. (2010).

to 30-year age range. This lower reported accretion rate is equivalent to a calcium accretion rate of only 6 mg/day. In addition to reporting only very small bone accretion for ages 19 through 30 years, Barger-Lux et al. (2005) also noted the possibility that there was no further effect on bone accretion above calcium intake levels of approximately 800 mg/day.

In short, bone accretion may continue during this early stage of adulthood, but at very low, almost indiscernible, levels. Interpretation of the data is further complicated by evidence from the Canadian Multicentre Osteoporosis Study (Berger et al., 2010), which demonstrates that attainment of peak bone mass depends upon which site is measured; peak bone mass is achieved by age 18 at some sites, but by age 25 or so at others. This newer population-based study is much larger than earlier studies, for example, Recker et al. (1992), and relies on the newer technique of DXA to estimate BMC. Tuck and Datta (2007) reported that maximal bone mass is attained in the second decade of life followed by a period of consolidation lasting 5 years, such that maximal levels are achieved in the early to mid 20s. Interestingly, peak trabecular bone mass is achieved earlier, at 15 to 18 years of age, is maintained for several years, and then begins to decline in young adulthood (Riggs et al., 2008).

Bone mineral content/bone mineral density: Calcium Measures of BMC and BMD in addition to calcium retention levels are also of interest as a measure of bone accretion. In a cross–sectional evaluation in 136 boys and men and 130 girls and women, including children beginning at the age of 4 years as well as adults through the age of 27 years, BMD of total body, lumbar spine, and femoral neck increased significantly with age until 17.5 years in boys and 15.8 years in girls (Lu et al., 1994). However, care must be taken in interpreting calcium intakes—specifically, calcium supplementation that results in total intakes above 1,500 mg/day for these groups—relative to BMC or BMD measures. Studies have suggested that increasing intakes of calcium in girls above their habitual intake of about 900 mg/day is associated with positive effects on bone mineral accretion and, in turn, BMD (Johnston et al., 1992; Lloyd et al., 1993; Chan et al., 1995). However, there is evidence that the bone mass gained through calcium or milk supplementation during childhood and adolescence is not retained post-intervention, suggesting that there is no benefit to intakes above that needed to ensure normal bone accretion (Fehily et al., 1992; Lee et al., 1996; Slemenda et al., 1997). A study conducted by Matkovic et al. (2004) evaluated BMD measures among female white adolescents 15 to 18 years of age in the United States, and reported that there was a positive influence of calcium supplementation and dairy products on BMD of the hip and forearm. The background level of calcium intake was approximately 833 mg/day, whereas the supplemented subjects had total calcium intakes of 1,586 mg/day. The Matkovic et al. (2004) study, however, did not follow the subjects after the intervention ceased in order to determine whether the bone mass was retained. Overall, it would appear that levels of calcium intake consistent with levels established as supportive of bone accretion are associated with a normal, healthy increase in BMD. However, calcium intake levels above those consistent with established bone accretion rates appear to offer no meaningful benefit.

Bone mineral content/bone mineral density: Vitamin D   Regarding vitamin D nutriture and very young children, virtually no data are available to link vitamin D intake or serum 25OHD level to bone accretion measures. However, for older children and adolescents, as described above, there was *fair evidence* from the AHRQ-Ottawa analyses of an association between 25OHD levels and baseline BMD and change in BMD or BMC indexes based on observational data. However, the results from the RCTs, as described above, did not confirm a consistent benefit on BMD or BMC across skeletal sites and age groups. Reasons for these differences may be due to the difficulty in controlling confounding variables for bone mass in observational studies.

Rickets   Although consideration of rickets provides only a starting point for considering nutrient reference values, AHRQ-Ottawa, as described above, analyzed serum 25OHD concentrations in the context of the onset of rickets in children up to 5 years of age. It identified serum concentrations below 27.5 nmol/L as consistently associated with rickets. However, many of the relevant studies were from developing countries where dietary calcium intake is low; therefore, for these studies the onset of rickets was associated with higher levels of serum 25OHD, likely due to low calcium intakes. Specker et al. (1992) concluded that serum 25OHD concentrations of below 27 to 30 nmol/L place the infant at an increased risk for developing rickets, although they indicated that the measure is not diagnostic of the disease. It is worth noting that there is very limited evidence of rickets due to calcium deficiency in the face of vitamin D sufficiency (Abrams, 2002). The minimum calcium intake needed to prevent calcium-deficiency rickets has not been precisely identified, and the available studies (all outside North America) reflect varying levels at which calcium-deficiency rickets occurred. Levels of intake between 200 and 300 mg of calcium per day in infants and small children have been associated with risk for rickets in these cases (Abrams, 2002).

Calcium absorption and serum 25OHD   As described above, life stages that experience bone accretion demonstrate a maximal calcium absorption associated with serum 25OHD levels of at least 30 nmol/L and closer to 40 to 50 nmol/L. Fractional calcium absorption does not appear to increase with serum 25OHD concentrations above 50 nmol/L. In addition, rickets in populations that are not calcium deficient does not occur until serum 25OHD levels drop below 30 nmol/L.

Summary of evidence for bone accretion   In summary, average calcium retention (100 to 140 mg/day) during periods of bone accretion provide critical evidence to support the development of DRIs for calcium for these life stages using the factorial method as outlined in the 1997 DRI report (IOM, 1997), based on the average calcium retention, the specific age period, fractional calcium absorption rate, urinary calcium losses, and other small calcium losses. Data of good quality have been made available in the past 10 to 15 years for ages 1 through 18 for average bone mineral calcium accretion or retention; these can be used to determine the EAR and Recommended Dietary Allowance (RDA) for calcium for these age groups. BMC is of less utility for developing the DRIs for calcium, as noted above, but intakes of calcium that support average calcium accretion are also associated with normal healthy BMC/BMD.

Neither rickets nor calcium absorption is informative for establishing DRIs for calcium. During bone accretion, low serum 25OHD levels (< 30 nmol/L) are associated with increased risk of rickets when calcium intakes are not limiting. Further, fractional calcium absorption may be impaired at low serum 25OHD levels (< 30 nmol/L) and does not appear to be enhanced further above serum 25OHD above 50 nmol/L. Although the AHRQ-Ottawa report found fair evidence of an association between serum 25OHD levels and BMC/BMD based on observational data, results from the RCTs did not confirm a consistent benefit on BMC/BMD across skeletal sites and age groups.

Bone maintenance   Whereas bone accretion ceases in early adulthood, bone continues to be remodeled throughout life. The goal—bone maintenance—is to provide adequate levels of calcium and vitamin D to support the process and maintain healthy bone and bone density. In turn, maintaining neutral calcium balance is the measure of interest—positive balance no longer occurs and negative calcium balance is to be avoided. In addition to highlighting the five key indicators relevant to bone maintenance, this section addresses pregnancy and lactation within the context of relevant indicators for DRI development.

Neutral calcium balance   An important body of evidence is contributed by a recent comprehensive analysis of metabolic studies, as reported by Hunt and Johnson (2007). Their work not only offers solutions for some of the confounding associated with the interpretation of data from calcium balance studies, as discussed in Chapter 2, but also it provides new information on the levels of calcium associated with neutral calcium balance.

Participants in the Hunt and Johnson (2007) study included 73 women 20 to 75 years of age (average 47 years) and 82 men 19 to 64 years of age (average 28 years). The analysis included 19 feeding studies conducted at one site in a metabolic unit under carefully controlled conditions. Balance data from the final 6 to 12 days of each dietary period were analyzed. For these studies, only healthy individuals participated, calcium intakes below and near the presumed required amounts were included, and adequate dietary adaptation was ensured by examining only dietary periods greater than or equal to 18 days. The statistical model used by Hunt and Johnson (2007) predicted neutral calcium balance at calcium intakes of 741 mg/day for healthy adults, regardless of age or gender. The upper limit of the 95 percent prediction interval around this estimate was 1,035 mg/day. Given the subjects, the outcomes are most readily applicable for adults up to the age of 50 years. These authors concluded that their data indicated tight control of calcium homeostasis in the range of typical calcium intakes and far above the point at which calcium balance is neutral (i.e., 741 mg/day). Moreover, they indicated that calcium balance is highly resistant to changes in calcium intake across a broad range of intakes—specifically, 414 to 1,740 mg/day, the approximate 25th and 99th percentiles from their studies.

Bone mineral density: Calcium   In the case of female subjects, there are observational studies relating calcium intake to bone mass in premenopausal women, but virtually all are confounded by the absence of data on vitamin D (either intake or serum 25OHD concentrations) and factors such as physical activity and hormonal status. In addition, there are only two randomized trials of calcium supplementation and bone mass in women (and none in men) from the fourth to the sixth decade of life, despite the relative importance of this period for the maintenance of skeletal health. Thus, overall, little information specifically for BMD and calcium is available, and there is no evidence that levels above that needed for neutral calcium balance are beneficial. Needless to say there are no fracture studies, in part because of the relative rarity of osteoporotic fractures in this age group. However, BMD is considered predictive of future fracture risk.

One recent observational study of 300 premenopausal Greek women demonstrated that those who had calcium intakes above 800 mg per day and were physically active had higher ultrasound bone mass measurements than those with lower calcium intakes, regardless of physical activity level (Dionyssiotis et al., 2010). Furthermore, a 10-year observational study of 133 premenopausal Finnish women demonstrated that those with high calcium intake had less trochanteric BMC loss than those with lower intake (Uusi-Rasi et al., 2008). A recent observational study from Bischoff-Ferrari et al. (2009b) examined NHANES data and calcium intake against the incidence of hip BMD and serum 25OHD level among individuals without previous fractures across a wide age range. These authors found that among premenopausal women, a higher calcium intake was associated with greater BMD only for those women with a serum 25OHD level below 50 nmol/L. No such association was found for men. The methodologies do not indicate whether the authors applied the prescribed weighting factors for NHANES data, which if not carried out could significantly impact the nature of the results.

Other observational data provide only marginal evidence to suggest that calcium intakes can have an impact on bone mass in men. One observational study of nearly 2,400 young Swedish men (mean age 18.4 years) suggested that physical activity level but not calcium intake was related to calcaneal BMD (Pettersson et al., 2010). Similarly, in a study of 131 men ages 20 to 75 years, calcium intake had no relationship to lumbar or femoral BMD at any age (Atalar et al., 2009). In the Amsterdam Growth and Health Longitudinal Study of 225 men 27 to 36 years of age during a 10-year period, calcium intake was not related to lumbar BMD. In contrast, in a study of 300 Greek men ages 18 to 30 years, only calcium intakes below 400 mg per day were associated with the lower BMD (Kyriazopoulous et al., 2006).

As mentioned, randomized trial data are few and underpowered. In one very small ($n = 37$) randomized trial of women 30 to 42 years of age, those who increased their dietary calcium intake by an average of 600 mg/day for 3 years exhibited no vertebral bone loss compared with the women with no calcium supplementation, who lost an average of 1 percent of their spine BMD per year (Baran et al., 1990). In another small randomized study of 300 women between 45 and 55 years of age who were considered "perimenopausal," Elders et al. (1991) demonstrated that supplemental calcium at 1,000 mg/day over 2 years prevented a relatively small degree of bone loss in the spine compared with placebo-treated controls.

Bone mineral density: Vitamin D   Regarding vitamin D and BMD measures, the AHRQ analyses incorporated largely studies that administered vitamin D in combination with calcium. Further, regarding the relationship between serum 25OHD levels and BMD measures for persons likely to be experiencing bone maintenance, very few studies for persons between the ages of 18 and 20 years were located. Regarding the intake of vitamin D with and without calcium supplementation, again most studies focused on postmenopausal women. In any case, bone density is known to vary among adults with age, gender, and race/ethnicity (Looker et al., 2009).

For studies of vitamin D nutriture and BMD, observational data are available. For example, Bischoff-Ferrari et al. (2009b) examined a cohort of men and women from NHANES III with average age of 47 years (20 to 69 years) and found that for both genders, there was a stepwise increase in BMD for higher serum 25OHD concentrations, even among individuals less than 50 years of age. The analysis is reported on the basis of cutoff point, and overall distributions were not provided; further it is not clear that the NHANES III sampling weights were applied. Van Dijk et al. (2009) studied vitamin D intake and BMD in 320 Dutch men and women at 36 years of age and found that vitamin D intake was positively associated with BMD at all sites in men but not in women. AHRQ-Tufts reported inconsistent outcomes for the measures of BMD relative to serum 25OHD. In any case, observational data are best used when causality has been demonstrated by RCTs, which does not appear to be the case for BMD and serum 25OHD.

One recent RCT that focused on vitamin D measures included persons between the ages of 18 and 64 years, the period at which bone maintenance is paramount. Andersen et al. (2008) analyzed 89 women and 83 men separately; subjects were Pakistani immigrants living in Copenhagen, Denmark. The men and women were assigned to receive either a daily dose of 400 or 800 IU of vitamin D_3 or placebo for 1 year. For women, the mean baseline dietary calcium intake was 495 mg/day, and mean serum 25OHD concentration was 12 nmol/L. For men, the mean baseline dietary calcium intake was 548 mg/day, and the mean serum 25OHD concentration was 21 nmol/L. At the end of the study, there was no significant difference in lumbar spine BMD changes regardless of the dose in both women or men.

Not unexpectedly, osteoporotic fractures are not a factor during the younger years of adulthood, a life stage not characterized by bone loss. In young adult women, stress fractures and overuse injuries in Navy recruits were examined in relation to calcium and vitamin D intake (Lappe et al., 2008). Supplementation with these two nutrients (2,000 mg of calcium per day and 800 IU of vitamin D per day) reduced the incidence of stress fractures. However, the generalizability of this study to the normal population is questionable.

Osteomalacia   Recent data on osteomalacia are illuminating. A study conducted by Priemel et al. (2010) provides useful information on serum 25OHD levels and osteomalacia. Postmortem bone biopsies and measurement of serum 25OHD levels were performed in 675 individuals between 20 and 100 years of age. Subjects had been residing in Germany and died for reasons not related to cancer, metabolic disorders, or bone diseases. The mean age of the persons biopsied was 58.7 years for the 401 men, and 68.3 years for the 274 women. The authors noted that unlike PTH or calcium, serum 25OHD level has been found to be stable in various experiments for at least 10 days postmortem; one question is the extent to which serum 25OHD levels at one point in time (death) correlate with levels during adulthood. This is the largest study to date examining vitamin D (in the form of serum 25OHD) and undermineralization of bone as reflected by pathological accumulation of osteoid.

The Priemel et al. (2010) group defined a mineralization defect as a value of greater than or equal to 2 percent for the ratio of osteoid volume (i.e., bone matrix that is not mineralized) to total bone volume, referred to as OV/BV. The authors pointed out that, based on their findings, no subject experienced the defect at serum 25OHD levels of 75 nmol/L. That is, 100 percent of the population could be considered "covered" by a serum 25OHD concentration of 75 nmol/L. However, this conclusion from Priemel et al. (2010) over-states the levels of 25OHD in serum consistent with population coverage akin to an RDA. The question for DRI development is not whether a maximal level provides benefit, but at what level can the vast majority of the population (97.5 percent) expect benefit.

The committee, therefore, examined the data provided in Panel D of Figure 4 (osteoid volume versus 25OHD scatterplot) from Priemel et al. (2010) in detail. Determination of the number of cases with serum 25OHD levels above 50 nmol/L and above 40 nmol/L was of interest. The number of data points above 50 nmol/L was counted by inspection of the data. At a serum 25OHD level of 50 nmol/L, there were seven data points reflecting persons who failed to achieve the prescribed bone mineralization (OV/BV > 2 percent). This suggested that a serum 25OHD level of 50 nmol/L met the needs of 99 percent of the persons in the study (that is, only 7 of 675 surpassed the measure). In fact, the analysis suggested that 97.5 percent of the population met the measure at a serum 25OHD level of approximately 45 nmol/L; however, as it could not be precisely calculated from the graphic, 50 nmol/L was selected to err on the side of caution. Thus, more than 97.5 percent of the cohort was protected from the defect (OV/BV of ≥ 2 percent) at a serum 25OHD concentration of 50 nmol/L. Further, it is noteworthy that a majority of subjects for whom serum 25OHD levels were below 40 nmol/L actually achieved adequate bone mineralization (OV/ BV < 2 percent) as measured by this study. In fact, even at levels lower than 25 nmol/L more than half of the subjects were below the threshold defect measure. Premortem calcium intakes were not available, and this remains a limitation of this study. It is apparent that calcium intake is an important variable in bone mineralization. Calcium intake in children can prevent rickets even in the face of low serum 25OHD levels or in the genetic conditions of absent calcitriol (VDDR I) and absent VDR (VDDR II). From this unique data set of Priemel et al. (2010) it is likely that higher calcium intake in adults can have a positive impact on the skeleton even in the face of lower vitamin D levels. In this regard, the observational data from Bischoff-Ferrari et al. (2009b) using NHANES II, is also noted. In short, the indication is that higher calcium intakes can compensate for lower intestinal calcium absorption as a result of low serum 25OHD levels. Conversely, higher serum 25OHD levels cannot compensate for inadequate calcium intake.

Earlier observational studies from the UK (Leeds, Cardiff) and the United States (New York) histologically examined the hips of first-time hip fracture patients and found that 30 to 40 percent had proven osteomalacia in the fractured hip (Jenkins et al., 1973; Aaron et al., 1974; Sokoloff, 1978; Doppelt, 1984). Additional studies have found serum 25OHD levels to be significantly lower, PTH levels higher, and biochemical or histological evidence of osteomalacia more likely in patients with hip fracture than those without hip fracture (Hoikka et al., 1982; Lips et al., 1982; von Knorring et al., 1982; Wilton et al., 1987; Diamond et al., 1998; LeBoff et al., 1999). Osteomalacia was also seen on bone biopsy in about 4 to 5 percent of general medical and geriatric patients who had not suffered a fracture (Anderson et al., 1966; Stacey and Daly, 1989). Of 111 women with postmenopausal vertebral compression fractures attributed to osteoporosis, 8 percent had evidence of osteomalacia (Avioli, 1978). Overall, these data suggest that the contribution of osteomalacia to fragility may be more significant than previously realized: 30 to 40 percent of hip fractures may be due to frank osteomalacia not osteoporosis; the remaining 60 to 70 percent of hip fractures may represent a spectrum that includes earlier stages of osteomalacia/demineralization due to inadequate calcium/vitamin D as well as osteoporosis. These data may also explain why vitamin D supplementation was found to effectively prevent hip fractures in an elderly population (Chapuy et al., 1992): it could be healing various degrees of underlying osteomalacia in the hip.

Calcium absorption and serum 25OHD   As described earlier, studies of serum 25OHD concentrations and calcium absorption in adults (mostly in postmenopausal women and older men) have suggested that adequate calcium absorption occurs in the range of 30 to 50 nmol/L serum 25OHD for most persons. Fractional calcium absorption generally does not appear to increase with serum 25OHD concentration levels above 50 nmol/L. In addition, osteomalacia as explored in one study is not found to be meaningfully present until levels of serum 25OHD are at least below 30 nmol/L.

POTENTIAL INDICATORS FOR PREGNANCY: CALCIUM   For the majority of women, pregnancy comes at a period of life when the mother's body is normally experiencing bone maintenance. Key physiological changes during pregnancy, mediated by hormonal action, assure delivery of adequate calcium to meet the needs of the fetus, as discussed earlier (e.g., Kovacs and Kronenberg, 1997; Prentice, 2003; and Kovacs, 2008). These key changes also affect the utility of the bone health indicators detailed above for assessing dietary calcium needs. Potential indicators for calcium requirements during pregnancy are discussed below.

- *Calcium absorption*   Absorption efficiency doubles during pregnancy in adults (Heaney and Skillman, 1971; Kent et al., 1991) and adolescents (O'Brien et al., 2003). Calcium absorption is, thus, informative in the DRI development for pregnancy.
- *Calcium balance*   Pregnant women are in positive calcium balance early in pregnancy as indicated by the measures of hypercalciuria and direct measurement (Heaney and Skillman, 1971). However,

the utility of calcium balance in DRI development in pregnancy is complex, because the positive calcium balance achieved early in pregnancy is reduced to a neutral calcium balance or a slightly negative calcium balance by term.

- *Maternal BMD/fetal BMC/maternal fracture risk* Neither AHRQ-Ottawa nor AHRQ-Tufts addressed calcium and bone health in pregnancy. Bone turnover is modestly increased from as early as the first trimester, and the analysis concludes there is inconsistent evidence that BMD may decrease between prepartum and postpartum measurements, as discussed above.

  Olausson et al. (2008) reported 1 to 4 percent decreases in whole-body, spine, and total hip BMC and BMD from before pregnancy to 2 weeks postpartum compared with a nonpregnant, nonlactating group, but calcium intake was not related to this skeletal change. Thus, it is conceivable that some calcium provided to the fetus derives from the maternal skeleton during pregnancy. Calcium supplementation among Gambian women with low calcium intakes (355 mg/day) during pregnancy resulted in significantly lower maternal hip BMC and BMD and greater loss of bone mineral in the lumbar spine and distal radius compared with that found in the placebo group (Jarjou et al., 2010). The rate of increase in whole-body BMC is also slower in the breast-fed offspring of calcium-supplemented women during the first year (Jarjou et al., 2006). These two RCTs suggest no benefit to the fetus and possibly an adverse effect on the mother and infant, at least in the short term, of calcium supplementation during pregnancy. Further, the majority of epidemiological and prospective studies report that parity is associated with a neutral or even a protective effect relative to maternal BMD or fracture risk later in life (Sowers, 1996; Kovacs and Kronenberg, 1997; O'Brien et al., 2003; Chantry et al., 2004).

  Thus, additional calcium intake during pregnancy does not appear necessary for maternal or fetal bone health. Similarly, pregnant adolescents, who are in an active period of bone accretion, do not have impaired BMD or increased fracture risk as reported in observational and large cohort studies (Sowers et al., 1985, 1992; Fox et al., 1993; Sowers, 1996; Kovacs and Kronenberg, 1997; Chantry et al., 2004). Thus, maternal and fetal BMD/BMC and maternal fracture risk have utility as an indicator for DRI development for pregnant adults and adolescents.

- *Hypercalciuria* Most pregnant women are hypercalciuric with typical intakes of calcium (Gertner et al., 1986; Dahlman et al., 1994; Cross et al., 1995; Seely et al., 1997). This suggests that increased intakes of calcium could aggravate hypercalciuria as well as the inherent risk of kidney stones associated with pregnancy. Thus, hypercalciuria may be of some utility in DRI development, in that it indicates that dietary intake of calcium is more than adequate.

In sum, although no studies have directly explored levels of calcium intake sufficient for pregnant women, indirect measures suggest that the maternal calcium requirement is not increased over the non-pregnant state because of the physiological changes in calcium absorption and possibly, to some extent, bone turnover during pregnancy. The majority of epidemiological and long-term prospective studies that have examined the effect of parity on BMD, risk of osteoporosis, and incidence of fracture have found that parity is associated with a neutral or even a protective effect relative to these outcomes (Sowers, 1996; Kovacs and Kronenberg, 1997). In short, pregnancy does not impair long-term BMD or skeletal health of the mother.

POTENTIAL INDICATORS FOR PREGNANCY: VITAMIN D Key physiologic changes that occur in pregnancy to assure delivery of adequate calcium to meet fetal needs are relevant for DRI development. Potential indicators for vitamin D requirements during pregnancy are described below.

- *Calcium absorption* Although the efficiency of calcium absorption doubles in pregnancy, evidence from studies in the *Vdr*-null mouse shows that this up-regulation occurs independently of vitamin D or calcitriol (Van Cromphaut et al., 2001; Fudge and Kovacs, 2010). Mechanistic evidence is not available from humans; indeed, if such data were available they would still be difficult to interpret because of the known concomitant physiological adaptations. Thus, this measure is not useful for an integrated bone health indicator for vitamin D in pregnancy.
- *Maternal, fetal, and childhood BMC/BMD* Regarding biological plausibility, fetal calcium homeostasis, skeletal development, and bone mineralization appear independent of vitamin D, the VDR, and calcitriol, based on animal models, and human genetic mutations, as discussed above. Regarding AHRQ-Ottawa, this analysis identified three cohort studies and found insufficient evidence on the association of serum 25OHD levels with maternal BMD during pregnancy. No additional studies were identified addressing vitamin D and maternal BMD. One RCT (Delvin et al., 1986) found no effect of vitamin D supplementation on fetal calcium homeostasis. One observational study (Akcakus et al., 2006) reported no relationship between maternal 25OHD level and fetal BMC or BMD. A number of observational studies found normal fetal skeletal devel-

opment and mineral content (Maxwell and Miles, 1925; Congdon et al., 1983) and no radiological evidence of rickets at birth (Pereira and Zucker, 1986; Campbell and Fleischman, 1988; Specker et al., 1992; Specker, 1994; Beck-Nielsen et al., 2009) in severe vitamin D deficiency, or even in the absence of 1α-hydroxylase or the VDR (Silver et al., 1985; Takeda et al., 1997; Teotia and Teotia, 1997; Kitanaka et al., 1998; Bouillon et al., 2006). In contrast, four associational studies reported lower maternal serum 25OHD levels associated with craniotabes (Reif et al., 1988), lower tibia BMC and cross–sectional area, maternal serum 25OHD level below 42.6 nmol/L (Viljakainen et al., 2010), and higher fetal femur metaphyseal cross–sectional area and splaying (Mahon et al., 2010).

Regarding the developmental programming of later skeletal health in older offspring, one observational study, using 33 percent of the initial infants in a cohort, reported an association of lower whole-body and lumbar spine BMC and areal BMD at age 9 years in children whose mothers had low serum 25OHD levels late in gestation, even though no skeletal parameters differed at birth or nine months of age (Javaid et al., 2006). In offspring of mothers whose serum 25OHD levels late in gestation were less than 27.5 nmol/L or between 27.5 and 50.0 nmol/L, whole-body BMC was reduced compared with those whose mothers had serum 25OHD levels above 50.0 nmol/L. The definition of developmental programming as an indicator per se is questionable; in any case, the evidence for developmental programming of offspring skeletal health outcomes is insufficient to permit the committee to draw any conclusions, but it may be considered within the larger context of fetal skeletal BMD.

Although the congruence of the limited RCT data and majority of the observational data in humans suggests that fetal skeletal outcomes are not adversely affected by maternal vitamin D intake or serum 25OHD concentrations, fetal BMD and related skeletal outcomes may still be of some utility for DRI development. Little evidence could be identified for maternal BMD, making it unclear as to this measure's utility for DRI development.

- *Neonatal rickets* The AHRQ-Ottawa report included neonatal rickets infants 0 to 6 months of age and young children 1 to 6 years of age and found fair evidence for an association between low serum 25OHD levels and rickets identified as early as 2 months, but inconsistent evidence about the threshold level of 25OHD in serum above which rickets does not occur. AHRQ-Tufts identified no additional studies. Generally, the available observational studies do not report the development of vitamin D–deficiency rickets until weeks or months after birth (Begum et al., 1968; Ford et al., 1973; Moncrieff and Fadahunsi, 1974; Sann et al., 1976; Pereira and Zucker, 1986; Park et al., 1987; Campbell and Fleischman, 1988; Specker, 1994; Teotia et al., 1995; Beck-Nielsen et al., 2009). Thus, neonatal rickets is of limited utility in the development of DRIs for pregnancy.

- *Maternal and cord blood 25OHD levels* Regarding pregnancy outcomes, maternal and cord blood 25OHD levels may be of interest. AHRQ-Ottawa reported inconsistent evidence on changes in serum 25OHD levels during pregnancy, with two studies reporting no change and one study reporting a decline. In a few other studies, maternal serum 25OHD levels have responded to supplemental vitamin D (Marya et al., 1981, 1988; Mallet et al., 1986; Yu et al., 2009). In observational studies, babies born of vitamin D–deficient mothers have the lowest serum 25OHD levels and are at higher risk for complications sooner after birth than are babies born of vitamin D–replete mothers. Maternal serum 25OHD levels were stable and largely unaffected by pregnancy (Hillman et al., 1978; Brooke et al., 1980; Ardawi et al., 1997; Morley et al., 2006), even when the baseline serum 25OHD level was very low (20.1 ± 1.9 nmol/L) (Brooke et al., 1980).

Overall, fetal BMC and related skeletal outcomes are informative for DRI development for pregnancy.

POTENTIAL INDICATORS FOR LACTATION: CALCIUM The key physiological changes to meet the calcium demands of lactation occur through increased bone resorption, and most of the calcium in human milk comes from the maternal skeleton (Kalkwarf, 1999; Prentice, 2003; Kovacs, 2005; Kovacs and Kronenberg, 2008). Thus, lactation is a period of transient bone mineral loss and not, per se, a period of bone maintenance, although BMD is restored post-weaning (Kalkwarf, 1999). However, lactation is included in the category of bone maintenance in order to discuss pregnancy and lactation contiguously, and because bone mineral is restored in the immediate period post-lactation. Potential indicators related to calcium requirements during lactation are outlined below.

- *Maternal BMD* The need to provide calcium to the infant—a need that is two to three times greater than the daily amount needed for fetal development during pregnancy—is met by the maternal adaptation of increased bone resorption (Specker et al., 1994; Kalkwarf et al., 1997), resulting in a 5 to 10 percent decline in BMD during the first 6 months of exclusive breastfeeding

(Kalkwarf et al., 1997). Neither of the AHRQ analyses addressed calcium and BMD during lactation. Both RCTs and observational studies indicate that increased dietary calcium intake does not suppress maternal bone resorption during lactation (Cross et al., 1995; Fairweather-Tait et al., 1995; Prentice et al., 1995; Kalkwarf et al., 1997; Laskey et al., 1998; Polatti et al., 1999) nor does it alter the calcium content of human milk (Kalkwarf et al., 1997; Jarjou et al., 2006). Further, the calcium content of human milk does not predict maternal BMD decline, but breast milk volume does (Laskey et al., 1998), although milk calcium content is known to vary within and between feeds, complicating interpretation. During the post-lactation period (6 to 12 months), maternal bone mineral is deposited; in turn, maternal BMD is restored to pre-lactation levels without any consistent evidence of a need for higher calcium intake compared with non-pregnant women (Sowers, 1996; Kovacs and Kronenberg, 1997; Kalkwarf, 1999). Two RCTs found no effect of calcium supplementation post-weaning (Cross et al., 1995; Prentice et al., 1995), although one RCT found a slightly greater (1.5 percent) increase in BMD in calcium-supplemented women post-weaning (Kalkwarf et al., 1997). Adolescents, like adults, resorb bone during lactation and recover fully afterward, with no evidence that lactation impairs achievement of peak bone mass (Chantry et al., 2004). Maternal BMD is therefore informative for DRI development.

- *Calcium balance* Although calcium balance is negative during lactation owing to the enhanced bone resorption discussed above, mothers are restored to a positive balance and net accretion of bone mineral immediately upon cessation of lactation, followed by BMD restoration. Notably, urinary calcium excretion decreases during lactation. Thus, during lactation, higher calcium intakes will be less well tolerated and may not be needed, because higher calcium intake does not suppress bone loss. Calcium balance in lactation can be informative for DRI development.

Overall, available evidence indicates that the maternal calcium requirement is not increased during lactation, and it may also not be increased during the post-weaning interval in which the skeleton recovers to its pre-pregnancy baseline BMC.

POTENTIAL INDICATORS FOR LACTATION: VITAMIN D   As noted above, lactation is a period of transient bone loss, but it is discussed here in order to consider pregnancy and lactation contiguously and because BMD is restored in the post-lactation period. Potential indicators for vitamin D requirements during lactation are discussed below.

- *Maternal BMD*   AHRQ-Ottawa found good evidence from one cohort study that there is no association between serum 25OHD level and maternal BMD during lactation. No studies have examined what level of maternal vitamin D intake is required for the maternal skeleton to recover lost mineral content after lactation, although one observational study (Ghannam et al., 1999) in Saudi women found no relationship between maternal serum 25OHD levels (including levels consistent with hypovitaminosis D) and lumbar or femoral neck BMD. There is no evidence that lactating adolescents require any more vitamin D or higher serum 25OHD levels than non-lactating adolescents. Thus, maternal BMD is of limited use in DRI development for lactation.

- *Maternal and infant serum 25OHD levels*   Regarding lactation, maternal and infant serum 25OHD levels are of limited use given the present lack of consistent data. AHRQ-Tufts identified only one RCT, which it graded C (i.e., the report from Wagner et al., 2006), that found no effect of maternal supplemental vitamin D (6,400 IU) during lactation on infants' weight or length. Eight other RCTs (Rothberg et al., 1982; Ala-Houhala, 1985; Ala-Houhala et al., 1988; Kalkwarf et al., 1996; Hollis and Wagner, 2004; Basile et al., 2006; Wagner et al., 2006; Saadi et al., 2007) suggest that maternal vitamin D supplementation increases maternal serum 25OHD levels but does not affect neonatal serum 25OHD levels unless the maternal intake of vitamin D is extremely high, in the range of 4,000 to 6,400 IU/day (Hollis and Wagner, 2004; Wagner et al., 2006). With respect to observational studies, maternal serum 25OHD levels are not affected by lactation (Kent et al., 1990; Sowers et al., 1998), although one study found an increase post-weaning (Cross et al., 1997). Observational studies (Cancela et al., 1986; Okonofua et al., 1987; Takeuchi et al., 1989; Kent et al., 1990; Alfaham et al. 1995; Sowers et al., 1998) also show little impact of maternal serum 25OHD levels. Thus, maternal and fetal serum 25OHD concentrations have limited utility for DRI development.

Summary of evidence for bone maintenance   During bone maintenance, calcium intakes that maintain a neutral calcium balance have been recently elucidated in an important 2007 study (Hunt and Johnson, 2007) and are informative for the development of an EAR as well as an RDA. The relationship of calcium intake to BMD is more difficult to discern given the limited, and often contradictory observational data and relatively few and small RCTs. There is little evidence that levels of calcium intake above that needed for neutral calcium balance are consistent with an improvement in BMD. Of note, the pregnancy-induced increase in fractional calcium absorption allows the needs of pregnancy to be met without an increase in calcium intake above normal requirements. Although it does result in bone resorption, lactation does not increase the risk of reduced BMD or osteoporosis.

Osteomalacia, as explored in one recent study, is not found to be meaningfully present until serum 25OHD levels are at or below at least 30 nmol/L and is rarely present when serum 25OHD levels are above 50 nmol/L, suggesting the possibility of a population distribution. Further, fractional calcium absorption is not additionally enhanced when serum 25OHD levels are above 50 nmol/L. Both osteomalacia and fractional calcium absorption are, thus, informative for the development of DRIs for vitamin D in periods of bone maintenance.

Finally, calcium and vitamin D requirements are not increased during pregnancy or lactation. Nor does vitamin D supplementation alter the development of the fetal, infant, or maternal skeletal health outcomes.

Bone loss   A sustained bone loss is associated with the normal aging process and with menopause, as discussed in Chapter 2. The older adult loses bone at an estimated 1 percent per year (Sowers et al., 2010), although the rate of loss varies. The loss is abrupt for women at menopause and is quite rapid until approximately the sixth or seventh year after the onset of menopause. For men, bone loss begins later in life and generally declines steadily over time. Although neutral calcium balance is desired, the realities focus on reducing bone loss and mitigating the degree of negative calcium balance to the extent possible.

Calcium balance   Bone loss is reflected by negative calcium balance, and ideally the degree of negative calcium balance would be reduced to the extent possible. Therefore, a reasonable starting point for considering the nutrient intake levels that may be relevant during the life stages associated with bone loss is information on calcium balance. However, relatively few data are available. The study conducted by Hunt and Johnson (2007), described previously, included a few older men up to the age of 64 years and some older women up to the age of 75 years. Specifically, information provided by the study authors[6] indicated that there were 2 men and 34 women between 51 and 70 years of age and 4 women more than 70 years of age. The Hunt and Johnson (2007) analysis suggested that, overall, per-

---

[6]Specific age breakdown for subjects in Hunt and Johnson (2007): ages 19 to 50 years (35 women, 80 men); ages 51 to 70 years (34 women, 2 men); ages > 70 years (4 women, 0 men). Personal communication, L. Johnson, June 30, 2010.

sons of any age in the study achieved neutral calcium balance at calcium intakes of 741 mg/day.

Although these data may be relevant for the younger aging male, the Hunt and Johnson (2007) analysis may not be adequate for considering specific issues of bone loss due to aging among men; there were only two men in the age range of 51 to 70 years and no men over the age of 70 years in the analysis. Further, it is uncertain what proportion of women in the Hunt and Johnson (2007) study were menopausal, although approximately half were over the age of 50 years.

Heaney et al. (1977), in examining 130 Catholic nuns as part of a longitudinal study, reported that neutral calcium balance during the perimenopausal state for these women (between the ages of 35 and 50 years) was achieved at 1,240 mg/day. This intake is notably higher than that reported by Hunt and Johnson (2007). In a second study of the same group of women ($n = 168$), Heaney et al. (1978) reported that perimenopausal and estrogen-treated women reached neutral calcium balance with calcium intakes of 990 mg/day, whereas untreated postmenopausal women required 1,504 mg of calcium per day for neutral calcium balance. This suggests, in contrast to the findings of Hunt and Johnson (2007), that menopausal state may be relevant to considerations of calcium requirements. In any case, because the indicator of interest is bone health, other measures, such as bone density and fracture risk are also considered.

Bone mineral density and fracture risk: Calcium   Fracture risk occurs in the later years of life and can be useful as an indicator of bone health, but fractures are less common in persons less than 70 years of age. Therefore, as an indicator, it is not particularly revealing as far as the effects of nutrient intake in slowing the bone loss of early menopause, when many women are in their 50s. It is also of questionable relevance to men less than 70 years of age who generally have yet to experience the full impact of bone loss due to aging. However, BMD measures are predictive of future fractures and can serve as a relevant indicator to ensure bone health to the extent possible during the onset of menopause and during the early aging process.

Regarding BMD measures and calcium intake among younger menopausal women, the AHRQ analyses are not specifically helpful in that the analyses used primarily studies that supplemented participants with both vitamin D and calcium, and neither AHRQ analysis addressed calcium alone relative to bone health. One report reviewed by AHRQ, which used a combination of calcium and vitamin D supplements, should be noted, especially given the large size of the cohort. The study (Jackson et al., 2006), stemming from the WHI, randomly assigned more than 36,000 postmenopausal women between the ages of 50 and 79 years (mean = 62 years) to a placebo or 1,000 mg of calcium with a supplement of 400 IU of vitamin D_3. Fractures were ascertained during a period of about 7 years, and

BMD was measured for some of the subjects. On average, the background intake of these women provided a relatively high intake of calcium (average 1,150 mg/day), compared with that typically reported for the general population. With the addition of the supplement given as part of the study protocol, calcium intakes approached 2,150 mg/day. Overall, following the intervention, the authors found a small, but significant, improvement in hip BMD; however, the study did not demonstrate a reduction in hip fracture. This appears to be consistent with the understanding that fracture risk is less prevalent under the age of 70 years, particularly among persons 50 to 60 years of age. On the basis of age stratification, women 50 to 59 years of age showed a hazard ratio for hip fracture of 2.17, whereas the HR for women 60 to 69 years of age was 0.74. It is notable that the vitamin D supplementation was relatively low, thereby enhancing the ability to consider the effects of calcium per se. Under these conditions, there is the suggestion that calcium intakes of 2,150 mg/day increased BMD slightly compared with intakes of 1,150 mg/day (placebo with background diet). However, the calcium–vitamin D treatment was associated with an increased risk of kidney stones.

Several studies (Table 4-15) are noted in the context of examining the effect of calcium on BMD at times when menopause occurs or is on-going. As shown in the table, the data suggest mixed results. None measured the nature of the dose–response relationship. Some indicate benefit at lower levels of calcium intake, whereas others show no effect at higher levels of intake. The benefits vary by bone site, but not consistently; and lifestyle factors, such as exercise, appear to be related to outcome. However, the meta-analysis of Shea et al. (2002), which examined calcium supplementation with minimal vitamin D intake, suggested a relatively small, but consistent, effect of calcium supplementation on BMD in postmenopausal women, many of whom were less than 70 years of age. The authors reported that the inference that calcium increases bone density for this group was strengthened by the consistency of the findings across four sites of measurement, but pointed out that loss to follow-up and unexplained heterogeneity confounded the conclusions. In a study of free-living menopausal women that measured total body calcium (by neutral activation analysis), a retardation of bone loss in the femoral neck in early menopause was reported with a calcium intake of 1,700 mg/day (Aloia et al., 1994). However, the study protocol combined the calcium supplementation with 400 IU of vitamin D per day. In contrast, in some studies focused on reducing bone loss in menopausal women using various treatments including increased calcium intake, it was found that the retardation of bone loss with calcium intake was not equivalent to that associated with hormone replacement therapy, but also that it appeared to have minimal effect on retarding that compo-

TABLE 4-15 Intervention Studies of Interest: Calcium Supplementation (without Vitamin D) and Bone Mineral Density Among Menopausal Women < 71 Years of Age

Reference; Study Type; Country	Population Description	Calcium Intake and BMD Measures
Dawson-Hughes et al., 1990 RCT United States	Healthy, postmenopausal women Average age = 58 years n = 301	500 mg with background diet (intakes grouped as < 400 mg or 400–650 mg) of 274 ± 80 mg/day and 513 ± 71 mg/day (early postmenopausal); 283 ± 89 mg/day and 530 ± 95 mg/day (late postmenopausal) If postmenopausal for 6+ years, maintenance of BMD at hip and radius, but loss at spine Bone loss from spine not affected by calcium supplementation if menopausal for 5 or fewer years
Reid et al., 1993 RCT New Zealand	Healthy, postmenopausal women (≥ 3 years postmenopause) Average age = 58 years n = 122	1,000 mg supplement with background diet of 750 ± 260 mg/day at 2 years (mean) Loss of total body BMD reduced by 43%
Prince et al., 1995 RCT Australia	Healthy, postmenopausal women (> 10 years postmenopause) Average age = 62 years n = 168	1,000 mg supplement with background diet of 822 ± 286 mg/day (Ca group) and 919 ± 411 mg/day (Ca + exercise group) (means) Cessation of bone loss at the intertrochanteric and trochanteric hip site; reduced bone loss of the tibias (ultradistal); no significant bone loss at the spine site in any group Exercise with calcium supplementation resulted in less bone loss at the femoral neck site compared with calcium supplementation alone
Riggs et al., 1998 RCT United States	Healthy, postmenopausal women Average age = 66 years n = 177	1,600 mg with background diet of 711 ± 276 mg/day Small retardation of rate of bone loss (total body BMD, lumbar spine, proximal femur), but significant difference

NOTE: BMD = bone mineral density; RCT = randomized controlled trials.

nent of bone loss that was due to estrogen withdrawal (Riis et al., 1987; Dawson-Hughes et al., 1990).

Although the meta-analysis of Tang et al. (2007) concluded that in addition to fracture risk reduction, calcium supplementation was associated with a larger reduction in the rate of bone loss when the supplemented dose was 1,200 mg/day, the analysis included both men and women, many of whom were over the age of 70 years. Further, the authors noted that the regimen was most effective for persons who were quite elderly, lived in institutions, had low body weight, and had low calcium intakes at the time of the study. Such persons are likely different from the younger menopausal women undergoing the rapid bone loss associated with the early stages of menopause.

Taken as a whole, the evidence suggests some benefit for BMD/bone loss related to calcium intake, but the minimum level of intake that is effective is difficult to ascertain, because dose–response relationships were not examined and there were many confounding variables. Most studies added a large supplemental dose to existing background calcium intakes of approximately 700 to 800 mg/day. Therefore, the benefit has been studied at calcium intakes ranging from about 750 mg/day to 1,700 to 1,800 mg/day.

Bone loss becomes more characteristic of both genders as age increases, and the risk of osteoporotic fracture becomes more common, along with decreased bone density. Although most evidence for fractures focuses on women, fracture rate for men has also been studied and is of concern. Overall, the question is whether and at what levels calcium intake can mitigate or reduce fracture risk in older persons.

Relative to calcium intake alone, the meta-analysis offered by Tang et al. (2007) and discussed previously, provides some information. While all subjects were over 50 years of age, many were in the age range of 70 years and above. The results suggested benefit for BMD and fracture risk reduction relative to calcium in combination with vitamin D *or* calcium alone. However, the number of calcium-alone studies was small, and the vitamin D status of those in the trials was not always evident. The authors' conclusion that a calcium intake of 1,200 mg/day was effective in demonstrating this benefit must be considered in light of the fact that most studies did not provide supplementation at lower levels, such as 1,000 mg/day.

Many of the same studies that were relevant at the time of the 1997 DRI review (IOM, 1997) remain relevant today, such as Chevalley et al. (1994) and Recker et al. (1996). The available studies in 1997 suggested that there was a favorable effect of calcium on reduction in fracture rate, but there were insufficient data to allow estimation of the magnitude of the impact of calcium intake on fracture rates. The Bischoff-Ferrari et al. (2007) meta-analysis of RCTs with calcium basically came to similar conclusions. In that paper, a summary of prospective cohort studies of calcium alone suggested

TABLE 4-16 Intervention Studies of Interest: Calcium Supplementation (without Vitamin D) and Fracture Risk and/or BMD in Persons > 70 Years of Age

Reference; Country	Subjects	Calcium Intake and Fracture Risk and/or BMD
Peacock et al., 2000 United States	Independent, mobile older men and women n = 316 women n = 122 men Average age = 75 years	750 mg/day Background diet of 670 ± 325 mg/day (men) and 564 ± 294 mg/day (women) [Note: Study protocol included a group receiving 25OHD₃] For hip, calcium supplement recipients had similar BMD compared with placebo (at the spine, both placebo and calcium supplementation increased BMD during the study)
Grant et al., 2005 UK	Older men and women with previous fracture; 85% women n = 5,292 Average age = 78 years	1,000 mg/day Background diet not reported [Note: Study protocol included a group receiving vitamin D₃ and a group receiving combination of calcium and vitamin D₃] Incidence of new fractures (26% were of the hip) did not differ significantly between participants allocated calcium and those who were not Compliance with tablets containing calcium was significantly low
Prince et al., 2006 Australia	Healthy, older women over age of 70 years n = 1,460 Average age = 75 years	1,200 mg/day Background diet of 897 mg/day (placebo, compliant with regimen), 915 mg/day (calcium, compliant with regimen), 950 mg/day (placebo, noncompliant with regimen), 903 mg/day (calcium, noncompliant with regimen) Supplementation overall did not significantly reduce fracture risk, but subanalysis on the basis of compliance showed significantly reduced fracture incidence with calcium supplementation Calcium recipients had improved quantitative ultrasonography findings of the heel, femoral neck, and whole-body DXA

NOTE: BMD = bone mineral density; DXA = dual-energy X-ray absorptiometry; UK = United Kingdom.

no effect on non-vertebral fracture risk. However, in a pooled meta-analysis of five RCTs of calcium alone, the authors found that risk reduction was 8 percent (HR = 0.92 [95% CI: 0.81-1.05]) for non-vertebral fractures. This is consistent with the committee's conclusion that calcium supplementation alone has a modest benefit for skeletal health, both in terms of increased

BMD and a suggestion of non-vertebral fracture risk reduction. Peacock et al. (2000) more recently reported no effect of calcium compared with placebo relative to hip BMD (see Table 4-16).

In summary, considering calcium alone, intakes at or above 1,200 mg/day, whether with supplements or diet, are not associated with a reduced fracture risk, although calcium supplementation can prevent bone loss from both the hip and spine in both young and older postmenopausal women. In contrast, there is evidence from several meta-analyses to suggest that sufficient calcium (≥ 1,200 mg/day) with vitamin D supplementation (800 IU/day) reduces fracture risk, particularly hip, in those over age 70 years and those institutionalized (Tang et al., 2007; Avenell et al., 2009b).

Bone mineral density and fracture risk: Vitamin D   The vast majority of the studies that consider bone health and the issues of bone loss, BMD, and fracture risk contain protocols that administered a combination of vitamin D with calcium. These are well described in the AHRQ analyses, which focused on postmenopausal women and older men. AHRQ-Tufts concluded that there is *good evidence* that vitamin D_3 plus calcium supplementation resulted in small increases in BMD of the spine, total body, femoral neck, and total hip. Based on included trials, it was less certain whether vitamin D_3 supplementation alone has a significant effect on BMD. Two of the three relevant new RCTs identified by AHRQ-Tufts showed a significant increase in hip or total BMD in postmenopausal women, supplemented with vitamin D_3 or vitamin D_2 (300 or 1,000 IU/day, respectively) plus calcium (1,200 mg/day), compared with placebo. Only one of these three trials did not combine calcium supplementation with vitamin D supplementation. AHRQ-Ottawa concluded that supplementation with vitamin D (most studies used vitamin D_3) plus calcium was effective in reducing fractures in institutionalized older populations, although the benefit in community-dwelling individuals was inconsistent. AHRQ-Tufts did not identify any new RCTs examining the combined effect of vitamin D plus calcium supplementation on fractures in postmenopausal women and older men. For vitamin D alone, the evidence was specified as inconsistent for a relationship with reduction in fracture risk. Three new RCTs identified by AHRQ-Tufts (Bunout et al., 2006; Burleigh et al., 2007; Lyons et al., 2007) did not show significant effects of either vitamin D_2 or vitamin D_3 (daily doses ranged from 400 to 822 IU) in reducing the risk of total fractures.

Avenell et al. (2009b) performed a meta-analysis comparing the effects of vitamin D alone with those of vitamin D plus calcium relative to fracture risk. In nine trials encompassing nearly 25,000 participants, vitamin D supplementation alone had no effect on risk reduction for hip, vertebral, or any fracture. In contrast, calcium plus vitamin D (typical intake range of 400 to 800 IU/day, but up to a high of 2,286 IU/day, as well as bolus doses on a weekly basis) suggested a 16 percent risk reduction for hip fractures, particularly among institutionalized elders.

The meta-analysis conducted by Tang et al. (2007) did not consider the effect of vitamin D independently, but is nonetheless of interest. These authors analyzed 17 trials that used calcium or calcium in combination with vitamin D supplementation and reported fracture as an outcome, concluding that a supplementation of 800 IU of vitamin D per day or greater in combination with a calcium intake of at least 1,200 mg per day is more effective for fracture risk reduction than supplementation with less than 800 IU of vitamin D per day with the same level of calcium supplementation.

Another meta-analysis with fewer studies (Bischoff-Ferrari et al., 2009c) examined the prevention of non-vertebral fractures with vitamin D supplementation alone. These authors concluded that non-vertebral fracture rate is reduced with vitamin D supplementation in a dose-dependent manner. The analysis, however, has some limitations. First, it did not take into account baseline vitamin D intake, which could have been as high as 250 to 300 IU/day, as was noted in a cohort study of older women (Jackson et al., 2006). Second, their approach to defining a dose–response relationship included a sensitivity analysis, based on analysis of a subgroup of women identified as having been the most compliant in taking their supplement. Finally, the regression line that produced a 75 nmol/L threshold serum 25OHD level at which fractures were prevented used an x-axis with irregularly spaced intervals of serum 25OHD level from 50 to 80 nmol/L. With this confounding as a limitation on the utility of the data, the Bischoff-Ferrari et al. (2009c) analysis may support the possibility that vitamin D intakes of approximately 400 IU/day provide some level of benefit relative to fracture risk reduction.

Two recent RCTs are now available that were not considered in the AHRQ analyses. Sanders et al. (2010) treated nearly 2,300 women 70 years of age or older with either placebo or 500,000 IU of vitamin D once yearly for 3 years. The mean serum 25OHD level in the treated group at baseline was 49 nmol/L and rose at 1 month to 120 nmol/L. Remarkably, the risk of any fracture was 25 percent higher in the treated group than in the placebo group, primarily during the first 3 months of treatment. Salovaara et al. (2010) performed a recent 3-year randomized trial of 3,432 free-living Finnish postmenopausal women ages 65 to 71 years, testing the effects of 1,000 mg of calcium per day plus 800 IU of vitamin D per day on incident fractures. Baseline average calcium intake was the same for treatment and control groups, approximately 950 mg/day likewise, serum 25OHD levels were 50 nmol/L for each. After 3 years, the serum 25OHD level in the treated group was 75 nmol/L compared with 55 nmol/L in controls. There was no statistically significant effect of the combination of calcium and vitamin D on incident fractures at any site, although as with other studies, there was a trend in overall fracture risk reduction for the treated group (adjusted HR = 0.83; 95% CI: 0.61–1.12).

Osteomalacia   The data from Priemel et al. (2010) as examined by the committee have been discussed above in the section on bone maintenance. Given that this study included persons from 20 to 100 years of age, with a majority between 60 and 100 years of age, the information from the study is relevant to considerations of bone loss. As determined by the committee, nearly all persons were free of the measure of osteomalacia used in the study when serum 25OHD levels were above 50 nmol/L; a significant increase in the number of people displaying the mineralization defect was not observed until the serum 25OHD level had decreased below 30 nmol/L. A number of subjects continued to achieve adequate bone mineralization even at very low levels of 25OHD.

Calcium absorption and serum 25OHD level   As described above, studies of serum 25OHD concentrations and calcium absorption in adults (most studies used postmenopausal women and older men) have suggested that ample calcium absorption occurs in the serum 25OHD concentration range of 30 to 50 nmol/L for most persons. Fractional calcium absorption generally does not appear to increase with serum 25OHD concentration above 50 nmol/L. In addition, osteomalacia as explored in one study, is not found to be meaningfully present until serum 25OHD levels are at least below 30 nmol/L 25OHD.

Integration of evidence for bone accretion, maintenance, and loss

Calcium   The indicator of bone health for calcium depends on the stage of bone health: accretion, maintenance, or loss. For the accretion stage, average bone calcium accretion/retention is informative when combined with a factorial approach (IOM, 1997) to develop an EAR and calculate an RDA. During bone maintenance, neutral calcium balance maintains bone health. For the bone loss stage, integrating BMD with neutral calcium balance may provide additional information for women in the early menopausal period, as discussed above. For younger men entering the same life stage, neutral calcium balance maintains bone health. In later menopause and with aging, fracture risk integrated with the limited information on BMD is informative. Of special note is the pregnancy-induced increase in fractional calcium absorption that precludes an increased calcium requirement during pregnancy. The period of transient but notable bone mineral loss during lactation is not affected by calcium intake and is remedied within a short period post-lactation without increased calcium intake.

Vitamin D   Specifying the indicator for vitamin D and bone health across the key stages of bone accretion, bone maintenance, and bone loss presents a challenge because of the limitations of the data and the desirable features of an indicator of effect. Serum 25OHD concentrations are often reported for a range of outcomes of interest, making this indicator of "exposure" useful, even though it is not a validated intermediate indicator of effect. Potentially further complicating the specification of an indicator is the public health interest in developing a reference value that addresses bone health beyond the impact of classic vitamin D deficiency, such as rickets. Of note is that existing evidence does not suggest a unique role for vitamin D during pregnancy or lactation beyond that which it plays during non-pregnant and non-lactating states.

As the committee considered the limitations and variability of the evidence across the stages of bone accretion, bone maintenance, and bone loss, a strong congruence of several indicators of bone health—no one of which was sufficiently informative to serve as a basis for a reference value—emerged in relation to serum 25OHD levels and, thus, vitamin D exposure. Integrating these indicators—BMC/BMD, fractional calcium absorption, rickets, osteomalacia, and fracture risk—revealed, as can be seen in the conceptual model in Figure 4-9, an increase in risk of rickets or osteomalacia, impaired fractional calcium absorption, and fractures in older persons when serum 25OHD levels were low, and no apparent benefit for these

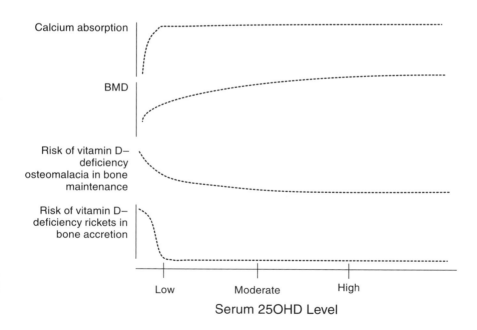

FIGURE 4-9 Conceptualization of integrated bone health outcomes and vitamin D exposure.

measures when serum 25OHD levels were higher. At moderate levels of serum 25OHD, risk was variable, depending on the specific measure. Collectively, however, the integration of these indicators, if used for DRI development, would support the development of an EAR within this moderate range in which risk for one or more of these bone health indicators may be increased in approximately 50 percent of the healthy population, but reduced in the remaining 50 percent of the population. Illustrated, then, in the companion Figure 4-10 is the consistency of this integrated conceptual model with the classical requirement distribution, or, more specifically, with a marker of exposure. As this is a conceptual model, specific values are not assigned in this figure for "low," "moderate," and "high."

CONSIDERATIONS RELATED TO
AFRICAN AMERICAN ANCESTRY

As a result of their greater skin pigmentation, African Americans as well as other dark-skinned groups have lower serum 25OHD concentrations throughout life—as discussed in the section below. However, despite lower serum 25OHD concentrations, African Americans have a superior "calcium economy" compared with whites in North America and have less risk for osteoporosis and fracture (Cohn et al., 1977; Anderson and Pollitzer, 1994; Bell et al., 1995; Aloia et al., 1996b, 1999, 2000; Finkelstein et al., 2002; Barrett-Connor et al., 2005; Cauley et al., 2005a; Tracy et al., 2006). Racial/ethnic differences have been sought to explain the paradox

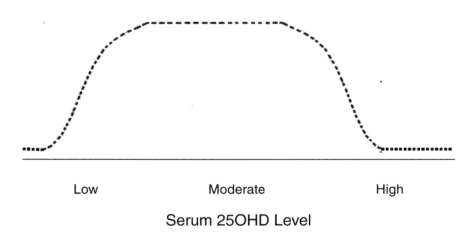

Low   Moderate   High

Serum 25OHD Level

FIGURE 4-10 Theoretical distribution of serum 25OHD level in healthy populations based on integrated bone health outcomes.

of a decreased incidence of osteoporosis in the presence of lower serum 25OHD levels (Aloia, 2008).

Initially, there is an important caution in considering available data. For many comparative studies, the derivation of the assignment of "race" is not clear. Detailed ancestry is not included in most studies, and socio-economic characteristics of the ethnic groups are not described. Usually, no genetic data are collected. When the approach has been to consider social and behavioral variables in relation to a single ethnic group, there have been studies suggesting that there is considerable variability in the black ethnic group (Melton et al., 2002; Nelson et al., 2004; Thandrayen et al., 2009). For instance, spinal BMD is lower in recent Sudanese im-migrants than in African Americans or whites (Gong et al., 2006). Thus, our interpretation of studies considering bone health in Americans of African heritage must be approached with caution. Moreover, the search for genomic explanations for bone mass variability has thus far not been rewarding (Fleet et al., 1995; Harris et al., 1997; Zmuda et al., 1997, 1999, 2003; Koller et al., 2000; Nelson et al., 2000; Peacock et al., 2002; Gong and Haynatzki, 2003; Edderkaoui et al., 2007; Shaffer et al., 2007; Wang et al., 2007; Engelman et al., 2008; Foroud et al., 2008; Eisman, 2010).

In any case, numerous studies have demonstrated that bone mass is higher in African Americans throughout the life cycle (Cohn et al., 1977; Li et al., 1989; Luckey et al., 1989; Bell et al., 1991; Gilsanz et al., 1991;

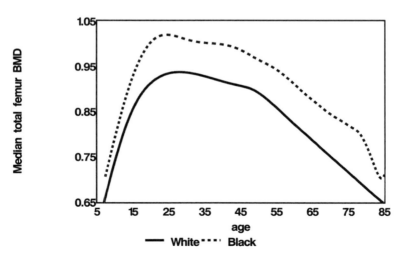

FIGURE 4-11 Bone density of the femur in the black and white population. SOURCE: Aloia, 2008. Reprinted with permission from the *American Journal of Clinical Nutrition* (2008; volume 88: 545S-550S), American Society for Nutrition.

Kleerekoper et al., 1994; Nelson et al., 1995, 1997; Aloia et al., 1996a, 1997). The evidence is illustrated in Figure 4-11, using data from one study (Kalkwarf et al., 2007). The advantage in bone mass is associated with one-half the prevalence of osteoporosis and one-half the fracture risk of whites (Barrett-Connor et al., 2005). Longitudinal BMD studies demonstrate that this skeletal advantage for African Americans is present before 6 years of age and increases during adolescence, a stage when the skeleton accrues 50 percent of its peak bone mass (Li et al., 1989; Gilsanz et al., 1991; Cromer et al., 2004; Kalkwarf et al., 2007). The skeletal advantage developed during adolescence is maintained throughout adult life, with African Americans having the same pattern of bone loss as whites in each life stage but at a slower rate (Meier et al., 1992; Bryant et al., 2003; Cauley et al., 2005b; Looker et al., 2009).

However, the Study of Osteoporotic Fractures has also demonstrated that for any given bone density value the risk for fracture is less in African Americans, indicating that bone mass is not the only protective factor against fracture (Cauley et al., 2005a). Other possible factors are lower bone turnover, the micro-architecture of bone, bone geometry, body composition, and heredity (Weinstein and Bell, 1988; Schnitzler et al., 1990; Faulkner et al., 1993; Cummings et al., 1994; Han et al., 1996; Wang et al., 1997; Nelson et al., 2000; Gundberg et al., 2002; Hanlon et al., 2002; Faulkner et al., 2005; Schnitzler and Mesquita, 2006; Travison et al., 2008). Bone biopsies in African Americans show an advantageous architecture with more osteocytes and a lower bone formation rate (Parfitt et al., 1997; Parisien et al., 1997; Qiu et al., 2006).

African American girls have higher calcium absorption efficiency, presumably because of their higher calcitriol levels, and lower urinary calcium excretion compared with white girls (Abrams et al., 1995; Bryant et al., 2003; Harkness and Cromer, 2005; Braun et al., 2007; Weaver et al., 2008) (Figure 4-12). There is no threshold for calcium retention at calcium intakes up to 2,000 mg/day, leading to the conclusion that calcium requirements should be the same in the two races.

African American adults retain superior renal calcium conservation and generally have higher serum PTH and calcitriol levels and lower urinary calcium excretion (Bell et al., 1985; Meier et al., 1991; Dawson-Hughes et al., 1993; Kleerekoper et al., 1994; Harris et al., 2000; Aloia et al., 2006a, b; Cosman et al., 2007). Skeletal resistance to PTH is also present in adult African Americans, demonstrated by lower bone turnover despite elevated PTH levels and by resistance of bone resorption to PTH infusion (Aloia et al., 1996a; Cosman et al., 1997; Han et al., 1997, 1999).

Older African Americans—similar to older persons in other population groups in the United States and Canada—develop secondary hyperparathyroidism and accelerated bone turnover and bone loss, but it is

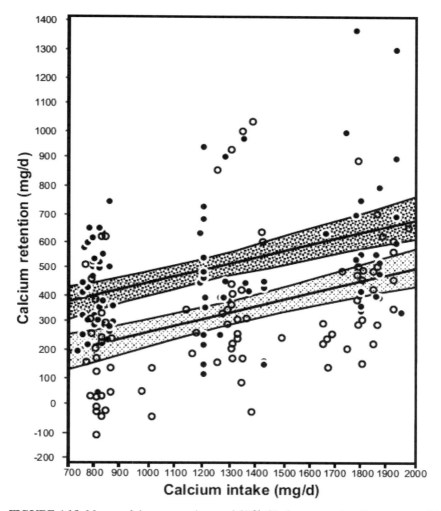

FIGURE 4-12 Mean calcium retention and 95% CIs for regression lines across different calcium intakes, by race. The darker shading represents African American girls (●, 84 observations in 55 girls), and the lighter shading represents white girls (○, 98 observations in 66 girls).

SOURCE: Braun et al., 2007. Reprinted with permission from the *American Journal of Clinical Nutrition* (2007, volume 85, pages 1657-63), American Society for Nutrition.

unknown if this is attenuated by increasing calcium or vitamin D intake (S. S. Harris et al., 2001; Cauley et al., 2005b; Tracy et al., 2005). There is limited information on the effect of calcium and vitamin D supplements on bone mass or fracture in older subjects, because African Americans have usually not been included in clinical trials in meaningful numbers. A 3-year randomized, double-blind, placebo-controlled vitamin D_3 intervention in postmenopausal black women showed no difference in rate of bone loss between treatment and control groups (Aloia et al., 2005). There was also no relationship between serum 25OHD and rates of bone loss. The WHI did include African American subjects, who took part in a calcium plus vitamin D trial. Hip fracture risk was not reduced by the intervention (Jackson et al., 2006). Changes in bone density in this trial were adjusted for race, but separate analyses by race for the positive outcome on BMD of the hip were not provided. However, a more recent meeting presentation using data from the WHI Observational Study (Cauley et al., 2009) has revealed the concerning finding that fracture risk was directly related to serum 25OHD level in the African American subgroup.

Thus, although the available, emerging evidence would suggest that there is perhaps a lower requirement for calcium and vitamin D among African Americans relative to ensuring bone health, at least compared with whites, there is a notable lack of high-quality and convincing evidence to act on this possibility or to set different requirements for persons of African American ancestry. See Chapter 6 for discussions related to race/ethnicity and estimation of the Tolerable Upper Intake Levels (ULs) for vitamin D.

SELECTION OF INDICATORS

As described in Chapter 1, following the examination of the relevance and quality of the data for the potential indicators of interest, the next step in the DRI development process is to select the indicator or indicators to be used for estimating average requirements or EARs, in this case for calcium and vitamin D. Overall, the selection of indicators is evidence-based; indicators for levels of dietary adequacy are selected based on the strength and quality of the evidence and their demonstrated public health significance, taking into consideration sources of uncertainty in the evidence.

The indicator of bone health is selected as to form the basis of the DRIs for calcium and vitamin D for all life stage groups. With the exception of measures related to bone health, the potential indicators examined are currently not associated with evidence that could be judged either compelling or sufficient in terms of cause and effect, nor informative regarding dose–response relationships for the purposes of determining nutrient requirements. Cancer/neoplasms, cardiovascular disease and hypertension, diabetes and metabolic syndrome, falls and physical performance, immune functioning and autoimmune disorder, infections, neuropsychological functioning, and preeclampsia could not be causally linked reliably or consistently with relevant outcomes as a function of calcium or vitamin D intake. Although the conclusions at this time do not preclude the possibility that future studies may specify the existence of such relationships, they are currently best described as hypotheses of emerging interest, and the conflicting nature of the available evidence means that it cannot be used to establish a positive impact on health outcomes with any level of confidence.

REFERENCES

Aaron, J. E., J. C. Gallagher, J. Anderson, L. Stasiak, E. B. Longton, B. E. Nordin and M. Nicholson. 1974. Frequency of osteomalacia and osteoporosis in fractures of the proximal femur. Lancet 1(7851): 229-33.

Abbasi, A. A., J. K. Chemplavil, S. Farah, B. F. Muller and A. R. Arnstein. 1979. Hypercalcemia in active pulmonary tuberculosis. Annals of Internal Medicine 90(3): 324-8.

Abrahams, B. S. and D. H. Geschwind. 2008. Advances in autism genetics: on the threshold of a new neurobiology. National Review of Genetics 9(5): 341-55.

Abrams, S. A., K. O. O'Brien, L. K. Liang and J. E. Stuff. 1995. Differences in calcium absorption and kinetics between black and white girls aged 5-16 years. Journal of Bone and Mineral Research 10(5): 829-33.

Abrams, S. A., K. C. Copeland, S. K. Gunn, J. E. Stuff, L. L. Clarke and K. J. Ellis. 1999. Calcium absorption and kinetics are similar in 7- and 8-year-old Mexican-American and Caucasian girls despite hormonal differences. Journal of Nutrition 129(3): 666-71.

Abrams, S. A. 2002. Nutritional rickets: an old disease returns. Nutrition Reviews 60(4): 111-5.

Abrams, S. A., I. J. Griffin, K. M. Hawthorne, S. K. Gunn, C. M. Gundberg and T. O. Carpenter. 2005. Relationships among vitamin D levels, parathyroid hormone, and calcium absorption in young adolescents. Journal of Clinical Endocrinology and Metabolism 90(10): 5576-81.

Abrams, S. A., P. D. Hicks and K. M. Hawthorne. 2009. Higher serum 25-hydroxyvitamin D levels in school-age children are inconsistently associated with increased calcium absorption. Journal of Clinical Endocrinology and Metabolism 94(7): 2421-7.

Abrams, S. A. 2010. Calcium absorption in infants and small children: methods of determination and recent findings. Nutrients 2(4): 474-80.

Adams, J. S., R. L. Modlin, M. M. Diz and P. F. Barnes. 1989. Potentiation of the macrophage 25-hydroxyvitamin D-1-hydroxylation reaction by human tuberculous pleural effusion fluid. Journal of Clinical Endocrinology and Metabolism 69(2): 457-60.

Ahonen, M. H., L. Tenkanen, L. Teppo, M. Hakama and P. Tuohimaa. 2000. Prostate cancer risk and prediagnostic serum 25-hydroxyvitamin D levels (Finland). Cancer Causes and Control 11(9): 847-52.

AHRQ. 2007. Methods reference guide for effectiveness and comparative effectiveness reviews, Version 1.0. Rockville, MD: Agency for Healthcare Research and Quality.

Aihara, K., H. Azuma, M. Akaike, Y. Ikeda, M. Yamashita, T. Sudo, H. Hayashi, Y. Yamada, F. Endoh, M. Fujimura, T. Yoshida, H. Yamaguchi, S. Hashizume, M. Kato, K. Yoshimura, Y. Yamamoto, S. Kato and T. Matsumoto. 2004. Disruption of nuclear vitamin D receptor gene causes enhanced thrombogenicity in mice. Journal of Biological Chemistry 279(34): 35798-802.

Akcakus, M., E. Koklu, N. Budak, M. Kula, S. Kurtoglu and S. Koklu. 2006. The relationship between birthweight, 25-hydroxyvitamin D concentrations and bone mineral status in neonates. Annals of Tropical Paediatrics 26(4): 267-75.

Akesson, A., M. Vahter, M. Berglund, T. Eklof, K. Bremme and P. Bjellerup. 2004. Bone turnover from early pregnancy to postweaning. Acta Obstetrica et Gynecologica Scandinavica 83(11): 1049-55.

Ala-Houhala, M. 1985. 25-hydroxyvitamin D levels during breast-feeding with or without maternal or infantile supplementation of vitamin D. Journal of Pediatric Gastroenterology and Nutrition 4(2): 220-6.

Ala-Houhala, M., T. Koskinen, M. Koskinen and J. K. Visakorpi. 1988. Double blind study on the need for vitamin D supplementation in prepubertal children. Acta Paediatrica Scandinavica 77(1): 89-93.

Al-Delaimy, W. K., E. Rimm, W. C. Willett, M. J. Stampfer and F. B. Hu. 2003. A prospective study of calcium intake from diet and supplements and risk of ischemic heart disease among men. American Journal of Clinical Nutrition 77(4): 814-8.

Alexianu, M. E., E. Robbins, S. Carswell and S. H. Appel. 1998. 1Alpha, 25 dihydroxyvitamin D_3-dependent up-regulation of calcium-binding proteins in motoneuron cells. Journal of Neuroscience Research 51(1): 58-66.

Alfaham, M., S. Woodhead, G. Pask and D. Davies. 1995. Vitamin D deficiency: a concern in pregnant Asian women. British Journal of Nutrition 73(6): 881-7.

Allen, J. C., R. P. Keller, P. Archer and M. C. Neville. 1991. Studies in human lactation: milk composition and daily secretion rates of macronutrients in the first year of lactation. American Journal of Clinical Nutrition 54(1): 69-80.

Al-oanzi, Z. H., S. P. Tuck, N. Raj, J. S. Harrop, G. D. Summers, D. B. Cook, R. M. Francis and H. K. Datta. 2006. Assessment of vitamin D status in male osteoporosis. Clinical Chemistry 52(2): 248-54.

Aloia, J. F., A. Vaswani, J. K. Yeh, P. L. Ross, E. Flaster and F. A. Dilmanian. 1994. Calcium supplementation with and without hormone replacement therapy to prevent postmenopausal bone loss. Annals of Internal Medicine 120(2): 97-103.

Aloia, J. F., A. Vaswani, R. Ma and E. Flaster. 1996a. Body composition in normal black women: the four-compartment model. Journal of Clinical Endocrinology and Metabolism 81(6): 2363-9.

Aloia, J. F., A. Vaswani, J. K. Yeh and E. Flaster. 1996b. Risk for osteoporosis in black women. Calcified Tissue International 59(6): 415-23.

Aloia, J. F., A. Vaswani, R. Ma and E. Flaster. 1997. Comparison of body composition in black and white premenopausal women. Journal of Laboratory and Clinical Medicine 129(3): 294-9.

Aloia, J. F., A. Vaswani, M. Mikhail and E. R. Flaster. 1999. Body composition by dual-energy X-ray absorptiometry in black compared with white women. Osteoporosis International 10(2): 114-9.

Aloia, J. F., A. Vaswani, M. Feuerman, M. Mikhail and R. Ma. 2000. Differences in skeletal and muscle mass with aging in black and white women. American Journal of Physiology, Endocrinology, and Metabolism 278(6): E1153-7.

Aloia, J. F., S. A. Talwar, S. Pollack and J. Yeh. 2005. A randomized controlled trial of vitamin D_3 supplementation in African American women. Archives of Internal Medicine 165(14): 1618-23.

Aloia, J. F., M. Feuerman and J. K. Yeh. 2006a. Reference range for serum parathyroid hormone. Endocrinology Practice 12(2): 137-44.

Aloia, J. F., S. A. Talwar, S. Pollack, M. Feuerman and J. K. Yeh. 2006b. Optimal vitamin D status and serum parathyroid hormone concentrations in African American women. American Journal of Clinical Nutrition 84(3): 602-9.

Aloia, J. F. 2008. African Americans, 25-hydroxyvitamin D, and osteoporosis: a paradox. American Journal of Clinical Nutrition 88(2): 545S-50S.

Aloia, J. F., D. G. Chen, J. K. Yeh and H. Chen. 2010. Serum vitamin D metabolites and intestinal calcium absorption efficiency in women. American Journal of Clinical Nutrition 92(4): 835-40.

Ames, S. K., K. J. Ellis, S. K. Gunn, K. C. Copeland and S. A. Abrams. 1999. Vitamin D receptor gene Fok1 polymorphism predicts calcium absorption and bone mineral density in children. Journal of Bone and Mineral Research 14(5): 740-6.

Amling, M., M. Priemel, T. Holzmann, K. Chapin, J. M. Rueger, R. Baron and M. B. Demay. 1999. Rescue of the skeletal phenotype of vitamin D receptor-ablated mice in the setting of normal mineral ion homeostasis: formal histomorphometric and biomechanical analyses. Endocrinology 140(11): 4982-7.

Andersen, R., C. Molgaard, L. T. Skovgaard, C. Brot, K. D. Cashman, J. Jakobsen, C. Lamberg-Allardt and L. Ovesen. 2008. Effect of vitamin D supplementation on bone and vitamin D status among Pakistani immigrants in Denmark: a randomised double-blinded placebo-controlled intervention study. British Journal of Nutrition 100(1): 197-207.

Anderson, I., A. E. R. Campbell, A. Dunn and J. B. M. Rumciman. 1966. Osteomalacia in elderly women. Scottish Medical Journal 11: 429-35.

Anderson, J. J. and W. S. Pollitzer. 1994. Ethnic and genetic differences in susceptibility to osteoporotic fractures. Advances in Nutritional Research 9: 129-49.

Anderson, F. H., H. E. Smith, H. M. Raphael and et al. 2004. Effect of annual intramuscular vitamin D_3 supplementation on fracture risk in 9440 community-living older people: the Wessex fracture prevention trial. [Abstract] ASBMR 26th Annual Meeting. Presentation #1220 10/5/2004.

Anderson, L. N., M. Cotterchio, R. Vieth and J. A. Knight. 2010. Vitamin D and calcium intakes and breast cancer risk in pre- and postmenopausal women. American Journal of Clinical Nutrition 91(6): 1699-707.

Annweiler, C., A. M. Schott, M. Montero-Odasso, G. Berrut, B. Fantino, F. R. Herrmann and O. Beauchet. 2010. Cross–sectional association between serum vitamin D concentration and walking speed measured at usual and fast pace among older women: The EPIDOS study. Journal of Bone and Mineral Research 25(8): 1858-66.

Apperley, F. 1941. The relation of solar radiation to cancer mortality in North America. Cancer Research 1: 191-5.

Ardawi, M. S., H. A. Nasrat and B. A. A. HS. 1997. Calcium-regulating hormones and parathyroid hormone-related peptide in normal human pregnancy and postpartum: a longitudinal study. European Journal of Endocrinology/European Federation of Endocrine Societies 137(4): 402-9.

Arden, N. K., P. Major, J. R. Poole, R. W. Keen, S. Vaja, R. Swaminathan, C. Cooper and T. D. Spector. 2002. Size at birth, adult intestinal calcium absorption and 1,25(OH)(2) vitamin D. Quarterly Journal of Medicine 95(1): 15-21.

Arnaud, S. B., G. B. Stickler and J. C. Haworth. 1976. Serum 25-hydroxyvitamin D in infantile rickets. Pediatrics 57(2): 221-5.

Aspray, T. J., L. Yan and A. Prentice. 2005. Parathyroid hormone and rates of bone formation are raised in perimenopausal rural Gambian women. Bone 36(4): 710-20.

Atalar, E., G. Aydin, I. Keles, E. Inal, G. Zog, A. Arslan and S. Orkun. 2009. Factors affecting bone mineral density in men. Rheumatology International 29(9): 1025-30.

August, P., B. Marcaccio, J. M. Gertner, M. L. Druzin, L. M. Resnick and J. H. Laragh. 1992. Abnormal 1,25-dihydroxyvitamin D metabolism in preeclampsia. American Journal of Obstetrics and Gynecology 166(4): 1295-9.

Avenell, A., J. A. Cook, G. S. MacLennan and G. C. McPherson. 2009a. Vitamin D supplementation and type 2 diabetes: a substudy of a randomised placebo-controlled trial in older people (RECORD trial, ISRCTN 51647438). Age and Ageing 38(5): 606-9.

Avenell, A., W. J. Gillespie, L. D. Gillespie and D. O'Connell. 2009b. Vitamin D and vitamin D analogues for preventing fractures associated with involutional and post-menopausal osteoporosis. Cochrane Database of Systematic Reviews(2): CD000227.

Avioli, L. V. 1978. What to do with "postmenopausal osteoporosis?". American Journal of Medicine 65(6): 881-4.

Baas, D., K. Prufer, M. E. Ittel, S. Kuchler-Bopp, G. Labourdette, L. L. Sarlieve and P. Brachet. 2000. Rat oligodendrocytes express the vitamin D(3) receptor and respond to 1,25-dihydroxyvitamin D(3). Glia 31(1): 59-68.

Baeksgaard, L., K. P. Andersen and L. Hyldstrup. 1998. Calcium and vitamin D supplementation increases spinal BMD in healthy, postmenopausal women. Osteoporosis International 8(3): 255-60.

Baker, S. G. and B. S. Kramer. 2008. Randomized trials for the real world: making as few and as reasonable assumptions as possible. Statistical Methods in Medical Research 17(3): 243-52.

Bakhtiyarova, S., O. Lesnyak, N. Kyznesova, M. A. Blankenstein and P. Lips. 2006. Vitamin D status among patients with hip fracture and elderly control subjects in Yekaterinburg, Russia. Osteoporosis International 17(3): 441-6.

Balasubramanian, K., J. Rajeswari, Gulab, Y. C. Govil, A. K. Agarwal, A. Kumar and V. Bhatia. 2003. Varying role of vitamin D deficiency in the etiology of rickets in young children vs. adolescents in northern India. Journal of Tropical Pediatrics 49(4): 201-6.

Balsan, S., M. Garabedian, M. Larchet, A. M. Gorski, G. Cournot, C. Tau, A. Bourdeau, C. Silve and C. Ricour. 1986. Long-term nocturnal calcium infusions can cure rickets and promote normal mineralization in hereditary resistance to 1,25-dihydroxyvitamin D. Journal of Clinical Investigation 77(5): 1661-7.

Baran, D., A. Sorensen, J. Grimes, R. Lew, A. Karellas, B. Johnson and J. Roche. 1990. Dietary modification with dairy products for preventing vertebral bone loss in premenopausal women: a three-year prospective study. Journal of Clinical Endocrinology and Metabolism 70(1): 264-70.

Barger-Lux, M. J. and R. P. Heaney. 2002. Effects of above average summer sun exposure on serum 25-hydroxyvitamin D and calcium absorption. Journal of Clinical Endocrinology and Metabolism 87(11): 4952-6.

Barger-Lux, M. J., K. M. Davies and R. P. Heaney. 2005. Calcium supplementation does not augment bone gain in young women consuming diets moderately low in calcium. Journal of Nutrition 135(10): 2362-6.

Barrett-Connor, E., E. S. Siris, L. E. Wehren, P. D. Miller, T. A. Abbott, M. L. Berger, A. C. Santora and L. M. Sherwood. 2005. Osteoporosis and fracture risk in women of different ethnic groups. Journal of Bone and Mineral Research 20(2): 185-94.

Bartley, J. 2010. Vitamin D, innate immunity and upper respiratory tract infection. Journal of Laryngology and Otology 124(5): 465-9.

Basile, L. A., S. N. Taylor, C. L. Wagner, R. L. Horst and B. W. Hollis. 2006. The effect of high-dose vitamin D supplementation on serum vitamin D levels and milk calcium concentration in lactating women and their infants. Breastfeed Medicine 1(1): 27-35.

Bates, C. J., G. D. Carter, G. D. Mishra, D. O'Shea, J. Jones and A. Prentice. 2003. In a population study, can parathyroid hormone aid the definition of adequate vitamin D status? A study of people aged 65 years and over from the British National Diet and Nutrition Survey. Osteoporosis International 14(2): 152-9.

Becker, A., D. W. Eyles, J. J. McGrath and G. Grecksch. 2005. Transient prenatal vitamin D deficiency is associated with subtle alterations in learning and memory functions in adult rats. Behavioural Brain Research 161(2): 306-12.

Beck-Nielsen, S. S., T. K. Jensen, J. Gram, K. Brixen and B. Brock-Jacobsen. 2009. Nutritional rickets in Denmark: a retrospective review of children's medical records from 1985 to 2005. European Journal of Pediatrics 168(8): 941-9.

Begum, R., M. L. Coutinho, T. L. Dormandy and S. Yudkin. 1968. Maternal malabsorption presenting as congenital rickets. Lancet 1(7551): 1048-52.

Bell, N. H., A. Greene, S. Epstein, M. J. Oexmann, S. Shaw and J. Shary. 1985. Evidence for alteration of the vitamin D-endocrine system in blacks. Journal of Clinical Investigation 76(2): 470-3.

Bell, N. H., J. Shary, J. Stevens, M. Garza, L. Gordon and J. Edwards. 1991. Demonstration that bone mass is greater in black than in white children. Journal of Bone and Mineral Research 6(7): 719-23.

Bell, N. H. 1995. 25-hydroxyvitamin D_3 reverses alteration of the vitamin D-endocrine system in blacks. American Journal of Medicine 99(6): 597-9.

Bell, N. H., L. Gordon, J. Stevens and J. R. Shary. 1995. Demonstration that bone mineral density of the lumbar spine, trochanter, and femoral neck is higher in black than in white young men. Calcified Tissue International 56(1): 11-3.

Bell, N. H. 1997. Bone and mineral metabolism in African Americans. Trends in Endocrinology Metabolism 8(6): 240-5.

Benjamin, A., A. Moriakova, N. Akhter, D. Rao, H. Xie, S. Kukreja and E. Barengolts. 2009. Determinants of 25-hydroxyvitamin D levels in African-American and Caucasian male veterans. Osteoporosis International 20(10): 1795-803.

Ben-Zvi, I., C. Aranow, M. Mackay, A. Stanevsky, D. L. Kamen, L. M. Marinescu, C. E. Collins, G. S. Gilkeson, B. Diamond and J. A. Hardin. 2010. The impact of vitamin D on dendritic cell function in patients with systemic lupus erythematosus. PLoS ONE [Electronic Resource] 5(2): e9193.

Berger, C., D. Goltzman, L. Langsetmo, L. Joseph, N. Kreiger, A. Tenenhouse, K. S. Davison, R. G. Josse, J. C. Prior and D. A. Hanley. 2010. Peak bone mass from longitudinal data: implications for the prevalence, pathophysiology, and diagnosis of osteoporosis. Journal of Bone and Mineral Research 25(9): 1948-57.

Bertone-Johnson, E. R., W. Y. Chen, M. F. Holick, B. W. Hollis, G. A. Colditz, W. C. Willett and S. E. Hankinson. 2005. Plasma 25-hydroxyvitamin D and 1,25-dihydroxyvitamin D and risk of breast cancer. Cancer Epidemiology, Biomarkers & Prevention 14(8): 1991-7.

Bertone-Johnson, E. R. 2009. Vitamin D and breast cancer. Annals of Epidemiology 19(7): 462-7.

Berube, S., C. Diorio, W. Verhoek-Oftedahl and J. Brisson. 2004. Vitamin D, calcium, and mammographic breast densities. Cancer Epidemiology, Biomarkers & Prevention 13(9): 1466-72.

Bhimma, R., J. M. Pettifor, H. M. Coovadia, M. Moodley and M. Adhikari. 1995. Rickets in black children beyond infancy in Natal. South African Medical Journal 85(7): 668-72.

Bikle, D. D., E. Gee, B. Halloran and J. G. Haddad. 1984. Free 1,25-dihydroxyvitamin D levels in serum from normal subjects, pregnant subjects, and subjects with liver disease. Journal of Clinical Investigation 74(6): 1966-71.

Billaudel, B., L. Barakat and A. Faure-Dussert. 1998. Vitamin D_3 deficiency and alterations of glucose metabolism in rat endocrine pancreas. Diabetes and Metabolism 24(4): 344-50.

Bischoff, H. A., H. B. Stahelin, W. Dick, R. Akos, M. Knecht, C. Salis, M. Nebiker, R. Theiler, M. Pfeifer, B. Begerow, R. A. Lew and M. Conzelmann. 2003. Effects of vitamin D and calcium supplementation on falls: a randomized controlled trial. Journal of Bone and Mineral Research 18(2): 343-51.

Bischoff-Ferrari, H. A., B. Dawson-Hughes, W. C. Willett, H. B. Staehelin, M. G. Bazemore, R. Y. Zee and J. B. Wong. 2004a. Effect of Vitamin D on falls: a meta-analysis. JAMA 291(16): 1999-2006.

Bischoff-Ferrari, H. A., T. Dietrich, E. J. Orav, F. B. Hu, Y. Zhang, E. W. Karlson and B. Dawson-Hughes. 2004b. Higher 25-hydroxyvitamin D concentrations are associated with better lower-extremity function in both active and inactive persons aged ≥60 y. American Journal of Clinical Nutrition 80(3): 752-8.

Bischoff-Ferrari, H. A., Y. Zhang, D. P. Kiel and D. T. Felson. 2005. Positive association between serum 25-hydroxyvitamin D level and bone density in osteoarthritis. Arthritis and Rheumatism 53(6): 821-6.

Bischoff-Ferrari, H. A., E. Giovannucci, W. C. Willett, T. Dietrich and B. Dawson-Hughes. 2006a. Estimation of optimal serum concentrations of 25-hydroxyvitamin D for multiple health outcomes. American Journal of Clinical Nutrition 84(1): 18-28.

Bischoff-Ferrari, H. A., E. J. Orav and B. Dawson-Hughes. 2006b. Effect of cholecalciferol plus calcium on falling in ambulatory older men and women: a 3-year randomized controlled trial. Archives of Internal Medicine 166(4): 424-30.

Bischoff-Ferrari, H. A., B. Dawson-Hughes, J. A. Baron, P. Burckhardt, R. Li, D. Spiegelman, B. Specker, J. E. Orav, J. B. Wong, H. B. Staehelin, E. O'Reilly, D. P. Kiel and W. C. Willett. 2007. Calcium intake and hip fracture risk in men and women: a meta-analysis of prospective cohort studies and randomized controlled trials. American Journal of Clinical Nutrition 86(6): 1780-90.

Bischoff-Ferrari, H. A., B. Dawson-Hughes, H. B. Staehelin, J. E. Orav, A. E. Stuck, R. Theiler, J. B. Wong, A. Egli, D. P. Kiel and J. Henschkowski. 2009a. Fall prevention with supplemental and active forms of vitamin D: a meta-analysis of randomised controlled trials. British Medical Journal 339: b3692.

Bischoff-Ferrari, H. A., D. P. Kiel, B. Dawson-Hughes, J. E. Orav, R. Li, D. Spiegelman, T. Dietrich and W. C. Willett. 2009b. Dietary calcium and serum 25-hydroxyvitamin D status in relation to BMD among U.S. adults. Journal of Bone and Mineral Research 24(5): 935-42.

Bischoff-Ferrari, H. A., W. C. Willett, J. B. Wong, A. E. Stuck, H. B. Staehelin, E. J. Orav, A. Thoma, D. P. Kiel and J. Henschkowski. 2009c. Prevention of nonvertebral fractures with oral vitamin D and dose dependency: a meta-analysis of randomized controlled trials. Archives of Internal Medicine 169(6): 551-61.

Bischoff-Ferrari, H. A., B. Dawson-Hughes, A. Platz, E. J. Orav, H. B. Stahelin, W. C. Willett, U. Can, A. Egli, N. J. Mueller, S. Looser, B. Bretscher, E. Minder, A. Vergopoulos and R. Theiler. 2010. Effect of high-dosage cholecalciferol and extended physiotherapy on complications after hip fracture: a randomized controlled trial. Archives of Internal Medicine 170(9): 813-20.

Black, A. J., J. Topping, B. Durham, R. G. Farquharson and W. D. Fraser. 2000. A detailed assessment of alterations in bone turnover, calcium homeostasis, and bone density in normal pregnancy. Journal of Bone and Mineral Research 15(3): 557-63.

Black, P. N. and S. Sharpe. 1997. Dietary fat and asthma: is there a connection? European Respiratory Journal 10(1): 6-12.

Boass, A., S. U. Toverud, J. W. Pike and M. R. Haussler. 1981. Calcium metabolism during lactation: enhanced intestinal calcium absorption in vitamin D-deprived, hypocalcemic rats. Endocrinology 109(3): 900-7.

Bodnar, L. M., H. N. Simhan, R. W. Powers, M. P. Frank, E. Cooperstein and J. M. Roberts. 2007. High prevalence of vitamin D insufficiency in black and white pregnant women residing in the northern United States and their neonates. Journal of Nutrition 137(2): 447-52.

Bodnar, L. M., M. A. Krohn and H. N. Simhan. 2009. Maternal vitamin D deficiency is associated with bacterial vaginosis in the first trimester of pregnancy. Journal of Nutrition 139(6): 1157-61.

Bodnar, L. M., J. M. Catov, J. M. Zmuda, M. E. Cooper, M. S. Parrott, J. M. Roberts, M. L. Marazita and H. N. Simhan. 2010. Maternal serum 25-hydroxyvitamin D concentrations are associated with small-for-gestational age births in white women. Journal of Nutrition 140(5): 999-1006.

Bolla, L. R., C. M. Filley and R. M. Palmer. 2000. Dementia DDx. Office diagnosis of the four major types of dementia. Geriatrics 55(1): 34-7, 41-2, 45-6.

Bolland, M. J., P. A. Barber, R. N. Doughty, B. Mason, A. Horne, R. Ames, G. D. Gamble, A. Grey and I. R. Reid. 2008. Vascular events in healthy older women receiving calcium supplementation: randomised controlled trial. British Medical Journal 336(7638): 262-6.

Bolland, M. J., A. Avenell, J. A. Baron, A. Grey, G. S. MacLennan, G. D. Gamble and I. R. Reid. 2010a. Effect of calcium supplements on risk of myocardial infarction and cardiovascular events: meta-analysis. British Medical Journal 341: 3691-9.

Bolland, M. J., C. J. Bacon, A. M. Horne, B. H. Mason, R. W. Ames, T. K. Wang, A. B. Grey, G. D. Gamble and I. R. Reid. 2010b. Vitamin D insufficiency and health outcomes over 5 y in older women. American Journal of Clinical Nutrition 91(1): 82-9.

Bolton-Smith, C., M. E. McMurdo, C. R. Paterson, P. A. Mole, J. M. Harvey, S. T. Fenton, C. J. Prynne, G. D. Mishra and M. J. Shearer. 2007. Two-year randomized controlled trial of vitamin K1 (phylloquinone) and vitamin D_3 plus calcium on the bone health of older women. Journal of Bone and Mineral Research 22(4): 509-19.

Boonen, S., X. G. Cheng, J. Nijs, P. H. Nicholson, G. Verbeke, E. Lesaffre, J. Aerssens and J. Dequeker. 1997. Factors associated with cortical and trabecular bone loss as quantified by peripheral computed tomography (pQCT) at the ultradistal radius in aging women. Calcified Tissue International 60(2): 164-70.

Boonen, S., S. Mohan, J. Dequeker, J. Aerssens, D. Vanderschueren, G. Verbeke, P. Broos, R. Bouillon and D. J. Baylink. 1999. Down-regulation of the serum stimulatory components of the insulin-like growth factor (IGF) system (IGF-I, IGF-II, IGF binding protein [BP]-3, and IGFBP-5) in age-related (type II) femoral neck osteoporosis. Journal of Bone and Mineral Research 14(12): 2150-8.

Boscoe, F. P. and M. J. Schymura. 2006. Solar ultraviolet-B exposure and cancer incidence and mortality in the United States, 1993-2002. BMC Cancer 6: 264.

Bougle, D., J. P. Sabatier, F. Bureau, D. Laroche, J. Brouard, B. Guillois and J. F. Duhamel. 1998. Relationship between bone mineralization and aluminium in the healthy infant. European Journal of Clinical Nutrition 52(6): 431-5.

Bouillon, R., A. Verstuyf, C. Mathieu, S. Van Cromphaut, R. Masuyama, P. Dehaes and G. Carmeliet. 2006. Vitamin D resistance. Best Practice Research Clinical Endocrinology Metabolism 20(4): 627-45.

Bouillon, R., G. Carmeliet, L. Verlinden, E. van Etten, A. Verstuyf, H. F. Luderer, L. Lieben, C. Mathieu and M. Demay. 2008. Vitamin D and human health: lessons from vitamin D receptor null mice. Endocrine Reviews 29(6): 726-76.

Bourlon, P. M., A. Faure-Dussert and B. Billaudel. 1999. The de novo synthesis of numerous proteins is decreased during vitamin D_3 deficiency and is gradually restored by 1, 25-dihydroxyvitamin D_3 repletion in the islets of langerhans of rats. Journal of Endocrinology 162(1): 101-9.

Boxer, R. S., D. A. Dauser, S. J. Walsh, W. D. Hager and A. M. Kenny. 2008. The association between vitamin D and inflammation with the 6-minute walk and frailty in patients with heart failure. Journal of the American Geriatrics Society 56(3): 454-61.

Brannon, P. M., E. A. Yetley, R. L. Bailey and M. F. Picciano. 2008. Vitamin D and health in the 21st century: an update. Proceedings of a conference held September 2007 in Bethesda, Maryland, USA. American Journal of Clinical Nutrition 88(2): 483S-592S.

Braun, M., C. Palacios, K. Wigertz, L. A. Jackman, R. J. Bryant, L. D. McCabe, B. R. Martin, G. P. McCabe, M. Peacock and C. M. Weaver. 2007. Racial differences in skeletal calcium retention in adolescent girls with varied controlled calcium intakes. American Journal of Clinical Nutrition 85(6): 1657-63.

Brazier, M., F. Grados, S. Kamel, M. Mathieu, A. Morel, M. Maamer, J. L. Sebert and P. Fardellone. 2005. Clinical and laboratory safety of one year's use of a combination calcium + vitamin D tablet in ambulatory elderly women with vitamin D insufficiency: results of a multicenter, randomized, double-blind, placebo-controlled study. Clinical Therapeutics 27(12): 1885-93.

Brehm, J. M., J. C. Celedon, M. E. Soto-Quiros, L. Avila, G. M. Hunninghake, E. Forno, D. Laskey, J. S. Sylvia, B. W. Hollis, S. T. Weiss and A. A. Litonjua. 2009. Serum vitamin D levels and markers of severity of childhood asthma in Costa Rica. American Journal of Respiratory and Critical Care Medicine 179(9): 765-71.

Brewer, L. D., N. M. Porter, D. S. Kerr, P. W. Landfield and O. Thibault. 2006. Chronic 1alpha,25-(OH)2 vitamin D_3 treatment reduces Ca2+-mediated hippocampal biomarkers of aging. Cell Calcium 40(3): 277-86.

Brisson, J., S. Berube, C. Diorio, M. Sinotte, M. Pollak and B. Masse. 2007. Synchronized seasonal variations of mammographic breast density and plasma 25-hydroxyvitamin D. Cancer Epidemiology, Biomarkers & Prevention 16(5): 929-33.

Britton, J., I. Pavord, K. Richards, A. Wisniewski, A. Knox, S. Lewis, A. Tattersfield and S. Weiss. 1994a. Dietary magnesium, lung function, wheezing, and airway hyperreactivity in a random adult population sample. Lancet 344(8919): 357-62.

Britton, J., I. Pavord, K. Richards, A. Knox, A. Wisniewski, S. Weiss and A. Tattersfield. 1994b. Dietary sodium intake and the risk of airway hyperreactivity in a random adult population. Thorax 49(9): 875-80.

Broe, K. E., T. C. Chen, J. Weinberg, H. A. Bischoff-Ferrari, M. F. Holick and D. P. Kiel. 2007. A higher dose of vitamin D reduces the risk of falls in nursing home residents: a randomized, multiple-dose study. Journal of the American Geriatrics Society 55(2): 234-9.

Brommage, R., D. C. Baxter and L. W. Gierke. 1990. Vitamin D-independent intestinal calcium and phosphorus absorption during reproduction. American Journal of Physiology 259(4 Pt 1): G631-8.

Brooke, O. G., I. R. Brown, C. D. Bone, N. D. Carter, H. J. Cleeve, J. D. Maxwell, V. P. Robinson and S. M. Winder. 1980. Vitamin D supplements in pregnant Asian women: effects on calcium status and fetal growth. British Medical Journal 280(6216): 751-4.

Brown, J., J. I. Bianco, J. J. McGrath and D. W. Eyles. 2003. 1,25-dihydroxyvitamin D_3 induces nerve growth factor, promotes neurite outgrowth and inhibits mitosis in embryonic rat hippocampal neurons. Neuroscience Letters 343(2): 139-43.

Brunvand, L., S. S. Shah, S. Bergstrom and E. Haug. 1998. Vitamin D deficiency in pregnancy is not associated with obstructed labor. A study among Pakistani women in Karachi. Acta Obstetricia et Gynecologica Scandinavica 77(3): 303-6.

Bryant, R. J., M. E. Wastney, B. R. Martin, O. Wood, G. P. McCabe, M. Morshidi, D. L. Smith, M. Peacock and C. M. Weaver. 2003. Racial differences in bone turnover and calcium metabolism in adolescent females. Journal of Clinical Endocrinology and Metabolism 88(3): 1043-7.

Buell, J. S. and B. Dawson-Hughes. 2008. Vitamin D and neurocognitive dysfunction: preventing "D"ecline? Molecular Aspects of Medicine 29(6): 415-22.

Buell, J. S., B. Dawson-Hughes, T. M. Scott, D. E. Weiner, G. E. Dallal, W. Q. Qui, P. Bergethon, I. H. Rosenberg, M. F. Folstein, S. Patz, R. A. Bhadelia and K. L. Tucker. 2010. 25-hydroxyvitamin D, dementia, and cerebrovascular pathology in elders receiving home services. Neurology 74(1): 18-26.

Bunout, D., G. Barrera, L. Leiva, V. Gattas, M. P. de la Maza, M. Avendano and S. Hirsch. 2006. Effects of vitamin D supplementation and exercise training on physical performance in Chilean vitamin D deficient elderly subjects. Experimental Gerontology 41(8): 746-52.

Burleigh, E., J. McColl and J. Potter. 2007. Does vitamin D stop inpatients falling? A randomised controlled trial. Age and Ageing 36(5): 507-13.

Burney, P. 1987. A diet rich in sodium may potentiate asthma. Epidemiologic evidence for a new hypothesis. Chest 91(Suppl 6): 143S-8S.

Cade, C. and A. W. Norman. 1986. Vitamin D_3 improves impaired glucose tolerance and insulin secretion in the vitamin D-deficient rat in vivo. Endocrinology 119(1): 84-90.

Cadranel, J. L., M. Garabedian, B. Milleron, H. Guillozzo, D. Valeyre, F. Paillard, G. Akoun and A. J. Hance. 1994. Vitamin D metabolism by alveolar immune cells in tuberculosis: correlation with calcium metabolism and clinical manifestations. European Respiratory Journal 7(6): 1103-10.

Camargo, C. A., Jr., S. L. Rifas-Shiman, A. A. Litonjua, J. W. Rich-Edwards, S. T. Weiss, D. R. Gold, K. Kleinman and M. W. Gillman. 2007. Maternal intake of vitamin D during pregnancy and risk of recurrent wheeze in children at 3 y of age. American Journal of Clinical Nutrition 85(3): 788-95.

Campbell, D. E. and A. R. Fleischman. 1988. Rickets of prematurity: controversies in causation and prevention. Clinics in Perinatology 15(4): 879-90.

Cancela, L., N. Le Boulch and L. Miravet. 1986. Relationship between the vitamin D content of maternal milk and the vitamin D status of nursing women and breast-fed infants. Journal of Endocrinology 110(1): 43-50.

Cannell, J. J., R. Vieth, J. C. Umhau, M. F. Holick, W. B. Grant, S. Madronich, C. F. Garland and E. Giovannucci. 2006. Epidemic influenza and vitamin D. Epidemiology and Infection 134(6): 1129-40.

Cantorna, M. T., C. E. Hayes and H. F. DeLuca. 1996. 1,25-dihydroxyvitamin D_3 reversibly blocks the progression of relapsing encephalomyelitis, a model of multiple sclerosis. Proceedings of the National Academy of Sciences of the United States of America 93(15): 7861-4.

Cantorna, M. T., C. E. Hayes and H. F. DeLuca. 1998. 1,25-dihydroxycholecalciferol inhibits the progression of arthritis in murine models of human arthritis. Journal of Nutrition 128(1): 68-72.

Cantorna, M. T. and B. D. Mahon. 2005. D-hormone and the immune system. Journal of Rheumatology (Suppl 76): 11-20.

Canzoniero, L. M. and B. J. Snider. 2005. Calcium in Alzheimer's disease pathogenesis: too much, too little or in the wrong place? Journal of Alzheimers Disease 8(2): 147-54; discussion 209-15.

Cauley, J. A., L. Y. Lui, K. E. Ensrud, J. M. Zmuda, K. L. Stone, M. C. Hochberg and S. R. Cummings. 2005a. Bone mineral density and the risk of incident nonspinal fractures in black and white women. JAMA 293(17): 2102-8.

Cauley, J. A., L. Y. Lui, K. L. Stone, T. A. Hillier, J. M. Zmuda, M. Hochberg, T. J. Beck and K. E. Ensrud. 2005b. Longitudinal study of changes in hip bone mineral density in Caucasian and African-American women. Journal of the American Geriatrics Society 53(2): 183-9.

Cauley, J. A., A. Z. Lacroix, L. Wu, M. Horwitz, M. E. Danielson, D. C. Bauer, J. S. Lee, R. D. Jackson, J. A. Robbins, C. Wu, F. Z. Stanczyk, M. S. LeBoff, J. Wactawski-Wende, G. Sarto, J. Ockene and S. R. Cummings. 2008. Serum 25-hydroxyvitamin D concentrations and risk for hip fractures. Annals of Internal Medicine 149(4): 242-50.

Cauley, J., et al. 2009. Serum 25 hydroxyvitamin (OH)D and fracture risk in multi-ethnic women: the Women's Health Initiative (WHI). Presented at ASBMR 31st Annual Meeting. Denver, CO.

Cauley, J. A., N. Parimi, K. E. Ensrud, D. C. Bauer, P. M. Cawthon, S. R. Cummings, A. R. Hoffman, J. M. Shikany, E. Barrett-Connor and E. Orwoll. 2010. Serum 25 hydroxyvitamin D and the risk of hip and non-spine fractures in older men. Journal of Bone and Mineral Research 25(3): 545.

Ceglia, L. 2008. Vitamin D and skeletal muscle tissue and function. Molecular Aspects of Medicine 29(6): 407-14.

Cesur, Y., H. Caksen, A. Gundem, E. Kirimi and D. Odabas. 2003. Comparison of low and high dose of vitamin D treatment in nutritional vitamin D deficiency rickets. Journal of Pediatric Endocrinology and Metabolism 16(8): 1105-9.

Chan, G. M., C. C. Roberts, D. Folland and R. Jackson. 1982. Growth and bone mineralization of normal breast-fed infants and the effects of lactation on maternal bone mineral status. American Journal of Clinical Nutrition 36(3): 438-43.

Chan, G. M., K. Hoffman and M. McMurry. 1995. Effects of dairy products on bone and body composition in pubertal girls. Journal of Pediatrics 126(4): 551-6.

Chan, T. Y., P. Poon, J. Pang, R. Swaminathan, C. H. Chan, M. Nisar, C. S. Williams and P. D. Davies. 1994. A study of calcium and vitamin D metabolism in Chinese patients with pulmonary tuberculosis. Journal of Tropical Medicine and Hygiene 97(1): 26-30.

Chantry, C. J., P. Auinger and R. S. Byrd. 2004. Lactation among adolescent mothers and subsequent bone mineral density. Archives of Pediatrics and Adolescent Medicine 158(7): 650-6.

Chapuy, M. C., M. E. Arlot, F. Duboeuf, J. Brun, B. Crouzet, S. Arnaud, P. D. Delmas and P. J. Meunier. 1992. Vitamin D_3 and calcium to prevent hip fractures in the elderly women. New England Journal of Medicine 327(23): 1637-42.

Chapuy, M. C., P. Preziosi, M. Maamer, S. Arnaud, P. Galan, S. Hercberg and P. J. Meunier. 1997. Prevalence of vitamin D insufficiency in an adult normal population. Osteoporosis International 7(5): 439-43.

Chapuy, M. C., R. Pamphile, E. Paris, C. Kempf, M. Schlichting, S. Arnaud, P. Garnero and P. J. Meunier. 2002. Combined calcium and vitamin D_3 supplementation in elderly women: confirmation of reversal of secondary hyperparathyroidism and hip fracture risk: the Decalyos II study. Osteoporosis International 13(3): 257-64.

Chen, P., P. Hu, D. Xie, Y. Qin, F. Wang and H. Wang. 2010. Meta-analysis of vitamin D, calcium and the prevention of breast cancer. Breast Cancer Research and Treatment 121(2): 469-77.

Cheng, S., A. Lyytikainen, H. Kroger, C. Lamberg-Allardt, M. Alen, A. Koistinen, Q. J. Wang, M. Suuriniemi, H. Suominen, A. Mahonen, P. H. Nicholson, K. K. Ivaska, R. Korpela, C. Ohlsson, K. H. Vaananen and F. Tylavsky. 2005. Effects of calcium, dairy product, and vitamin D supplementation on bone mass accrual and body composition in 10-12-y-old girls: a 2-y randomized trial. American Journal of Clinical Nutrition 82(5): 1115-26; quiz 1147-8.

Chertow, B. S., W. I. Sivitz, N. G. Baranetsky, S. A. Clark, A. Waite and H. F. Deluca. 1983. Cellular mechanisms of insulin release: the effects of vitamin D deficiency and repletion on rat insulin secretion. Endocrinology 113(4): 1511-8.

Chevalley, T., R. Rizzoli, V. Nydegger, D. Slosman, C. H. Rapin, J. P. Michel, H. Vasey and J. P. Bonjour. 1994. Effects of calcium supplements on femoral bone mineral density and vertebral fracture rate in vitamin-D-replete elderly patients. Osteoporosis International 4(5): 245-52.

Chlebowski, R. T., K. C. Johnson, C. Kooperberg, M. Pettinger, J. Wactawski-Wende, T. Rohan, J. Rossouw, D. Lane, M. J. O'Sullivan, S. Yasmeen, R. A. Hiatt, J. M. Shikany, M. Vitolins, J. Khandekar and F. A. Hubbell. 2008. Calcium plus vitamin D supplementation and the risk of breast cancer. Journal of the National Cancer Institute 100(22): 1581-91.

Chonchol, M., M. Cigolini and G. Targher. 2008. Association between 25-hydroxyvitamin D deficiency and cardiovascular disease in type 2 diabetic patients with mild kidney dysfunction. Nephrology, Dialysis, Transplantation 23(1): 269-74.

Chung M., E. M. Balk, M. Brendel, S. Ip, J. Lau, J. Lee, A. Lichtenstein, K. Patel, G. Raman, A. Tatsioni, T. Terasawa and T. A. Trikalinos. 2009. Vitamin D and calcium: a systematic review of health outcomes. Evidence Report No. 183. (Prepared by the Tufts Evidence-based Practice Center under Contract No. HHSA 290-2007-10055-I.) AHRQ Publication No. 09-E015. Rockville, MD: Agency for Healthcare Research and Quality.

Cigolini, M., M. P. Iagulli, V. Miconi, M. Galiotto, S. Lombardi and G. Targher. 2006. Serum 25-hydroxyvitamin D_3 concentrations and prevalence of cardiovascular disease among type 2 diabetic patients. Diabetes Care 29(3): 722-4.

Clark, S. A., W. E. Stumpf and M. Sar. 1981. Effect of 1,25 dihydroxyvitamin D_3 on insulin secretion. Diabetes 30(5): 382-6.

Cohn, S. H., C. Abesamis, S. Yasumura, J. F. Aloia, I. Zanzi and K. J. Ellis. 1977. Comparative skeletal mass and radial bone mineral content in black and white women. Metabolism 26(2): 171-8.

Congdon, P., A. Horsman, P. A. Kirby, J. Dibble and T. Bashir. 1983. Mineral content of the forearms of babies born to Asian and white mothers. British Medical Journal (Clinical Research Edition) 286(6373): 1233-5.

Cooper, C., M. McLaren, P. J. Wood, L. Coulton and J. A. Kanis. 1989. Indices of calcium metabolism in women with hip fractures. Bone and Mineral 5(2): 193-200.

Cooper, L., P. B. Clifton-Bligh, M. L. Nery, G. Figtree, S. Twigg, E. Hibbert and B. G. Robinson. 2003. Vitamin D supplementation and bone mineral density in early postmenopausal women. American Journal of Clinical Nutrition 77(5): 1324-9.

Cooper, C., K. Javaid, S. Westlake, N. Harvey and E. Dennison. 2005. Developmental origins of osteoporotic fracture: the role of maternal vitamin D insufficiency. Journal of Nutrition 135(11): 2728S-34S.

Cosman, F., D. C. Morgan, J. W. Nieves, V. Shen, M. M. Luckey, D. W. Dempster, R. Lindsay and M. Parisien. 1997. Resistance to bone resorbing effects of PTH in black women. Journal of Bone and Mineral Research 12(6): 958-66.

Cosman, F., J. Nieves, D. Dempster and R. Lindsay. 2007. Vitamin D economy in blacks. Journal of Bone and Mineral Research 22 (Suppl 2): V34-8.

Costenbader, K. H., D. Feskanich, M. Holmes, E. W. Karlson and E. Benito-Garcia. 2008. Vitamin D intake and risks of systemic lupus erythematosus and rheumatoid arthritis in women. Annals of the Rheumatic Diseases 67(4): 530-5.

Cranney A., T. Horsley, S. O'Donnell, H. A. Weiler, L. Puil, D. S. Ooi, S. A. Atkinson, L. M. Ward, D. Moher, D. A. Hanley, M. Fang, F. Yazdi, C. Garritty, M. Sampson, N. Barrowman, A. Tsertsvadze and V. Mamaladze. 2007. Effectiveness and safety of vitamin D in relation to bone health. Evidence Report/Technology Assessment No. 158. (Prepared by the University of Ottawa Evidence-based Practice Center (UO-EPC) under Contract No. 290-02-0021.) AHRQ Publication No. 07-E013. Rockville, MD: Agency for Healthcare Research and Quality.

Cromer, B. A., L. Binkovitz, J. Ziegler, R. Harvey and S. M. Debanne. 2004. Reference values for bone mineral density in 12- to 18-year-old girls categorized by weight, race, and age. Pediatric Radiology 34(10): 787-92.

Cross, N. A., L. S. Hillman, S. H. Allen, G. F. Krause and N. E. Vieira. 1995. Calcium homeostasis and bone metabolism during pregnancy, lactation, and postweaning: a longitudinal study. American Journal of Clinical Nutrition 61(3): 514-23.

Cross, H. S., M. Peterlik, G. S. Reddy and I. Schuster. 1997. Vitamin D metabolism in human colon adenocarcinoma-derived Caco-2 cells: expression of 25-hydroxyvitamin D_3-1alpha-hydroxylase activity and regulation of side-chain metabolism. Journal of Steroid Biochemistry and Molecular Biology 62(1): 21-8.

Croswell, J. M. and B. S. Kramer. 2009. Clinical trial design and evidence-based outcomes in the study of liver diseases. Journal of Hepatology 50(4): 817-26.

Cummings, S. R., J. A. Cauley, L. Palermo, P. D. Ross, R. D. Wasnich, D. Black and K. G. Faulkner. 1994. Racial differences in hip axis lengths might explain racial differences in rates of hip fracture. Study of Osteoporotic Fractures Research Group. Osteoporosis International 4(4): 226-9.

Cummings, S. R., W. S. Browner, D. Bauer, K. Stone, K. Ensrud, S. Jamal and B. Ettinger. 1998. Endogenous hormones and the risk of hip and vertebral fractures among older women. Study of Osteoporotic Fractures Research Group. New England Journal of Medicine 339(11): 733-8.

Dahlman, T., H. E. Sjoberg and E. Bucht. 1994. Calcium homeostasis in normal pregnancy and puerperium. A longitudinal study. Acta Obstetrica et Gynecologica Scandinavica 73(5): 393-8.

Dardenne, O., J. Prud'homme, A. Arabian, F. H. Glorieux and R. St-Arnaud. 2001. Targeted inactivation of the 25-hydroxyvitamin D(3)-1(alpha)-hydroxylase gene (CYP27B1) creates an animal model of pseudovitamin D-deficiency rickets. Endocrinology 142(7): 3135-41.

Dardenne, O., J. Prudhomme, S. A. Hacking, F. H. Glorieux and R. St-Arnaud. 2003. Rescue of the pseudo-vitamin D deficiency rickets phenotype of CYP27B1-deficient mice by treatment with 1,25-dihydroxyvitamin D_3: biochemical, histomorphometric, and biomechanical analyses. Journal of Bone and Mineral Research 18(4): 637-43.

Davis, C. D. 2008. Vitamin D and cancer: current dilemmas and future research needs. American Journal of Clinical Nutrition 88(2): 565S-9.

Dawodu, A., M. Agarwal, M. Sankarankutty, D. Hardy, J. Kochiyil and P. Badrinath. 2005. Higher prevalence of vitamin D deficiency in mothers of rachitic than nonrachitic children. Journal of Pediatrics 147(1): 109-11.

Dawson-Hughes, B., G. E. Dallal, E. A. Krall, L. Sadowski, N. Sahyoun and S. Tannenbaum. 1990. A controlled trial of the effect of calcium supplementation on bone density in postmenopausal women. New England Journal of Medicine 323(13): 878-83.

Dawson-Hughes, B., G. E. Dallal, E. A. Krall, S. Harris, L. J. Sokoll and G. Falconer. 1991. Effect of vitamin D supplementation on wintertime and overall bone loss in healthy postmenopausal women. Annals of Internal Medicine 115(7): 505-12.

Dawson-Hughes, B., S. Harris, C. Kramich, G. Dallal and H. M. Rasmussen. 1993. Calcium retention and hormone levels in black and white women on high- and low-calcium diets. Journal of Bone and Mineral Research 8(7): 779-87.

Dawson-Hughes, B., S. S. Harris, E. A. Krall, G. E. Dallal, G. Falconer and C. L. Green. 1995. Rates of bone loss in postmenopausal women randomly assigned to one of two dosages of vitamin D. American Journal of Clinical Nutrition 61(5): 1140-5.

Dawson-Hughes, B., S. S. Harris and G. E. Dallal. 1997a. Plasma calcidiol, season, and serum parathyroid hormone concentrations in healthy elderly men and women. American Journal of Clinical Nutrition 65(1): 67-71.

Dawson-Hughes, B., S. S. Harris, E. A. Krall and G. E. Dallal. 1997b. Effect of calcium and vitamin D supplementation on bone density in men and women 65 years of age or older. New England Journal of Medicine 337(10): 670-6.

de Abreu, D. A., E. Nivet, N. Baril, M. Khrestchatisky, F. Roman and F. Feron. 2010. Developmental vitamin D deficiency alters learning in C57Bl/6J mice. Behavioural Brain Research 208(2): 603-8.

de Viragh, P. A., K. G. Haglid and M. R. Celio. 1989. Parvalbumin increases in the caudate putamen of rats with vitamin D hypervitaminosis. Proceedings of the National Academy of Sciences of the United States of America 86(10): 3887-90.

Deeb, K. K., D. L. Trump and C. S. Johnson. 2007. Vitamin D signalling pathways in cancer: potential for anticancer therapeutics. Nature Reviews Cancer 7(9): 684-700.

del Puente, A., A. Esposito, S. Savastano, A. Carpinelli, L. Postiglione and P. Oriente. 2002. Dietary calcium intake and serum vitamin D are major determinants of bone mass variations in women. A longitudinal study. Aging Clinical Experimental Research 14(5): 382-8.

Delvin, E. E., B. L. Salle, F. H. Glorieux, P. Adeleine and L. S. David. 1986. Vitamin D supplementation during pregnancy: effect on neonatal calcium homeostasis. Journal of Pediatrics 109(2): 328-34.

Dennison, E., R. Eastell, C. H. Fall, S. Kellingray, P. J. Wood and C. Cooper. 1999. Determinants of bone loss in elderly men and women: a prospective population-based study. Osteoporosis International 10(5): 384-91.

Deth, R., C. Muratore, J. Benzecry, V. A. Power-Charnitsky and M. Waly. 2008. How environmental and genetic factors combine to cause autism: a redox/methylation hypothesis. Neurotoxicology 29(1): 190-201.

Devereux, G., G. McNeill, G. Newman, S. Turner, L. Craig, S. Martindale, P. Helms and A. Seaton. 2007. Early childhood wheezing symptoms in relation to plasma selenium in pregnant mothers and neonates. Clinical and Experimental Allergy 37(7): 1000-8.

Devine, A., S. G. Wilson, I. M. Dick and R. L. Prince. 2002. Effects of vitamin D metabolites on intestinal calcium absorption and bone turnover in elderly women. American Journal of Clinical Nutrition 75(2): 283-8.

Dhesi, J. K., S. H. Jackson, L. M. Bearne, C. Moniz, M. V. Hurley, C. G. Swift and T. J. Allain. 2004. Vitamin D supplementation improves neuromuscular function in older people who fall. Age and Ageing 33(6): 589-95.

Diamond, T., P. Smerdely, N. Kormas, R. Sekel, T. Vu and P. Day. 1998. Hip fracture in elderly men: the importance of subclinical vitamin D deficiency and hypogonadism. Medical Journal of Australia 169(3): 138-41.

Diaz, V. A., A. G. Mainous, 3rd, P. J. Carek, A. M. Wessell and C. J. Everett. 2009. The association of vitamin D deficiency and insufficiency with diabetic nephropathy: implications for health disparities. Journal of the American Board of Family Medicine 22(5): 521-7.

Dickinson, J. L., D. I. Perera, A. F. van der Mei, A. L. Ponsonby, A. M. Polanowski, R. J. Thomson, B. V. Taylor, J. D. McKay, J. Stankovich and T. Dwyer. 2009. Past environmental sun exposure and risk of multiple sclerosis: a role for the Cdx-2 vitamin D receptor variant in this interaction. Multiple Sclerosis 15(5): 563-70.

Dietel, M. 2010. Hormone replacement therapy (HRT), breast cancer and tumor pathology. Maturitas 65(3): 183-9.

Dionyssiotis, Y., I. Paspati, G. Trovas, A. Galanos and G. P. Lyritis. 2010. Association of physical exercise and calcium intake with bone mass measured by quantitative ultrasound. BMC Women's Health 10: 12.

Dobnig, H., F. Kainer, V. Stepan, R. Winter, R. Lipp, M. Schaffer, A. Kahr, S. Nocnik, G. Patterer and G. Leb. 1995. Elevated parathyroid hormone-related peptide levels after human gestation: relationship to changes in bone and mineral metabolism. Journal of Clinical Endocrinology and Metabolism 80(12): 3699-707.

Dobnig, H., S. Pilz, H. Scharnagl, W. Renner, U. Seelhorst, B. Wellnitz, J. Kinkeldei, B. O. Boehm, G. Weihrauch and W. Maerz. 2008. Independent association of low serum 25-hydroxyvitamin d and 1,25-dihydroxyvitamin d levels with all-cause and cardiovascular mortality. Archives of Internal Medicine 168(12): 1340-9.

Doppelt, S. H. 1984. Vitamin D, rickets, and osteomalacia. Orthopedic Clinics of North America 15(4): 671-86.

Durazo-Arvizu, R. A., B. Dawson-Hughes, C. T. Sempos, E. A. Yetley, A. C. Looker, G. Cao, S. S. Harris, V. L. Burt, A. L. Carriquiry and M. F. Picciano. 2010. Three-phase model harmonizes estimates of the maximal suppression of parathyroid hormone by 25-hydroxyvitamin D in persons 65 years of age and older. Journal of Nutrition 140(3): 595-9.

Dwyer, T., I. van der Mei, A. L. Ponsonby, B. V. Taylor, J. Stankovich, J. D. McKay, R. J. Thomson, A. M. Polanowski and J. L. Dickinson. 2008. Melanocortin 1 receptor genotype, past environmental sun exposure, and risk of multiple sclerosis. Neurology 71(8): 583-9.

Edderkaoui, B., D. J. Baylink, W. G. Beamer, J. E. Wergedal, R. Porte, A. Chaudhuri and S. Mohan. 2007. Identification of mouse Duffy antigen receptor for chemokines (Darc) as a BMD QTL gene. Genome Research 17(5): 577-85.

Eisman, J. 2010. Is the genomics glass half empty or almost completely empty? International Bone & Mineral Society BoneKEy 27-31.

Elders, P. J., J. C. Netelenbos, P. Lips, F. C. van Ginkel, E. Khoe, O. R. Leeuwenkamp, W. H. Hackeng and P. F. van der Stelt. 1991. Calcium supplementation reduces vertebral bone loss in perimenopausal women: a controlled trial in 248 women between 46 and 55 years of age. Journal of Clinical Endocrinology and Metabolism 73(3): 533-40.

El-Hajj Fuleihan, G., M. Nabulsi, H. Tamim, J. Maalouf, M. Salamoun, H. Khalife, M. Choucair, A. Arabi and R. Vieth. 2006. Effect of vitamin D replacement on musculoskeletal parameters in school children: a randomized controlled trial. Journal of Clinical Endocrinology and Metabolism 91(2): 405-12.

Ellis, K. J., R. J. Shypailo, A. Hergenroeder, M. Perez and S. Abrams. 1996. Total body calcium and bone mineral content: comparison of dual-energy X-ray absorptiometry with neutron activation analysis. Journal of Bone and Mineral Research 11(6): 843-8.

Elzouki, A. Y., T. Markestad, M. Elgarrah, N. Elhoni and L. Aksnes. 1989. Serum concentrations of vitamin D metabolites in rachitic Libyan children. Journal of Pediatric Gastroenterology and Nutrition 9(4): 507-12.

Engelman, C. D., T. E. Fingerlin, C. D. Langefeld, P. J. Hicks, S. S. Rich, L. E. Wagenknecht, D. W. Bowden and J. M. Norris. 2008. Genetic and environmental determinants of 25-hydroxyvitamin D and 1,25-dihydroxyvitamin D levels in Hispanic and African Americans. Journal of Clinical Endocrinology and Metabolism 93(9): 3381-8.

Ensrud, K. E., B. C. Taylor, M. L. Paudel, J. A. Cauley, P. M. Cawthon, S. R. Cummings, H. A. Fink, E. Barrett-Connor, J. M. Zmuda, J. M. Shikany and E. S. Orwoll. 2009. Serum 25-hydroxyvitamin D levels and rate of hip bone loss in older men. Journal of Clinical Endocrinology and Metabolism 94(8): 2773-80.

Erem, C., R. Tanakol, F. Alagol, B. Omer and O. Cetin. 2002. Relationship of bone turnover parameters, endogenous hormones and vit D deficiency to hip fracture in elderly postmenopausal women. International Journal of Clinical Practice 56(5): 333-7.

Eskandari, F., P. E. Martinez, S. Torvik, T. M. Phillips, E. M. Sternberg, S. Mistry, D. Ronsaville, R. Wesley, C. Toomey, N. G. Sebring, J. C. Reynolds, M. R. Blackman, K. A. Calis, P. W. Gold and G. Cizza. 2007. Low bone mass in premenopausal women with depression. Archives of Internal Medicine 167(21): 2329-36.

Evans, K. N., L. Nguyen, J. Chan, B. A. Innes, J. N. Bulmer, M. D. Kilby and M. Hewison. 2006. Effects of 25-hydroxyvitamin D_3 and 1,25-dihydroxyvitamin D_3 on cytokine production by human decidual cells. Biology of Reproduction 75(6): 816-22.

Evers, I. M., H. W. de Valk and G. H. Visser. 2004. Risk of complications of pregnancy in women with type 1 diabetes: nationwide prospective study in the Netherlands. BMJ 328(7445): 915.

Fairweather-Tait, S., A. Prentice, K. G. Heumann, L. M. Jarjou, D. M. Stirling, S. G. Wharf and J. R. Turnlund. 1995. Effect of calcium supplements and stage of lactation on the calcium absorption efficiency of lactating women accustomed to low calcium intakes. American Journal of Clinical Nutrition 62(6): 1188-92.

Farrant, H. J., G. V. Krishnaveni, J. C. Hill, B. J. Boucher, D. J. Fisher, K. Noonan, C. Osmond, S. R. Veena and C. H. Fall. 2009. Vitamin D insufficiency is common in Indian mothers but is not associated with gestational diabetes or variation in newborn size. European Journal of Clinical Nutrition 63(5): 646-52.

Faulkner, K. G., S. R. Cummings, D. Black, L. Palermo, C. C. Gluer and H. K. Genant. 1993. Simple measurement of femoral geometry predicts hip fracture: the study of osteoporotic fractures. Journal of Bone and Mineral Research 8(10): 1211-7.

Faulkner, K. A., J. A. Cauley, J. M. Zmuda, D. P. Landsittel, M. C. Nevitt, A. B. Newman, S. A. Studenski and M. S. Redfern. 2005. Ethnic differences in the frequency and circumstances of falling in older community-dwelling women. Journal of the American Geriatrics Society 53(10): 1774-9.

Faupel-Badger, J. M., L. Diaw, D. Albanes, J. Virtamo, K. Woodson and J. A. Tangrea. 2007. Lack of association between serum levels of 25-hydroxyvitamin D and the subsequent risk of prostate cancer in Finnish men. Cancer Epidemiology, Biomarkers & Prevention 16(12): 2784-6.

Faure, A., B. C. Sutter and B. Billaudel. 1991. Is 1,25-dihydroxyvitamin D_3 the specific vitamin D_3 metabolite active on insulin release and calcium handling by islets from vitamin D_3-deprived rats? Diabete Metabolism 17(2): 271-8.

Fehily, A. M., R. J. Coles, W. D. Evans and P. C. Elwood. 1992. Factors affecting bone density in young adults. American Journal of Clinical Nutrition 56(3): 579-86.

Fentiman, I. S. 2002. 20. Oral contraceptives, hormone replacement therapy and breast cancer. International Journal of Clinical Practice 56(10): 755-9.

Fernell, E. and C. Gillberg. 2010. Autism spectrum disorder diagnoses in Stockholm preschoolers. Research in Developmental Disabilities 31(3): 680-5.

Feron, F., T. H. Burne, J. Brown, E. Smith, J. J. McGrath, A. Mackay-Sim and D. W. Eyles. 2005. Developmental vitamin D_3 deficiency alters the adult rat brain. Brain Research Bulletin 65(2): 141-8.

Finch, S. L., F. Rauch and H. A. Weiler. 2010. Postnatal vitamin D supplementation following maternal dietary vitamin D deficiency does not affect bone mass in weanling guinea pigs. Journal of Nutrition 140(9): 1574-81.

Finkelstein, J. S., M. L. Lee, M. Sowers, B. Ettinger, R. M. Neer, J. L. Kelsey, J. A. Cauley, M. H. Huang and G. A. Greendale. 2002. Ethnic variation in bone density in premenopausal and early perimenopausal women: effects of anthropometric and lifestyle factors. Journal of Clinical Endocrinology and Metabolism 87(7): 3057-67.

Fleet, J. C., S. S. Harris, R. J. Wood and B. Dawson-Hughes. 1995. The BsmI vitamin D receptor restriction fragment length polymorphism (BB) predicts low bone density in premenopausal black and white women. Journal of Bone and Mineral Research 10(6): 985-90.

Flicker, L., R. J. MacInnis, M. S. Stein, S. C. Scherer, K. E. Mead, C. A. Nowson, J. Thomas, C. Lowndes, J. L. Hopper and J. D. Wark. 2005. Should older people in residential care receive vitamin D to prevent falls? Results of a randomized trial. Journal of the American Geriatrics Society 53(11): 1881-8.

Fomon, S. J. and S. E. Nelson. 1993. Calcium, phosphorus, magnesium, and sulfur. In *Nutrition of Normal Infants*, edited by S. J. Fomon. St. Louis: Mosby-Year Book, Inc. Pp. 192-216.

Ford, J. A., D. C. Davidson, W. B. McIntosh, W. M. Fyfe and M. G. Dunnigan. 1973. Neonatal rickets in Asian immigrant population. British Medical Journal 3(5873): 211-2.

Forman, J. P., E. Giovannucci, M. D. Holmes, H. A. Bischoff-Ferrari, S. S. Tworoger, W. C. Willett and G. C. Curhan. 2007. Plasma 25-hydroxyvitamin D levels and risk of incident hypertension. Hypertension 49(5): 1063-9.

Foroud, T., S. Ichikawa, D. Koller, D. Lai, L. Curry, X. Xuei, H. J. Edenberg, S. Hui, M. Peacock and M. J. Econs. 2008. Association studies of ALOX5 and bone mineral density in healthy adults. Osteoporosis International 19(5): 637-43.

Fox, K. M., J. Magaziner, R. Sherwin, J. C. Scott, C. C. Plato, M. Nevitt and S. Cummings. 1993. Reproductive correlates of bone mass in elderly women. Study of Osteoporotic Fractures Research Group. Journal of Bone and Mineral Research 8(8): 901-8.

Francis, R. M., I. T. Boyle, C. Moniz, A. M. Sutcliffe, B. S. Davis, G. H. Beastall, R. A. Cowan and N. Downes. 1996. A comparison of the effects of alfacalcidol treatment and vitamin D₂ supplementation on calcium absorption in elderly women with vertebral fractures. Osteoporosis International 6(4): 284-90.

Frankel, B. J., J. Sehlin and I. B. Taljedal. 1985. Vitamin D₃ stimulates calcium-45 uptake by isolated mouse islets in vitro. Acta Physiologica Scandinavica 123(1): 61-6.

Fraser, W. D., A. M. Ahmad and J. P. Vora. 2004. The physiology of the circadian rhythm of parathyroid hormone and its potential as a treatment for osteoporosis. Current Opinion in Nephrology and Hypertension 13(4): 437-44.

Freedman, D. M., A. C. Looker, S. C. Chang and B. I. Graubard. 2007. Prospective study of serum vitamin D and cancer mortality in the United States. Journal of the National Cancer Institute 99(21): 1594-602.

Freedman, D. M., S. C. Chang, R. T. Falk, M. P. Purdue, W. Y. Huang, C. A. McCarty, B. W. Hollis, B. I. Graubard, C. D. Berg and R. G. Ziegler. 2008. Serum levels of vitamin D metabolites and breast cancer risk in the prostate, lung, colorectal, and ovarian cancer screening trial. Cancer Epidemiology, Biomarkers & Prevention 17(4): 889-94.

Frolich, A., M. Rudnicki, T. Storm, N. Rasmussen and L. Hegedus. 1992. Impaired 1,25-dihydroxyvitamin D production in pregnancy-induced hypertension. European Journal of Obstetrics, Gynecology, and Reproductive Biology 47(1): 25-9.

Fudge, N. J., J. P. Woodrow and C. S. Kovacs. 2006. Pregnancy rescues low bone mass and normalizes intestinal calcium absorption in Vdr null mice. Journal of Bone and Mineral Research 21(S1): S52.

Fudge, N. J. and C. S. Kovacs. 2010. Pregnancy up-regulates intestinal calcium absorption and skeletal mineralization independently of the vitamin D receptor. Endocrinology 151(3): 886-95.

Gale, C. R., S. M. Robinson, N. C. Harvey, M. K. Javaid, B. Jiang, C. N. Martyn, K. M. Godfrey and C. Cooper. 2008. Maternal vitamin D status during pregnancy and child outcomes. European Journal of Clinical Nutrition 62(1): 68-77.

Garabedian, M., M. Vainsel, E. Mallet, H. Guillozo, M. Toppet, R. Grimberg, T. M. Nguyen and S. Balsan. 1983. Circulating vitamin D metabolite concentrations in children with nutritional rickets. Journal of Pediatrics 103(3): 381-6.

Garcion, E., S. Nataf, A. Berod, F. Darcy and P. Brachet. 1997. 1,25-dihydroxyvitamin D₃ inhibits the expression of inducible nitric oxide synthase in rat central nervous system during experimental allergic encephalomyelitis. Brain Research. Molecular Brain Research 45(2): 255-67.

Garn, S. M. 1972. The course of bone gain and the phases of bone loss. Orthopedic Clinics of North America 3(3): 503-20.

Gerdhem, P., K. A. Ringsberg, K. J. Obrant and K. Akesson. 2005. Association between 25-hydroxy vitamin D levels, physical activity, muscle strength and fractures in the prospective population-based OPRA Study of Elderly Women. Osteoporosis International 16(11): 1425-31.

Gertner, J. M., D. R. Coustan, A. S. Kliger, L. E. Mallette, N. Ravin and A. E. Broadus. 1986. Pregnancy as state of physiologic absorptive hypercalciuria. American Journal of Medicine 81(3): 451-6.

Ghannam, N. N., M. M. Hammami, S. M. Bakheet and B. A. Khan. 1999. Bone mineral density of the spine and femur in healthy Saudi females: relation to vitamin D status, pregnancy, and lactation. Calcified Tissue International 65(1): 23-8.

Ghishan, F. K., J. T. Jenkins and M. K. Younoszai. 1980. Maturation of calcium transport in the rat small and large intestine. Journal of Nutrition 110(8): 1622-8.

Ghishan, F. K., P. Parker, S. Nichols and A. Hoyumpa. 1984. Kinetics of intestinal calcium transport during maturation in rats. Pediatric Research 18(3): 235-9.

Gibney, K. B., L. MacGregor, K. Leder, J. Torresi, C. Marshall, P. R. Ebeling and B. A. Biggs. 2008. Vitamin D deficiency is associated with tuberculosis and latent tuberculosis infection in immigrants from sub-Saharan Africa. Clinical Infectious Diseases 46(3): 443-6.

Gilsanz, V., T. F. Roe, S. Mora, G. Costin and W. G. Goodman. 1991. Changes in vertebral bone density in black girls and white girls during childhood and puberty. New England Journal of Medicine 325(23): 1597-600.

Giovannucci, E., E. B. Rimm, A. Wolk, A. Ascherio, M. J. Stampfer, G. A. Colditz and W. C. Willett. 1998. Calcium and fructose intake in relation to risk of prostate cancer. Cancer Research 58(3): 442-7.

Giovannucci, E., Y. Liu, E. B. Rimm, B. W. Hollis, C. S. Fuchs, M. J. Stampfer and W. C. Willett. 2006. Prospective study of predictors of vitamin D status and cancer incidence and mortality in men. Journal of the National Cancer Institute 98(7): 451-9.

Giovannucci, E., Y. Liu, B. W. Hollis and E. B. Rimm. 2008. 25-hydroxyvitamin D and risk of myocardial infarction in men: a prospective study. Archives of Internal Medicine 168(11): 1174-80.

Giulietti, A., C. Gysemans, K. Stoffels, E. van Etten, B. Decallonne, L. Overbergh, R. Bouillon and C. Mathieu. 2004. Vitamin D deficiency in early life accelerates Type 1 diabetes in non-obese diabetic mice. Diabetologia 47(3): 451-62.

Givens, M. H. and I. G. Macy. 1933. The chemical composition of the human fetus. Journal of Biological Chemistry 102(1): 7-17.

Gloth, F. M., 3rd, W. Alam and B. Hollis. 1999. Vitamin D vs broad spectrum phototherapy in the treatment of seasonal affective disorder. Journal of Nutrition, Health, and Aging 3(1): 5-7.

Gong, G. and G. Haynatzki. 2003. Association between bone mineral density and candidate genes in different ethnic populations and its implications. Calcified Tissue International 72(2): 113-23.

Gong, G., G. Haynatzki, V. Haynatzka, S. Kosoko-Lasaki, R. Howell, Y. X. Fu, J. C. Gallagher and M. R. Wilson. 2006. Bone mineral density of recent African immigrants in the United States. Journal of the National Medical Association 98(5): 746-52.

Gordis, L. 2009. Epidemiology, 4th Edition. Philadelphia, PA: Saunders Elsevier.

Graafmans, W. C., M. E. Ooms, H. M. Hofstee, P. D. Bezemer, L. M. Bouter and P. Lips. 1996. Falls in the elderly: a prospective study of risk factors and risk profiles. American Journal of Epidemiology 143(11): 1129-36.

Grados, F., M. Brazier, S. Kamel, S. Duver, N. Heurtebize, M. Maamer, M. Mathieu, M. Garabedian, J. L. Sebert and P. Fardellone. 2003a. Effects on bone mineral density of calcium and vitamin D supplementation in elderly women with vitamin D deficiency. Joint, Bone, Spine: Revue du Rhumatisme 70(3): 203-8.

Grados, F., M. Brazier, S. Kamel, M. Mathieu, N. Hurtebize, M. Maamer, M. Garabedian, J. L. Sebert and P. Fardellone. 2003b. Prediction of bone mass density variation by bone remodeling markers in postmenopausal women with vitamin D insufficiency treated with calcium and vitamin D supplementation. Journal of Clinical Endocrinology and Metabolism 88(11): 5175-9.

Graff, M., T. D. Thacher, P. R. Fischer, D. Stadler, S. D. Pam, J. M. Pettifor, C. O. Isichei and S. A. Abrams. 2004. Calcium absorption in Nigerian children with rickets. American Journal of Clinical Nutrition 80(5): 1415-21.

Grant, A. M., A. Avenell, M. K. Campbell, A. M. McDonald, G. S. MacLennan, G. C. McPherson, F. H. Anderson, C. Cooper, R. M. Francis, C. Donaldson, W. J. Gillespie, C. M. Robinson, D. J. Torgerson and W. A. Wallace. 2005. Oral vitamin D_3 and calcium for secondary prevention of low-trauma fractures in elderly people (Randomised Evaluation of Calcium Or vitamin D, RECORD): a randomised placebo-controlled trial. Lancet 365(9471): 1621-8.

Greer, F. R., J. E. Searcy, R. S. Levin, J. J. Steichen, P. S. Steichen-Asche and R. C. Tsang. 1982. Bone mineral content and serum 25-hydroxyvitamin D concentrations in breast-fed infants with and without supplemental vitamin D: one-year follow-up. Journal of Pediatrics 100(6): 919-22.

Greer, F. R., J. Lane and M. Ho. 1984. Elevated serum parathyroid hormone, calcitonin, and 1,25-dihydroxyvitamin D in lactating women nursing twins. American Journal of Clinical Nutrition 40(3): 562-8.

Greer, F. R. and S. Marshall. 1989. Bone mineral content, serum vitamin D metabolite concentrations, and ultraviolet B light exposure in infants fed human milk with and without vitamin D_2 supplements. Journal of Pediatrics 114(2): 204-12.

Grossman, H., C. Bergmann and S. Parker. 2006. Dementia: a brief review. Mount Sinai Journal of Medicine 73(7): 985-92.

Guillemant, J., P. Taupin, H. T. Le, N. Taright, A. Allemandou, G. Peres and S. Guillemant. 1999. Vitamin D status during puberty in French healthy male adolescents. Osteoporosis International 10(3): 222-5.

Gundberg, C. M., A. C. Looker, S. D. Nieman and M. S. Calvo. 2002. Patterns of osteocalcin and bone specific alkaline phosphatase by age, gender, and race or ethnicity. Bone 31(6): 703-8.

Gysemans, C., E. van Etten, L. Overbergh, A. Giulietti, G. Eelen, M. Waer, A. Verstuyf, R. Bouillon and C. Mathieu. 2008. Unaltered diabetes presentation in NOD mice lacking the vitamin D receptor. Diabetes 57(1): 269-75.

Haddad, J. G., Jr., V. Boisseau and L. V. Avioli. 1971. Placental transfer of vitamin D_3 and 25-hydroxycholecalciferol in the rat. Journal of Laboratory and Clinical Medicine 77(6): 908-15.

Halloran, B. P., E. N. Barthell and H. F. DeLuca. 1979. Vitamin D metabolism during pregnancy and lactation in the rat. Proceedings of the National Academy of Sciences of the United States of America 76(11): 5549-53.

Halloran, B. P. and H. F. DeLuca. 1979. Vitamin D deficiency and reproduction in rats. Science 204(4388): 73-4.

Halloran, B. P. and H. F. DeLuca. 1980a. Calcium transport in small intestine during pregnancy and lactation. American Journal of Physiology 239(1): E64-8.

Halloran, B. P. and H. F. DeLuca. 1980b. Skeletal changes during pregnancy and lactation: the role of vitamin D. Endocrinology 107(6): 1923-9.

Halloran, B. P. and H. F. DeLuca. 1980c. Calcium transport in small intestine during early development: role of vitamin D. American Journal of Physiology 239(6): G473-9.

Halloran, B. P. and H. F. De Luca. 1981. Effect of vitamin D deficiency on skeletal development during early growth in the rat. Archives of Biochemistry and Biophysics 209(1): 7-14.

Han, Z. H., S. Palnitkar, D. S. Rao, D. Nelson and A. M. Parfitt. 1996. Effect of ethnicity and age or menopause on the structure and geometry of iliac bone. Journal of Bone and Mineral Research 11(12): 1967-75.

Han, Z. H., S. Palnitkar, D. S. Rao, D. Nelson and A. M. Parfitt. 1997. Effects of ethnicity and age or menopause on the remodeling and turnover of iliac bone: implications for mechanisms of bone loss. Journal of Bone and Mineral Research 12(4): 498-508.

Hanahan, D. and R. A. Weinberg. 2000. The hallmarks of cancer. Cell 100(1): 57-70.

Hanlon, J. T., L. R. Landerman, G. G. Fillenbaum and S. Studenski. 2002. Falls in African American and white community-dwelling elderly residents. Journals of Gerontology. Series A, Biological Sciences and Medical Sciences 57(7): M473-8.

Hansen, K. E., A. N. Jones, M. J. Lindstrom, L. A. Davis, J. A. Engelke and M. M. Shafer. 2008. Vitamin D insufficiency: disease or no disease? Journal of Bone and Mineral Research 23(7): 1052-60.

Harkness, L. and B. Cromer. 2005. Low levels of 25-hydroxy vitamin D are associated with elevated parathyroid hormone in healthy adolescent females. Osteoporosis International 16(1): 109-13.

Harms, L. R., D. W. Eyles, J. J. McGrath, A. Mackay-Sim and T. H. Burne. 2008. Developmental vitamin D deficiency alters adult behaviour in 129/SvJ and C57BL/6J mice. Behavioural Brain Research 187(2): 343-50.

Harris, D. M. and V. L. Go. 2004. Vitamin D and colon carcinogenesis. Journal of Nutrition 134(12 Suppl): 3463S-71S.

Harris, R. P., M. Helfand, S. H. Woolf, K. N. Lohr, C. D. Mulrow, S. M. Teutsch and D. Atkins. 2001. Current methods of the US Preventive Services Task Force: a review of the process. American Journal of Preventive Medicine 20(3 Suppl): 21-35.

Harris, S. and B. Dawson-Hughes. 1993. Seasonal mood changes in 250 normal women. Psychiatry Research 49(1): 77-87.

Harris, S. S., T. R. Eccleshall, C. Gross, B. Dawson-Hughes and D. Feldman. 1997. The vitamin D receptor start codon polymorphism (FokI) and bone mineral density in premenopausal American black and white women. Journal of Bone and Mineral Research 12(7): 1043-8.

Harris, S. S., E. Soteriades, J. A. Coolidge, S. Mudgal and B. Dawson-Hughes. 2000. Vitamin D insufficiency and hyperparathyroidism in a low income, multiracial, elderly population. Journal of Clinical Endocrinology and Metabolism 85(11): 4125-30.

Harris, S. S., E. Soteriades and B. Dawson-Hughes. 2001. Secondary hyperparathyroidism and bone turnover in elderly blacks and whites. Journal of Clinical Endocrinology and Metabolism 86(8): 3801-4.

Harwood, R. H., O. Sahota, K. Gaynor, T. Masud and D. J. Hosking. 2004. A randomised, controlled comparison of different calcium and vitamin D supplementation regimens in elderly women after hip fracture: The Nottingham Neck of Femur (NONOF) Study. Age and Ageing 33(1): 45-51.

Hatton, D. C., H. Xue, J. A. DeMerritt and D. A. McCarron. 1994. 1,25(OH)2 vitamin D_3-induced alterations in vascular reactivity in the spontaneously hypertensive rat. American Journal of the Medical Sciences 307 (Suppl 1): S154-8.

Haugen, M., A. L. Brantsaeter, L. Trogstad, J. Alexander, C. Roth, P. Magnus and H. M. Meltzer. 2009. Vitamin D supplementation and reduced risk of preeclampsia in nulliparous women. Epidemiology 20(5): 720-6.

Hawa, M. I., M. G. Valorani, L. R. Buckley, P. E. Beales, A. Afeltra, F. Cacciapaglia, R. D. Leslie and P. Pozzilli. 2004. Lack of effect of vitamin D administration during pregnancy and early life on diabetes incidence in the non-obese diabetic mouse. Hormone and Metabolic Research 36(9): 620-4.

Hayes, D. P. 2009. Influenza pandemics, solar activity cycles, and vitamin D. Medical Hypotheses 74(5): 831-4.

Heaney, R. P. and T. G. Skillman. 1971. Calcium metabolism in normal human pregnancy. Journal of Clinical Endocrinology and Metabolism 33(4): 661-70.

Heaney, R. P., R. R. Recker and P. D. Saville. 1977. Calcium balance and calcium requirements in middle-aged women. American Journal of Clinical Nutrition 30(10): 1603-11.

Heaney, R. P., R. R. Recker and P. D. Saville. 1978. Menopausal changes in calcium balance performance. Journal of Laboratory and Clinical Medicine 92(6): 953-63.

Heaney, R. P., M. S. Dowell, C. A. Hale and A. Bendich. 2003. Calcium absorption varies within the reference range for serum 25-hydroxyvitamin D. Journal of the American College of Nutrition 22(2): 142-6.

Heaney, R. P. 2005. The vitamin D requirement in health and disease. Journal of Steroid Biochemistry and Molecular Biology 97(1-2): 13-9.

Herndon, A. C., C. DiGuiseppi, S. L. Johnson, J. Leiferman and A. Reynolds. 2009. Does nutritional intake differ between children with autism spectrum disorders and children with typical development? Journal of Autism and Developmental Disorders 39(2): 212-22.

Herran, A., J. A. Amado, M. T. Garcia-Unzueta, J. L. Vazquez-Barquero, L. Perera and J. Gonzalez-Macias. 2000. Increased bone remodeling in first-episode major depressive disorder. Psychosomatic Medicine 62(6): 779-82.

Hiller, J. E., C. A. Crowther, V. A. Moore, K. Willson and J. S. Robinson. 2007. Calcium supplementation in pregnancy and its impact on blood pressure in children and women: follow up of a randomised controlled trial. Australian and New Zealand Journal of Obstetrics and Gynaecology 47(2): 115-21.

Hillman, L. S., E. Slatopolsky and J. G. Haddad. 1978. Perinatal vitamin D metabolism. IV. Maternal and cord serum 24,25-dihydroxyvitamin D concentrations. Journal of Clinical Endocrinology and Metabolism 47(5): 1073-7.

Hillman, L., S. Sateesha, M. Haussler, W. Wiest, E. Slatopolsky and J. Haddad. 1981. Control of mineral homeostasis during lactation: interrelationships of 25-hydroxyvitamin D, 24,25-dihydroxyvitamin D, 1,25-dihydroxyvitamin D, parathyroid hormone, calcitonin, prolactin, and estradiol. American Journal of Obstetrics and Gynecology 139(4): 471-6.

Hochberg, Z., D. Tiosano and L. Even. 1992. Calcium therapy for calcitriol-resistant rickets. Journal of Pediatrics 121(5 Pt 1): 803-8.

Hodsman, A. B., D. A. Hanley, P. H. Watson and L. J. Fraher. 2002. Parathyroid hormone. In Principles of Bone Biology, edited by J. P. Bilezikian, L. G. Raisz and G. A. Rodan. New York: Academic Press. Pp. 1305-24.

Hoenderop, J. G., O. Dardenne, M. Van Abel, A. W. Van Der Kemp, C. H. Van Os, R. St-Arnaud and R. J. Bindels. 2002. Modulation of renal Ca2+ transport protein genes by dietary Ca2+ and 1,25-dihydroxyvitamin D_3 in 25-hydroxyvitamin D_3-1alpha-hydroxylase knockout mice. FASEB Journal 16(11): 1398-406.

Hofmeyr, G. J., A. N. Atallah and L. Duley. 2006. Calcium supplementation during pregnancy for preventing hypertensive disorders and related problems. Cochrane Database System Review 3: CD001059.

Hofmeyr, G. J., L. Duley and A. Atallah. 2007. Dietary calcium supplementation for prevention of pre-eclampsia and related problems: a systematic review and commentary. British Journal of Obstetrics and Gynaecology 114(8): 933-43.

Hoikka, V., E. M. Alhava, K. Savolainen and M. Parviainen. 1982. Osteomalacia in fractures of the proximal femur. Acta Orthopaedica Scandinavica 53(2): 255-60.

Holick, M. F., E. S. Siris, N. Binkley, M. K. Beard, A. Khan, J. T. Katzer, R. A. Petruschke, E. Chen and A. E. de Papp. 2005. Prevalence of vitamin D inadequacy among postmenopausal North American women receiving osteoporosis therapy. Journal of Clinical Endocrinology and Metabolism 90(6): 3215-24.

Hollis, B. W. and C. L. Wagner. 2004. Vitamin D requirements during lactation: high-dose maternal supplementation as therapy to prevent hypovitaminosis D for both the mother and the nursing infant. American Journal of Clinical Nutrition 80(Suppl 6): 1752S-8S.

Holt, P. R., N. Arber, B. Halmos, K. Forde, H. Kissileff, K. A. McGlynn, S. F. Moss, N. Kurihara, K. Fan, K. Yang and M. Lipkin. 2002. Colonic epithelial cell proliferation decreases with increasing levels of serum 25-hydroxy vitamin D. Cancer Epidemiology, Biomarkers & Prevention 11(1): 113-9.

Hoogendijk, W. J., P. Lips, M. G. Dik, D. J. Deeg, A. T. Beekman and B. W. Penninx. 2008. Depression is associated with decreased 25-hydroxyvitamin D and increased parathyroid hormone levels in older adults. Archives of General Psychiatry 65(5): 508-12.

Hsia, J., G. Heiss, H. Ren, M. Allison, N. C. Dolan, P. Greenland, S. R. Heckbert, K. C. Johnson, J. E. Manson, S. Sidney and M. Trevisan. 2007. Calcium/vitamin D supplementation and cardiovascular events. Circulation 115(7): 846-54.

Huisman, A. M., K. P. White, A. Algra, M. Harth, R. Vieth, J. W. Jacobs, J. W. Bijlsma and D. A. Bell. 2001. Vitamin D levels in women with systemic lupus erythematosus and fibromyalgia. Journal of Rheumatology 28(11): 2535-9.

Humble, M. B., S. Gustafsson and S. Bejerot. 2010. Low serum levels of 25-hydroxyvitamin D (25-OHD) among psychiatric out-patients in Sweden: relations with season, age, ethnic origin and psychiatric diagnosis. Journal of Steroid Biochemistry and Molecular Biology 121(1-2): 467-70.

Huncharek, M., J. Muscat and B. Kupelnick. 2008. Dairy products, dietary calcium and vitamin D intake as risk factors for prostate cancer: a meta-analysis of 26,769 cases from 45 observational studies. Nutrition and Cancer 60(4): 421-41.

Hunt, C. D. and L. K. Johnson. 2007. Calcium requirements: new estimations for men and women by cross–sectional statistical analyses of calcium balance data from metabolic studies. American Journal of Clinical Nutrition 86(4): 1054-63.

Hunter, D., P. Major, N. Arden, R. Swaminathan, T. Andrew, A. J. MacGregor, R. Keen, H. Snieder and T. D. Spector. 2000. A randomized controlled trial of vitamin D supplementation on preventing postmenopausal bone loss and modifying bone metabolism using identical twin pairs. Journal of Bone and Mineral Research 15(11): 2276-83.

Hypponen, E., U. Sovio, M. Wjst, S. Patel, J. Pekkanen, A. L. Hartikainen and M. R. Jarvelinb. 2004. Infant vitamin d supplementation and allergic conditions in adulthood: northern Finland birth cohort 1966. Annals of the New York Academy of Sciences 1037: 84-95.

Hypponen, E., A. L. Hartikainen, U. Sovio, M. R. Jarvelin and A. Pouta. 2007. Does vitamin D supplementation in infancy reduce the risk of pre-eclampsia? European Journal of Clinical Nutrition 61(9): 1136-9.

IARC (International Agency for Research on Cancer). 1992. Monographs on the Evaluation of Carcinogenic Risks to Humans, Volume 55, Solar and Ultraviolet Radiation. Lyon: World Health Organization.

IARC (International Agency for Research on Cancer). 2008. Vitamin D and Cancer. IARC Working Group Reports, Volume 5. Lyon: World Health Organization.

Innes, A. M., M. M. Seshia, C. Prasad, S. Al Saif, F. R. Friesen, A. E. Chudley, M. Reed, L. A. Dilling, J. C. Haworth and C. R. Greenberg. 2002. Congenital rickets caused by maternal vitamin D deficiency. Paediatric Child Health 7(7): 455-8.

Inui, N., A. Murayama, S. Sasaki, T. Suda, K. Chida, S. Kato and H. Nakamura. 2001. Correlation between 25-hydroxyvitamin D_3 1 alpha-hydroxylase gene expression in alveolar macrophages and the activity of sarcoidosis. American Journal of Medicine 110(9): 687-93.

IOM. 1997. *Dietary Reference Intakes for Calcium, Phosphorus, Magnesium, Vitamin D, and Fluoride.* Washington, DC, National Academy Press.

Isaia, G., R. Giorgino and S. Adami. 2001. High prevalence of hypovitaminosis D in female type 2 diabetic population. Diabetes Care 24(8): 1496.

Israni, N., R. Goswami, A. Kumar and R. Rani. 2009. Interaction of vitamin D receptor with HLA DRB1 0301 in type 1 diabetes patients from North India. PLoS One 4(12): e8023.

Ito, M., H. Koyama, A. Ohshige, T. Maeda, T. Yoshimura and H. Okamura. 1994. Prevention of preeclampsia with calcium supplementation and vitamin D_3 in an antenatal protocol. International Journal of Gynaecology and Obstetrics 47(2): 115-20.

Jackson, R. D., A. Z. LaCroix, M. Gass, R. B. Wallace, J. Robbins, C. E. Lewis, T. Bassford, S. A. Beresford, H. R. Black, P. Blanchette, D. E. Bonds, R. L. Brunner, R. G. Brzyski, B. Caan, J. A. Cauley, R. T. Chlebowski, S. R. Cummings, I. Granek, J. Hays, G. Heiss, S. L. Hendrix, B. V. Howard, J. Hsia, F. A. Hubbell, K. C. Johnson, H. Judd, J. M. Kotchen, L. H. Kuller, R. D. Langer, N. L. Lasser, M. C. Limacher, S. Ludlam, J. E. Manson, K. L. Margolis, J. McGowan, J. K. Ockene, M. J. O'Sullivan, L. Phillips, R. L. Prentice, G. E. Sarto, M. L. Stefanick, L. Van Horn, J. Wactawski-Wende, E. Whitlock, G. L. Anderson, A. R. Assaf and D. Barad. 2006. Calcium plus vitamin D supplementation and the risk of fractures. New England Journal of Medicine 354(7): 669-83.

Jadad, A. R., R. A. Moore, D. Carroll, C. Jenkinson, D. J. M. Reynolds, D. J. Gavaghan and H. J. McQuay. 1996. Assessing the quality of reports of randomized clinical trials: is blinding necessary? Controlled Clinical Trials 17(1): 1-12.

Jahnsen, J., J. A. Falch, P. Mowinckel and E. Aadland. 2002. Vitamin D status, parathyroid hormone and bone mineral density in patients with inflammatory bowel disease. Scandinavian Journal of Gastroenterology 37(2): 192-9.

Jarjou, L. M., A. Prentice, Y. Sawo, M. A. Laskey, J. Bennett, G. R. Goldberg and T. J. Cole. 2006. Randomized, placebo-controlled, calcium supplementation study in pregnant Gambian women: effects on breast-milk calcium concentrations and infant birth weight, growth, and bone mineral accretion in the first year of life. American Journal of Clinical Nutrition 83(3): 657-66.

Jarjou, L. M., M. A. Laskey, Y. Sawo, G. R. Goldberg, T. J. Cole and A. Prentice. 2010. Effect of calcium supplementation in pregnancy on maternal bone outcomes in women with a low calcium intake. American Journal of Clinical Nutrition 92(2): 450-7.

Javaid, M. K., S. R. Crozier, N. C. Harvey, C. R. Gale, E. M. Dennison, B. J. Boucher, N. K. Arden, K. M. Godfrey and C. Cooper. 2006. Maternal vitamin D status during pregnancy and childhood bone mass at age 9 years: a longitudinal study. Lancet 367(9504): 36-43.

Jenab, M., H. B. Bueno-de-Mesquita, P. Ferrari, F. J. van Duijnhoven, T. Norat, T. Pischon, E. H. Jansen, N. Slimani, G. Byrnes, S. Rinaldi, A. Tjonneland, A. Olsen, K. Overvad, M. C. Boutron-Ruault, F. Clavel-Chapelon, S. Morois, R. Kaaks, J. Linseisen, H. Boeing, M. M. Bergmann, A. Trichopoulou, G. Misirli, D. Trichopoulos, F. Berrino, P. Vineis, S. Panico, D. Palli, R. Tumino, M. M. Ros, C. H. van Gils, P. H. Peeters, M. Brustad, E. Lund, M. J. Tormo, E. Ardanaz, L. Rodriguez, M. J. Sanchez, M. Dorronsoro, C. A. Gonzalez, G. Hallmans, R. Palmqvist, A. Roddam, T. J. Key, K. T. Khaw, P. Autier, P. Hainaut and E. Riboli. 2010. Association between pre-diagnostic circulating vitamin D concentration and risk of colorectal cancer in European populations: a nested case–control study. BMJ 340: b5500.

Jenkins, D. H., J. G. Roberts, D. Webster and E. O. Williams. 1973. Osteomalacia in elderly patients with fracture of the femoral neck. A clinico-pathological study. Journal of Bone and Joint Surgery. British Volume 55(3): 575-80.

Jensen, C., L. Holloway, G. Block, G. Spiller, G. Gildengorin, E. Gunderson, G. Butterfield and R. Marcus. 2002. Long-term effects of nutrient intervention on markers of bone remodeling and calciotropic hormones in late-postmenopausal women. American Journal of Clinical Nutrition 75(6): 1114-20.

Johnston, C. C., Jr., J. Z. Miller, C. W. Slemenda, T. K. Reister, S. Hui, J. C. Christian and M. Peacock. 1992. Calcium supplementation and increases in bone mineral density in children. New England Journal of Medicine 327(2): 82-7.

Jorde, R., M. Sneve, Y. Figenschau, J. Svartberg and K. Waterloo. 2008. Effects of vitamin D supplementation on symptoms of depression in overweight and obese subjects: randomized double blind trial. Journal of Internal Medicine 264(6): 599-609.

Jorde, R., M. Sneve, P. Torjesen and Y. Figenschau. 2010. No improvement in cardiovascular risk factors in overweight and obese subjects after supplementation with vitamin D₃ for 1 year. Journal of Internal Medicine 267(5): 462-72.

Kalkwarf, H. J., B. L. Specker, J. E. Heubi, N. E. Vieira and A. L. Yergey. 1996. Intestinal calcium absorption of women during lactation and after weaning. American Journal of Clinical Nutrition 63(4): 526-31.

Kalkwarf, H. J., B. L. Specker, D. C. Bianchi, J. Ranz and M. Ho. 1997. The effect of calcium supplementation on bone density during lactation and after weaning. New England Journal of Medicine 337(8): 523-8.

Kalkwarf, H. J. 1999. Hormonal and dietary regulation of changes in bone density during lactation and after weaning in women. Journal of Mammary Gland Biology and Neoplasia 4(3): 319-29.

Kalkwarf, H. J., B. S. Zemel, V. Gilsanz, J. M. Lappe, M. Horlick, S. Oberfield, S. Mahboubi, B. Fan, M. M. Frederick, K. Winer and J. A. Shepherd. 2007. The bone mineral density in childhood study: bone mineral content and density according to age, sex, and race. Journal of Clinical Endocrinology and Metabolism 92(6): 2087-99.

Kamen, D. L., G. S. Cooper, H. Bouali, S. R. Shaftman, B. W. Hollis and G. S. Gilkeson. 2006. Vitamin D deficiency in systemic lupus erythematosus. Autoimmune Reviews 5(2): 114-7.

Karakelides, H., J. L. Geller, A. L. Schroeter, H. Chen, P. S. Behn, J. S. Adams, M. Hewison and R. A. Wermers. 2006. Vitamin D-mediated hypercalcemia in slack skin disease: evidence for involvement of extrarenal 25-hydroxyvitamin D 1alpha-hydroxylase. Journal of Bone and Mineral Research 21(9): 1496-9.

Kaur, M., D. Pearson, I. Godber, N. Lawson, P. Baker and D. Hosking. 2003. Longitudinal changes in bone mineral density during normal pregnancy. Bone 32(4): 449-54.

Kent, G. N., R. I. Price, D. H. Gutteridge, M. Smith, J. R. Allen, C. I. Bhagat, M. P. Barnes, C. J. Hickling, R. W. Retallack, S. G. Wilson and et al. 1990. Human lactation: forearm trabecular bone loss, increased bone turnover, and renal conservation of calcium and inorganic phosphate with recovery of bone mass following weaning. Journal of Bone and Mineral Research 5(4): 361-9.

Kent, G. N., R. I. Price, D. H. Gutteridge, K. J. Rosman, M. Smith, J. R. Allen, C. J. Hickling and S. L. Blakeman. 1991. The efficiency of intestinal calcium absorption is increased in late pregnancy but not in established lactation. Calcified Tissue International 48(4): 293-5.

Kinyamu, H. K., J. C. Gallagher, K. A. Rafferty and K. E. Balhorn. 1998. Dietary calcium and vitamin D intake in elderly women: effect on serum parathyroid hormone and vitamin D metabolites. American Journal of Clinical Nutrition 67(2): 342-8.

Kitanaka, S., K. Takeyama, A. Murayama, T. Sato, K. Okumura, M. Nogami, Y. Hasegawa, H. Niimi, J. Yanagisawa, T. Tanaka and S. Kato. 1998. Inactivating mutations in the 25-hydroxyvitamin D₃ 1alpha-hydroxylase gene in patients with pseudovitamin D-deficiency rickets. New England Journal of Medicine 338(10): 653-61.

Kivineva, M., M. Blauer, H. Syvala, T. Tammela and P. Tuohimaa. 1998. Localization of 1,25-dihydroxyvitamin D₃ receptor (VDR) expression in human prostate. Journal of Steroid Biochemistry and Molecular Biology 66(3): 121-7.

Kleerekoper, M., D. A. Nelson, E. L. Peterson, M. J. Flynn, A. S. Pawluszka, G. Jacobsen and P. Wilson. 1994. Reference data for bone mass, calciotropic hormones, and biochemical markers of bone remodeling in older (55-75) postmenopausal white and black women. Journal of Bone and Mineral Research 9(8): 1267-76.

Ko, P., R. Burkert, J. McGrath and D. Eyles. 2004. Maternal vitamin D₃ deprivation and the regulation of apoptosis and cell cycle during rat brain development. Brain Research. Developmental Brain Research 153(1): 61-8.

Koeffler, H. P., H. Reichel, J. E. Bishop and A. W. Norman. 1985. gamma-Interferon stimulates production of 1,25-dihydroxyvitamin D$_3$ by normal human macrophages. Biochemical and Biophysical Research Communications 127(2): 596-603.

Koller, D. L., M. J. Econs, P. A. Morin, J. C. Christian, S. L. Hui, P. Parry, M. E. Curran, L. A. Rodriguez, P. M. Conneally, G. Joslyn, M. Peacock, C. C. Johnston and T. Foroud. 2000. Genome screen for QTLs contributing to normal variation in bone mineral density and osteoporosis. Journal of Clinical Endocrinology and Metabolism 85(9): 3116-20.

Komulainen, M. H., H. Kroger, M. T. Tuppurainen, A. M. Heikkinen, E. Alhava, R. Honkanen and S. Saarikoski. 1998. HRT and vit D in prevention of non-vertebral fractures in postmenopausal women; a 5 year randomized trial. Maturitas 31(1): 45-54.

Koo, W. and R. Tsang. 1997. Calcium, magnesium, phosphorus, and vitamin D. In Nutrition During Infancy, 2nd Edition, edited by Cincinnati: Digital Education. Pp. 175-89.

Koo, W. W., J. C. Walters, J. Esterlitz, R. J. Levine, A. J. Bush and B. Sibai. 1999. Maternal calcium supplementation and fetal bone mineralization. Obstetrics and Gynecology 94(4): 577-82.

Kovacs, C. S. and C. L. Chik. 1995. Hyperprolactinemia caused by lactation and pituitary adenomas is associated with altered serum calcium, phosphate, parathyroid hormone (PTH), and PTH-related peptide levels. Journal of Clinical Endocrinology and Metabolism 80(10): 3036-42.

Kovacs, C. S. and H. M. Kronenberg. 1997. Maternal-fetal calcium and bone metabolism during pregnancy, puerperium, and lactation. Endocrine Reviews 18(6): 832-72.

Kovacs, C. S. 2005. Calcium and bone metabolism during pregnancy and lactation. Journal of Mammary Gland Biology and Neoplasia 10(2): 105-18.

Kovacs, C. S., M. L. Woodland, N. J. Fudge and J. K. Friel. 2005. The vitamin D receptor is not required for fetal mineral homeostasis or for the regulation of placental calcium transfer in mice. American Journal of Physiology Endocrinology Metabolism 289(1): E133-44.

Kovacs, C. S. and H. Fuleihan Gel. 2006. Calcium and bone disorders during pregnancy and lactation. Endocrinology and Metabolism Clinics of North America 35(1): 21-51, v.

Kovacs, C. S. 2008. Vitamin D in pregnancy and lactation: maternal, fetal, and neonatal outcomes from human and animal studies. American Journal of Clinical Nutrition 88(2): 520S-8S.

Kovacs, C. S. and H. M. Kronenberg. 2008. Pregnancy and lactation. In Primer on the Metabolic Bone Diseases and Disorders of Mineral Metabolism, 7th Edition, edited by C. J. Rosen. Washington, DC: ASBMR Press. Pp. 90-5.

Kovalenko, P. L., Z. Zhang, M. Cui, S. K. Clinton and J. C. Fleet. 2010. 1,25 dihydroxyvitamin D-mediated orchestration of anticancer, transcript-level effects in the immortalized, non-transformed prostate epithelial cell line, RWPE1. BMC Genomics 11: 26.

Krall, E. A., N. Sahyoun, S. Tannenbaum, G. E. Dallal and B. Dawson-Hughes. 1989. Effect of vitamin D intake on seasonal variations in parathyroid hormone secretion in postmenopausal women. New England Journal of Medicine 321(26): 1777-83.

Krause, R., M. Buhring, W. Hopfenmuller, M. F. Holick and A. M. Sharma. 1998. Ultraviolet B and blood pressure. Lancet 352(9129): 709-10.

Krishnan, A. V., R. Shinghal, N. Raghavachari, J. D. Brooks, D. M. Peehl and D. Feldman. 2004. Analysis of vitamin D-regulated gene expression in LNCaP human prostate cancer cells using cDNA microarrays. Prostate 59(3): 243-51.

Kumar, A., S. G. Devi, S. Batra, C. Singh and D. K. Shukla. 2009. Calcium supplementation for the prevention of pre-eclampsia. International Journal of Gynaecology and Obstetrics 104(1): 32-6.

Kyriazopoulos, P., G. Trovas, J. Charopoulos, E. Antonogiannakis, A. Galanos and G. Lyritis. 2006. Lifestyle factors and forearm bone density in young Greek men. Clinical Endocrinology 65(2): 234-8.

Lachenmaier-Currle, U. and J. Harmeyer. 1989. Placental transport of calcium and phosphorus in pigs. Journal of Perinatal Medicine 17(2): 127-36.

Lacroix, A. Z., J. Kotchen, G. Anderson, R. Brzyski, J. A. Cauley, S. R. Cummings, M. Gass, K. C. Johnson, M. Ko, J. Larson, J. E. Manson, M. L. Stefanick and J. Wactawski-Wende. 2009. Calcium plus vitamin D supplementation and mortality in postmenopausal women: the Women's Health Initiative Calcium-Vitamin D Randomized Controlled Trial. Journals of Gerontology. Series A, Biological Sciences and Medical Sciences 64(5): 559-67.

Lalau, J. D., I. Jans, N. el Esper, R. Bouillon and A. Fournier. 1993. Calcium metabolism, plasma parathyroid hormone, and calcitriol in transient hypertension of pregnancy. American Journal of Hypertension 6(6 Pt 1): 522-7.

Landin-Wilhelmsen, K., L. Wilhelmsen and B. A. Bengtsson. 1999. Postmenopausal osteoporosis is more related to hormonal aberrations than to lifestyle factors. Clinical Endocrinology 51(4): 387-94.

Lansdowne, A. T. and S. C. Provost. 1998. Vitamin D_3 enhances mood in healthy subjects during winter. Psychopharmacology 135(4): 319-23.

Lappe, J. M., K. M. Davies, D. Travers-Gustafson and R. P. Heaney. 2006. Vitamin D status in a rural postmenopausal female population. Journal of the American College of Nutrition 25(5): 395-402.

Lappe, J. M., D. Travers-Gustafson, K. M. Davies, R. R. Recker and R. P. Heaney. 2007. Vitamin D and calcium supplementation reduces cancer risk: results of a randomized trial. American Journal of Clinical Nutrition 85(6): 1586-91.

Lappe, J., D. Cullen, G. Haynatzki, R. Recker, R. Ahlf and K. Thompson. 2008. Calcium and vitamin d supplementation decreases incidence of stress fractures in female navy recruits. Journal of Bone and Mineral Research 23(5): 741-9.

Larsen, E. R., L. Mosekilde and A. Foldspang. 2004. Vitamin D and calcium supplementation prevents osteoporotic fractures in elderly community dwelling residents: a pragmatic population-based 3-year intervention study. Journal of Bone and Mineral Research 19(3): 370-8.

Larsen, E. R., L. Mosekilde and A. Foldspang. 2005. Vitamin D and calcium supplementation prevents severe falls in elderly community-dwelling women: a pragmatic population-based 3-year intervention study. Aging Clinical Experimental Research 17(2): 125-32.

Laskey, M. A., A. Prentice, L. A. Hanratty, L. M. Jarjou, B. Dibba, S. R. Beavan and T. J. Cole. 1998. Bone changes after 3 mo of lactation: influence of calcium intake, breast-milk output, and vitamin D-receptor genotype. American Journal of Clinical Nutrition 67(4): 685-92.

Latham, N. K., C. S. Anderson, A. Lee, D. A. Bennett, A. Moseley and I. D. Cameron. 2003. A randomized, controlled trial of quadriceps resistance exercise and vitamin D in frail older people: the Frailty Interventions Trial in Elderly Subjects (FITNESS). Journal of the American Geriatrics Society 51(3): 291-9.

Lau, E. M., J. Woo, R. Swaminathan, D. MacDonald and S. P. Donnan. 1989. Plasma 25-hydroxyvitamin D concentration in patients with hip fracture in Hong Kong. Gerontology 35(4): 198-204.

Law, M., H. Withers, J. Morris and F. Anderson. 2006. Vitamin D supplementation and the prevention of fractures and falls: results of a randomised trial in elderly people in residential accommodation. Age and Ageing 35(5): 482-6.

LeBoff, M. S., L. Kohlmeier, S. Hurwitz, J. Franklin, J. Wright and J. Glowacki. 1999. Occult vitamin D deficiency in postmenopausal US women with acute hip fracture. JAMA 281(16): 1505-11.

Lee, D. M., A. Tajar, A. Ulubaev, N. Pendleton, T. W. O'Neill, D. B. O'Connor, G. Bartfai, S. Boonen, R. Bouillon, F. F. Casanueva, J. D. Finn, G. Forti, A. Giwercman, T. S. Han, I. T. Huhtaniemi, K. Kula, M. E. J. Lean, M. Punab, A. J. Silman, D. Vanderschueren, F. C. W. Wu and Emas study group. 2009. Association between 25-hydroxyvitamin D levels and cognitive performance in middle-aged and older European men. Journal of Neurology, Neurosurgery and Psychiatry 80(7): 722-9.

Lee, L., S. A. Kang, H. O. Lee, B. H. Lee, J. S. Park, J. H. Kim, I. K. Jung, Y. J. Park and J. E. Lee. 2001. Relationships between dietary intake and cognitive function level in Korean elderly people. Public Health 115(2): 133-8.

Lee, W. T., S. S. Leung, D. M. Leung and J. C. Cheng. 1996. A follow-up study on the effects of calcium-supplement withdrawal and puberty on bone acquisition of children. American Journal of Clinical Nutrition 64(1): 71-7.

Leffelaar, E. R., T. G. Vrijkotte and M. van Eijsden. 2010. Maternal early pregnancy vitamin D status in relation to fetal and neonatal growth: results of the multi-ethnic Amsterdam Born Children and their Development cohort. British Journal of Nutrition 104(1): 108-17.

Lehtonen-Veromaa, M. K., T. T. Mottonen, I. O. Nuotio, K. M. Irjala, A. E. Leino and J. S. Viikari. 2002. Vitamin D and attainment of peak bone mass among peripubertal Finnish girls: a 3-y prospective study. American Journal of Clinical Nutrition 76(6): 1446-53.

Leitch, I. and F. C. Aitken. 1959. The estimation of calcium requirement: a re-examination. Nutrition Abstracts and Reviews. Series A: Human and Experimental 29(2): 393-411.

Lemire, J. M., A. Ince and M. Takashima. 1992. 1,25-dihydroxyvitamin D_3 attenuates the expression of experimental murine lupus of MRL/1 mice. Autoimmunity 12(2): 143-8.

Levis, S., A. Gomez, C. Jimenez, L. Veras, F. Ma, S. Lai, B. Hollis and B. A. Roos. 2005. Vitamin D deficiency and seasonal variation in an adult South Florida population. Journal of Clinical Endocrinology and Metabolism 90(3): 1557-62.

Li, J. Y., B. L. Specker, M. L. Ho and R. C. Tsang. 1989. Bone mineral content in black and white children 1 to 6 years of age. Early appearance of race and sex differences. American Journal of Diseases of Children 143(11): 1346-9.

Li, Y. C., A. E. Pirro, M. Amling, G. Delling, R. Baron, R. Bronson and M. B. Demay. 1997. Targeted ablation of the vitamin D receptor: an animal model of vitamin D-dependent rickets type II with alopecia. Proceedings of the National Academy of Sciences of the United States of America 94(18): 9831-5.

Li, Y. C., M. Amling, A. E. Pirro, M. Priemel, J. Meuse, R. Baron, G. Delling and M. B. Demay. 1998. Normalization of mineral ion homeostasis by dietary means prevents hyperparathyroidism, rickets, and osteomalacia, but not alopecia in vitamin D receptor-ablated mice. Endocrinology 139(10): 4391-6.

Li, Y. C., G. Qiao, M. Uskokovic, W. Xiang, W. Zheng and J. Kong. 2004. Vitamin D: a negative endocrine regulator of the renin-angiotensin system and blood pressure. Journal of Steroid Biochemistry and Molecular Biology 89-90(1-5): 387-92.

Linday, L. A., R. D. Shindledecker, J. N. Dolitsky, T. C. Chen and M. F. Holick. 2008. Plasma 25-hydroxyvitamin D levels in young children undergoing placement of tympanostomy tubes. Annals of Otology, Rhinology and Laryngology 117(10): 740-4.

Li-Ng, M., J. F. Aloia, S. Pollack, B. A. Cunha, M. Mikhail, J. Yeh and N. Berbari. 2009. A randomized controlled trial of vitamin D_3 supplementation for the prevention of symptomatic upper respiratory tract infections. Epidemiology and Infection 137(10): 1396-404.

Lips, P., J. C. Netelenbos, M. J. Jongen, F. C. van Ginkel, A. L. Althuis, C. L. van Schaik, W. J. van der Vijgh, J. P. Vermeiden and C. van der Meer. 1982. Histomorphometric profile and vitamin D status in patients with femoral neck fracture. Metabolic Bone Disease and Related Research 4(2): 85-93.

Lips, P., W. H. Hackeng, M. J. Jongen, F. C. van Ginkel and J. C. Netelenbos. 1983. Seasonal variation in serum concentrations of parathyroid hormone in elderly people. Journal of Clinical Endocrinology and Metabolism 57(1): 204-6.

Lips, P., F. C. van Ginkel, M. J. Jongen, F. Rubertus, W. J. van der Vijgh and J. C. Netelenbos. 1987. Determinants of vitamin D status in patients with hip fracture and in elderly control subjects. American Journal of Clinical Nutrition 46(6): 1005-10.

Lips, P., W. C. Graafmans, M. E. Ooms, P. D. Bezemer and L. M. Bouter. 1996. Vitamin D supplementation and fracture incidence in elderly persons. A randomized, placebo-controlled clinical trial. Annals of Internal Medicine 124(4): 400-6.

Litonjua, A. A. and S. T. Weiss. 2007. Is vitamin D deficiency to blame for the asthma epidemic? Journal of Allergy and Clinical Immunology 120(5): 1031-5.

Liu, P. T., S. Stenger, H. Li, L. Wenzel, B. H. Tan, S. R. Krutzik, M. T. Ochoa, J. Schauber, K. Wu, C. Meinken, D. L. Kamen, M. Wagner, R. Bals, A. Steinmeyer, U. Zugel, R. L. Gallo, D. Eisenberg, M. Hewison, B. W. Hollis, J. S. Adams, B. R. Bloom and R. L. Modlin. 2006. Toll-like receptor triggering of a vitamin D-mediated human antimicrobial response. Science 311(5768): 1770-3.

Liu, S., Y. Song, E. S. Ford, J. E. Manson, J. E. Buring and P. M. Ridker. 2005. Dietary calcium, vitamin D, and the prevalence of metabolic syndrome in middle-aged and older U.S. women. Diabetes Care 28(12): 2926-32.

Llewellyn, D. J., K. M. Langa and I. A. Lang. 2009. Serum 25-hydroxyvitamin D concentration and cognitive impairment. Journal of Geriatric Psychiatry and Neurology 22(3): 188-95.

Lloyd, T., M. B. Andon, N. Rollings, J. K. Martel, R. Landis, L. M. Demers, D. F. Eggli, K. Kieselhorst and H. E. Kulin. 1993. Calcium supplementation and bone mineral density in adolescent girls. Journal of the American Medical Association 270: 841-4.

Lobaugh, B., A. Boass, G. E. Lester and S. U. Toverud. 1990. Regulation of serum 1,25-dihydroxyvitamin D_3 in lactating rats. American Journal of Physiology 259(5 Pt 1): E665-71.

Lobaugh, B., A. Boass, S. C. Garner and S. U. Toverud. 1992. Intensity of lactation modulates renal 1 alpha-hydroxylase and serum 1,25(OH)2D in rats. American Journal of Physiology 262(6 Pt 1): E840-4.

Looker, A. C. and M. E. Mussolino. 2008. Serum 25-hydroxyvitamin D and hip fracture risk in older U.S. white adults. Journal of Bone and Mineral Research 23(1): 143-50.

Looker, A. C., L. J. Melton, 3rd, T. Harris, L. Borrud, J. Shepherd and J. McGowan. 2009. Age, gender, and race/ethnic differences in total body and subregional bone density. Osteoporosis International 20(7): 1141-9.

Lu, P. W., J. N. Briody, G. D. Ogle, K. Morley, I. R. Humphries, J. Allen, R. Howman-Giles, D. Sillence and C. T. Cowell. 1994. Bone mineral density of total body, spine, and femoral neck in children and young adults: A cross-sectional and longitudinal study. Journal of Bone and Mineral Research 9(9): 1451-8.

Luckey, M. M., D. E. Meier, J. P. Mandeli, M. C. DaCosta, M. L. Hubbard and S. J. Goldsmith. 1989. Radial and vertebral bone density in white and black women: evidence for racial differences in premenopausal bone homeostasis. Journal of Clinical Endocrinology and Metabolism 69(4): 762-70.

Lund, B., O. H. Sorensen and A. B. Christensen. 1975. 25-hydroxycholecaliferol and fractures of the proximal. Lancet 2(7929): 300-2.

Lynch, M. F., I. J. Griffin, K. M. Hawthorne, Z. Chen, M. Hamzo and S. A. Abrams. 2007. Calcium balance in 1-4-y-old children. American Journal of Clinical Nutrition 85(3): 750-4.

Lyons, R. A., A. Johansen, S. Brophy, R. G. Newcombe, C. J. Phillips, B. Lervy, R. Evans, K. Wareham and M. D. Stone. 2007. Preventing fractures among older people living in institutional care: a pragmatic randomised double blind placebo controlled trial of vitamin D supplementation. Osteoporosis International 18(6): 811-8.

Mahon, P., N. Harvey, S. Crozier, H. Inskip, S. Robinson, N. Arden, R. Swaminathan, C. Cooper and K. Godfrey. 2010. Low maternal vitamin D status and fetal bone development: cohort study. Journal of Bone and Mineral Research 25(1): 14-9.

Majid Molla, A., M. H. Badawi, S. al-Yaish, P. Sharma, R. S. el-Salam and A. M. Molla. 2000. Risk factors for nutritional rickets among children in Kuwait. Pediatrics International 42(3): 280-4.

Major, G. C., F. Alarie, J. Dore, S. Phouttama and A. Tremblay. 2007. Supplementation with calcium + vitamin D enhances the beneficial effect of weight loss on plasma lipid and lipoprotein concentrations. American Journal of Clinical Nutrition 85(1): 54-9.

Malabanan, A., I. E. Veronikis and M. F. Holick. 1998. Redefining vitamin D insufficiency. Lancet 351(9105): 805-6.

Mallet, E., B. Gugi, P. Brunelle, A. Henocq, J. P. Basuyau and H. Lemeur. 1986. Vitamin D supplementation in pregnancy: a controlled trial of two methods. Obstetrics and Gynecology 68(3): 300-4.

Malloy, P. J., T. R. Eccleshall, C. Gross, L. Van Maldergem, R. Bouillon and D. Feldman. 1997. Hereditary vitamin D resistant rickets caused by a novel mutation in the vitamin D receptor that results in decreased affinity for hormone and cellular hyporesponsiveness. Journal of Clinical Investigation 99(2): 297-304.

Manson, J. E., M. A. Allison, J. J. Carr, R. D. Langer, B. B. Cochrane, S. L. Hendrix, J. Hsia, J. R. Hunt, C. E. Lewis, K. L. Margolis, J. G. Robinson, R. J. Rodabough and A. M. Thomas. 2010. Calcium/vitamin D supplementation and coronary artery calcification in the Women's Health Initiative. Menopause 17(4): 683-91.

Margolis, K. L., R. M. Ray, L. Van Horn, J. E. Manson, M. A. Allison, H. R. Black, S. A. Beresford, S. A. Connelly, J. D. Curb, R. H. Grimm, Jr., T. A. Kotchen, L. H. Kuller, S. Wassertheil-Smoller, C. A. Thomson and J. C. Torner. 2008. Effect of calcium and vitamin D supplementation on blood pressure: the Women's Health Initiative Randomized Trial. Hypertension 52(5): 847-55.

Marie, P. J., L. Cancela, N. Le Boulch and L. Miravet. 1986. Bone changes due to pregnancy and lactation: influence of vitamin D status. American Journal of Physiology 251(4 Pt 1): E400-6.

Marjamaki, L., S. Niinisto, M. G. Kenward, L. Uusitalo, U. Uusitalo, M. L. Ovaskainen, C. Kronberg-Kippila, O. Simell, R. Veijola, J. Ilonen, M. Knip and S. M. Virtanen. 2010. Maternal intake of vitamin D during pregnancy and risk of advanced beta cell autoimmunity and type 1 diabetes in offspring. Diabetologia 53(8): 1599-607.

Markestad, T., S. Halvorsen, K. S. Halvorsen, L. Aksnes and D. Aarskog. 1984. Plasma concentrations of vitamin D metabolites before and during treatment of vitamin D deficiency rickets in children. Acta Paediatrica Scandinavica 73(2): 225-31.

Marniemi, J., E. Alanen, O. Impivaara, R. Seppanen, P. Hakala, T. Rajala and T. Ronnemaa. 2005. Dietary and serum vitamins and minerals as predictors of myocardial infarction and stroke in elderly subjects. Nutrition, Metabolism, and Cardiovascular Diseases 15(3): 188-97.

Martineau, A. R., F. U. Honecker, R. J. Wilkinson and C. J. Griffiths. 2007a. Vitamin D in the treatment of pulmonary tuberculosis. Journal of Steroid Biochemistry and Molecular Biology 103(3-5): 793-8.

Martineau, A. R., R. J. Wilkinson, K. A. Wilkinson, S. M. Newton, B. Kampmann, B. M. Hall, G. E. Packe, R. N. Davidson, S. M. Eldridge, Z. J. Maunsell, S. J. Rainbow, J. L. Berry and C. J. Griffiths. 2007b. A single dose of vitamin D enhances immunity to mycobacteria. American Journal of Respiratory and Critical Care Medicine 176(2): 208-13.

Maruotti, N. and F. P. Cantatore. 2010. Vitamin D and the immune system. Journal of Rheumatology 37(3): 491-5.

Marwaha, R. K., N. Tandon, D. R. Reddy, R. Aggarwal, R. Singh, R. C. Sawhney, B. Saluja, M. A. Ganie and S. Singh. 2005. Vitamin D and bone mineral density status of healthy schoolchildren in northern India. American Journal of Clinical Nutrition 82(2): 477-82.

Marya, R. K., S. Rathee, V. Lata and S. Mudgil. 1981. Effects of vitamin D supplementation in pregnancy. Gynecologic and Obstetric Investigation 12(3): 155-61.

Marya, R. K., S. Rathee and M. Manrow. 1987. Effect of calcium and vitamin D supplementation on toxaemia of pregnancy. Gynecologic and Obstetric Investigation 24(1): 38-42.

Marya, R. K., S. Rathee, V. Dua and K. Sangwan. 1988. Effect of vitamin D supplementation during pregnancy on foetal growth. Indian Journal of Medical Research 88: 488-92.

Matkovic, V., J. D. Landoll, N. E. Badenhop-Stevens, E. Y. Ha, Z. Crncevic-Orlic, B. Li and P. Goel. 2004. Nutrition influences skeletal development from childhood to adulthood: a study of hip, spine, and forearm in adolescent females. Journal of Nutrition 134(3): 701S-5S.

Matthews, D., E. Laporta, G. M. Zinser, C. J. Narvaez and J. Welsh. 2010. Genomic vitamin D signaling in breast cancer: Insights from animal models and human cells. Journal of Steroid Biochemistry and Molecular Biology 121(1-2): 362-7.

Mattila, C., P. Knekt, S. Mannisto, H. Rissanen, M. A. Laaksonen, J. Montonen and A. Reunanen. 2007. Serum 25-hydroxyvitamin D concentration and subsequent risk of type 2 diabetes. Diabetes Care 30(10): 2569-70.

Mattson, M. P. 2007. Calcium and neurodegeneration. Aging Cell 6(3): 337-50.

Maxwell, J. D., L. Ang, O. G. Brooke and I. R. Brown. 1981. Vitamin D supplements enhance weight gain and nutritional status in pregnant Asians. British Journal of Obstetrics and Gynaecology 88(10): 987-91.

Maxwell, J. P. and L. M. Miles. 1925. Osteomalacia in China. Proceedings of the Royal Society of Medicine 18: 48-66.

McCann, J. C. and B. N. Ames. 2008. Is there convincing biological or behavioral evidence linking vitamin D deficiency to brain dysfunction? FASEB Journal 22(4): 982-1001.

McCarthy, D., P. Duggan, M. O'Brien, M. Kiely, J. McCarthy, F. Shanahan and K. D. Cashman. 2005. Seasonality of vitamin D status and bone turnover in patients with Crohn's disease. Alimentary Pharmacology and Therapeutics 21(9): 1073-83.

McCullough, M. L., C. Rodriguez, W. R. Diver, H. S. Feigelson, V. L. Stevens, M. J. Thun and E. E. Calle. 2005. Dairy, calcium, and vitamin D intake and postmenopausal breast cancer risk in the Cancer Prevention Study II Nutrition Cohort. Cancer Epidemiology, Biomarkers & Prevention 14(12): 2898-904.

McGill, A. T., J. M. Stewart, F. E. Lithander, C. M. Strik and S. D. Poppitt. 2008. Relationships of low serum vitamin D_3 with anthropometry and markers of the metabolic syndrome and diabetes in overweight and obesity. Nutrition Journal 7: 4.

McGrath, J. J., F. P. Feron, T. H. Burne, A. Mackay-Sim and D. W. Eyles. 2004. Vitamin D_3-implications for brain development. Journal of Steroid Biochemistry and Molecular Biology 89-90(1-5): 557-60.

McGrath, J., R. Scragg, D. Chant, D. Eyles, T. Burne and D. Obradovic. 2007. No association between serum 25-hydroxyvitamin D_3 level and performance on psychometric tests in NHANES III. Neuroepidemiology 29(1-2): 49-54.

McKay, J. D., M. L. McCullough, R. G. Ziegler, P. Kraft, B. S. Saltzman, E. Riboli, A. Barricarte, C. D. Berg, G. Bergland, S. Bingham, M. Brustad, H. B. Bueno-de-Mesquita, L. Burdette, J. Buring, E. E. Calle, S. J. Chanock, F. Clavel-Chapelon, D. G. Cox, L. Dossus, H. S. Feigelson, C. A. Haiman, S. E. Hankinson, R. N. Hoover, D. J. Hunter, A. Husing, R. Kaaks, L. N. Kolonel, L. Le Marchand, J. Linseisen, C. A. McCarty, K. Overvad, S. Panico, M. P. Purdue, D. O. Stram, V. L. Stevens, D. Trichopoulos, W. C. Willett, J. Yuenger and M. J. Thun. 2009. Vitamin D receptor polymorphisms and breast cancer risk: results from the National Cancer Institute Breast and Prostate Cancer Cohort Consortium. Cancer Epidemiology, Biomarkers & Prevention 18(1): 297-305.

Meehan, T. F. and H. F. DeLuca. 2002. The vitamin D receptor is necessary for 1alpha,25-dihydroxyvitamin D(3) to suppress experimental autoimmune encephalomyelitis in mice. Archives of Biochemistry and Biophysics 408(2): 200-4.

Meier, C., H. W. Woitge, K. Witte, B. Lemmer and M. J. Seibel. 2004. Supplementation with oral vitamin D_3 and calcium during winter prevents seasonal bone loss: a randomized controlled open-label prospective trial. Journal of Bone and Mineral Research 19(8): 1221-30.

Meier, D. E., M. M. Luckey, S. Wallenstein, T. L. Clemens, E. S. Orwoll and C. I. Waslien. 1991. Calcium, vitamin D, and parathyroid hormone status in young white and black women: association with racial differences in bone mass. Journal of Clinical Endocrinology and Metabolism 72(3): 703-10.

Meier, D. E., M. M. Luckey, S. Wallenstein, R. H. Lapinski and B. Catherwood. 1992. Racial differences in pre- and postmenopausal bone homeostasis: association with bone density. Journal of Bone and Mineral Research 7(10): 1181-9.

Melamed, M. L., P. Muntner, E. D. Michos, J. Uribarri, C. Weber, J. Sharma and P. Raggi. 2008. Serum 25-hydroxyvitamin D levels and the prevalence of peripheral arterial disease: results from NHANES 2001 to 2004. Arteriosclerosis, Thrombosis, and Vascular Biology 28(6): 1179-85.

Melhus, H., G. Snellman, R. Gedeborg, L. Byberg, L. Berglund, H. Mallmin, P. Hellman, R. Blomhoff, E. Hagstrom, J. Arnlov and K. Michaelsson. 2010. Plasma 25-hydroxyvitamin D levels and fracture risk in a community-based cohort of elderly men in Sweden. Journal of Clinical Endocrinology and Metabolism 95(6): 2637-45.

Melin, A., J. Wilske, H. Ringertz and M. Saaf. 2001. Seasonal variations in serum levels of 25-hydroxyvitamin D and parathyroid hormone but no detectable change in femoral neck bone density in an older population with regular outdoor exposure. Journal of the American Geriatrics Society 49(9): 1190-6.

Melton, I. L., M. A. Marquez, S. J. Achenbach, A. Tefferi, M. K. O'Connor, W. M. O'Fallon and B. L. Riggs. 2002. Variations in bone density among persons of African heritage. Osteoporosis International 13(7): 551-9.

Merewood, A., S. D. Mehta, T. C. Chen, H. Bauchner and M. F. Holick. 2009. Association between vitamin D deficiency and primary cesarean section. Journal of Clinical Endocrinology and Metabolism 94(3): 940-5.

Merlino, L. A., J. Curtis, T. R. Mikuls, J. R. Cerhan, L. A. Criswell and K. G. Saag. 2004. Vitamin D intake is inversely associated with rheumatoid arthritis: results from the Iowa Women's Health Study. Arthritis & Rheumatism 50(1): 72-7.

Michelson, D., C. Stratakis, L. Hill, J. Reynolds, E. Galliven, G. Chrousos and P. Gold. 1996. Bone mineral density in women with depression. New England Journal of Medicine 335(16): 1176-81.

Miller, S. C., B. P. Halloran, H. F. DeLuca and W. S. Jee. 1982. Role of vitamin D in maternal skeletal changes during pregnancy and lactation: a histomorphometric study. Calcified Tissue International 34(3): 245-52.

Miller, S. C., B. P. Halloran, H. F. DeLuca and W. S. Jee. 1983. Studies on the role of vitamin D in early skeletal development, mineralization, and growth in rats. Calcified Tissue International 35(4-5): 455-60.

Minasyan, A., T. Keisala, Y. R. Lou, A. V. Kalueff and P. Tuohimaa. 2007. Neophobia, sensory and cognitive functions, and hedonic responses in vitamin D receptor mutant mice. Journal of Steroid Biochemistry and Molecular Biology 104(3-5): 274-80.

Miyake, Y., S. Sasaki, K. Tanaka and Y. Hirota. 2009. Dairy food, calcium, and vitamin D intake in pregnancy and wheeze and eczema in infants. European Respiratory Journal 35(6): 1128-34.

Mohr, S. B., C. F. Garland, E. D. Gorham and F. C. Garland. 2008. The association between ultraviolet B irradiance, vitamin D status and incidence rates of type 1 diabetes in 51 regions worldwide. Diabetologia 51(8): 1391-8.

Moncrieff, M. and T. O. Fadahunsi. 1974. Congenital rickets due to maternal vitamin D deficiency. Archives of Disease in Childhood 49(10): 810-1.

Monkawa, T., T. Yoshida, M. Hayashi and T. Saruta. 2000. Identification of 25-hydroxyvitamin D_3 1alpha-hydroxylase gene expression in macrophages. Kidney International 58(2): 559-68.

Moore, T. B., H. P. Koeffler, J. M. Yamashiro and R. K. Wada. 1996. Vitamin D_3 analogs inhibit growth and induce differentiation in LA-N-5 human neuroblastoma cells. Clinical and Experimental Metastasis 14(3): 239-45.

More, C., P. Bettembuk, H. P. Bhattoa and A. Balogh. 2001. The effects of pregnancy and lactation on bone mineral density. Osteoporosis International 12(9): 732-7.

Morley, R., J. B. Carlin, J. A. Pasco and J. D. Wark. 2006. Maternal 25-hydroxyvitamin D and parathyroid hormone concentrations and offspring birth size. Journal of Clinical Endocrinology and Metabolism 91(3): 906-12.

Moschonis, G. and Y. Manios. 2006. Skeletal site-dependent response of bone mineral density and quantitative ultrasound parameters following a 12-month dietary intervention using dairy products fortified with calcium and vitamin D: the Postmenopausal Health Study. British Journal of Nutrition 96(6): 1140-8.

Muller, K., N. J. Kriegbaum, B. Baslund, O. H. Sorensen, M. Thymann and K. Bentzen. 1995. Vitamin D_3 metabolism in patients with rheumatic diseases: low serum levels of 25-hydroxyvitamin D_3 in patients with systemic lupus erythematosus. Clinical Rheumatology 14(4): 397-400.

Munger, K. L., L. I. Levin, B. W. Hollis, N. S. Howard and A. Ascherio. 2006. Serum 25-hydroxyvitamin D levels and risk of multiple sclerosis. Journal of the American Medical Association 296(23): 2832-8.

Nagpal, J., J. N. Pande and A. Bhartia. 2009. A double-blind, randomized, placebo-controlled trial of the short-term effect of vitamin D_3 supplementation on insulin sensitivity in apparently healthy, middle-aged, centrally obese men. Diabetic Medicine 26(1): 19-27.

Namgung, R., R. C. Tsang, C. Lee, D. G. Han, M. L. Ho and R. I. Sierra. 1998. Low total body bone mineral content and high bone resorption in Korean winter-born versus summer-born newborn infants. Journal of Pediatrics 132(3 Pt 1): 421-5.

Narod, S. A. 2006. Modifiers of risk of hereditary breast cancer. Oncogene 25(43): 5832-6.

Naveilhan, P., I. Neveu, D. Wion and P. Brachet. 1996. 1,25-dihydroxyvitamin D_3, an inducer of glial cell line-derived neurotrophic factor. Neuroreport 7(13): 2171-5.

Naylor, K. E., P. Iqbal, C. Fledelius, R. B. Fraser and R. Eastell. 2000. The effect of pregnancy on bone density and bone turnover. Journal of Bone and Mineral Research 15(1): 129-37.

Need, A. G. and P. J. Phillips. 1979. Pulmonary tuberculosis and hypercalcaemia. Annals of Internal Medicine 91(4): 652-3.

Need, A. G., P. D. O'Loughlin, H. A. Morris, P. S. Coates, M. Horowitz and B. E. Nordin. 2008. Vitamin D metabolites and calcium absorption in severe vitamin D deficiency. Journal of Bone and Mineral Research 23(11): 1859-63.

Nelson, D. A., G. Jacobsen, D. A. Barondess and A. M. Parfitt. 1995. Ethnic differences in regional bone density, hip axis length, and lifestyle variables among healthy black and white men. Journal of Bone and Mineral Research 10(5): 782-7.

Nelson, D. A., P. M. Simpson, C. C. Johnson, D. A. Barondess and M. Kleerekoper. 1997. The accumulation of whole body skeletal mass in third- and fourth-grade children: effects of age, gender, ethnicity, and body composition. Bone 20(1): 73-8.

Nelson, D. A., D. A. Barondess, S. L. Hendrix and T. J. Beck. 2000. Cross–sectional geometry, bone strength, and bone mass in the proximal femur in black and white postmenopausal women. Journal of Bone and Mineral Research 15(10): 1992-7.

Nelson, D. A., J. M. Pettifor, D. A. Barondess, D. D. Cody, K. Uusi-Rasi and T. J. Beck. 2004. Comparison of cross–sectional geometry of the proximal femur in white and black women from Detroit and Johannesburg. Journal of Bone and Mineral Research 19(4): 560-5.

Newmark, H. L., K. Yang, N. Kurihara, K. Fan, L. H. Augenlicht and M. Lipkin. 2009. Western-style diet-induced colonic tumors and their modulation by calcium and vitamin D in C57Bl/6 mice: a preclinical model for human sporadic colon cancer. Carcinogenesis 30(1): 88-92.

Nnoaham, K. E. and A. Clarke. 2008. Low serum vitamin D levels and tuberculosis: a systematic review and meta-analysis. International Journal of Epidemiology 37(1): 113-9.

Noff, D. and S. Edelstein. 1978. Vitamin D and its hydroxylated metabolites in the rat. Placental and lacteal transport, subsequent metabolic pathways and tissue distribution. Hormone Research 9(5): 292-300.

Norman, A. W., J. B. Frankel, A. M. Heldt and G. M. Grodsky. 1980. Vitamin D deficiency inhibits pancreatic secretion of insulin. Science 209(4458): 823-5.

Nwaru, B. I., S. Ahonen, M. Kaila, M. Erkkola, A. M. Haapala, C. Kronberg-Kippila, R. Veijola, J. Ilonen, O. Simell, M. Knip and S. M. Virtanen. 2010. Maternal diet during pregnancy and allergic sensitization in the offspring by 5 yrs of age: a prospective cohort study. Pediatric Allergy and Immunology 21(1 Pt 1): 29-37.

Obradovic, D., H. Gronemeyer, B. Lutz and T. Rein. 2006. Cross-talk of vitamin D and glucocorticoids in hippocampal cells. Journal of Neurochemistry 96(2): 500-9.

O'Brien, K. O., M. S. Nathanson, J. Mancini and F. R. Witter. 2003. Calcium absorption is significantly higher in adolescents during pregnancy than in the early postpartum period. American Journal of Clinical Nutrition 78(6): 1188-93.

O'Brien, K. O., C. M. Donangelo, C. L. Zapata, S. A. Abrams, E. M. Spencer and J. C. King. 2006. Bone calcium turnover during pregnancy and lactation in women with low calcium diets is associated with calcium intake and circulating insulin-like growth factor 1 concentrations. American Journal of Clinical Nutrition 83(2): 317-23.

Oginni, L. M., M. Worsfold, O. A. Oyelami, C. A. Sharp, D. E. Powell and M. W. Davie. 1996. Etiology of rickets in Nigerian children. Journal of Pediatrics 128(5 Pt 1): 692-4.

Okonofua, F., R. K. Menon, S. Houlder, M. Thomas, D. Robinson, S. O'Brien and P. Dandona. 1986. Parathyroid hormone and neonatal calcium homeostasis: evidence for secondary hyperparathyroidism in the Asian neonate. Metabolism 35(9): 803-6.

Okonofua, F., R. K. Menon, S. Houlder, M. Thomas, D. Robinson, S. O'Brien and P. Dandona. 1987. Calcium, vitamin D and parathyroid hormone relationships in pregnant Caucasian and Asian women and their neonates. Annals of Clinical Biochemistry 24(Pt 1): 22-8.

Olausson, H., M. A. Laskey, G. R. Goldberg and A. Prentice. 2008. Changes in bone mineral status and bone size during pregnancy and the influences of body weight and calcium intake. American Journal of Clinical Nutrition 88(4): 1032-9.

Ooms, M. E., P. Lips, J. C. Roos, W. J. van der Vijgh, C. Popp-Snijders, P. D. Bezemer and L. M. Bouter. 1995a. Vitamin D status and sex hormone binding globulin: determinants of bone turnover and bone mineral density in elderly women. Journal of Bone and Mineral Research 10(8): 1177-84.

Ooms, M. E., J. C. Roos, P. D. Bezemer, W. J. van der Vijgh, L. M. Bouter and P. Lips. 1995b. Prevention of bone loss by vitamin D supplementation in elderly women: a randomized double-blind trial. Journal of Clinical Endocrinology and Metabolism 80(4): 1052-8.

Pan, A., L. Lu, O. H. Franco, Z. Yu, H. Li and X. Lin. 2009. Association between depressive symptoms and 25-hydroxyvitamin D in middle-aged and elderly Chinese. Journal of Affective Disorders 118(1-3): 240-3.

Panda, D. K., D. Miao, M. L. Tremblay, J. Sirois, R. Farookhi, G. N. Hendy and D. Goltzman. 2001. Targeted ablation of the 25-hydroxyvitamin D 1alpha-hydroxylase enzyme: evidence for skeletal, reproductive, and immune dysfunction. Proceedings of the National Academy of Sciences of the United States of America 98(13): 7498-503.

Papapetrou, P. D. 2010. The interrelationship of serum 1,25-dihydroxyvitamin D, 25-hydroxyvitamin D and 24,25-dihydroxyvitamin D in pregnancy at term: a meta-analysis. Hormones (Athens) 9(2): 136-44.

Pappa, H. M., C. M. Gordon, T. M. Saslowsky, A. Zholudev, B. Horr, M. C. Shih and R. J. Grand. 2006. Vitamin D status in children and young adults with inflammatory bowel disease. Pediatrics 118(5): 1950-61.

Parfitt, A. M., Z. H. Han, S. Palnitkar, D. S. Rao, M. S. Shih and D. Nelson. 1997. Effects of ethnicity and age or menopause on osteoblast function, bone mineralization, and osteoid accumulation in iliac bone. Journal of Bone and Mineral Research 12(11): 1864-73.

Parisien, M., F. Cosman, D. Morgan, M. Schnitzer, X. Liang, J. Nieves, L. Forese, M. Luckey, D. Meier, V. Shen, R. Lindsay and D. W. Dempster. 1997. Histomorphometric assessment of bone mass, structure, and remodeling: a comparison between healthy black and white premenopausal women. Journal of Bone and Mineral Research 12(6): 948-57.

Park, M. J., R. Namgung, D. H. Kim and R. C. Tsang. 1998. Bone mineral content is not reduced despite low vitamin D status in breast milk-fed infants versus cow's milk based formula-fed infants. Journal of Pediatrics 132(4): 641-5.

Park, W., H. Paust, H. J. Kaufmann and G. Offermann. 1987. Osteomalacia of the mother—rickets of the newborn. European Journal of Pediatrics 146(3): 292-3.

Park, Y., M. F. Leitzmann, A. F. Subar, A. Hollenbeck and A. Schatzkin. 2009. Dairy food, calcium, and risk of cancer in the NIH-AARP Diet and Health Study. Archives of Internal Medicine 169(4): 391-401.

Parsa, P. and B. Parsa. 2009. Effects of reproductive factors on risk of breast cancer: a literature review. Asian Pacific Journal of Cancer Prevention 10(4): 545-50.

Partridge, J. M., S. J. Weatherby, J. A. Woolmore, D. J. Highland, A. A. Fryer, C. L. Mann, M. D. Boggild, W. E. Ollier, R. C. Strange and C. P. Hawkins. 2004. Susceptibility and outcome in MS: associations with polymorphisms in pigmentation-related genes. Neurology 62(12): 2323-5.

Patel, R., D. Collins, S. Bullock, R. Swaminathan, G. M. Blake and I. Fogelman. 2001. The effect of season and vitamin D supplementation on bone mineral density in healthy women: a double-masked crossover study. Osteoporosis International 12(4): 319-25.

Patel, S., S. Hyer and J. Barron. 2007. Glomerular filtration rate is a major determinant of the relationship between 25-hydroxyvitamin D and parathyroid hormone. Calcified Tissue International 80(4): 221-6.

Peacock, M., G. Liu, M. Carey, R. McClintock, W. Ambrosius, S. Hui and C. C. Johnston. 2000. Effect of calcium or 25OH vitamin D_3 dietary supplementation on bone loss at the hip in men and women over the age of 60. Journal of Clinical Endocrinology and Metabolism 85(9): 3011-9.

Peacock, M., C. H. Turner, M. J. Econs and T. Foroud. 2002. Genetics of osteoporosis. Endocrine Reviews 23(3): 303-26.

Pearson, D., M. Kaur, P. San, N. Lawson, P. Baker and D. Hosking. 2004. Recovery of pregnancy mediated bone loss during lactation. Bone 34(3): 570-8.

Pedersen, E. B., P. Johannesen, S. Kristensen, A. B. Rasmussen, K. Emmertsen, J. Moller, J. G. Lauritsen and M. Wohlert. 1984. Calcium, parathyroid hormone and calcitonin in normal pregnancy and preeclampsia. Gynecologic and Obstetric Investigation 18(3): 156-64.

Peehl, D. M., R. Shinghal, L. Nonn, E. Seto, A. V. Krishnan, J. D. Brooks and D. Feldman. 2004. Molecular activity of 1,25-dihydroxyvitamin D_3 in primary cultures of human prostatic epithelial cells revealed by cDNA microarray analysis. Journal of Steroid Biochemistry and Molecular Biology 92(3): 131-41.

Pereira, G. R. and A. H. Zucker. 1986. Nutritional deficiencies in the neonate. Clinics in Perinatology 13(1): 175-89.

Pettersson, U., M. Nilsson, V. Sundh, D. Mellstrom and M. Lorentzon. 2010. Physical activity is the strongest predictor of calcaneal peak bone mass in young Swedish men. Osteoporosis International 21(3): 447-55.

Peyrin-Biroulet, L., A. Oussalah and M. A. Bigard. 2009. Crohn's disease: the hot hypothesis. Medical Hypotheses 73(1): 94-6.

Pfeifer, M., B. Begerow, H. W. Minne, C. Abrams, D. Nachtigall and C. Hansen. 2000. Effects of a short-term vitamin D and calcium supplementation on body sway and secondary hyperparathyroidism in elderly women. Journal of Bone and Mineral Research 15(6): 1113-8.

Pfeifer, M., B. Begerow, H. W. Minne, D. Nachtigall and C. Hansen. 2001. Effects of a short-term vitamin D(3) and calcium supplementation on blood pressure and parathyroid hormone levels in elderly women. Journal of Clinical Endocrinology and Metabolism 86(4): 1633-7.

Pfeifer, M., B. Begerow, H. W. Minne, K. Suppan, A. Fahrleitner-Pammer and H. Dobnig. 2009. Effects of a long-term vitamin D and calcium supplementation on falls and parameters of muscle function in community-dwelling older individuals. Osteoporosis International 20(2): 315-22.

Pilz, S., H. Dobnig, B. Winklhofer-Roob, G. Riedmuller, J. E. Fischer, U. Seelhorst, B. Wellnitz, B. O. Boehm and W. Marz. 2008. Low serum levels of 25-hydroxyvitamin D predict fatal cancer in patients referred to coronary angiography. Cancer Epidemiology, Biomarkers & Prevention 17(5): 1228-33.

Pittas, A. G., B. Dawson-Hughes, T. Li, R. M. Van Dam, W. C. Willett, J. E. Manson and F. B. Hu. 2006. Vitamin D and calcium intake in relation to type 2 diabetes in women. Diabetes Care 29(3): 650-6.

Pittas, A. G., S. S. Harris, P. C. Stark and B. Dawson-Hughes. 2007a. The effects of calcium and vitamin D supplementation on blood glucose and markers of inflammation in nondiabetic adults. Diabetes Care 30(4): 980-6.

Pittas, A. G., J. Lau, F. B. Hu and B. Dawson-Hughes. 2007b. The role of vitamin D and calcium in type 2 diabetes. A systematic review and meta-analysis. Journal of Clinical Endocrinology and Metabolism 92(6): 2017-29.

Polatti, F., E. Capuzzo, F. Viazzo, R. Colleoni and C. Klersy. 1999. Bone mineral changes during and after lactation. Obstetrics and Gynecology 94(1): 52-6.

Poole, K. E., N. Loveridge, P. J. Barker, D. J. Halsall, C. Rose, J. Reeve and E. A. Warburton. 2006. Reduced vitamin D in acute stroke. Stroke 37(1): 243-5.

Poon, A. H., C. Laprise, M. Lemire, A. Montpetit, D. Sinnett, E. Schurr and T. J. Hudson. 2004. Association of vitamin D receptor genetic variants with susceptibility to asthma and atopy. American Journal of Respiratory and Critical Care Medicine 170(9): 967-73.

Porthouse, J., S. Cockayne, C. King, L. Saxon, E. Steele, T. Aspray, M. Baverstock, Y. Birks, J. Dumville, R. Francis, C. Iglesias, S. Puffer, A. Sutcliffe, I. Watt and D. J. Torgerson. 2005. Randomised controlled trial of calcium and supplementation with cholecalciferol (vitamin D3) for prevention of fractures in primary care. British Medical Journal 330(7498): 1003.

Prentice, A., L. M. Jarjou, T. J. Cole, D. M. Stirling, B. Dibba and S. Fairweather-Tait. 1995. Calcium requirements of lactating Gambian mothers: effects of a calcium supplement on breast-milk calcium concentration, maternal bone mineral content, and urinary calcium excretion. American Journal of Clinical Nutrition 62(1): 58-67.

Prentice, A., L. Yan, L. M. Jarjou, B. Dibba, M. A. Laskey, D. M. Stirling and S. Fairweather-Tait. 1997. Vitamin D status does not influence the breast-milk calcium concentration of lactating mothers accustomed to a low calcium intake. Acta Paediatrica 86(9): 1006-8.

Prentice, A. 2003. Micronutrients and the bone mineral content of the mother, fetus and newborn. Journal of Nutrition 133(5 Suppl 2): 1693S-9S.

Prentice, A. 2008. Vitamin D deficiency: a global perspective. Nutrition Reviews 66(10 Suppl 2): S153-64.

Prentice, A., G. R. Goldberg and I. Schoenmakers. 2008. Vitamin D across the lifecycle: physiology and biomarkers. American Journal of Clinical Nutrition 88(2): 500S-6S.

Priemel, M., C. von Domarus, T. O. Klatte, S. Kessler, J. Schlie, S. Meier, N. Proksch, F. Pastor, C. Netter, T. Streichert, K. Puschel and M. Amling. 2010. Bone mineralization defects and vitamin D deficiency: histomorphometric analysis of iliac crest bone biopsies and circulating 25-hydroxyvitamin D in 675 patients. Journal of Bone and Mineral Research 25(2): 305-12.

Prince, R., A. Devine, I. Dick, A. Criddle, D. Kerr, N. Kent, R. Price and A. Randell. 1995. The effects of calcium supplementation (milk powder or tablets) and exercise on bone density in postmenopausal women. Journal of Bone and Mineral Research 10(7): 1068-75.

Prince, R. L., A. Devine, S. S. Dhaliwal and I. M. Dick. 2006. Effects of calcium supplementation on clinical fracture and bone structure: results of a 5-year, double-blind, placebo-controlled trial in elderly women. Archives of Internal Medicine 166(8): 869-75.

Prince, R. L., N. Austin, A. Devine, I. M. Dick, D. Bruce and K. Zhu. 2008. Effects of ergo-calciferol added to calcium on the risk of falls in elderly high-risk women. Archives of Internal Medicine 168(1): 103-8.

Prineas, J. W., A. S. Mason and R. A. Henson. 1965. Mypopathy in metabolic bone disease. British Medical Journal 1(5441): 1034-6.

Punnonen, R., J. Salmi, R. Tuimala, M. Jarvinen and P. Pystynen. 1986. Vitamin D deficiency in women with femoral neck fracture. Maturitas 8(4): 291-5.

Qiu, S., D. S. Rao, S. Palnitkar and A. M. Parfitt. 2006. Differences in osteocyte and lacunar density between black and white American women. Bone 38(1): 130-5.

Rajakumar, K., J. D. Fernstrom, J. E. Janosky and S. L. Greenspan. 2005. Vitamin D insufficiency in preadolescent African-American children. Clinical Pediatrics 44(8): 683-92.

Recker, R. R., K. M. Davies, S. M. Hinders, R. P. Heaney, M. R. Stegman and D. B. Kimmel. 1992. Bone gain in young adult women. Journal of the American Medical Association 268(17): 2403-8.

Recker, R. R., S. Hinders, K. M. Davies, R. P. Heaney, M. R. Stegman, J. M. Lappe and D. B. Kimmel. 1996. Correcting calcium nutritional deficiency prevents spine fractures in elderly women. Journal of Bone and Mineral Research 11(12): 1961-6.

Reichel, H., H. P. Koeffler and A. W. Norman. 1987. Synthesis in vitro of 1,25-dihydroxyvitamin D_3 and 24,25-dihydroxyvitamin D_3 by interferon-gamma-stimulated normal human bone marrow and alveolar macrophages. Journal of Biological Chemistry 262(23): 10931-7.

Reid, I. R., R. W. Ames, M. C. Evans, G. D. Gamble and S. J. Sharpe. 1993. Effect of calcium supplementation on bone loss in postmenopausal women. New England Journal of Medicine 328(7): 460-4.

Reid, I. R., R. Ames, B. Mason, H. E. Reid, C. J. Bacon, M. J. Bolland, G. D. Gamble, A. Grey and A. Horne. 2008. Randomized controlled trial of calcium supplementation in healthy, nonosteoporotic, older men. Archives of Internal Medicine 168(20): 2276-82.

Reif, S., Y. Katzir, Z. Eisenberg and Y. Weisman. 1988. Serum 25-hydroxyvitamin D levels in congenital craniotabes. Acta Paediatrica Scandinavica 77(1): 167-8.

Rhodes, S. G., L. A. Terry, J. Hope, R. G. Hewinson and H. M. Vordermeier. 2003. 1,25-dihydroxyvitamin D_3 and development of tuberculosis in cattle. Clinical and Diagnostic Laboratory Immunology 10(6): 1129-35.

Riggs, B. L., W. M. O'Fallon, J. Muhs, M. K. O'Connor, R. Kumar and L. J. Melton, 3rd. 1998. Long-term effects of calcium supplementation on serum parathyroid hormone level, bone turnover, and bone loss in elderly women. Journal of Bone and Mineral Research 13(2): 168-74.

Riggs, B. L., L. J. Melton, R. A. Robb, J. J. Camp, E. J. Atkinson, L. McDaniel, S. Amin, P. A. Rouleau and S. Khosla. 2008. A population-based assessment of rates of bone loss at multiple skeletal sites: evidence for substantial trabecular bone loss in young adult women and men. Journal of Bone and Mineral Research 23(2): 205-14.

Riis, B., K. Thomsen and C. Christiansen. 1987. Does calcium supplementation prevent postmenopausal bone loss? A double-blind, controlled clinical study. New England Journal of Medicine 316(4): 173-7.

Ritchie, L. D., E. B. Fung, B. P. Halloran, J. R. Turnlund, M. D. Van Loan, C. E. Cann and J. C. King. 1998. A longitudinal study of calcium homeostasis during human pregnancy and lactation and after resumption of menses. American Journal of Clinical Nutrition 67(4): 693-701.

Rohan, T. E., A. Negassa, R. T. Chlebowski, C. D. Ceria-Ulep, B. B. Cochrane, D. S. Lane, M. Ginsberg, S. Wassertheil-Smoller and D. L. Page. 2009. A randomized controlled trial of calcium plus vitamin D supplementation and risk of benign proliferative breast disease. Breast Cancer Research and Treatment 116(2): 339-50.

Ron, M., M. Levitz, J. Chuba and J. Dancis. 1984. Transfer of 25-hydroxyvitamin D_3 and 1,25-dihydroxyvitamin D_3 across the perfused human placenta. American Journal of Obstetrics and Gynecology 148(4): 370-4.

Rosen, C. J., A. Morrison, H. Zhou, D. Storm, S. J. Hunter, K. Musgrave, T. Chen, W. Wei and M. F. Holick. 1994. Elderly women in northern New England exhibit seasonal changes in bone mineral density and calciotropic hormones. Bone and Mineral 25(2): 83-92.

Rossi, M., J. K. McLaughlin, P. Lagiou, C. Bosetti, R. Talamini, L. Lipworth, A. Giacosa, M. Montella, S. Franceschi, E. Negri and C. La Vecchia. 2009. Vitamin D intake and breast cancer risk: a case–control study in Italy. Annals of Oncology 20(2): 374-8.

Rothberg, A. D., J. M. Pettifor, D. F. Cohen, E. W. Sonnendecker and F. P. Ross. 1982. Maternal-infant vitamin D relationships during breast-feeding. Journal of Pediatrics 101(4): 500-3.

Rowling, M. J., C. Gliniak, J. Welsh and J. C. Fleet. 2007. High dietary vitamin D prevents hypocalcemia and osteomalacia in CYP27B1 knockout mice. Journal of Nutrition 137(12): 2608-15.

Rucker, D., J. A. Allan, G. H. Fick and D. A. Hanley. 2002. Vitamin D insufficiency in a population of healthy western Canadians. Canadian Medical Association Journal 166(12): 1517-24.

Ruiz-Irastorza, G., M. V. Egurbide, N. Olivares, A. Martinez-Berriotxoa and C. Aguirre. 2008. Vitamin D deficiency in systemic lupus erythematosus: prevalence, predictors and clinical consequences. Rheumatology 47(6): 920-3.

Rummens, K., R. van Bree, E. Van Herck, Z. Zaman, R. Bouillon, F. A. Van Assche and J. Verhaeghe. 2002. Vitamin D deficiency in guinea pigs: exacerbation of bone phenotype during pregnancy and disturbed fetal mineralization, with recovery by 1,25(OH)2D3 infusion or dietary calcium-phosphate supplementation. Calcified Tissue International 71(4): 364-75.

Russell, R., M. Chung, E. M. Balk, S. Atkinson, E. L. Giovannucci, S. Ip, A. H. Lichtenstein, S. T. Mayne, G. Raman, A. C. Ross, T. A. Trikalinos, K. P. West, Jr. and J. Lau. 2009. Opportunities and challenges in conducting systematic reviews to support the development of nutrient reference values: vitamin A as an example. American Journal of Clinical Nutrition 89(3): 728-33.

Saadi, H. F., A. Dawodu, B. O. Afandi, R. Zayed, S. Benedict and N. Nagelkerke. 2007. Efficacy of daily and monthly high-dose calciferol in vitamin D-deficient nulliparous and lactating women. American Journal of Clinical Nutrition 85(6): 1565-71.

Salovaara, K., M. Tuppurainen, M. Karkkainen, T. Rikkonen, L. Sandini, J. Sirola, R. Honkanen, E. Alhava and H. Kroger. 2010. Effect of vitamin D(3) and calcium on fracture risk in 65- to 71-year-old women: a population-based 3-year randomized, controlled trial—the OSTPRE-FPS. Journal of Bone and Mineral Research 25(7): 1487-95.

Sanchez, B., E. Lopez-Martin, C. Segura, J. L. Labandeira-Garcia and R. Perez-Fernandez. 2002. 1,25-dihydroxyvitamin D(3) increases striatal GDNF mRNA and protein expression in adult rats. Brain Research. Molecular Brain Research 108(1-2): 143-6.

Sanders, K. M., A. L. Stuart, E. J. Williamson, J. A. Simpson, M. A. Kotowicz, D. Young and G. C. Nicholson. 2010. Annual high-dose oral vitamin D and falls and fractures in older women: a randomized controlled trial. Journal of the American Medical Association 303(18): 1815-22.

Sann, L., L. David, A. Thomas, A. Frederich, M. C. Chapuy and R. Francois. 1976. Congenital hyperparathyroidism and vitamin D deficiency secondary to maternal hypoparathyroidism. Acta Paediatrica Scandinavica 65(3): 381-5.

Sarkis, K. S., M. B. Salvador, M. M. Pinheiro, R. G. Silva, C. A. Zerbini and L. A. Martini. 2009. Association between osteoporosis and rheumatoid arthritis in women: a cross–sectional study. Sao Paulo Medical Journal 127(4): 216-22.

Sayers, A. and J. H. Tobias. 2009. Estimated maternal ultraviolet B exposure levels in pregnancy influence skeletal development of the child. Journal of Clinical Endocrinology and Metabolism 94(3): 765-71.

Schaafsma, A., J. J. van Doormaal, F. A. Muskiet, G. J. Hofstede, I. Pakan and E. van der Veer. 2002. Positive effects of a chicken eggshell powder-enriched vitamin-mineral supplement on femoral neck bone mineral density in healthy late post-menopausal Dutch women. British Journal of Nutrition 87(3): 267-75.

Schauber, J., R. A. Dorschner, K. Yamasaki, B. Brouha and R. L. Gallo. 2006. Control of the innate epithelial antimicrobial response is cell-type specific and dependent on relevant microenvironmental stimuli. Immunology 118(4): 509-19.

Schleithoff, S. S., A. Zittermann, G. Tenderich, H. K. Berthold, P. Stehle and R. Koerfer. 2006. Vitamin D supplementation improves cytokine profiles in patients with congestive heart failure: a double-blind, randomized, placebo-controlled trial. American Journal of Clinical Nutrition 83(4): 754-9.

Schneider, B., B. Weber, A. Frensch, J. Stein and J. Fritz. 2000. Vitamin D in schizophrenia, major depression and alcoholism. Journal of Neural Transmission 107(7): 839-42.

Schnitzler, C. M., J. M. Pettifor, J. M. Mesquita, M. D. Bird, E. Schnaid and A. E. Smyth. 1990. Histomorphometry of iliac crest bone in 346 normal black and white South African adults. Bone and Mineral 10(3): 183-99.

Schnitzler, C. M. and J. M. Mesquita. 2006. Cortical bone histomorphometry of the iliac crest in normal black and white South African adults. Calcified Tissue International 79(6): 373-82.

Scholl, T. O. and X. Chen. 2009. Vitamin D intake during pregnancy: association with maternal characteristics and infant birth weight. Early Human Development 85(4): 231-4.

Schwartz, G. G. and B. S. Hulka. 1990. Is vitamin D deficiency a risk factor for prostate cancer? (Hypothesis). Anticancer Research 10(5A): 1307-11.

Scragg, R., R. Jackson, I. M. Holdaway, T. Lim and R. Beaglehole. 1990. Myocardial infarction is inversely associated with plasma 25-hydroxyvitamin D_3 levels: a community-based study. International Journal of Epidemiology 19(3): 559-63.

Scragg, R., I. Holdaway, V. Singh, P. Metcalf, J. Baker and E. Dryson. 1995. Serum 25-hydroxyvitamin D_3 levels decreased in impaired glucose tolerance and diabetes mellitus. Diabetes Research and Clinical Practice 27(3): 181-8.

Seely, E. W., R. J. Wood, E. M. Brown and S. W. Graves. 1992. Lower serum ionized calcium and abnormal calciotropic hormone levels in preeclampsia. Journal of Clinical Endocrinology and Metabolism 74(6): 1436-40.

Seely, E. W., E. M. Brown, D. M. DeMaggio, D. K. Weldon and S. W. Graves. 1997. A prospective study of calciotropic hormones in pregnancy and post partum: reciprocal changes in serum intact parathyroid hormone and 1,25-dihydroxyvitamin D. American Journal of Obstetrics and Gynecology 176(1 Pt 1): 214-7.

Seino, Y., M. Ishida, K. Yamaoka, T. Ishii, T. Hiejima, C. Ikehara, Y. Tanaka, S. Matsuda, T. Shimotsuji, H. Yabuuchi, S. Morimoto and T. Onishi. 1982. Serum calcium regulating hormones in the perinatal period. Calcified Tissue International 34(2): 131-5.

Selvaraj, P., M. Vidyarani, K. Alagarasu, S. Prabhu Anand and P. R. Narayanan. 2008. Regulatory role of promoter and 3' UTR variants of vitamin D receptor gene on cytokine response in pulmonary tuberculosis. Journal of Clinical Immunology 28(4): 306-13.

Sergeev, I. N. and W. B. Rhoten. 1995. 1,25-dihydroxyvitamin D_3 evokes oscillations of intracellular calcium in a pancreatic beta-cell line. Endocrinology 136(7): 2852-61.

Shaffer, J. R., C. M. Kammerer, D. Reich, G. McDonald, N. Patterson, B. Goodpaster, D. C. Bauer, J. Li, A. B. Newman, J. A. Cauley, T. B. Harris, F. Tylavsky, R. E. Ferrell and J. M. Zmuda. 2007. Genetic markers for ancestry are correlated with body composition traits in older African Americans. Osteoporosis International 18(6): 733-41.

Sharma, O. P., J. Lamon and D. Winsor. 1972. Hypercalcemia and tuberculosis. Journal of the American Medical Association 222(5): 582.

Sharma, S. C. 1981. Serum calcium in pulmonary tuberculosis. Postgraduate Medical Journal 57(673): 694-6.

Shea, B., G. Wells, A. Cranney, N. Zytaruk, V. Robinson, L. Griffith, Z. Ortiz, J. Peterson, J. Adachi, P. Tugwell and G. Guyatt. 2002. Meta-analyses of therapies for postmenopausal osteoporosis. VII. Meta-analysis of calcium supplementation for the prevention of postmenopausal osteoporosis. Endocrine Reviews 23(4): 552-9.

Shea, M. K., S. L. Booth, J. M. Massaro, P. F. Jacques, R. B. D'Agostino, Sr., B. Dawson-Hughes, J. M. Ordovas, C. J. O'Donnell, S. Kathiresan, J. F. Keaney, Jr., R. S. Vasan and E. J. Benjamin. 2008. Vitamin K and vitamin D status: associations with inflammatory markers in the Framingham Offspring Study. American Journal of Epidemiology 167(3): 313-20.

Shin, M. H., M. D. Holmes, S. E. Hankinson, K. Wu, G. A. Colditz and W. C. Willett. 2002. Intake of dairy products, calcium, and vitamin D and risk of breast cancer. Journal of the National Cancer Institute 94(17): 1301-11.

Silver, J., H. Landau, I. Bab, Y. Shvil, M. M. Friedlaender, D. Rubinger and M. M. Popovtzer. 1985. Vitamin D-dependent rickets types I and II. Diagnosis and response to therapy. Israel Journal of Medical Sciences 21(1): 53-6.

Simmons, J. D., C. Mullighan, K. I. Welsh and D. P. Jewell. 2000. Vitamin D receptor gene polymorphism: association with Crohn's disease susceptibility. Gut 47(2): 211-4.

Sita-Lumsden, A., G. Lapthorn, R. Swaminathan and H. J. Milburn. 2007. Reactivation of tuberculosis and vitamin D deficiency: the contribution of diet and exposure to sunlight. Thorax 62(11): 1003-7.

Skaria, J., B. C. Katiyar, T. P. Srivastava and B. Dube. 1975. Myopathy and neuropathy associated with osteomalacia. Acta Neurologica Scandinavica 51(1): 37-58.

Slack, J. H., L. Hang, J. Barkley, R. J. Fulton, L. D'Hoostelaere, A. Robinson and F. J. Dixon. 1984. Isotypes of spontaneous and mitogen-induced autoantibodies in SLE-prone mice. Journal of Immunology 132(3): 1271-5.

Slemenda, C. W., M. Peacock, S. Hui, L. Zhou and C. C. Johnston. 1997. Reduced rates of skeletal remodeling are associated with increased bone mineral density during the development of peak skeletal mass. Journal of Bone and Mineral Research 12(4): 676-82.

Slinin, Y., M. L. Paudel, B. C. Taylor, H. A. Fink, A. Ishani, M. T. Canales, K. Yaffe, E. Barrett-Connor, E. S. Orwoll, J. M. Shikany, E. S. Leblanc, J. A. Cauley and K. E. Ensrud. 2010. 25-hydroxyvitamin D levels and cognitive performance and decline in elderly men. Neurology 74(1): 33-41.

Sloka, J. S., W. E. Pryse-Phillips and M. Stefanelli. 2008. The relation of ultraviolet radiation and multiple sclerosis in Newfoundland. Canadian Journal of Neurological Sciences 35(1): 69-74.

Sloka, S., J. Stokes, E. Randell and L. A. Newhook. 2009. Seasonal variation of maternal serum vitamin D in Newfoundland and Labrador. Journal of Obstetrics and Gynaecology Canada 31(4): 313-21.

Sloka, S., M. Grant and L. A. Newhook. 2010. The geospatial relation between UV solar radiation and type 1 diabetes in Newfoundland. Acta Diabetologica 47(1): 73-8.

Slovik, D. M., J. S. Adams, R. M. Neer, M. F. Holick and J. T. Potts, Jr. 1981. Deficient production of 1,25-dihydroxyvitamin D in elderly osteoporotic patients. New England Journal of Medicine 305(7): 372-4.

Smith, H., F. Anderson, H. Raphael, P. Maslin, S. Crozier and C. Cooper. 2007. Effect of annual intramuscular vitamin D on fracture risk in elderly men and women—a population-based, randomized, double-blind, placebo-controlled trial. Rheumatology 46(12): 1852-7.

Smith, S. J., M. E. Hayes, P. L. Selby and E. B. Mawer. 1999. Autocrine control of vitamin D metabolism in synovial cells from arthritic patients. Annals of the Rheumatic Diseases 58(6): 372-8.

Smolders, J., P. Menheere, A. Kessels, J. Damoiseaux and R. Hupperts. 2008. Association of vitamin D metabolite levels with relapse rate and disability in multiple sclerosis. Multiple Sclerosis 14(9): 1220-4.

Smolders, J., J. Damoiseaux, P. Menheere, J. W. Tervaert and R. Hupperts. 2009. Association study on two vitamin D receptor gene polymorphisms and vitamin D metabolites in multiple sclerosis. Annals of the New York Academy of Sciences 1173: 515-20.

Snijder, M. B., N. M. van Schoor, S. M. Pluijm, R. M. van Dam, M. Visser and P. Lips. 2006. Vitamin D status in relation to one-year risk of recurrent falling in older men and women. Journal of Clinical Endocrinology and Metabolism 91(8): 2980-5.

Soilu-Hanninen, M., M. Laaksonen, I. Laitinen, J. P. Eralinna, E. M. Lilius and I. Mononen. 2008. A longitudinal study of serum 25-hydroxyvitamin D and intact parathyroid hormone levels indicate the importance of vitamin D and calcium homeostasis regulation in multiple sclerosis. Journal of Neurology, Neurosurgery and Psychiatry 79(2): 152-7.

Sokoloff, L. 1978. Occult osteomalacia in American (U.S.A.) patients with fracture of the hip. American Journal of Surgical Pathology 2(1): 21-30.

Song, Y. and J. C. Fleet. 2007. Intestinal resistance to 1,25 dihydroxyvitamin D in mice heterozygous for the vitamin D receptor knockout allele. Endocrinology 148(3): 1396-402.

Sowers, M., R. B. Wallace and J. H. Lemke. 1985. Correlates of forearm bone mass among women during maximal bone mineralization. Preventive Medicine 14(5): 585-96.

Sowers, M. R., M. K. Clark, B. Hollis, R. B. Wallace and M. Jannausch. 1992. Radial bone mineral density in pre- and perimenopausal women: a prospective study of rates and risk factors for loss. Journal of Bone and Mineral Research 7(6): 647-57.

Sowers, M. 1996. Pregnancy and lactation as risk factors for subsequent bone loss and osteoporosis. Journal of Bone and Mineral Research 11(8): 1052-60.

Sowers, M., D. Zhang, B. W. Hollis, B. Shapiro, C. A. Janney, M. Crutchfield, M. A. Schork, F. Stanczyk and J. Randolph. 1998. Role of calciotrophic hormones in calcium mobilization of lactation. American Journal of Clinical Nutrition 67(2): 284-91.

Sowers, M. R., H. Zheng, M. L. Jannausch, D. McConnell, B. Nan, S. Harlow and J. F. Randolph, Jr. 2010. Amount of bone loss in relation to time around the final menstrual period and follicle-stimulating hormone staging of the transmenopause. Journal of Clinical Endocrinology and Metabolism 95(5): 2155-62.

Specker, B. L., R. C. Tsang and M. L. Ho. 1991. Changes in calcium homeostasis over the first year postpartum: effect of lactation and weaning. Obstetrics and Gynecology 78(1): 56-62.

Specker, B. L., M. L. Ho, A. Oestreich, T. A. Yin, Q. M. Shui, X. C. Chen and R. C. Tsang. 1992. Prospective study of vitamin D supplementation and rickets in China. Journal of Pediatrics 120(5): 733-9.

Specker, B. L. 1994. Do North American women need supplemental vitamin D during pregnancy or lactation? American Journal of Clinical Nutrition 59(Suppl 2): 484S-90S; discussion 490S-1S.

Specker, B. L., N. E. Vieira, K. O. O'Brien, M. L. Ho, J. E. Heubi, S. A. Abrams and A. L. Yergey. 1994. Calcium kinetics in lactating women with low and high calcium intakes. American Journal of Clinical Nutrition 59(3): 593-9.

Specker, B. 2004. Vitamin D requirements during pregnancy. American Journal of Clinical Nutrition 80(Suppl 6): 1740S-7S.

Stacey, J. and C. Daly. 1989. Osteomalacia in the elderly: biochemical screening in general practice. Irish Medical Journal 82(2): 72-3.

St-Arnaud, R., S. Messerlian, J. M. Moir, J. L. Omdahl and F. H. Glorieux. 1997. The 25-hydroxyvitamin D 1-alpha-hydroxylase gene maps to the pseudovitamin D-deficiency rickets (PDDR) disease locus. Journal of Bone and Mineral Research 12(10): 1552-9.

Steingrimsdottir, L., O. Gunnarsson, O. S. Indridason, L. Franzson and G. Sigurdsson. 2005. Relationship between serum parathyroid hormone levels, vitamin D sufficiency, and calcium intake. Journal of the American Medical Association 294(18): 2336-41.

Stewart, J. W., D. L. Alekel, L. M. Ritland, M. Van Loan, E. Gertz and U. Genschel. 2009. Serum 25-hydroxyvitamin D is related to indicators of overall physical fitness in healthy postmenopausal women. Menopause 16(6): 1093-101.

Stio, M., B. Lunghi, T. Iantomasi, M. T. Vincenzini and C. Treves. 1993. Effect of vitamin D deficiency and 1,25-dihydroxyvitamin D_3 on metabolism and D-glucose transport in rat cerebral cortex. Journal of Neuroscience Research 35(5): 559-66.

Stone, K., D. C. Bauer, D. M. Black, P. Sklarin, K. E. Ensrud and S. R. Cummings. 1998. Hormonal predictors of bone loss in elderly women: a prospective study. The Study of Osteoporotic Fractures Research Group. Journal of Bone and Mineral Research 13(7): 1167-74.

Storm, D., R. Eslin, E. S. Porter, K. Musgrave, D. Vereault, C. Patton, C. Kessenich, S. Mohan, T. Chen, M. F. Holick and C. J. Rosen. 1998. Calcium supplementation prevents seasonal bone loss and changes in biochemical markers of bone turnover in elderly New England women: a randomized placebo-controlled trial. Journal of Clinical Endocrinology and Metabolism 83(11): 3817-25.

Strachan, D. P., K. J. Powell, A. Thaker, F. J. Millard and J. D. Maxwell. 1995. Vegetarian diet as a risk factor for tuberculosis in immigrant south London Asians. Thorax 50(2): 175-80.

Swami, S., N. Raghavachari, U. R. Muller, Y. P. Bao and D. Feldman. 2003. Vitamin D growth inhibition of breast cancer cells: gene expression patterns assessed by cDNA microarray. Breast Cancer Research and Treatment 80(1): 49-62.

Szodoray, P., B. Nakken, J. Gaal, R. Jonsson, A. Szegedi, E. Zold, G. Szegedi, J. G. Brun, R. Gesztelyi, M. Zeher and E. Bodolay. 2008. The complex role of vitamin D in autoimmune diseases. Scandinavian Journal of Immunology 68(3): 261-9.

Takeda, E., H. Yamamoto, Y. Taketani and K. Miyamoto. 1997. Vitamin D-dependent rickets type I and type II. Acta Paediatrica Japonica 39(4): 508-13.

Takeuchi, A., T. Okano, N. Tsugawa, Y. Tasaka, T. Kobayashi, S. Kodama and T. Matsuo. 1989. Effects of ergocalciferol supplementation on the concentration of vitamin D and its metabolites in human milk. Journal of Nutrition 119(11): 1639-46.

Tang, B. M., G. D. Eslick, C. Nowson, C. Smith and A. Bensoussan. 2007. Use of calcium or calcium in combination with vitamin D supplementation to prevent fractures and bone loss in people aged 50 years and older: a meta-analysis. Lancet 370(9588): 657-66.

Taniura, H., M. Ito, N. Sanada, N. Kuramoto, Y. Ohno, N. Nakamichi and Y. Yoneda. 2006. Chronic vitamin D_3 treatment protects against neurotoxicity by glutamate in association with upregulation of vitamin D receptor mRNA expression in cultured rat cortical neurons. Journal of Neuroscience Research 83(7): 1179-89.

Targher, G., L. Bertolini, R. Padovani, L. Zenari, L. Scala, M. Cigolini and G. Arcaro. 2006. Serum 25-hydroxyvitamin D_3 concentrations and carotid artery intima-media thickness among type 2 diabetic patients. Clinical Endocrinology 65(5): 593-7.

Teotia, M., S. P. Teotia and M. Nath. 1995. Metabolic studies in congenital vitamin D deficiency rickets. Indian Journal of Pediatrics 62(1): 55-61.

Teotia, M. and S. P. Teotia. 1997. Nutritional and metabolic rickets. Indian Journal of Pediatrics 64(2): 153-7.

Tetlow, L. C. and D. E. Woolley. 1999. The effects of 1 alpha,25-dihydroxyvitamin D(3) on matrix metalloproteinase and prostaglandin E(2) production by cells of the rheumatoid lesion. Arthritis Research 1(1): 63-70.

Thacher, T. D. 1997. Rickets without vitamin D deficiency in Nigerian children. Ambulatory Child Health 3(1 Pt 1): 56-64.

Thacher, T. D., P. R. Fischer, J. M. Pettifor, J. O. Lawson, C. O. Isichei and G. M. Chan. 2000. Case–control study of factors associated with nutritional rickets in Nigerian children. Journal of Pediatrics 137(3): 367-73.

Thacher, T. D., M. O. Obadofin, K. O. O'Brien and S. A. Abrams. 2009. The effect of vitamin D_2 and vitamin D_3 on intestinal calcium absorption in Nigerian children with rickets. Journal of Clinical Endocrinology and Metabolism 94(9): 3314-21.

Thandrayen, K., S. A. Norris and J. M. Pettifor. 2009. Fracture rates in urban South African children of different ethnic origins: the Birth to Twenty cohort. Osteoporosis International 20(1): 47-52.

Thiebaud, D., P. Burckhardt, M. Costanza, D. Sloutskis, D. Gilliard, F. Quinodoz, A. F. Jacquet and B. Burnand. 1997. Importance of albumin, 25(OH)-vitamin D and IGFBP-3 as risk factors in elderly women and men with hip fracture. Osteoporosis International 7(5): 457-62.

Thorne, J. and M. J. Campbell. 2008. The vitamin D receptor in cancer. Proceedings of the Nutrition Society 67(2): 115-27.

Thys-Jacobs, S., P. Starkey, D. Bernstein and J. Tian. 1998. Calcium carbonate and the premenstrual syndrome: effects on premenstrual and menstrual symptoms. Premenstrual Syndrome Study Group. American Journal of Obstetrics and Gynecology 179(2): 444-52.

Timms, P. M., N. Mannan, G. A. Hitman, K. Noonan, P. G. Mills, D. Syndercombe-Court, E. Aganna, C. P. Price and B. J. Boucher. 2002. Circulating MMP9, vitamin D and variation in the TIMP-1 response with VDR genotype: mechanisms for inflammatory damage in chronic disorders? Quarterly Journal of Medicine 95(12): 787-96.

Toescu, E. C. and A. Verkhratsky. 2007. Role of calcium in normal aging and neurodegeneration. Aging Cell 6(3): 265.

Towler, D. 2009. Adverse health effects of excessive vitamin D and calcium intake: considerations relevant to cardiovascular disease and nephrocalcinosis. A white paper commissioned for the Committee to Review Dietary Reference Intakes for Vitamin D and Calcium. Washington, DC.

Tracy, J. K., W. A. Meyer, R. H. Flores, P. D. Wilson and M. C. Hochberg. 2005. Racial differences in rate of decline in bone mass in older men: the Baltimore men's osteoporosis study. Journal of Bone and Mineral Research 20(7): 1228-34.

Tracy, J. K., W. A. Meyer, M. Grigoryan, B. Fan, R. H. Flores, H. K. Genant, C. Resnik and M. C. Hochberg. 2006. Racial differences in the prevalence of vertebral fractures in older men: the Baltimore Men's Osteoporosis Study. Osteoporosis International 17(1): 99-104.

Travison, T. G., T. J. Beck, G. R. Esche, A. B. Araujo and J. B. McKinlay. 2008. Age trends in proximal femur geometry in men: variation by race and ethnicity. Osteoporosis International 19(3): 277-87.

Trivedi, D. P., R. Doll and K. T. Khaw. 2003. Effect of four monthly oral vitamin D_3 (cholecalciferol) supplementation on fractures and mortality in men and women living in the community: randomised double blind controlled trial. British Medical Journal 326(7387): 469.

Trotter, M. and B. B. Hixon. 1974. Sequential changes in weight, density, and percentage ash weight of human skeletons from an early fetal period through old age. Anatomical Record 179(1): 1-18.

Tuck, S. P. and H. K. Datta. 2007. Osteoporosis in the aging male: treatment options. Clinical Intervention Aging 2(4): 521-36.

Turner, M., P. E. Barre, A. Benjamin, D. Goltzman and M. Gascon-Barre. 1988. Does the maternal kidney contribute to the increased circulating 1,25-dihydroxyvitamin D concentrations during pregnancy? Mineral and Electrolyte Metabolism 14(4): 246-52.

Tylavsky, F. A., K. A. Ryder, A. Lyytikainen and S. Cheng. 2005. Vitamin D, parathyroid hormone, and bone mass in adolescents. Journal of Nutrition 135(11): 2735S-8S.

Ulrich, U., P. B. Miller, D. R. Eyre, C. H. Chesnut, 3rd, H. Schlebusch and M. R. Soules. 2003. Bone remodeling and bone mineral density during pregnancy. Archives of Gynecology and Obstetrics 268(4): 309-16.

Underdahl, N. R. and G. A. Young. 1956. Effect of dietary intake of fat-soluble vitamins on intensity of experimental swine influenza virus infection in mice. Virology 2(3): 415-29.

Urashima, M., T. Segawa, M. Okazaki, M. Kurihara, Y. Wada and H. Ida. 2010. Randomized trial of vitamin D supplementation to prevent seasonal influenza A in schoolchildren. American Journal of Clinical Nutrition 91(5): 1255-60.

Uusi-Rasi, K., H. Sievanen, M. Pasanen, T. J. Beck and P. Kannus. 2008. Influence of calcium intake and physical activity on proximal femur bone mass and structure among pre- and postmenopausal women. A 10-year prospective study. Calcified Tissue International 82(3): 171-81.

Vaisberg, M. W., R. Kaneno, M. F. Franco and N. F. Mendes. 2000. Influence of cholecalciferol (vitamin D_3) on the course of experimental systemic lupus erythematosus in F1 (NZBxW) mice. Journal of Clinical Laboratory Analysis 14(3): 91-6.

Van Cromphaut, S. J., M. Dewerchin, J. G. Hoenderop, I. Stockmans, E. Van Herck, S. Kato, R. J. Bindels, D. Collen, P. Carmeliet, R. Bouillon and G. Carmeliet. 2001. Duodenal calcium absorption in vitamin D receptor-knockout mice: functional and molecular aspects. Proceedings of the National Academy of Sciences of the United States of America 98(23): 13324-9.

van der Mei, I. A., A. L. Ponsonby, T. Dwyer, L. Blizzard, B. V. Taylor, T. Kilpatrick, H. Butzkueven and A. J. McMichael. 2007. Vitamin D levels in people with multiple sclerosis and community controls in Tasmania, Australia. Journal of Neurology 254(5): 581-90.

van der Wiel, H. E., P. Lips, J. Nauta, J. C. Netelenbos and G. J. Hazenberg. 1991. Biochemical parameters of bone turnover during ten days of bed rest and subsequent mobilization. Bone and Mineral 13(2): 123-9.

van Dijk, C. E., M. R. de Boer, L. L. Koppes, J. C. Roos, P. Lips and J. W. Twisk. 2009. Positive association between the course of vitamin D intake and bone mineral density at 36 years in men. Bone 44(3): 437-41.

van Schoor, N. M., M. Visser, S. M. Pluijm, N. Kuchuk, J. H. Smit and P. Lips. 2008. Vitamin D deficiency as a risk factor for osteoporotic fractures. Bone 42(2): 260-6.

Vatanparast, H., D. A. Bailey, A. D. Baxter-Jones and S. J. Whiting. 2010. Calcium requirements for bone growth in Canadian boys and girls during adolescence. British Journal of Nutrition: 1-6.

Velho, S., P. Marques-Vidal, F. Baptista and M. E. Camilo. 2008. Dietary intake adequacy and cognitive function in free-living active elderly: a cross–sectional and short-term prospective study. Clinical Nutrition 27(1): 77-86.

Velie, E. M., S. Nechuta and J. R. Osuch. 2005. Lifetime reproductive and anthropometric risk factors for breast cancer in postmenopausal women. Breast Disease 24: 17-35.

Vieth, R., Y. Ladak and P. G. Walfish. 2003. Age-related changes in the 25-hydroxyvitamin D versus parathyroid hormone relationship suggest a different reason why older adults require more vitamin D. Journal of Clinical Endocrinology and Metabolism 88(1): 185-91.

Vieth, R., S. Kimball, A. Hu and P. G. Walfish. 2004. Randomized comparison of the effects of the vitamin D_3 adequate intake versus 100 mcg (4000 IU) per day on biochemical responses and the wellbeing of patients. Nutrition Journal 3: 8.

Viljakainen, H. T., E. Saarnio, T. Hytinantti, M. Miettinen, H. Surcel, O. Makitie, S. Andersson, K. Laitinen and C. Lamberg-Allardt. 2010. Maternal vitamin D status determines bone variables in the newborn. Journal of Clinical Endocrinology and Metabolism 95(4): 1749-57.

Villar, J., H. Abdel-Aleem, M. Merialdi, M. Mathai, M. M. Ali, N. Zavaleta, M. Purwar, J. Hofmeyr, T. N. Nguyen, L. Campodonico, S. Landoulsi, G. Carroli and M. Lindheimer. 2006. World Health Organization randomized trial of calcium supplementation among low calcium intake pregnant women. American Journal of Obstetrics and Gynecology 194(3): 639-49.

Villareal, D. T., R. Civitelli, A. Chines and L. V. Avioli. 1991. Subclinical vitamin D deficiency in postmenopausal women with low vertebral bone mass. Journal of Clinical Endocrinology and Metabolism 72(3): 628-34.

von Hurst, P. R., W. Stonehouse and J. Coad. 2010. Vitamin D supplementation reduces insulin resistance in South Asian women living in New Zealand who are insulin resistant and vitamin D deficient—a randomised, placebo-controlled trial. British Journal of Nutrition 103(4): 549-55.

von Knorring, J., P. Slatis, T. H. Weber and T. Helenius. 1982. Serum levels of 25-hydroxyvitamin D, 24,25-dihydroxyvitamin D and parathyroid hormone in patients with femoral neck fracture in southern Finland. Clinical Endocrinology 17(2): 189-94.

Wagner, C. L., T. C. Hulsey, D. Fanning, M. Ebeling and B. W. Hollis. 2006. High-dose vitamin D_3 supplementation in a cohort of breastfeeding mothers and their infants: a 6-month follow-up pilot study. Breastfeeding Medicine 1(2): 59-70.

Wagner, C. L. and F. R. Greer. 2008. Prevention of rickets and vitamin D deficiency in infants, children, and adolescents. Pediatrics 122(5): 1142-52.

Wagner, C. L., D. Johnson, T. C. Hulsey, M. Ebeling, J. Shary, P. G. Smith, B. B. Bivens and B. W. Hollis. 2010a. Vitamin D Supplementation during Pregnancy Part 2 NICHD/CTSA Randomized Clinical Trial (RCT): Outcomes. PAS Abstract.

Wagner, C. L., D. Johnson, T. C. Hulsey, M. Ebeling, J. Shary, P. G. Smith, B. B. Bivens and B. W. Hollis. 2010b. Vitamin D Supplementation during Pregnancy Part 1 NICHD/CTSA Randomized Clinical Trial (RCT): Safety Consideration. PAS Abstract.

Wang, L., J. E. Manson, J. E. Buring, I. M. Lee and H. D. Sesso. 2008. Dietary intake of dairy products, calcium, and vitamin D and the risk of hypertension in middle-aged and older women. Hypertension 51(4): 1073-9.

Wang, L., J. E. Manson, Y. Song and H. D. Sesso. 2010. Systematic review: vitamin D and calcium supplementation in prevention of cardiovascular events. Annals of Internal Medicine 152(5): 315-23.

Wang, M. C., M. Aguirre, G. S. Bhudhikanok, C. G. Kendall, S. Kirsch, R. Marcus and L. K. Bachrach. 1997. Bone mass and hip axis length in healthy Asian, black, Hispanic, and white American youths. Journal of Bone and Mineral Research 12(11): 1922-35.

Wang, T. J., M. J. Pencina, S. L. Booth, P. F. Jacques, E. Ingelsson, K. Lanier, E. J. Benjamin, R. B. D'Agostino, M. Wolf and R. S. Vasan. 2008. Vitamin D deficiency and risk of cardiovascular disease. Circulation 117(4): 503-11.

Wang, X., C. M. Kammerer, V. W. Wheeler, A. L. Patrick, C. H. Bunker and J. M. Zmuda. 2007. Genetic and environmental determinants of volumetric and areal BMD in multi-generational families of African ancestry: the Tobago Family Health Study. Journal of Bone and Mineral Research 22(4): 527-36.

Washington, M. N. and N. L. Weigel. 2010. 1{alpha},25-dihydroxyvitamin D_3 inhibits growth of VCaP prostate cancer cells despite inducing the growth-promoting TMPRSS2:ERG gene fusion. Endocrinology 151(4): 1409-17.

Waters, W. R., M. V. Palmer, B. J. Nonnecke, D. L. Whipple and R. L. Horst. 2004. Mycobacterium bovis infection of vitamin D-deficient NOS2-/- mice. Microbial Pathogenesis 36(1): 11-7.

Watson, K. E., M. L. Abrolat, L. L. Malone, J. M. Hoeg, T. Doherty, R. Detrano and L. L. Demer. 1997. Active serum vitamin D levels are inversely correlated with coronary calcification. Circulation 96(6): 1755-60.

WCRF (World Cancer Research Fund)/AICR (American Institute for Cancer Research). 2007. Food, Nutrition, Physical Activity, and the Prevention of Cancer: A Global Perspective. Washington, DC: AICR.

Weaver, C. M. 1994. Age related calcium requirements due to changes in absorption and utilization. Journal of Nutrition 124(Suppl 8): 1418S-25S.

Weaver, C. M., L. D. McCabe, G. P. McCabe, M. Braun, B. R. Martin, L. A. Dimeglio and M. Peacock. 2008. Vitamin D status and calcium metabolism in adolescent black and white girls on a range of controlled calcium intakes. Journal of Clinical Endocrinology and Metabolism 93(10): 3907-14.

Wei, M. Y., C. F. Garland, E. D. Gorham, S. B. Mohr and E. Giovannucci. 2008. Vitamin D and prevention of colorectal adenoma: a meta-analysis. Cancer Epidemiology, Biomarkers & Prevention 17(11): 2958-69.

Weingarten, M. A., A. Zalmanovici and J. Yaphe. 2008. Dietary calcium supplementation for preventing colorectal cancer and adenomatous polyps. Cochrane Database System Review (1): CD003548.

Weinstein, R. S. and N. H. Bell. 1988. Diminished rates of bone formation in normal black adults. New England Journal of Medicine 319(26): 1698-701.

Wejse, C., V. F. Gomes, P. Rabna, P. Gustafson, P. Aaby, I. M. Lisse, P. L. Andersen, H. Glerup and M. Sodemann. 2009. Vitamin D as supplementary treatment for tuberculosis: a double-blind, randomized, placebo-controlled trial.[see comment]. American Journal of Respiratory and Critical Care Medicine 179(9): 843-50.

Welsh, J. 2004. Vitamin D and breast cancer: insights from animal models. American Journal of Clinical Nutrition 80(Suppl 6): 1721S-4S.

Welsh, J. 2007. Vitamin D and prevention of breast cancer. Acta Pharmacologica Sinica 28(9): 1373-82.

Wicherts, I. S., N. M. van Schoor, A. J. Boeke, M. Visser, D. J. Deeg, J. Smit, D. L. Knol and P. Lips. 2007. Vitamin D status predicts physical performance and its decline in older persons. Journal of Clinical Endocrinology and Metabolism 92(6): 2058-65.

Widdowson, E. M., R. A. McCance and C. M. Spray. 1951. The chemical composition of the human body. Clinical Science 10: 113-25.

Wilkins, C. H., S. J. Birge, Y. I. Sheline and J. C. Morris. 2009. Vitamin D deficiency is associated with worse cognitive performance and lower bone density in older African Americans. Journal of the National Medical Association 101(4): 349-54.

Wilton, T., D. Hosking, E. Pawley, A. Stevens and L. Harvey. 1987. Osteomalacia and femoral neck fractures in the elderly patient. Journal of Bone and Joint Surgery. British Volume 69-B(3): 388-90.

Wjst, M. 2005. Variants in the vitamin D receptor gene and asthma. BMC Genetics 6: 2.

Wjst, M. and E. Hypponen. 2007. Vitamin D serum levels and allergic rhinitis. Allergy 62(9): 1085-6.

Wolfberg, A. J., A. Lee-Parritz, A. J. Peller and E. S. Lieberman. 2004. Association of rheumatologic disease with preeclampsia. Obstetrics and Gynecology 103(6): 1190-3.

Woo, J., E. Lau, R. Swaminathan, C. P. Pang and D. MacDonald. 1990. Biochemical predictors for osteoporotic fractures in elderly Chinese—a longitudinal study. Gerontology 36(1): 55-8.

Wu, L., B. R. Martin, M. M. Braun, M. E. Wastney, G. P. McCabe, L. D. McCabe, L. A. DiMeglio, M. Peacock and C. M. Weaver. 2010. Calcium requirements and metabolism in Chinese-American boys and girls. Journal of Bone and Mineral Research 25(8): 1842-9.

Xue, Y. and J. C. Fleet. 2009. Intestinal vitamin D receptor is required for normal calcium and bone metabolism in mice. Gastroenterology 136(4): 1317-27, e1-2.

Yan, J., J. Feng, N. Craddock, I. R. Jones, E. H. Cook, Jr., D. Goldman, L. L. Heston, J. Chen, P. Burkhart, W. Li, A. Shibayama and S. S. Sommer. 2005. Vitamin D receptor variants in 192 patients with schizophrenia and other psychiatric diseases. Neuroscience Letters 380(1-2): 37-41.

Yan, L., B. Zhou, X. Wang, S. D'Ath, A. Laidlaw, M. A. Laskey and A. Prentice. 2003. Older people in China and the United Kingdom differ in the relationships among parathyroid hormone, vitamin D, and bone mineral status. Bone 33(4): 620-7.

Yang, K., M. Lipkin, H. Newmark, B. Rigas, C. Daroqui, S. Maier and L. Augenlicht. 2007. Molecular targets of calcium and vitamin D in mouse genetic models of intestinal cancer. Nutrition Reviews 65(8 Pt 2): S134-7.

Yang, K., N. Kurihara, K. Fan, H. Newmark, B. Rigas, L. Bancroft, G. Corner, E. Livote, M. Lesser, W. Edelmann, A. Velcich, M. Lipkin and L. Augenlicht. 2008. Dietary induction of colonic tumors in a mouse model of sporadic colon cancer. Cancer Research 68(19): 7803-10.

Yang, Z., K. Wang, T. Li, W. Sun, Y. Li, Y. F. Chang, J. S. Dorman and R. E. LaPorte. 1998. Childhood diabetes in China. Enormous variation by place and ethnic group. Diabetes Care 21(4): 525-9.

Yesudian, P. D., J. L. Berry, S. Wiles, S. Hoyle, D. B. Young, A. K. Haylett, L. E. Rhodes and P. Davies. 2008. The effect of ultraviolet B-induced vitamin D levels on host resistance to Mycobacterium tuberculosis: a pilot study in immigrant Asian adults living in the United Kingdom. Photodermatology, Photoimmunology and Photomedicine 24(2): 97-8.

Yetley, E. A., D. Brule, M. C. Cheney, C. D. Davis, K. A. Esslinger, P. W. Fischer, K. E. Friedl, L. S. Greene-Finestone, P. M. Guenther, D. M. Klurfeld, M. R. L'Abbe, K. Y. McMurry, P. E. Starke-Reed and P. R. Trumbo. 2009. Dietary reference intakes for vitamin D: justification for a review of the 1997 values. American Journal of Clinical Nutrition 89(3): 719-27.

Yokomura, K., T. Suda, S. Sasaki, N. Inui, K. Chida and H. Nakamura. 2003. Increased expression of the 25-hydroxyvitamin D(3)-1alpha-hydroxylase gene in alveolar macrophages of patients with lung cancer. Journal of Clinical Endocrinology and Metabolism 88(12): 5704-9.

Yoshikawa, S., T. Nakamura, H. Tanabe and T. Imamura. 1979. Osteomalacic myopathy. Endocrinologia Japonica 26(Suppl): 65-72.

Young, G. A., Jr., N. R. Underdahl and L. E. Carpenter. 1949. Vitamin D intake and susceptibility of mice to experimental swine influenza virus infection. Proceedings of the Society for Experimental Biology and Medicine 72(3): 695-7.

Yu, C. K. H., L. Sykes, M. Sethi, T. G. Teoh and S. Robinson. 2009. Vitamin D deficiency and supplementation during pregnancy. Clinical Endocrinology 70(5): 685-90.

Zeghoud, F., C. Vervel, H. Guillozo, O. Walrant-Debray, H. Boutignon and M. Garabedian. 1997. Subclinical vitamin D deficiency in neonates: definition and response to vitamin D supplements. American Journal of Clinical Nutrition 65(3): 771-8.

Zhu, K., D. Bruce, N. Austin, A. Devine, P. R. Ebeling and R. L. Prince. 2008a. Randomized controlled trial of the effects of calcium with or without vitamin D on bone structure and bone-related chemistry in elderly women with vitamin D insufficiency. Journal of Bone and Mineral Research 23(8): 1343-8.

Zhu, K., A. Devine, I. M. Dick, S. G. Wilson and R. L. Prince. 2008b. Effects of calcium and vitamin D supplementation on hip bone mineral density and calcium-related analytes in elderly ambulatory Australian women: a five-year randomized controlled trial. Journal of Clinical Endocrinology and Metabolism 93(3): 743-9.

Zipitis, C. S. and A. K. Akobeng. 2008. Vitamin D supplementation in early childhood and risk of type 1 diabetes: a systematic review and meta-analysis. Archives of Disease in Childhood 93(6): 512-7.

Zittermann, A., S. S. Schleithoff, G. Tenderich, H. K. Berthold, R. Korfer and P. Stehle. 2003. Low vitamin D status: a contributing factor in the pathogenesis of congestive heart failure? Journal of the American College of Cardiology 41(1): 105-12.

Zittermann, A., S. S. Schleithoff and R. Koerfer. 2005. Putting cardiovascular disease and vitamin D insufficiency into perspective. British Journal of Nutrition 94(4): 483-92.

Zittermann, A., S. Frisch, H. K. Berthold, C. Gotting, J. Kuhn, K. Kleesiek, P. Stehle, H. Koertke and R. Koerfer. 2009. Vitamin D supplementation enhances the beneficial effects of weight loss on cardiovascular disease risk markers. American Journal of Clinical Nutrition 89(5): 1321-7.

Zmuda, J. M., J. A. Cauley, M. E. Danielson, R. L. Wolf and R. E. Ferrell. 1997. Vitamin D receptor gene polymorphisms, bone turnover, and rates of bone loss in older African-American women. Journal of Bone and Mineral Research 12(9): 1446-52.

Zmuda, J. M., J. A. Cauley, M. E. Danielson, T. M. Theobald and R. E. Ferrell. 1999. Vitamin D receptor translation initiation codon polymorphism and markers of osteoporotic risk in older African-American women. Osteoporosis International 9(3): 214-9.

Zmuda, J. M., J. A. Cauley, M. E. Danielson and R. E. Ferrell. 2003. Vitamin D receptor and aromatase gene interaction and bone mass in older African-American women. Metabolism 52(5): 521-3.

5

Dietary Reference Intakes for Adequacy: Calcium and Vitamin D

OVERVIEW

Bone health has been selected as the indicator to serve as the basis of the Dietary Reference Intakes (DRIs) for calcium and vitamin D. The review that underpins this conclusion has been described in Chapter 4, the component of this report addressing the hazard identification step of risk assessment and specifying the selected indicator. The next step in the risk assessment approach for DRI development—the hazard characterization component of risk assessment—is contained in this chapter. The dose–response relationship between the nutrient intake and bone health is examined and dietary reference values for adequacy are specified. In the case of DRIs for calcium and vitamin D, such values take the form of Estimated Average Requirements (EARs) and Recommended Dietary Allowances (RDAs) or, alternatively, Adequate Intakes (AIs). The discussions related to the Tolerable Upper Intake Level (UL), which is also a DRI value, are contained in Chapter 6.

Currently available data on bone health outcomes—when considered as an integrated body of evidence—can be used to derive EARs and RDAs for calcium and vitamin D for all life stages except infants. Bone health measures associated with bone accretion, bone maintenance, and bone loss are relevant to different DRI life stages, and thus the indicator of bone health has been reflected by different bone health measures depending upon the life stage. With respect to infants 0 to 12 months of age, for whom data were very sparse, an AI can be specified for each nutrient based on the available evidence concerning levels of intake observed to be adequate.

The DRIs for calcium and vitamin D established in 1997 (IOM, 1997) also relied on bone health as the indicator in setting reference values for adequacy. However, the 1997 report established an AI for all life stage groups; no EARs or RDAs were specified. Newer data plus an integration of data have allowed the estimation of EARs and RDAs for all life stages except infants. Quantitative comparisons between AIs and EARs and RDAs are not appropriate.

In 1997, AIs were established for calcium in lieu of EARs and RDAs as a result of uncertainties associated with balance studies, lack of concordance between observational and experimental data, and lack of longitudinal data to verify the relationship between calcium intake, calcium retention and bone loss (IOM, 1997). In the past 10 years, newer evidence on skeletal health has emerged from a combination of large-scale randomized trials and calcium balance studies as described in Chapter 4. Further, there are now data relative to a number of life stage groups, and these help to avoid reliance on extrapolating or scaling data from one life stage to another unstudied life stage.

In the case of vitamin D, the 1997 report concluded that there were inadequate data available for EARs and RDAs as a result of uncertainties about sun exposure, the vitamin D content of the diet, and vitamin D stores (IOM, 1997). In the intervening years data have emerged that allow a requirement distribution to be simulated for vitamin D, which, in turn, has been found to be concordant with other available data. This analysis unexpectedly indicated that the dose–response relationship regarding median requirements is not significantly affected by age. Further, several newer studies can be used to elucidate the contributions made by sun exposure and to help separate total intake contributions from contributions stemming from cutaneous synthesis. Strides have been made in estimating the vitamin D content of foods as well as the amounts of vitamin D consumed by the U.S. and Canadian populations.

Despite new data since the earlier Institute of Medicine (IOM) report (IOM, 1997), there remain a number of uncertainties that have caused challenges in estimating DRI values for calcium and vitamin D. Notable among these is the absence of intervention trials that study dose–response relationships for the nutrients. Rather, most of the evidence is derived from a single dose that is often relatively high. Further, some studies fail to specify information about the background diet and hence the total level of intake is lacking. When this is the case, the mean population requirement may be below the dose used in the study, but cannot be further specified. In addition, there is the common practice of designing studies to examine calcium and vitamin D in combination, thereby precluding the ability to discern the effects of each nutrient alone, which is of interest when establishing a reference value for a nutrient.

As discussed in Chapter 4, there are very limited data to suggest that there may be some biological differences in the way in which different ethnic/racial groups respond to calcium and vitamin D, most notably among those of African American ancestry. The extent to which such observations may affect requirements for the nutrients is unknown at this time. Although it is important to take into account biological differences where they may exist among, for example, African Americans, Hispanics, and those of Asian descent, the available data are too limited to permit the committee to assess whether separate, quantitative reference values for such groups are required. The DRIs established in this report are based on the current understanding of the biological needs for calcium and vitamin D across the North American population. Other factors may come into play in terms of ensuring adequate intakes of these nutrients—for example, lactose intolerance or food choices—but as far as is known these factors do not affect the basic biological need for these nutrients. Rather, they are discussed in Chapter 8 as issues relevant to the application of the DRIs by dietary practitioners.

Described in this chapter is the committee's decision-making regarding the dose–response relationships for calcium and bone health, and for vitamin D and bone health. From these conclusions, DRI values for adequacy are specified. A significant underlying assumption made by the committee is that the DRIs for calcium are predicated on intakes that meet requirements for vitamin D and that the DRIs for vitamin D rest on the assumption of intakes that meet requirements for calcium. In other words, the requirement for one nutrient assumes that the need for the other nutrient is being met. This is an essential assumption, for three reasons:

1. Given that reference values are intended to act in concert for the purposes of planning diets, health policy makers would be working to meet all nutritional needs; therefore it would be inappropriate to establish requirements for such purposes on the basis that one or more related nutrients would be consumed by the population in inadequate amounts.
2. An inadequacy in one of the nutrients could cause changes in the efficient handling of or physiological response to the other nutrient that might not otherwise be present. For example, in vitamin D–deficient states with minimal calcium intake, absorption of calcium from the gut cannot be enhanced. The compensatory metabolic response to this scenario is the accelerated conversion of 25-hydroxyvitamin D (25OHD) to its active form (calcitriol) through an increase in parathyroid hormone (PTH) levels. Such perturbations confound the estimation of the true requirement under neutral circumstances.

3. No amount of vitamin D is able to compensate for inadequate total calcium intake; thus, setting a realistic DRI value for vitamin D requires that calcium is available in the diet in adequate amounts.

However, the committee has also commented on the consequences for one nutrient when the other is inadequate, in order to be transparent regarding the science underpinning the determination of reference values for these two nutrients.

CALCIUM: DIETARY REFERENCE INTAKES FOR ADEQUACY

The EARs, RDAs, and AIs for calcium are shown in Table 5-1 by life stage group. The studies used to estimate these values have been included in the review of potential indicators contained in Chapter 4. Therefore, in the discussions below, the relevant data are highlighted but not specifically critiqued again.

Infants 0 to 12 Months of Age

| Infants 0 to 6 Months of Age | AI 200 mg/day Calcium |
| Infants 6 to 12 Months of Age | AI 260 mg/day Calcium |

Data are not sufficient to establish an EAR for infants 0 to 6 and 7 to 12 months of age, and therefore AIs have been developed based on the available evidence. An AI value is not intended to signify an average requirement, but instead reflects an intake level based on approximations or estimates of nutrient intakes that are assumed to be adequate. Whether and how much the AI values for infants could be lowered and still meet the physiological needs for human milk-fed infants are unknown because mechanisms for adaptation to lower intakes of calcium are not well described for the infant population, and experimental data with overall relevance to estimating average requirements are extremely limited.

Calcium requirements for infants are presumed to be met by human milk (IOM, 1997). There are no functional criteria for calcium status that reflect response to calcium intake in infants (IOM, 1997). Rather, human milk is recognized as the optimal source of nourishment for infants (IOM, 1991; Gartner et al., 2005). There are no reports of any full-term, vitamin D–replete infants developing calcium deficiency when exclusively fed human milk (Mimouni et al., 1993; Abrams, 2006). Therefore, AIs for calcium

TABLE 5-1 Calcium Dietary Reference Intakes (DRIs) for Adequacy (amount/day)

Life Stage Group	AI	EAR	RDA
Infants			
0 to 6 mo	200 mg	—	—
6 to 12 mo	260 mg	—	—
Children			
1–3 y	—	500 mg	700 mg
4–8 y	—	800 mg	1,000 mg
Males			
9–13 y	—	1,100 mg	1,300 mg
14–18 y	—	1,100 mg	1,300 mg
19–30 y	—	800 mg	1,000 mg
31–50 y	—	800 mg	1,000 mg
51–70 y	—	800 mg	1,000 mg
> 70 y	—	1,000 mg	1,200 mg
Females			
9–13 y	—	1,100 mg	1,300 mg
14–18 y	—	1,100 mg	1,300 mg
19–30 y	—	800 mg	1,000 mg
31–50 y	—	800 mg	1,000 mg
51–70 y	—	1,000 mg	1,200 mg
> 70 y	—	1,000 mg	1,200 mg
Pregnancy			
14–18 y	—	1,100 mg	1,300 mg
19–30 y	—	800 mg	1,000 mg
31–50 y	—	800 mg	1,000 mg
Lactation			
14–18 y	—	1,100 mg	1,300 mg
19–30 y	—	800 mg	1,000 mg
31–50 y	—	800 mg	1,000 mg

NOTE: AI = Adequate Intake; EAR = Estimated Average Requirement; RDA = Recommended Dietary Allowance.

for infants are based on mean intake data from infants fed human milk as the principal fluid during the first year of life and on the studies that have determined the mean calcium content of breast milk. Additionally, information on calcium absorption and calcium accretion is taken into account.

With respect to estimating AIs for calcium for infants, studies reviewed previously in this report have provided the following information:

- Based on infant weighing studies, a reasonable average amount of breast milk consumed is 780 mL/day. The average level of calcium within a liter of breast milk is 259 mg (± 59 mg). It is therefore estimated that the intake of calcium for infants fed exclusively human milk is 202 mg/day. This number is rounded to 200 mg/day.

- Calcium absorption for this age group ranges somewhat above and below 60 percent depending upon the total amount of calcium consumed. For development of the AI, a 60 percent calcium absorption rate was assumed.
- The usual accretion rate for calcium in infants can be estimated using the approximation of 100 mg/day overall during the first year of life, with the recognition that the available literature contains reports of varying rates above and below that level.

Infants 0 to 6 Months of Age

Using the estimates described above for the calcium content of breast milk and the amount of milk consumed per day, the AI for calcium for infants 0 to 6 months of age is 200 mg/day, a value reflective of the calcium provided to exclusively breast-fed infants. The expected net retention of calcium from human milk assuming 60 percent absorption would be 120 mg/day, which is in excess of the values predicted from calcium accretion based on cadaver and metacarpal analysis. An AI of 200 mg/day is expected, therefore, to result in retention of sufficient amounts of calcium to meet growth needs.

Further, for infants in the first 4 months of life, balance studies suggest that 40 to 70 percent of the daily calcium intake is retained by the human milk-fed infant (Widdowson, 1965; Fomon and Nelson, 1993). In balance studies using human milk–fed infants, the mean calcium intake was 327 mg/day, and calcium retention was 172 mg/day on average (Fomon and Nelson, 1993). If infants consume calcium at the AI daily, they would achieve similar or greater calcium retention even if the efficiency of absorption was at the lower observed value of 30 percent. Thus, the AI should meet most infants' needs.

The AI established here of 200 mg/day is similar to the AI of 210 mg/day derived by the 1997 report (IOM, 1997). The difference is extremely small—only 10 mg/day—and likely within measurement error; however, the new AI reflects the current best estimate for calcium levels obtained exclusively from human milk

Infants 6 to 12 Months of Age

Estimation of the AI for infants 6 to 12 months of age takes into account the additional intake of calcium from food. From 6 to 12 months of age, the intake of solid foods becomes more significant, and calcium intakes may increase substantially from these sources. Only extremely limited data are available for typical calcium intakes from foods by older milk-fed infants, and mean calcium intake from solid foods has been approximated as 140 mg/day for formula-fed infants (personal communication, Dr. Steven Abrams, February 22, 2010).

For the purpose of developing an AI for this age group, it is assumed that infants who are fed human milk have intakes of solid food similar to those of formula-fed infants of the same age (Specker et al., 1997). Based on data from Dewey et al. (1984), mean human milk intake during the second 6 months of life would be 600 mL/day. Thus, calcium intake from human milk with a calcium concentration of about 200 mg/L during this age span (Atkinson et al., 1995) would be approximately 120 mg/day. Adding the estimated intake from food (140 mg/day) to the estimated intake from human milk (120 mg/day) gives a total intake of 260 mg/day. Again, this AI is slightly and probably insignificantly less than the 1997 AI (IOM, 1997) but is the current best estimate.

Children and Adolescents 1 Through 18 Years of Age

Children 1 Through 3 Years of Age

> EAR 500 mg/day Calcium
> RDA 700 mg/day Calcium

Children 4 Through 8 Years of Age

> EAR 800 mg/day Calcium
> RDA 1,000 mg/day Calcium

Children 9 Through 13 Years of Age
Adolescents 14 Through 18 Years of Age

> EAR 1,100 mg/day Calcium
> RDA 1,300 mg/day Calcium

For these life stage groups, the focus is the level of calcium intake consistent with bone accretion and positive calcium balance. Studies conducted primarily between 1999 and 2009 (see Table 5-2) provide a basis for estimating EARs and calculating RDAs. In contrast to earlier reference value deliberations for which there were virtually no available studies focused on children and adolescents, this committee benefited from several recent studies that used children as subjects.

The approach used for children was to determine average calcium accretion through bone measures such as DXA and average calcium retention as estimated by calcium balance studies (i.e., positive balance). Next, the factorial method (IOM, 1997) was used with these two data sets to estimate the intake needed to achieve the bone accretion. Average bone calcium accretion is used rather than peak calcium accretion because the committee judged this value to be more consistent with meeting the needs

TABLE 5-2 Calcium Intake Estimated to Achieve Average Bone Calcium Accretion for Children and Adolescents Using the Factorial Method

Study Author, Year	Age/ Gender	Average Calcium Accretion (mg/day)	Urinary Losses (mg/day)	Endogenous Fecal Calcium Losses (mg/day)	Sweat Losses (mg/day)	Total Needed (mg/day)	Absorption (percent)	Estimated Total Intake (Adjusted for Absorption)
Lynch et al., 2007	1–3 Male/Female	142	34	40	—	216	45.6	474
Abrams et al., 1999; Ames et al., 1999	4–8 Male/Female	140–160	40	50	—	240	30.0	800
Vatanparast et al., 2010	9–13 Female	151	106	112	55	424	38.0	1,116
	9–13 Male	141	127	108	55	465	38.0	1,224
	14–18 Female	92	106	112	55	365	38.0	961
	14–18 Male	210	127	105	55	500	38.0	1,316
	9–18 Female	121	106	112	55	394	38.0	1,037
	9–18 Male	175	127	108	55	465	38.0	1,224

of 50 percent of this population, and hence an EAR (rather than an AI). Moreover, as discussed in Chapter 2, peak calcium accretion with higher total calcium intakes is likely transitory and, thus, not consistent with DRI development.

The application of the factorial method using average bone calcium accretion allows an estimate of the calcium intake required to support bone accretion and net calcium retention, as shown in Table 5-2. The approach is described below, specifically for each life stage for children and adolescents.

Children 1 Through 3 Years of Age

The data are very limited for children 1 through 3 years of age given the challenges in studying young children. However, a report by Lynch et al. (2007) provides relevant data. Linear and non-linear modeling in this study suggested a target average calcium retention level of 142 mg/day, consistent with the growth needs of this life stage group. Through the factorial method, a calcium intake of 474 mg/day is estimated to meet this need (see Table 5-2). Given that these data are derived from mean estimates and are assumed to be normally distributed, the mean value is very likely the median value. An estimated EAR is, therefore, established as 500 mg of calcium per day, rounded from 474 mg/day.

An assumption specified by Lynch et al. (2007) is that an additional 30 percent calcium retention would meet the needs of 97.5 percent of this age group. This was calculated as 180 mg/day and is based on calcium absorptive efficiency for young children, and it is judged reasonable. This results in an estimated RDA for calcium of 700 mg/day calcium, with rounding.

Clearly, there are uncertainties when reliance is placed on a single study. The ability to study calcium requirements in a controlled study, however, does offer the ability to estimate an average requirement rather than an AI. The study is of high quality, and the reference values specified are in line with those specified for younger and older children.

Children 4 Through 8 Years of Age

The work of Abrams et al. (1999) and Ames et al. (1999) has indicated that, like that for younger children, an average calcium retention level of approximately 140 mg/day is consistent with the needs of bone accretion. However, there is evidence of a small increase during pre-puberty, yielding a calcium retention range of approximately 140 to 160 mg/day to allow for bone accretion across this age group of which a portion will be pre-pubertal. Using the factorial method (see Table 5-2) and from the non-linear dose–response relationship identified by the work of Ames et al.(1999) and Abrams et al. (1999), a calcium intake of 800 mg/day could be expected to achieve the levels of calcium needed for bone accretion. Again, the assumption that another approximately 30 percent is needed to cover about 97.5 percent of the population—through derivation as mean estimates and the assumption of normal distribution—results in a calculated and rounded RDA value for calcium of 1,000 mg/day.

Again, as with younger children, there are relatively few studies available and most have small sample sizes. While the studies included some ethnic/racial diversity, they focused on girls. These limitations cannot be remedied at this time. However, the data are sufficiently robust to support an estimation of an average requirement of 800 mg/day calcium.

Children 9 Through 13 Years of Age and Adolescents 14 Through 18 Years of Age

As reviewed in Chapter 4, data from a recent study (Vatanparast et al., 2010) have provided bone calcium accretion levels for children and adolescents ranging from 92 to 210 mg/day. Average bone calcium accretion was included in the factorial method, and the intake levels can be estimated as shown in Table 5-2.

While the committee was aware of data suggesting that calcium retention may vary by gender among children, these differences between girls and boys and between the 9- to 13- and 14- to 18-year age groups are relatively small quantitatively, and the limited nature of the data do not allow further specification of these differences to the extent they are real. Given the application of DRI values in real world settings such as school meal planning, recommending that boys receive a small amount more calcium than girls is not practicable, but it is also not warranted given the limited nature of the data suggesting this possibility. Additionally, there is wide variability in the onset of puberty and the pubertal growth spurt, and it is reasonable to conclude that increases in calcium intake may be needed early in puberty at times when children may be only 9 or 10 years old. Thus, for reference values for both boys and girls in the 9- to 13- and 14- to 18-year life stages, the differences in calcium intake to achieve mean bone calcium accretion as elucidated by Vatanparast et al. (2010) have been interpolated between 9- to 18-year old girls (1,037) and boys (1,224). This interpolation yields an estimated mean need for calcium for boys and girls of 1,100 mg/day with rounding, a value approximately at the midpoint between the two groups. Again, assuming a normal distribution, this estimate to achieve a mean calcium accretion represents the median and, thus, an EAR. The EAR is therefore set at 1,100 mg for both boys and girls for both life stages encompassed by the 9 through 18 year age range. In order to cover 97.5 percent of the population, an estimated RDA value for calcium of 1,300 mg/day is established.

The uncertainties surrounding the reference value stem from reliance on primarily a single study. Although carefully carried out, the study included only white children. These newer data, however, provide the opportunity to identify an average requirement.

Adults 19 Through 50 Years of Age

Adults 19 Through 30 Years of Age
Adults 31 Through 50 Years of Age
EAR 800 mg/day Calcium
RDA 1,000 mg/day Calcium

While there is evidence of minor bone accretion into early adulthood, the levels required to achieve this accretion—which appears to be site dependent—are very low. The goal, therefore, is intakes of calcium that promote bone maintenance and neutral calcium balance.

The report from Hunt and Johnson (2007) provides virtually the only evidence for these life stage groups. Based on a series of controlled calcium balance studies, they have established a calcium intake level of 741 mg/day to maintain neutral calcium balance. They further provide the 95 percent prediction interval around the level required for neutral calcium balance.

Other available measures that relate to bone maintenance include bone mineral density (BMD), but studies that measured bone mass concomitant to calcium intake are highly confounded by failures to control for other variables that impact bone mass and to specify a dose–response relationship. There is no evidence that intakes of calcium higher than those specified by Hunt and Johnson (2007) offer benefit for bone health in the context of bone maintenance for adults 19 to 50 years of age. Osteoporotic fracture is not a relevant measure for this life stage, therefore extrapolating from the more prevalent data focused on older adults is not appropriate, nor is extrapolating from the data for younger persons for whom the concern is bone accretion.

Therefore, the Hunt and Johnson (2007) data, which reflect the outcomes of a series of metabolic studies, provide a reasonable basis for an EAR for calcium of 800 mg/day calcium. That is, the observed value of 741 mg/day is rounded, but rounded up to 800 mg/day given the uncertainty. The upper limit of the 95 percent prediction interval around this estimate (1,035 mg/day) is appropriate as the basis for an RDA for calcium and rounded to 1,000 mg/day. As is the case with younger life stage groups, there is now the 2007 Hunt and Johnson study on the topic of calcium and bone health, which has allowed the estimation of an average requirement.

However, the data are still very sparse, and the DRI for this age group relies on one study, albeit a well-controlled and carefully analyzed study.

Adults 51 Years of Age and Older

Men 51 Through 70 Years of Age	EAR 800 mg/day Calcium
	RDA 1,000 mg/day Calcium
Women 51 Through 70 Years of Age	EAR 1,000 mg/day Calcium
	RDA 1,200 mg/day Calcium
Adults >70 Years of Age	EAR 1,000 mg/day Calcium
	RDA 1,200 mg/day Calcium

Men and Women 51 Through 70 Years of Age

The natural process of bone loss begins to manifest itself in the latter stages of adulthood. It begins earlier for women than for men as a result of the onset of menopause, which usually occurs when women reach 50 to 55 years of age. By the time both men and women have reached 70 or more years of age, each are experiencing bone loss. However, women— who have been undergoing the loss longer—are more at risk for adverse consequences. It is important to underscore that the goal of calcium intake during these life stages is to lessen the degree of bone loss; calcium intake at any level is not known to prevent bone loss.

Although calcium absorption (active calcium transport) has been reported to decrease with age (Avioli et al., 1965; Bullamore et al., 1970; Alevizaki et al., 1973; Gallagher et al., 1979; Tsai et al., 1984), it is challenging to consider higher calcium intake as a remedy given that calcium intake must be extremely high to have an effect on calcium uptake via passive absorption (i.e., paracellular transport, see Chapter 2).

The relative lack of data pertaining to bone changes in men as they age has received comment (Orwoll et al., 1990). It has been pointed out that cross–sectional data suggest that, overall, the rate of bone loss in men is substantially slower than that in women, and men have a lower incidence of fractures (Khosla et al., 2008); perhaps this accounts for the lack of research focused on this group. The limited available trials and observation studies (e.g., Osteoporotic Fractures in Men [MrOS] study) concerning bone health focus on men older than the 5 through 70 year age range (usually > 65 years) and typically include vitamin D administration. Likewise, organizations such as the National Osteoporosis Foundation have issued guidelines that do not stipulate BMD testing for men until the age of 70 years (NOF, 2008), whereas they recommend BMD testing at an earlier age for women. Given this context, the data from Hunt and Johnson (2007) with respect to neutral calcium balance among adults can provide some information for specifying requirements among men between the ages of 51 and 70 years. Although there were only two men over the age of 50 years in the Hunt and Johnson (2007) study, the absence of evidence that significant changes occur in skeletal maintenance for men in their 50s and 60s results in the assumption that their needs are akin to those of younger men. Therefore, the calcium EAR and RDA for men 51 to 70 years of age are set at the same levels as for persons 31 to 50 years of age: the EAR for calcium is established as 800 mg/day, and the RDA for calcium is 1,000 mg/day. The newer calcium balance data are used with caution, given its limitations for this purpose.

Women 51 through 70 years of age are considered separately from men. Although it is evident that calcium intake does not prevent bone less during the first few years of menopause, there is the question of whether or to what extent calcium intake can mitigate the loss of bone during and immediately following the onset of menopause. Although about half of the women in the Hunt and Johnson (2007) study were over the age of 50, the authors did not stratify on the basis of menopausal status. Therefore, there are some uncertainties surrounding the use of these newer calcium balance data for the purposes of determining an EAR and RDA for women. However, other information is available that can be useful. Absolute hip fracture rates are lower than for women in this age rang than for women over the age 70 but still greater than for premenopausal women. Moreover, BMD is a reliable predictor for fracture risk later in life and therefore becomes a useful measure for DRI purposes.

The available data for BMD among women 51 through 70 years of age provide mixed results concerning the relationship between BMD and calcium intake in menopausal women. This may be due in part to study protocols—which usually have relied on a single dose of 1,000 mg or more daily—that have failed to clarify background diet or estimate total intake. On balance, there is somewhat more evidence for a benefit of higher calcium intake among women over the age of 60 years, a group that is likely about half of the DRI life stage of women 51 through 70 years of age. Specifically, the meta-analysis conducted by Tang et al. (2007), which included studies in women ranging in mean age from 50 to 85 years, indicated that total calcium intake alone equal to 1,200 mg or more per day had a positive effect on BMD as well as a modest (relative risk [RR] = 0.88; 95%

confidence interval [CI]:0.83–0.95), but significant, effect on fracture risk reduction. In breaking down the meta-analysis further, there were six studies of more than 1,100 women with a mean age of 60 years who received additional calcium without vitamin D compared with placebo. The average calcium supplementation was 1,100 mg/day in the treated group, and those women had risk reduction for hip fracture and significant increases in both hip and spine BMD.

Further, evidence from the Women's Health Initiative trial (WHI) (Jackson et al., 2006) conducted using 36,282 women ages 50 to 79 years indicated that participants who were randomized to 1,000 mg of calcium plus 400 International Units (IU) of vitamin D per day experienced a small, but significant, improvement in hip bone density and a modest reduction in hip fractures, although the change in hip fracture risk was not statistically significant. A subgroup analysis indicated that women over the age of 60 years also experienced a small but statistically non-significant reduction in hip fracture risk (hazard ratio [HR] = 0.74; 95 percent CI 0.52–1.06) compared with those randomized to placebo. These data are taken into account cautiously for several reasons. The WHI study may be confounded by both hormone replacement therapy considerations as well as the inclusion of vitamin D, although the supplementation level of vitamin D was relatively low. The appropriateness of conducting a subgroup analysis for fracture risk, although interesting, is always considered questionable. Further, the same subgroup analysis revealed that women between the ages of 50 and 60 years experienced a greater hip fracture risk when they were supplemented with calcium and vitamin D. The absolute risk of hip fractures for women 50 to 60 years of age is derived from a small number of fractures per total cohort (i.e., 13 fractures in 6,694 women 50 to 60 years of age). The Tang et al. (2007) meta-analysis is compromised by the inability to study a true dose–response relationship; many studies were grouped at the 1,200 mg/day level of intake and could not be used to reveal the effects at lower levels of intake.

Within the confines of these limitations, there is nonetheless the emerging conclusion that in regard to the relevant indicator for this group, that is, BMD, a somewhat higher intake of calcium than required by men or suggested by the newer calcium balance data is justified for all postmenopausal women within the life stage 51 through 70 years. Not unexpectedly, absolute hip fracture rates are very low in the 50- to 60-year age group (e.g., 0.03 percent per year in WHI), and therefore fracture risk is not a particularly relevant factor, although to the extent that a subgroup analysis can be relied upon, women greater than 60 years of age appear to experience some benefit from calcium intake relevant to fracture risk reduction.

It would appear that the life stage consisting of women 51 through

70 years of age reflects a diverse set of physiological conditions—notably premenopausal, perimenopausal, and postmenopausal—with respect to the condition of bone health, and cannot be reliably characterized as a homogeneous single group for the purpose of deriving EARs and RDAs for calcium. Some may benefit from increased calcium, and some may not. Further, there is considerable variability in the age of onset of menopause, and so assumptions about the proportion of this age group that may or may not benefit cannot be made. Therefore, to ensure public health protection and to err on the side of caution, preference is given to covering the apparent benefit for BMD with higher intakes of calcium for postmenopausal women within this group. The EAR for women 51 through 70 years is set at 1,000 mg calcium per day. The addition of 200 mg/day to the estimates provided by Hunt and Johnson (2007) gives a reasonable margin of safety for lessening bone loss to the extent that is possible and is reasonably consistent with data from the existing intervention trials. Further, the value of 1,000 mg/ day is still within the 95 percent prediction interval offered by Hunt and Johnson (2007) for a value that encompasses a wider range of persons than younger menopausal women. Although this does result in a different DRI for women than for men in the 51 through 70 year age group, the physiological differences and apparent response to increased calcium intake evidenced from randomized trials warrants this difference.

As there is no reason to assume that requirements for this life stage are not normally distributed, the approximate 20 to 30 percent addition to achieve the level needed to cover 97.5 percent of the population results in an estimated RDA of 1,200 mg/day. The level errs in the direction of a lower value given concerns about an upper level of intake (see Chapter 6).

This reference value for women 51 to 70 years of age is notably uncertain and reflects a decision to provide public health protection in the face of inconsistent data. It also identifies menopausal women between the ages of 51 and 70 years as the basis for the reference value, rather than non-menopausal women, on the assumption that during this life stage many and eventually all will become menopausal. The value cannot be more certain until such time as there is information on calcium balance specifically for women experiencing the early stages of menopause, as well as well-controlled trials that more clearly elucidate dose–response measures for menopausal younger women relative to calcium intake and bone health.

Adults >70 Years of Age

Bone loss and the resulting osteoporotic fractures are the predominant bone health concern for persons >70 years of age. Although measures to ascertain fracture risk are often self-reported and can be challenging to verify, fracture risk represents the best measure for bone health for this life stage. One important caution is that the estimation of the effect of fracture risk is greatly complicated by the limited evidence concerning dose–response data relative to calcium intake. Importantly, calcium balance studies to determine the levels of calcium that result in neutral calcium balance are lacking in the literature for persons over the age of 70 years. Hunt and Johnson (2007) were able to incorporate only two women over the age of 70 years.

The analysis of Tang et al. (2007) is limited by the nature of the studies available, in that most studies tested intervention levels at or above 1,200 mg/day and often did not report total calcium intake. Those studies in the Tang et al. (2007) analysis that examined calcium alone, without vitamin D supplementation, were few. The authors' conclusion that 1,200 mg/ day was beneficial relative to reduced fracture risk is relevant, but may be compromised by the inability to examine the effectiveness at other levels. In contrast to the Tang et al. (2007) analysis, Peacock et al. (2000), Grant et al. (2005), and Prince et al. (2006), who studied calcium intake alone, were unable to demonstrate benefits for bone health among persons over 70 years of age with supplemental calcium intakes (750 to 1,200 mg/day); however, a compliance sub-analysis conducted by Prince et al. (2006) suggested reduced fracture incidence with calcium supplementation of 1,200 mg/day.

The data available do not clearly elucidate a requirement for calcium and primarily suggest values that may result in covering nearly all of the population group in terms of reduced fracture risk. That is, the available studies were not examining the levels of calcium intake that were effective, but rather were examining whether their administered calcium intake was effective. Further, the benefit of calcium supplementation was evident in the case of sub-analysis on the basis of compliance, which, while informative, are not ideal data sets. In addition, the populations studied varied considerably, many could be considered at high risk (such as institutionalized older persons and persons with low body weight), and the effect of calcium supplementation was usually not taken into account in the context of vitamin D status or existing calcium nutriture.

For this reason, public health protection was considered, and it was determined that a requirement somewhat above that established by calcium balance studies for bone maintenance was appropriate despite the unknowns and the inability to clearly estimate a dose–response for calcium relative to fracture risk. As with those estimates used for postmenopausal women, a 200 mg/day calcium increment was added to the estimated requirements for younger persons, resulting in an EAR value of 1,000 mg of calcium per day. It is assumed that the rapid and notable bone loss observed for early menopause has ceased, and the bone loss for women in this life stage group is similar to that experienced by men. The estimation of an RDA to cover more than 97.5 percent of the life stage group consistent with normally distributed data results in an RDA of 1,200 mg/day, again in the face of concerns about high levels of intake (see Chapter 6).

Pregnancy and Lactation

Pregnant 14 Through 18 Years of Age

EAR 1,100 mg/day Calcium
RDA 1,300 mg/day Calcium

Pregnant 19 Through 30 Years of Age
Pregnant 31 Through 50 Years of Age

EAR 800 mg/day Calcium
RDA 1,000 mg/day Calcium

Lactating 14 Through 18 Years of Age

EAR 1,100 mg/day Calcium
RDA 1,300 mg/day Calcium

Lactating 19 Through 30 Years of Age
Lactating 31 Through 50 Years of Age

EAR 800 mg/day Calcium
RDA 1,000 mg/day Calcium

Pregnancy

The EAR for non-pregnant women and adolescents is appropriate for pregnant women and adolescents based on the randomized controlled trials (RCTs) of calcium supplementation during pregnancy that reveal no evidence that additional calcium intake beyond normal non-pregnant requirements has any benefit to mother or fetus (Koo et al., 1999; Jarjou et al., 2010). Consistent with the RCT data indicating the appropriateness of the non-pregnant EAR and RDA for the pregnant woman is (1) the epidemiologic evidence suggesting that parity is associated with a neutral or even a protective effect relative to maternal BMD or fracture risk (Sowers, 1996; Kovacs and Kronenberg, 1997; O'Brien et al., 2003; Chantry et al., 2004), and (2) the physiologic evidence that maternal calcium needs are met through key changes resulting in a doubling of the intestinal fractional calcium absorption, which compensates for the increased calcium transferred to the fetus (200 to 250 mg/day) and potentially some transient mobilization of maternal bone mineral, particularly in the late third trimester.

Overall, it appears that pregnant adolescents make the same adaptations as pregnant women, and there is no evidence of adverse effects of pregnancy on BMD measures among adolescents.

The EARs are thus 800 mg/day for pregnant women and 1,100 mg/day for pregnant adolescents. Likewise, the RDA values for non-pregnant women and adolescents are applicable, providing RDAs of 1,000 mg/day and 1,300 mg/day, respectively.

Lactation

The EAR for non-lactating women and adolescents is appropriate for lactating women and adolescents based on (1) the strong evidence of physiologic changes resulting in a transient maternal bone resorption to provide the infant with calcium (Kalkwarf et al., 1997; Specker et al. 1997; Kalkwarf, 1999) and (2) evidence from RCTs and observational studies that increased total calcium intake does not suppress this maternal bone resorption (Cross et al., 1995; Fairweather-Tait et al., 1995; Prentice et al., 1995; Kalkwarf et al., 1997; Laskey et al., 1998; Polatti et al., 1999) or alter the calcium content of human milk (Kalkwarf et al., 1997; Jarjou et al., 2006). Post-lactation maternal bone mineral is restored without consistent evidence that higher calcium intake is required, as based on two RCTs (Cross et al., 1995; Prentice et al., 1995) and several observational studies (Sowers, 1996; Kovacs and Kronenberg 1997; Kalkwarf, 1999).

Adolescents, like adults, resorb bone during lactation and recover fully afterward with no evidence that lactation impairs achievement of peak bone mass (Chantry et al., 2004).

The EARs are thus 800 for lactating women and 1,100 mg/day for lactating adolescents. Likewise, the RDA values for non-lactating women and adolescents are applicable, providing RDAs of 1,000 and 1,300 mg/day, respectively.

VITAMIN D: DIETARY REFERENCE INTAKES FOR ADEQUACY

The EARs, RDAs, and AIs for vitamin D are shown in Table 5-3 by life stage group. The identical EARs across age groups are notable and, as discussed below, reflect the concordance of serum 25OHD levels with the integrated bone health outcomes as well as the lack of an age effect on the simulated dose–response. Studies used to estimate these values have been included in Chapter 4 in the review of potential indicators.

While at the outset the consideration of vitamin D requirements recognizes that humans are physiologically capable of obtaining vitamin D

TABLE 5-3 Vitamin D Dietary Reference Intakes (DRIs) for Adequacy (amount/day)

Life Stage Group	AI	EAR	RDA
Infants			
0 to 6 mo	400 IU (10 µg)	—	—
6 to 12 mo	400 IU (10 µg)	—	—
Children			
1–3 y	—	400 IU (10 µg)	600 IU (15 µg)
4–8 y	—	400 IU (10 µg)	600 IU (15 µg)
Males			
9–13 y	—	400 IU (10 µg)	600 IU (15 µg)
14–18 y	—	400 IU (10 µg)	600 IU (15 µg)
19–30 y	—	400 IU (10 µg)	600 IU (15 µg)
31–50 y	—	400 IU (10 µg)	600 IU (15 µg)
51–70 y	—	400 IU (10 µg)	600 IU (15 µg)
> 70 y	—	400 IU (10 µg)	800 IU (20 µg)
Females			
9–13 y	—	400 IU (10 µg)	600 IU (15 µg)
14–18 y	—	400 IU (10 µg)	600 IU (15 µg)
19–30 y	—	400 IU (10 µg)	600 IU (15 µg)
31–50 y	—	400 IU (10 µg)	600 IU (15 µg)
51–70 y	—	400 IU (10 µg)	600 IU (15 µg)
> 70 y	—	400 IU (10 µg)	800 IU (20 µg)
Pregnancy			
14–18 y	—	400 IU (10 µg)	600 IU (15 µg)
19–30 y	—	400 IU (10 µg)	600 IU (15 µg)
31–50 y	—	400 IU (10 µg)	600 IU (15 µg)
Lactation			
14–18 y	—	400 IU (10 µg)	600 IU (15 µg)
19–30 y	—	400 IU (10 µg)	600 IU (15 µg)
31–50 y	—	400 IU (10 µg)	600 IU (15 µg)

NOTE: AI = Adequate Intake; EAR = Estimated Average Requirement; IU = International Unit; RDA = Recommended Dietary Allowance.

through exposure to sunlight, the estimation of DRIs for vitamin D immediately requires a plethora of related considerations ranging from factors that affect and alter sun exposure and vitamin D synthesis, to public health recommendations regarding the need to limit sun exposure to avoid cancer risk. Just as importantly, the available data have not sufficiently explored the relationship between total intake of vitamin D per se and health outcomes. In short, a dose–response relationship between vitamin D intake and bone health is lacking. Rather, measures of serum 25OHD levels as a biomarker of exposure (i.e., intake) are more prevalent.

After considering the available evidence, including data published after the 2009 analysis by the Agency for Healthcare Research and Quality (Chung et al., 2009), hereafter referred to as AHRQ-Tufts, the committee concluded:

- A dose–response relationship can be simulated based on serum 25OHD measures. That is, serum 25OHD levels can reflect intake, and there are studies that relate bone health outcomes to serum 25OHD levels, as described in Chapter 4.
- Newer data provide the ability to link vitamin D intakes to the change in serum 25OHD level under conditions of minimal sun exposure, thereby reducing the confounding introduced by the effect of sun exposure on serum 25OHD concentrations. These data also provide an approach for estimating dietary reference values related to intakes that will achieve targeted serum 25OHD concentrations, albeit without regard to the contributions from sun exposure.

Generally, association studies that use a biomarker of exposure in relation to health outcomes can present challenges when establishing reference values. Such measures are not necessarily valid or reliable markers, and they can be subject to considerable confounding by a host of variables. In the case of vitamin D, there are certain factors that allow more confidence in using this measure in the estimation of reference values. Specific deficiencies of vitamin D lead to recognized, measurable deficiency states with adverse effects on the indicator of interest, in this case bone health as evidenced by rickets and osteomalacia. The next consideration is whether the biomarker is an accurate reflection of intake. In the case of serum 25OHD concentrations, despite the lack of clarity about the impact of a number of variables on serum 25OHD concentrations, the measure can be reasonably associated with total intake when sunlight exposure is minimal.

On this basis, serum 25OHD concentrations were used to simulate a dose–response relationship for bone health. Next, the available data—notably those obtained under conditions of limited sun exposure—were integrated in order to estimate a total intake that would result in the desired serum 25OHD relative to measures of bone health. This step-wise process for simulating a dose–response relationship for vitamin D considered, first, the relevance to this study of the confounding introduced by 25OHD assay methodologies and related measurement problems, including "assay drift." Next, the data from three bodies of evidence described in Chapter 3—the relationship between calcium absorption and serum 25OHD levels; serum 25OHD levels and bone health in children; and serum 25OHD levels and bone health in older adults—were summarized and used to specify a dose–response curve for serum 25OHD. Interestingly, concordance of serum 25OHD levels and bone health for median requirements emerged across all age groups. Finally, the relationship between changes in vitamin D intake and changes in serum 25OHD concentrations was considered.

Simulation of a Dose–Response Relationship for Vitamin D Intake and Bone Health

"Assay Drift" and Implications for Interpretation of
Serum 25OHD Data in the Literature

In considering serum 25OHD levels as reported by various studies, the committee was aware of the so-called "assay drift" associated with longitudinal comparison of assay results collected in the National Health and Nutrition Examination Survey (NHANES), as well as the large inter-laboratory variation worldwide (Carter et al., 2010) and the differences in performance characteristics between the various antibody-based and liquid chromatography (LC)-based assays. Although it was reported that a consistent assay bias was recognized within the NHANES data for certain time periods (2000–2006)[1], this assay drift as described in Chapter 3 is small in comparison with the inter-laboratory variation or the methodological differences observed in data from the Vitamin D External Quality Assurance Scheme (DEQAS) (Carter et al., 2010).

Accordingly, for the purposes of this study, a correction of data based on knowledge of assay drift was neither practical nor necessary for the determination of DRI values. The NHANES assay drift applies to certain data analyzed within a known time frame (2004–2006), but at the same time other data using similar methods might have experienced drift that was unknown and therefore could not be accounted for or corrected. Moreover, the dispersion of serum 25OHD levels across the range of vitamin D intakes is very large, as exemplified by data from Millen et al. (2010).

Although methodological issues contribute to uncertainty in comparing data among studies, the differences in serum 25OHD over time due to assay drift are relatively small and thus inconsequential when viewed relative to other sources of biological variation. In essence, assay drift is considered to be a component of the noise within the signal, and one of the contributors to uncertainty. But for DRI purposes it did not require re-evaluation or normalization of data. Regarding NHANES data specifically as they were used by the committee as a basis for the intake assessment (Chapter 7), the ramifications of "assay drift" are more significant

---

[1] Centers for Disease Control and Prevention (CDC). Available online at http://www.cdc.gov/nchs/data/nhanes/nhanes3/VitaminDanalyticnote.pdf (accessed July 8, 2010).

for longitudinal comparisons, which were not a component of the intake assessment.

Conclusions Regarding Data for Serum 25OHD and Bone Health

The evidence presented in Chapter 4 allows the following conclusions about serum 25OHD concentrations relative to DRI development:

- *Calcium absorption*
  Given that an identified key role of vitamin D is to enhance calcium absorption, evidence regarding the level of serum 25OHD associated with maximal calcium absorption is relevant to establishing a dose–response relationship for serum 25OHD level and bone health outcomes. As outlined in Chapter 4, for both children and adults there was a trend toward maximal calcium absorption between serum 25OHD levels of 30 and 50 nmol/L, with no clear evidence of further benefit above 50 nmol/L.

- *Rickets*
  In the face of adequate calcium, the risk of rickets increases below a serum 25OHD level of 30 nmol/L and is minimal when serum 25OHD levels range between 30 and 50 nmol/L. Moreover, when calcium intakes are inadequate, vitamin D supplementation to the point of serum 25OHD concentrations up to and beyond 75 nmol/L has no effect.

- *Serum 25OHD level and fracture risk: Randomized clinical trials using adults*
  Because available trials often administered relatively high doses of vitamin D, serum 25OHD concentrations varied considerably. Although some studies suggested that serum 25OHD concentrations of approximately 40 nmol/L are sufficient to meet bone health requirements for most people, findings from other studies suggested that levels of 50 nmol/L and higher were consistent with bone health. Given that causality has been established between changes in serum 25OHD levels and bone health outcomes, information from observational studies can be useful in determining the dose–response relationship.

- *Serum 25OHD level and fracture risk: Observational studies using adults*
  Melhus et al. (2010) found that serum 25OHD levels below 40 nmol/L predicted modestly increased risk of fracture in elderly men, but there was no additional risk reduction above 40 nmol/L,

suggesting maximum population coverage at 40 nmol/L. In contrast, Ensrud et al. (2009) observed that men with 25OHD levels below 50 nmol/L had greater subsequent rates of femoral bone loss, and there was no additional benefit from serum 25OHD concentrations higher than 50 nmol/L, suggesting maximum population coverage at 50 nmol/L. Still other studies suggested that somewhat higher serum 25OHD concentrations were needed to provide maximum population coverage. For example, Cauley et al. (2008), in a prospective cohort study, reported that serum 25OHD concentrations in the range of 60 to 70 nmol/L were associated with the lowest risk of hip fracture; above this level, risk was reported to increase, but not significantly. Looker and Mussolino (2008), using NHANES data, found that, among individuals with serum 25OHD levels above 60 nmol/L, the risk of hip fracture was reduced by one-third. The van Schoor et al. (2008) study reported that in more than 1,300 community-dwelling men and women ages 65 to 75 years, serum 25OHD levels less than or equal to 30 nmol/L were associated with a greater risk of fracture. Cauley et al. (2010) noted that men in the MrOs cohort with levels of serum 25OHD less than 50 nmol/L experienced a significant increase in hip fracture risk that was attenuated somewhat when considering hip BMD.

- *Osteomalacia from postmortem observational study*
  Data from the work of Priemel et al. (2010) have been used by the committee to support a serum 25OHD level of 50 nmol/L as providing coverage for at least 97.5 percent of the population. The data, however, do not allow specification of serum 25OHD levels above which half of the population is protected from osteomalacia and half is at risk; rather the evidence indicated that even relatively low serum 25OHD levels were not associated with the specified measures of osteomalacia, mostly likely owing to the impact of calcium intake. This is consistent with a number of studies, both from trials and from observational work, indicating that vitamin D alone appears to have little effect on bone health outcomes; it is most effective when coupled with calcium.

The wide variation in the precise relationship of serum 25OHD levels to any specific outcome for bone health is evident in the discussion above and the conclusion of the 2007 AHRQ report (Cranney et al., 2007; hereafter referred to as AHRQ-Ottawa) that a specific threshold serum 25OHD level could not be established for rickets. Nonetheless, the committee found a striking concordance of the data surrounding serum 25OHD levels across several of the specific outcomes and across age groups, which, in turn, allows an estimation of serum 25OHD concentrations that are consistent with an EAR- and RDA-type reference value when the indicators of bone health are integrated (see Figure 5-1). As shown above, the levels range between 30 and 50 nmol/L, respectively, for the EAR and the RDA. Further, the higher level of 75 nmol/L proposed by some as "optimal" and hence consistent with an RDA-type reference value is not well supported.

The congruence of the data links serum 25OHD levels below 30 nmol/L with the following outcomes: increased risk of rickets, impaired fractional calcium absorption, and decreased bone mineral content (BMC) in children and adolescents; increased risk of osteomalacia and impaired fetal skeletal outcomes; impaired fractional calcium absorption and an increased risk of osteomalacia in young and middle-aged adults; and impaired fractional calcium absorption and fracture risk in older adults. Similarly, for all age groups, there appears to be little causal evidence of additional benefit to any of these indicators of bone health at serum 25OHD levels above 50 nmol/L, suggesting that this level is consistent with an RDA-type reference value in that this value appears to cover the needs of 97.5 percent of the population. For some bone health outcomes, such as BMD

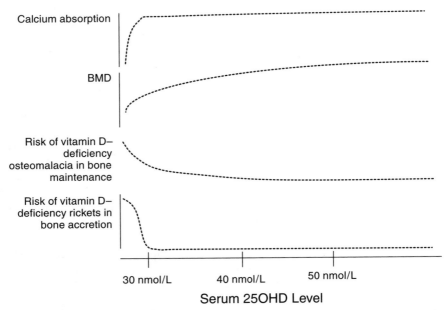

FIGURE 5-1 Conceptualization of integrated bone health outcomes and vitamin D exposure.

in adults, the results of the available RCT(s) show a negative relationship between serum 25OHD level and outcome, and the available observational studies yield mixed results. In addition, for several of these specific outcomes, the RCTs that show benefit for what is generally a single tested dose of supplemental vitamin D do not allow inference of intermediate levels of 25OHD in serum between the placebo and dose. When evaluating the congruence of the data, the committee, therefore, looked at the lowest effective dose and the achieved serum 25OHD level. Uncertainty does exist for the selected serum 25OHD levels consistent with an EAR- and RDA-type level; this uncertainty stems from the wide range of effects and relationships and the lack of a relevant dose–response relationship.

Overall, when the data are examined for an EAR-type of serum 25OHD concentration—that is, a median type of value, a level above which approximately half the population might meet requirements and below which one-half might not—the data do not specifically provide such information, although this value can be concluded to lie between 30 and 50 nmol/L for all age groups. This is likely due to the unique inter-relationship between calcium and vitamin D. At lower levels of vitamin D, there appears to be a compensation on the part of calcium, and calcium intake can overcome the marginal levels of vitamin D. Calcium appears to be the more critical nutrient in the case of bone health, and therefore has an impact the dose–response relationship. Therefore, calcium or lack thereof may "drive" the need for vitamin D.

In the case of vitamin D—or more precisely serum 25OHD concentrations—the data, especially for adults, do not lend themselves readily to the usual DRI model, which is based on the assumption that data concerning a median intake will be as available or even more prevalent than data concerning coverage for most of the population. The standard model specifies, based on the assumption of a normal distribution for requirements, that the average or median requirement (i.e., the EAR) is used to calculate the RDA. This unanticipated situation is primarily evident for adults for whom it is not possible to estimate the level of 25OHD in serum at which 50 percent of the population is at increased risk of osteomalacia. Rather, in this case, the data allow a better estimation of the serum 25OHD level that likely covers most persons in the population. In children and adolescents, however, and to some extent in adults, the integration of these indicators as shown in Figure 5-1 enables an approximation of a level of serum 25OHD at which the risk of adverse bone health outcomes increases; however, there is uncertainty associated with this value given the limitations of the data at present. Thus, for children and adolescents, a serum 25OHD level of 40 nmol/L from the middle of the range of 30 to 50 nmol/L, at which risk to the population is increasing, was selected to serve as the targeted level for a median dietary requirements. For adults, the evidence that most are covered by a serum 25OHD level of 50 nmol/L is used as the starting point, and a value of 40 nmol/L is estimated as the targeted level for a median dietary requirement.

Overall, as shown in Figure 5-1, the data suggest that 50 nmol/L can be set as the serum 25OHD level that coincides with the level that would cover the needs of 97.5 percent of the population. The serum 25OHD level of 40 nmol/L serum 25OHD is consistent with the median requirement. The lower end of the requirement range is consistent with 30 nmol/L, and deficiency symptoms may appear at levels less than 30 nmol/L depending upon a range of factors. What remains is to ascertain the level of vitamin D intake that would achieve these levels of 25OHD in serum.

Integration of Data to Estimate Vitamin D Intakes to
Achieve Serum 25OHD Concentrations

As diet is not necessarily the only source of vitamin D for the body, it would be ideal if the relative contribution made by sunlight to the overall serum 25OHD levels could be quantified, thereby clearing the path to better estimate total intakes of the nutrient needed to maintain a specified serum 25OHD level associated with the health outcome. In fact, however, the examination of data related to dietary recommendations about vitamin D is complicated by the confounding that sun exposure introduces, especially because the factors that affect sun exposure—such as skin pigmentation, genetics, latitude, use of sunscreens, cultural differences in dress, etc.—are not clearly measured and controlled for in research studies and in some cases not fully understood. Further, and just as critically, vitamin D requirements cannot be based on an accepted or "recommended" level of sun exposure as a means to meet vitamin D requirements, because existing public health concerns about sun exposure and skin cancer preclude this possibility. The absence of studies to explore whether a minimal-risk ultraviolet B (UVB) exposure relative to skin cancer exists to enable vitamin D production has been noted (Brannon et al., 2008).

Instead, the best remaining approach is to describe the relationship between total intake and serum 25OHD levels under conditions of minimal sun exposure. In doing so, the committee made the assumption that the outcomes, therefore, would reflect only a very small component attributable to sun exposure as would occur naturally in free-living individuals in winter in the northern hemisphere. This approach to DRI development requires that persons who use the DRI values for health policy or public health applications adjust their considerations relative to adequacy of the diet based on whether the population of interest is minimally, moderately, or highly exposed to sunlight. As mentioned previously, the potential contribution from body stores remains unknown and thus introduces uncertainty. Further, the application of the DRIs relative to assessing the adequacy of vitamin D intake/exposure for the population (foods, supplements, and sun exposure) would benefit from consideration of the serum 25OHD concentrations in the population of interest.

The committee examined information from controlled trials in younger and older adults and in children that could be used in the simulation to describe the relationship between vitamin D intake and changes in serum 25OHD concentrations. Of interest was the condition of minimal sun exposure, which occurs in northern latitudes and in Antarctica during their respective winters. The focus was clinical trials in Europeans or North Americans in which baseline total intake was measured or could be reliably estimated using peer-reviewed published data on baseline intakes of the population studied. In this way, the total intake of vitamin D (baseline plus supplement) was known or could be reliably estimated at latitudes greater than 50°N during late fall (October) through early spring (April) or in Antarctica during its fall (March) through its winter (October). These studies are summarized in Table 5-4. Studies needed to report measured serum 25OHD levels as means or medians with estimates of variance (standard deviation [SD], CI, or inter-quartile ranges) are included. Some studies in the United State at 40°N to 46°N were identified that met all inclusion criteria except that of latitude. These are also included in Table 5-4.

In reviewing these studies, most of which were published in the past 2 years, the committee noted the variability in the declines in serum 25OHD levels during the winter seasons in the respective hemispheres and the existence of a non-linear response to doses of vitamin D. These are discussed below prior to the description of the simulated dose–response analysis.

Winter season change in serum 25OHD levels across age groups As shown in Figure 5-2, the serum 25OHD levels of the placebo groups in the studies conducted with children (Viljakainen et al., 2006) and with younger, middle-aged, and older adults (Cashman et al., 2008, 2009; Smith et al., 2009) decreased over a wide range during the winter season at each latitude. In one study where participants started the season with lower baseline serum 25OHD levels (i.e., 36 nmol/L), the concentrations decreased only slightly (i.e., to 34 nmol/L) (Smith et al., 2009). However, in other studies where participants began the season with higher baseline serum 25OHD levels (i.e., 57 to 66 nmol/L, respectively) the serum 25OHD levels decreased more (i.e., to 34 and 43 nmol/L, respectively) (Viljakainen et al., 2006; Cashman et al., 2008, 2009), compared with those participants with lower baseline levels. In short, the decline in serum 25OHD levels in the placebo arm of these studies appears to be greatest when initial serum 25OHD levels are higher. Slightly higher intake of vitamin D (of approximately 10 to 150 IU/day, compared with other studies) in the study with

TABLE 5-4 Key Studies on the Response of Serum 25OHD Levels to Total Dietary Vitamin D Intake in Children and Adolescents, Young and Middle-Aged Adults, and Older Adults During the Winter at High Northern Latitudes and in Antarctica When Sun Exposure Is Minimal and at Lower Northern Latitudes When Sun Exposure Is Reduced

Reference; Type of Study	Location (Latitude)	Season (Duration)	Population Description	Baseline Vitamin D Intake (IU/day)	Baseline 25OHD Level (nmol/L)	Vitamin D Dose (IU/day)	Total Vitamin D Intake (IU/day)	Achieved 25OHD Level (nmol/L)
Children and adolescents								
Latitude ≥ 50°N								
Ala-Houhala et al., 1988 *RCT*	Finland (61°N)	February–March (1 y)	8–10 y boys/girls n = 60	200[a]	46.0 ± 15.5 (n = 27); 49.3 ± 19.0 (n = 24)	0; 400	200[a]; 600[a]	43.3 ± 19.5; 71.3 ± 23.8
Schou et al., 2003 *Double-blind RCT/crossover*	Denmark (55°N)	November–January (4 wk)	6–14 y boys/girls n = 20	96[a]	—	0; 600	96; 696[b]	33.7 ± 3.3 (n = 10); 32.3 ± 4.1 (n = 10); 50.2 ± 4.5 (n = 10); 43.4 ± 2.9 (n = 10)
Viljakainen et al., 2006 *RCT*	Finland (61°N)	September–March (1 y)	11 y girls n = 212	200; 188; 196 (FFQ; 10–14% using unspecified supplement)	47.8 ± 18.2 (n = 73); 46.3 ± 17.4 (n = 65); 46.7 ± 15.2 (n = 64)	0; 200; 400	200; 388; 596	42.8; 51.7; 58.8

Study	Location	Season (duration)	Population	Baseline (method)	Baseline value	Dose (IU)	Total intake	Final value
Latitude 40–49° N								
Rajakumar et al., 2008 *Non-RCT*	Pittsburgh, PA (40°N)	December–April (1 mo)	6–10 y boys/girls African American obese and nonobese n = 41	218 (obese) 339 (nonobese) (FFQ)	55.5 ± 24.0 64.8 ± 24.3	400 400	618 738	65.5 ± 20.3 72.8 ± 16.8

Young and middle-aged adults

Latitudes ≥ 50°N and Antarctica

Study	Location	Season (duration)	Population	Baseline (method)	Baseline value	Dose (IU)	Total intake	Final value
Cashman et al., 2009 *Double-blind RCT*	Cork, Ireland (51°N) Cochrane, Northern Ireland (55°N)	October/ November– February/ April (22 wk)	mean 29.9 ± 6.2 y range 20–40 y men/women	135 (80–200) 172 (88–228) 140 (92–188) 144 (72–232) (FFQ)	65.7 (58.4–94.1) (n = 57) 60.0 (50.0–89.7) (n = 48) 72.2 (55.7–81.9) (n = 57) 76.9 (55.9–89.3) (n = 53)	0 200 400 600	135 372 540 744	37.4 (31.4–47.9) 49.7 (44.6–60.9) 60.0 (51.0–69.1) 69.0 (59.1–84.2)
Smith et al., 2009 *Double-blind RCT*	Antarctica (78°S)	June/July– August (5 mo with 0, 18 wk, and 25 wk samples)	39–44 y men/women	302 (235–302) 329 (328–352) 356 (276–356) (Diet questionnaire)	44 ± 18 (n = 18) 44 ± 19 (n = 19) 45 ± 14 (n = 18)	400 1,000 2,000	659 1,342 2,305	55 ± 19 (18 wk) 57 ± 15 (25 wk) 63 ± 20 (18 wk) 63 ± 25 (25 wk) 71 ± 20 (18 wk) 71 ± 23 (25 wk)

continued

TABLE 5-4 Continued

Reference; Type of Study	Location (Latitude)	Season (Duration)	Population Description	Baseline Vitamin D Intake (IU/day)	Baseline 25OHD Level (nmol/L)	Vitamin D Dose (IU/day)	Total Vitamin D Intake (IU/day)	Achieved 25OHD Level (nmol/L)
Viljakainen et al., 2009 *Double-blind RCT*	Helsinki, Finland (61°N)	November–April (25 wk)	21–49 y men	264 ± 112	64.7 ± 18.5 ($n = 16$)	0	264	52.2 (Δ −12.5 ± 9.1)
				304 ± 2,202	60.3 ± 11.6 ($n = 16$)	412	716	75.4 (Δ +15.3 ± 2.3)
				344 ± 252 (FFQ)	62.3 ± 13.6 ($n = 16$)	760	1,104	90.1 (Δ +27.8 ± 17.5)
Latitudes 40–49°N								
Biancuzzo et al., 2010 *Double-blind RCT*	Boston, MA (42°N)	February–May (11 wk)	mean 29–41 y range 18–79 y men and women including European Americans, Asian Americans, African Americans, North Americans, Hispanic Americans	200[c]	49.5 ± 24 ($n = 15$)	0	200	45.3 ± 16.0
					49.0 ± 27.8 ($n = 20$)	1,000 D_3	1,200	70.0 ± 27.5
					41.5 ± 24.8 ($n = 16$)	1,000 D_2	1,200	68.5 ± 26.3
Harris and Dawson-Hughes, 2002 *RCT*	Boston, MA (42°N)	December–April (8 wk)	18–35 y	132	48.9 ± 17.2	0	132	53.5 (Δ −4.6 ± 6.5) ($n = 13$)
				71 (FFQ)	59.9 ± 16.4	800	871	82.4 (Δ 22.5 ± 14.7) ($n = 14$)
Heaney et al., 2003[d] *RCT*	Omaha, NE (41.2°N)	October–March (120–140 d)	38.7 ± 11.2 y	< 200 (estimated from milk consumed)	70.1 ± 5.8	0	< 200	52
					72.0 ± 4.0	1,000	< 1,200	77.1
					69.3 ± 4.2	5,000	< 5,200	150
					65.6 ± 6.3	10,000	< 10,200	212

Reference / Design	Location (Latitude)	Season (Duration)	Subjects	Baseline intake	Baseline value (n)	Dose	Total	Final value
Holick et al., 2008 *Double-blind RCT*	Boston, MA (42°N)	February–May (11 wk)	mean 35.5–40.5 y men and women	316[c] (Diet questionnaire used, but baseline intakes not reported)	46.5 ± 22.2 (n = 55)	0	316	47.0 ± 19.8
					49.0 ± 27.8 (n = 20)	1,000 (D$_3$)	1,316	72.3 ± 27.5
					42.3 ± 26.3 (n = 16)	1,000 (D$_2$)	1,316	67.0 ± 24.0
					50.5 ± 26.0 (n = 18)	500 D$_2$ + 500 D$_2$	1,316	71.0 ± 19.3
Li-Ng et al., 2009 *Double-blind RCT*	Long Island, NY (40.7°N)	December–March (3 mo)	mean 58.1–59.3 y range 18–80 y including European Americans, African Americans, Asian Americans	168.0 ± 146.5	63.0 ± 25.8 (n = 70)	0	168	61.9 (Δ −2.1)
				147.3 ± 182.3 (FFQ)	64.3 ± 25.4 (n = 78)	2,000	2,147	88.5 ± 23.2
Nelson et al., 2009 *Double-blind RCT*	Bangor, ME (44.5°N)	September–February	19–35 y women	140 ± 104	61.9 ± 22.5	0	140	72.7 ± 27.8
				140 ± 124 (4 d food records)	62.1 ± 24.0 (n = 31)	800	940	97.4 ± 31.3

Older adults

Latitude ≥ 50°N

Reference / Design	Location (Latitude)	Season (Duration)	Subjects	Baseline intake	Baseline value (n)	Dose	Total	Final value
Cashman et al., 2009 *Double-blind RCT*	Cork, Ireland (51°N) Cochrane, Northern Ireland (55°N)	September/November–February/April (22 wk)	mean 70.7 ± 5.4 y > 64 y men/women	188	58.8 (43.6, 78.5) (n = 55)	0	188	41.6 (28.0–55.4)
				164	51.8 (41.3, 68.7) (n = 48)	200	364	53.2 (45.6–68.7)
				168	54.3 (42.6, 72.0) (n = 53)	400	568	69.5 (58.0–81.4)
				192 (7 d diet record)	55.1 (39.6, 70.4) (n = 48)	600	792	73.8 (62.0–89.2)

continued

TABLE 5-4 Continued

Reference; Type of Study	Location (Latitude)	Season (Duration)	Population Description	Baseline Vitamin D Intake (IU/day)	Baseline 25OHD Level (nmol/L)	Vitamin D Dose (IU/day)	Total Vitamin D Intake (IU/day)	Achieved 25OHD Level (nmol/L)
Honkanen et al., 1990 RCT	Kuopio, Finland (62.9°N)	November/December–February/March (11 wk)	67–72 y women	380[a]	36.2 ± 2.7 (n = 26)	0	380	23.3 (18–28, CI)
					42.8 ± 3.5 (n = 25)	1,800	2,180	80.7 (75–86, CI)
Larsen et al., 2004 RCT	Randers, Denmark (56°N)	January–June (1 mo)	mean 74–74.9 y range 65–103 y men/women	136[a] for women	33 ± 19 (n = 37)	0	136	34 ± 19
					37 ± 19 (n = 67)	400	536	46 ± 17
					49.0 ± 14.2 (n = 22)	350	414	59 ± 20 (combined 350–400 IU)
					50.0 ± 15.9 (n = 23)	400	464	
Van Der Klis et al., 1996 RCT	Groningen, Netherlands (53.2°N)	April–May (5 wk)	61 y Dutch women	64[e] (n = 20)	61.2 ± 2.4	0	64	NS from baseline 87.9 ± 26.9 (n = 19)
						400	464	
						800	864	87.9 ± 26.9 (n = 19)
Viljakainen et al., 2006 RCT	Helsinki, Finland (61°N)	January–April (12 wk)	65–85 y women	436	52.2 ± 19.9 (n = 12)	0	436	43.9 (Δ −8.3 ± 13.2)
				388	46.0 ± 14.3 (n = 13)	200	588	56.9 (Δ +10.9 ± 8.9)
				424	46.5 ± 10.2 (n = 11)	400	824	60.9 (Δ +14.4 ± 4)
				388 (FFQ)	44.1 ± 13.5 (n = 13)	800	1,188	67.8 (Δ 23.7 ± 11.9)

Latitudes 40–49°N

Study	Location	Season	Age	Baseline intake	Supplement dose	Achieved intake	Baseline serum 25OHD	Achieved serum 25OHD
Dawson-Hughes et al., 1991 *Double-blind RCT*	Boston, MA (42°N)	February–May (winter period of 12-mo study)	mean 61–62 y women	90 / 110 (FFQ)	0 / 400	90 / 510		60.6 (55.6–65.6, CI) (n = 125) / 92.1 (87.9–96.3, CI) (n = 121)
Harris and Dawson-Hughes, 2002 *RCT*	Boston, MA (42°N)	December–April (8 wk)	62–79 y	115 / 142 (FFQ)	0 / 800	115 / 942	53.8 ± 18.2 / 61.5 ± 15.7	49.3 (Δ −4.5 ± 6.5) (n = 11) / 83.6 (Δ −22.1 ± 13.4) (Δ + 22.1 ± 13.4) (n = 14)

NOTE: BMD = bone mineral density; FFQ = food frequency questionnaire; IU = International Units; mo = month(s); NS = not significant; RCT = randomized controlled trial; wk = week(s); y = year(s).

[a] Baseline intakes from Andersen et al. (2005).

[b] Baseline intake from Ambroszkiewicz et al. (2007).

[c] NHANES intake data for 2005–2006.

[d] Achieved serum 25OHD levels for Heaney et al. (2003) were extracted from their graphic presentation in the article, and no variance could be extracted.

[e] Bergink et al. (2009).

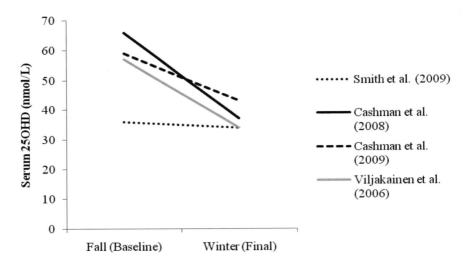

FIGURE 5-2 Fall (baseline) and winter (final) values of serum 25OHD concentrations in non-supplemented placebo (or no pills) groups measured during minimal sun and UVB exposure (Cashman et al., 2008, 2009; Smith et al., 2009) or at the same season for the year-long trials in children (Viljakainen et al., 2006) at latitudes above 50°N or in Antarctica.
NOTE: Values in the graph from Viljakainen et al. (2006) differ from values listed in Table 5-4 due to the use of a subgroup (6-month values for girls recruited in the fall) for graphing purposes.

the lowest baseline serum 25OHD levels (Smith et al., 2009) may have accounted for the attenuated reduction in serum 25OHD level.

A similar trend exists across many of the studies with a placebo group, as summarized in Table 5-4. Declines of 3 to 13 nmol/L in serum 25OHD level are reported for those with baseline levels from 36 to 47 nmol/L. Larger declines in serum 25OHD levels of 8 to 62 nmol/L are reported for those with baseline levels of 64 to 96 nmol/L. However, considerable variability exists in the seasonal decline in serum 25OHD level in winter months, as demonstrated by the increases of 1 nmol/L in some participants with baseline serum 25OHD levels of 33 nmol/L at latitudes above 50°N (Larsen et al., 2004), and increases of 4.6 to 10.8 nmol/L from a baseline of 48.9 to 61.9 nmol/L in some participants at latitudes above 42°N (Harris et al., 2002; Nelson et al., 2009).

These observations suggest that the assumption of minimal sun exposure was met. Further, they suggest that during the winter season small intakes of vitamin D may play a role in attenuating the winter decline in serum 25OHD levels in those with lower baseline serum 25OHD levels. They also suggest that the kinetics of vitamin D turnover or mobilization from stores may differ in those who have lower baseline serum 25OHD levels. Further, it is possible that the greater decline of serum 25OHD levels in those with higher baseline levels could, perhaps, also represent regression to the mean, at least in part. At this time, it is not possible to clarify which of these possibilities occur.

Non-linear response to vitamin D dosing　　The available data suggest a non-linear response of serum 25OHD above baseline levels to doses of vitamin D for all age groups. Non-linear response to doses of vitamin D (total or IU/kg) is also reported in mice (Fleet et al., 2008) and rats (Anderson et al., 2008; Fleet et al., 2008), demonstrating the biological plausibility of a non-linear response of serum 25OHD concentrations to vitamin D intake. It is noted that AHRQ-Ottawa and Heaney et al. (2003) reported a linear relationship between serum 25OHD levels and vitamin D dosing that ranges from 0.7 nmol/L per 40 IU (Heaney et al., 2003) to 1 to 2 nmol/L per 100 IU (AHRQ-Ottawa). Notably, AHRQ-Ottawa found heterogeneity that remained after adjusting for dose. However, in the studies considered by the committee, there is a steeper rise in serum 25OHD levels when vitamin D dosing is less than 1,000 IU/day of vitamin D. A slower, more flattened response is seen when doses of 1,000 IU/day or higher are administered. In short, regardless of baseline intakes or serum 25OHD levels, under conditions of dosing the increment in serum 25OHD above baseline differs depending upon whether the dose was above or below 1,000 IU/day. This is evidenced by examining several studies in young, middle-aged and older adults.

　　Smith et al. (2009) in Antarctica found a low serum 25OHD level of 37 nmol/L in men and women during the winter season (June to September). The rise in serum 25OHD levels with doses of 400, 1,000, and 2,000 IU/day after 13 and 20 weeks was 2.1, 0.8 and 0.54 nmol/L per 40 IU/day, respectively. In two other studies at latitudes of 52°N to 55°N during winter, the rise in serum 25OHD levels in response to 200, 400, or 600 IU of vitamin D per day with serum 25OHD baseline levels of 37 to 42 nmol/L was examined in young and older individuals. The average rise in serum 25OHD levels was equivalent to approximately 2.3 nmol/L for an intake of 40 IU vitamin D_3 per day without a difference due to age (Cashman et al., 2008, 2009). Others also found that age does not influence the change in serum 25OHD level in response to vitamin D intake (Harris and Dawson-Hughes, 2002). When the dose is 1,000 IU/day or higher, the rise in serum 25OHD level in individuals of all ages is approximately 1 nmol/L for a 40 IU/day intake, which is similar to the response to vitamin D intake found in the AHRQ-Ottawa analysis.

Analysis and Outcomes

A regression analysis of the relationship between serum 25OHD level and total intake of vitamin D during the winter season at latitudes above 49.5°N or in Antarctica, a period of low sun and UVB exposure, was carried out for each of three age groups—children and adolescents, young and middle-aged adults, and older adults. This approach differs from the others such as the study reported by Heaney et al. (2003) in that total vitamin D intake and not just a supplemental dose of vitamin D was considered, and because we show a non-linear response to total intake rather than the linear response published previously. The interest for this report was an approach that would be relevant to determining the intake needed to achieve the serum 25OHD levels consistent with an EAR- and RDA-type value. The regression analysis using a mixed effect model was preceded by a log transformation of the total vitamin D intake data because the log transformation was the best curvilinear fit. The model controlled for the effect of study clustering by including study as a random effect. Controlling for study effect using a random effect was needed because the interclass correlation of the variance due to study effect compared with the total variance was very high, approximately 95 percent overall, with about 88 percent for children and adolescents, 95 percent for young and middle-aged adults, and 96 percent for older adults. The regression was set for a y_0 intercept of 0 nmol of 25OHD per liter of serum, consistent with the biological reality preventing a negative value for achieved serum 25OHD levels. Baseline serum 25OHD levels did not have significant effect, and was, therefore, not included in the analysis.

The outcome is presented in Figure 5-3. Importantly, age did not significantly affect the response of serum 25OHD level to log vitamin D intake. Neither the main effect of age ($p = 0.162$) nor the interaction term between age and the log of total vitamin D intake ($p = 0.142$) was significant. Thus, there was no effect of age in the response of serum 25OHD level to total intake among the three age groups—children and adolescents, young and middle-aged adults, or older adults. This finding suggests that across ages under conditions of minimal sun exposure, similar intakes of vitamin D result in similar serum 25OHD concentrations, as shown in Figure 5-4.

Because there was no age effect in the response of serum 25OHD level to total intake of vitamin D, a single, combined regression analysis with study as a random effect was carried out. This resulted in the predictive equation of achieved 25OHD in nmol/L = 9.9 ln (total vitamin D intake) with predicted CIs of $y = 8.7$ ln total vitamin D intake) and upper interval of $y = 11.2$ ln (total vitamin intake), as specified in Figure 5-4.

The committee also analyzed the achieved 25OHD with total vitamin D intake at latitudes between 40°N to 49°N during the winter (data shown in Table 5-4 above) for which assumption of minimal sun exposure may not be as fully met as at latitudes above 49.5°N or in Antarctica during the winter. The approach was the same as described above for the simulated dose–response in which achieved serum 25OHD level was analyzed at latitudes above 49.5°S. The interclass correlation was large, approximately 80 percent, and study effect was again included as a random effect in the mixed effects model. Age did not affect achieved serum 25OHD level relative to log total vitamin D intake ($p = 0.09$ for main effect and $p = 0.6$ for the interaction of age and log total vitamin D intake), although the data available for children was limited to one study. Therefore, a combined analysis of all age groups at the lower latitudes was conducted. The predicted achieved serum 25OHD level was $y = 12.3$ ln (total vitamin D intake), which explained 45 percent of the within-study variability and 96.6 percent of the between-study variability. The predicted upper and lower CIs for achieved serum 25OHD levels were $y = 10.1$ ln (total vitamin D intake) and $y = 14.5$ ln (total vitamin D intake). There was a significant difference between lower and higher latitudes ($p = 0.000$ for the main effect and $p = 0.021$) for the interaction of latitude and ln (total vitamin D intake). Compared to the simulated dose–response at higher latitudes, the achieved serum 25OHD level at lower latitudes was 24 percent greater for the same total intake as that achieved at higher latitudes. Of note, less of the within-study variance at lower latitudes was explained by the total vitamin D intake (45 percent) compared to that explained (72 percent) for the higher latitudes. Taken together, these results suggest that sun exposure may be more than minimal at lower latitudes, as anticipated. Thus, the committee used the simulated dose–response at the higher latitudes to ensure minimal sun exposure to ensure as little contribution from endogenous production as the evidence allows.

Given the lack of an age effect in the response of the achieved serum 25OHD levels to any total intake of vitamin D, the intake to achieve the EAR-type value of 40 nmol/L was the same across all groups. An intake of 400 IU is associated with a predicted mean circulating 25OHD level of 59 nmol/L in children and adolescents, young and middle-aged adults, and older adults with a lower predicted CI of approximately 52 nmol/L. An intake of 600 IU/day predicts a mean serum 25OHD level of 63 nmol/L in children, adults, and older adults with a lower predicted CI of 56 nmol/L. Although this suggests that intakes of 400 and 600 IU would over-shoot the targeted serum 25OHD concentrations, there is considerable uncertainty in this simulated dose–response relationship that needs to be taken into account. This includes: (1) the large inter-study variance, which is most pronounced in older persons; (2) predicted lower CIs for each age group resulting in an achieved serum 25OHD level of 36 to 46 nmol/L for a 400 IU/day intake and a 38 to 49 nmol/L for a 600 IU/day intake (as

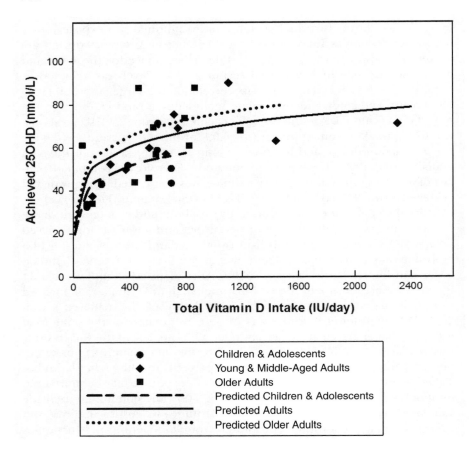

FIGURE 5-3 Response of serum 25OHD level to total intake of vitamin D in northern latitudes in Europe and Antarctica during their respective winter seasons

shown in Figure 5-4), even though there is no significant age effect; (3) the uncertainties in the comparability of the serum 25OHD levels measured with different assays across these studies; and (4) the uncertainty surrounding the predicted CIs of this relationship. Given these limitations and the uncertainties, the committee selected the estimated intakes needed in a fashion that would err on the side of the specified intake "overshooting" the targeted serum value to ensure that the specified levels of intake achieved the desired serum 25OHD levels of 40 and 50 nmol/L. This approach is used despite possible contributions to serum 25OHD from sun exposure that could not be taken into account.

when effective sun exposure for endogenous vitamin D synthesis is minimal. Mean or median responses of serum 25OHD level to total intake in the winter seasons at northern latitudes (> 49.5°N) and in Antarctica (78°S) (summarized in Table 5-4) were analyzed using a mixed effect model by regression following log transformation with study in a random effects model to control for the large study residual variability for: (1) children and adolescents (boys and girls) ages 6 to 14 years in Finland (Ala-Houhala et al., 1988); (2) young and middle-aged adults ages 19 to 59 years from men in Antarctica (Smith et al., 2009), Ireland (Cashman et al., 2008, 2009), and Finland (Viljakainen et al., 2006, 2009), and Denmark (Schou et al., 2003); and (3) older adult women and men > 60 years of age in Ireland (Cashman et al., 2009), the Netherlands (Van Der Klis et al., 1996), Finland (Viljakainen et al., 2006), and Denmark (Larsen et al., 2004). The relationship of serum 25OHD level to total intake of vitamin D is:

- For children and adolescents: achieved serum 25OHD = 8.6 ln(total vitamin D intake), which explains 68.8 percent of the within-subject variability and 98.3 percent of the between-study variability. Predicted CIs were $y = 6.0$ ln (total vitamin D intake) for lower limit, and $y = 11.3$ ln (total vitamin D intake) for upper limit.
- For young and middle-aged adults: achieved serum 25OHD = 10.1 ln (total vitamin D intake), which explained 70.3 percent of the within-study variability and 98.4 percent of the between-study variability. Predicted CIs were $y = 6.3$ ln (total vitamin D intake) for lower limit, and $y = 13.8$ ln (total vitamin D intake) for upper limit.
- For older adults > 71 years: achieved serum 25OHD = 10.9 ln (total vitamin D intake), which explains 77.5 percent of the within-study variability and 92.2 percent of the between-study variability. Predicted CIs were $y = 7.7$ ln (total vitamin D intake) for lower limit and $y = 14.2$ ln (total vitamin D intake) for upper limit.
- The interaction term between age and the log of total vitamin D intake ($p = 0.142$), as well as the main effect of age ($p = 0.162$) were not significant.

NOTE: log(total vitamin D) has been back-transformed to total vitamin D for presentation in this figure.

Specification of Vitamin D Dietary Reference Intakes for Adequacy

The DRIs for adequacy for vitamin D have been introduced previously in Table 5-3. The rationale for each is presented in the discussions below.

Infants 0 to 12 Months of Age

Infants 0 to 6 Months of Age
Infants 6 to 12 Months of Age

AI 400 IU (10 µg)/day Vitamin D

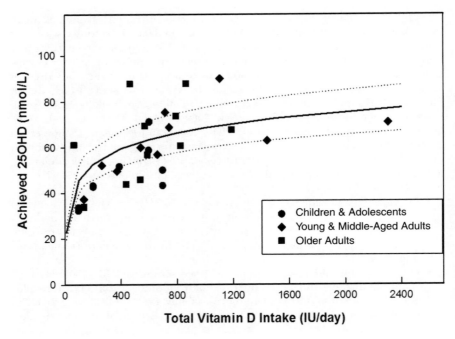

Total Vitamin D Intake (IU/day)

FIGURE 5-4 Response of serum 25OHD level to total intake of vitamin D in all age groups in northern latitudes in Europe and Antarctica during their respective winter seasons when effective sun exposure for endogenous vitamin D synthesis is minimal. Mean responses of serum 25OHD level to total vitamin D intake in the winter seasons at latitudes 49.5°N (Europe) and 78°S (Antarctica) for ages 6 to > 60 years (Ala-Houhala et al., 1988; Van Der Klis et al., 1996; Schou et al., 2003; Larsen et al., 2004; Viljakainen et al., 2006, 2009; Cashman et al., 2008, 2009; Smith et al., 2009; see Table 5-4 for summary of studies) were analyzed by regression using mixed effect model following log transformation controlling for study effect by a random effects model because there was no effect of age on the response of serum 25OHD level to total intake of vitamin D. The relationship for achieved vitamin D is y achieved 25OHD in nmol/L = 9.9 ln (total vitamin D intake) (shown as solid line) with predicted CIs (shown as two dashed lines) for lower interval of $y = 8.7$ ln (total vitamin D intake) and upper interval of $y = 11.2$ ln (total vitamin D intake). This regression explains 72 percent of the within-study variability and 96.4 percent of the between-subject variability.

NOTE: Log (total vitamin D intake) was back-transformed to total vitamin D intake for presentation in this figure.

Data are not sufficient to establish an EAR for infants less than 1 year of age, and therefore an AI has been developed. Unlike the case for calcium, the content of human milk does not shed light on the vitamin D requirements of infants, as breast milk is not a meaningful source of vitamin D.

The AI for the 0 to 6 months and 6 to 12 months life stage groups is set at 400 IU of vitamin D per day. There are very limited data beyond the conclusion that maintaining serum 25OHD concentrations in this life stage group above 30 nmol/L, and more likely closer to 50 nmol/L, appears to cover adequately the needs of the majority of the infants and support normal bone accretion. There are no data to suggest that older infants would benefit from higher intakes.

Intakes in the range of 400 IU/day appear consistent with maintenance of the desirable serum 25OHD concentrations. There are no reports of a clinical deficiency in infants receiving 400 IU of vitamin D per day, and an intake of 400 IU/day appears to maintain a serum 25OHD level generally above 50 nmol/L in infants (Greer et al., 1982; Rothberg et al., 1982; Ala-Houhala, 1985; Ala-Houhala et al., 1988; Greer and Marshall, 1989; Hollis and Wagner, 2004). There are differences in the volume of milk or formula intake during this 12-month period, with newborns taking in less than older infants. The AI of 400 IU/day, therefore, represents an overall intake for the first year of life, and may vary across the life stages; it also assumes early introduction of a supplement for breast-fed babies. In the case of exclusive formula feeding, there is an assumption of a gradual increase in intake to 800 to 1,000 mL/day during infancy, which for most standard formulas provides about 400 IU/day. Note is made of the case reports concerning the development of rickets among dark-skinned infants who are exclusively breast-fed and not provided a vitamin D supplement (see Chapter 8).

Children and Adolescents 1 Through 18 Years of Age

Children 1 Through 3 Years of Age		
Children 4 Through 8 Years of Age		
Children 9 Through 13 Years of Age		
Adolescents 14 Through 18 Years of Age		
	EAR 400 IU (10 µg)/day Vitamin D	
	RDA 600 IU (15 µg)/day Vitamin D	

For these life stage groups, ensuring normal, healthy bone accretion is central to the DRI values. The requirement distribution developed using serum 25OHD concentrations and the intakes estimated to achieve such concentrations are the basis for the reference values.

For very young children in this life stage group, virtually no data are available to link vitamin D nutriture directly to measures related to bone health outcomes. AHRQ-Ottawa examined the relationship between vitamin D and rickets in children 0 to 5 years of age but found no studies that evaluated BMC, BMD, or fractures in comparison with measures of vitamin D intake. Likewise, AHRQ-Tufts found no studies that update AHRQ-Ottawa.

AHRQ-Ottawa did consider serum 25OHD concentrations in the context of the onset of rickets in newborns through children 5 years of age and identified serum concentrations below 27.5 nmol/L as being consistently associated with rickets. However, many of the relevant studies were from developing countries where calcium intake is low; therefore, for these studies, the onset of rickets was associated with higher levels of 25OHD in serum, likely due to low calcium intakes. Specker et al. (1992) has concluded that serum concentrations of approximately 27 to 30 nmol/L places the infant at an increased risk for developing rickets, although the measure is not diagnostic of the disease.

Although the prevention of rickets can be a factor in establishing reference values, it is important to seek measures that are consistent with favorable bone health outcomes. Maximizing calcium absorption, especially for this life stage group, is therefore a reasonable parameter to take into account. Here, as with rickets, serum 25OHD measures are the only data available and there are no direct measures of vitamin D intake. Abrams et al. (2009) conducted calcium absorption studies in 251 children ranging in age from 4.9 to 16.7 years and found that children with serum 25OHD levels of 28 to 50 nmol/L had higher fractional calcium absorption than children with serum 25OHD levels at or greater than 50 nmol/L, suggesting again at the least that maximal calcium absorption is reached at 50 nmol/L. Fractional calcium absorption did not increase with serum 25OHD concentration levels above 50 nmol/L. The findings are consistent with the conclusions reached previously concerning serum 25OHD levels associated with maximum population coverage. Further, as rickets in populations that are not calcium deficient occurs at serum 25OHD levels below 30 nmol/L, it is reasonable to assume that 40 nmol/L is associated with an average requirement.

Serum 25OHD concentrations of 40 to 50 nmol/L would ideally coincide with bone health benefits such as positive effects on BMC and BMD. AHRQ-Ottawa found that there was *fair evidence* that circulating 25OHD levels are associated with a positive change in BMD and BMC in studies in older children and adolescents. The serum 25OHD concentrations varied from 30 to 83 nmol/L. A study conducted by Viljakainen et al. (2006) reported that vitamin D intakes of 200 and 400 IU/day in adolescent girls were associated with positive BMC measures at serum 25OHD levels of 50 nmol/L and above. This is consistent with conclusions inferred from calcium absorption studies and, in turn, with the ability to cover the requirements for nearly all in the population. A relatively wide range of total vitamin D intakes reportedly achieved serum 25OHD concentrations between approximately 40 and 60 nmol/L, but most intakes were between about 350 and 600 IU/day. The variability in the data cannot be readily attributed to differences in sun exposure because the studies were all conducted in northern locations during primarily winter months.

Taken as a body of evidence and in the absence of measures that directly relate total intake to health outcomes, the information concerning serum 25OHD concentrations associated with rickets prevention, calcium absorption, and positive effects on BMC measures are consistent with discussions above concerning a requirement distribution based on serum 25OHD concentrations. They support the conclusion that an average requirement for vitamin D for these life stage groups is associated with the achievement of concentrations of 25OHD in serum of 40 nmol/L. Further, they support the conclusion that the requirements for nearly all children and adolescents are covered when serum 25OHD concentrations reach 50 nmol/L. These findings are universally applicable across all children and adolescents from 1 to 18 years of age.

The analysis conducted, described above, indicates that an intake of vitamin D of 400 IU/day achieves serum concentrations of 40 nmol/L, and this intake is therefore set as the EAR for persons 1 to 3 years, 4 to 8 years, 9 to 13 years, and 14 to 18 years of age. As this requirement distribution appears to be normally distributed, the assumption of another 30 percent to cover nearly all the population (i.e., 97.5 percent) is appropriate and consistent with a serum 25OHD level of approximately 50 nmol/L as the target for an RDA value. Based on the same analysis relating serum 25OHD levels to intake, an intake of 600 IU/day is set as the RDA. These reference values assume minimal sun exposure.

Adults 19 Through 50 Years of Age

Adults 19 Through 30 Years of Age
Adults 31 Through 50 Years of Age
EAR 400 IU (10 µg)/day Vitamin D
RDA 600 IU (15 µg)/day Vitamin D

For these life stage groups, bone maintenance is the focus. The requirement distribution based on serum 25OHD concentrations and the intakes estimated to achieve such concentrations are the basis for the reference values. As described below, the available data have provided more information about intakes and serum 25OHD levels consistent with an RDA value than they have for an EAR value.

Data relating bone health outcomes to vitamin D intake are generally limited for adults 19 to 50 years of ages. Although bone mass measures are, of course, studied in this population, consideration of the dose–response relationship between vitamin D and bone health are not usually included in such studies. In fact, there are no randomized trials in this age group, and whatever data are available come from association studies. The results are inconsistent, in part because the confounding inherent in observational studies.

Serum 25OHD concentrations relative to calcium absorption, therefore, provide an important basis for DRI development for vitamin D for these life stage groups. The conclusions described above indicating that calcium absorption is maximal at serum 25OHD concentrations between 30 and 50 nmol/L with no consistent increase in calcium absorption above approximately 50 nmol/L are informative in estimating the relevant EAR and RDA values for vitamin D for these life stage groups.

In contrast, although data from a very recent study (Priemel et al., 2010) based on post-mortem analysis of the relationship between serum 25OHD levels and osteomalacia and re-examined by the committee (as described above) suggest a serum 25OHD level that would cover the needs of approximately 97.5 percent of the population, they also reveal that a level of serum 25OHD consistent with an average requirement is somewhat elusive. That is, serum 25OHD levels of approximately 40 nmol/L to even 30 nmol/L might be expected to be consistent with coverage for no more than half of the population (i.e., a mean/median value). But, in the Priemel et al. (2010) report, even at serum 25OHD levels well below 30 nmol/L more than half of the population studied failed to demonstrate osteomalacia as defined histologically in the study. In essence, these data, which admittedly have limitations, suggest that for some adults the need for vitamin D is extremely low. This is likely due to the very strong interrelationship between calcium and vitamin D; it may even suggest that calcium is the "driver" nutrient relative to bone health, and that calcium is able to more readily overcome lower levels of vitamin D for the purposes of bone health, while vitamin D is likely unable to compensate for a lack of calcium. This finding underscores the uncertainties that are introduced by the calcium-vitamin D interrelationship.

For the purposes of ensuring public health in the face of uncertainty and providing a reference value for stakeholders, a prudent approach is to begin the consideration of the DRIs for these age groups with the level of 25OHD in serum that is consistent with coverage of the requirement of nearly all adults in this age range, that is, 50 nmol/L. Taken together with calcium absorption and BMD, and assuming a normal distribution of requirements, given no evidence that the distribution is not normal, a serum level of 40 nmol/L can be set as consistent with a median requirement. This modified approach is bolstered by—and consistent with—the relationship between serum 25OHD levels and calcium absorption, in which serum 25OHD levels of between 30 and 50 nmol/L were consistent with maximal calcium absorption. Based on these considerations as well as the intake versus serum response analysis described above, an EAR of 400 IU/day and an RDA of 600 IU/day are established for adults 19 to 50 years of age. These DRI values assume minimal sun exposure.

Adults 51 Years of Age and Older

Adults 51 Through 70 Years of Age		
	EAR 400 IU (10 µg)/day Vitamin D	
	RDA 600 IU (15 µg)/day Vitamin D	
Adults >70 Years of Age		
	EAR 400 IU (10 µg)/day Vitamin D	
	RDA 800 IU (20 µg)/day Vitamin D	

For persons in these life stage groups of 51 through 70 years and >70 years, the ability to maintain bone mass and reduce the level of bone loss is the primary focus for DRI development. Evidence related to fracture risk becomes central. For this reason, DRIs for adults >70 years of age are discussed first, followed by DRIs for adults 51 through 70 years of age.

Adults 70 Years of Age and Older

The discussions above concerning serum 25OHD levels in relation to bone health indicate that several newer studies have helped to elucidate a relationship between serum 25OHD concentrations and bone health benefits based on measures of calcium absorption and osteomalacia for a wide age range of adults. These data when used for the purposes of DRI development—coupled with the approximation of intake associated with serum 25OHD concentrations derived from the simulation analysis carried out by the committee—provide a basis for an EAR for young and middle-aged adults of 400 IU/day vitamin D consistent with a serum 25OHD concentration of 40 nmol/L, and for an RDA of 600 IU/day consistent with a serum 25OHD concentration of 50 nmol/L. However, for adults more than 70 years of age, the number of unknowns associated with the physiology of normal aging, coupled with the level of variability around the average requirement for this group that such factors may introduce, all of which may affect the estimation of the RDA (the level of intake needed to cover

97.5 percent of the population) causes a closer examination of the level of intake appropriate for an RDA value.

For this life stage group (> 70 years), the reduction in fracture risk is the most important indicator of interest, not only because of the actual event, but also because of the high mortality and morbidity associated with fractures. The factors that may have an impact on fracture risk range from functional status to neurological, metabolic, and physical determinants. Such factors enhance uncertainties about vitamin D nutriture. Changes such as impaired renal function, less efficient synthesis of vitamin D in skin, lower endogenous production of active vitamin D, increased PTH as well as age-related changes in body composition affect the daily requirement of vitamin D. Moreover, a sizeable proportion of this population can be categorized as frail compared with other age groups, and the concerns for bone health are increased. Factors of increased institutionalization also come into play. Although there is insufficient evidence to point to any one of these factors as a contributor to increasing the variability at which 97.5 percent coverage of the population occurs, when taken as a group of unknowns, it would be inappropriate to ignore the concern when considering the level of vitamin D commensurate with an RDA for this group.

For this reason, the level of uncertainty should be taken into account during the specification of the RDA for vitamin D for persons more than 70 years of age. There are very few data that are relevant to adjusting for such uncertainty. There are no dose–response data that would allow comparisons for adults more than 70 years of age regarding the effects of intakes of 600 IU of vitamin D per day with that of a higher level of intake such as 800 or 1,000 IU/day. Moreover, the evidence for fracture risk in relation to vitamin D intake for this older life stage is confounded by study protocols that do not allow separation of the effect of calcium from vitamin D; as discussed previously there is reasonably compelling evidence that calcium alone in this age group can modestly reduce the risk of fracture. Therefore, it is not surprising that the inclusion of calcium with vitamin D treatment generally, albeit not consistently, reduces the risk of fractures among the oldest adults, especially when vitamin D nutriture is considered in the context of serum 25OHD concentrations (Tang et al., 2007; Avenell et al., 2009; AHRQ-Tufts, Tang et al., 2007). Even the 10 trials that examined vitamin D alone (Lips et al., 1996; Peacock et al., 2000; Meyer et al., 2002; Trivedi et al., 2003; Avenell et al., 2004; Harwood et al., 2004; Grant et al., 2005; Law et al., 2006; Lyons et al., 2007; Smith et al., 2007), when pooled by Avenell et al. (2009), showed no statistically significant effect on fracture risk. As shown in Table 5-5, which is focused on studies with subjects more than 70 years of age and vitamin D intakes as opposed to serum 25OHD concentrations, such studies are generally non-significant for fracture risk on the basis of both vitamin D alone and vitamin D with

TABLE 5-5 Randomized Trials on Fracture Risk Associated with Vitamin D and Calcium or Vitamin D Alone in Older Men and Women

Author, Date	Gender/ Mean Age	Vitamin D Dose (IU/day)	Calcium Dose (mg/day)	Relative Risk of Fracture
Vitamin D plus Calcium				
Chapuy et al., 2002	F, 85 y	800	1,200	0.85 NS
Harwood et al., 2004	F, 81 y	800	1,000	0.49 NS
Grant et al., 2005	M/F, 77 y	800	1,000	0.94 NS
Porthouse et al., 2005	F, 77 y	800	1,000	0.96 NS
Vitamin D Alone				
Lips et al., 1996	M/F, 80 y	400	—	1.1 NS
Meyer et al., 2002	M/F, 85 y	400	—	0.92 NS
Trivedi et al., 2003*	M/F, 75 y	800	—	0.67 Significant
Lyons et al., 200)	M/F, 84 y	800	—	0.96 NS

*100,000 IU every four months.
NOTE: NS = Non-significant

calcium. The exception is Trivedi et al. (2003), which examined vitamin D supplementation and fracture risk in a population of men and women of average age 75 years. In any case, interpretation of these data is complicated by the unknowns surrounding the background intake of vitamin D over and above the supplemented dose.

The large study ($n = 2,686$) carried out by Trivedi et al. (2003) included more men than women (suggesting that the included population was actually at lower risk for fracture than would have been the case if the study had focused predominantly on women) and was longitudinal (5 years), including repeat measures on the same individual. The amount of vitamin D used for treatment was the equivalent of 800 IU/day, although it was administered as a 100,000 IU dose every 4 months for the duration of the study. Although this may limit somewhat the applicability of the study for DRI purposes, it is not as large as the 500,000 IU dose once yearly used by others (e.g., Sanders et al., 2010). Under these circumstances, the work of Trivedi et al. (2003) is helpful in taking uncertainty into account.

The reason not to dismiss the effect of 800 IU of vitamin D per day as an aberration because of a lack of dose–response data, even in the face of data generally not supportive of an effect of vitamin D alone regarding reduced fracture risk for the oldest adults, is that persons more than 70 years are a very diverse group. This group is undergoing a number of physiological changes with aging that could have an impact on and increase the variability around an average requirement, particularly in light of the known and high variability of these physiological changes among aging individuals. If this is assumed to be the case, then it is likely that the

RDA for persons more than 70 years of age would be higher due to this variability. In addition, there is insufficient evidence to provide assurances that 600 IU/day vitamin D is as effective as 800 IU/day. By comparing the projected RDA based on the simulation analysis (600 IU/day) with the available evidence indicating benefit at 800 IU of vitamin D per day, taking into account the uncertainties would result in an estimation of an RDA of approximately one-third higher than the simulation analysis suggests. Over-all, this is a small increase that is not known to increase the possibility of adverse events while providing a certain level of caution for this particularly vulnerable and potentially frail segment of the population. This approach is predicated on caution in the face of uncertainties, and it is anticipated that newer data in the future will help to clarify the uncertainties surround-ing the level of intake of vitamin D that could be expected to cover 97.5 percent of persons over the age of 70 years.

The EAR of 400 IU/day and RDA of 800 IU/day for this life stage group, consistent with the DRIs for other life stage groups, assume minimal sun exposure.

Adults 51 Through 70 Years of Age

A question in establishing an EAR and RDA for this life stage group is the relevance of vitamin D in affecting bone loss due to the onset of menopause. Men in this life stage group have not yet reached the levels of bone loss and fracture rates associated with aging as manifested in persons more than 70 years of age and, unlike their female counterparts, they are not experiencing significant bone loss due to menopause. However, a portion—in fact perhaps the majority—of women in this life stage group are likely to be experiencing some degree of bone loss due to menopause.

As discussed above for adults more than 70 years of age, the available data do not suggest that median requirements increase with aging, result-ing in support for an EAR of 400 IU/day, the same as for younger adults. Likewise, the EAR for both women and men in the 51 through 70 year life stage group is set at 400 IU of vitamin D per day.

With respect to women 51 through 70 years of age, fracture risk is lower than it is later in life; and as such, it is not entirely congruent with the situation for adults more than 70 years of age. Further, findings for this age group are at best mixed, but are generally not supportive of an effect of vitamin D alone on bone health. Although the AHRQ analyses of studies using vitamin D alone found the results to be inconsistent for a relationship with reduction in fracture risk, more recent studies have trended toward no significant effects (Bunout et al., 2006; Burleigh et al., 2007; Lyons et al., 2007; Avenell et al., 2009b). For those studies showing benefit for BMD with a vitamin D and calcium combination, interpretation is confounded by the effects of calcium especially since calcium alone appears to have at least a modest effect on BMD. The report from the WHI (Jackson et al., 2006), a very large cohort study, has limited applicability to the question of the effect of vitamin D on bone health among women because of relatively high levels of calcium intake (baseline mean calcium intake of approximately 1,150 mg/day at randomization plus 1,000 mg/day supplement) and the confounding due to hormone replacement therapy. Given these data plus the inability to extrapolate the variability seen in the requirements surrounding persons 70 or more years of age to this life stage group, the RDA for women 51 through 70 years of age is set at 600 IU of vitamin D per day, the same level as that for younger adults. With respect to men 51 through 70 years of age, there is also no basis to deviate from the RDA set for younger adults. The available evidence for men is extremely limited, and there are not data to suggest that bone health is enhanced by vitamin D intake among men in this life stage group. An RDA of 600 IU/day is established for these men.

The DRIs for these two life stage groups assume minimal sun exposure.

Pregnancy and Lactation

Pregnant 14 Through 18 Years of Age
Pregnant 19 Through 30 Years of Age
Pregnant 31 Through 50 Years of Age
                    EAR 400 IU (10 μg)/day Vitamin D
                    RDA 600 IU (15 μg)/day Vitamin D
Lactating 14 Through 18 Years of Age
Lactating 19 Through 30 Years of Age
Lactating 31 Through 50 Years of Age
                    EAR 400 IU (10 μg)/day Vitamin D
                    RDA 600 IU (15 μg)/day Vitamin D

Pregnancy The EAR for non-pregnant women and adolescents is appropriate for pregnant women and adolescents based on: (1) AHRQ-Ottawa's finding of insufficient evidence on the association of serum 25OHD level with maternal BMD during pregnancy and (2) the 1 available RCT (Delvin et al., 1986) and 14 observational studies reviewed in Chapter 4 regarding vitamin D deficiency and genetic absence of the vitamin D receptor (VDR) or 1α-hydroxyalase, which all demonstrate no effect of maternal 25OHD level on fetal calcium homeostasis or skeletal outcomes. Of the limited number (i.e., four) of observational studies that suggest an influence of maternal serum 25OHD levels on the offspring's skeletal outcomes later in life (so-called developmental programming), one study reports associations consistent with an EAR-type value of approximately 40 nmol/L below which negative fetal skeletal outcomes were reported (Viljakainen et al., 2010), and another reports an RDA-type value of 50 nmol/L late in gestation above which reduced skeletal BMC was not seen in offspring at 9 years of age (Javaid et al., 2006). In addition, development of the fetal skeleton without dependence on maternal vitamin D is also biologically plausible as indicated by the studies in animal models in rats, mice, pigs, and sheep (see review in Chapter 3). Finally, there is no evidence that the vitamin D requirements of pregnant adolescents differ from those of non-pregnant adolescents.

The EAR is thus 400 IU of vitamin D per day for pregnant women and adolescents. Likewise, the RDA values for non-pregnant women and adolescents are applicable, providing an RDA of 600 IU/day for each group.

Lactation   The EAR for non-lactating women and adolescents is appropriate for lactating women and adolescents based on evidence from RCTs (Rothberg et al., 1982; Ala-Houhala, 1985; Ala-Houhala et al., 1988; Kalkwarf et al., 1996; Hollis and Wagner, 2004; Basile et al., 2006; Wagner et al., 2006; Saadi et al., 2007), which are consistent with observational data (Cancela et al., 1986; Okonofua et al., 1987; Takeuchi et al., 1989; Kent et al., 1990; Alfaham et al., 1995; Sowers et al., 1998) that increased maternal vitamin D intakes increase maternal serum 25OHD levels, with no effect on the neonatal serum 25OHD levels of breast-fed infants unless the maternal intake of vitamin D is extremely high (i.e., 4,000 to 6,400 IU/day) (Wagner et al., 2006). Observational studies report no relationship between maternal serum 25OHD levels and BMD (Ghannam et al., 1999) or breast milk calcium content (Prentice et al., 1997). Also, there is no evidence that lactating adolescents require any more vitamin D or higher serum 25OHD levels than non-lactating adolescents. The EAR is thus 400 IU of vitamin D per day for lactating women and adolescents. Likewise, the RDA values for non-lactating women and adolescents are applicable, providing an RDA of 600 IU/day for each group.

REFERENCES

Abrams, S. A., K. C. Copeland, S. K. Gunn, J. E. Stuff, L. L. Clarke and K. J. Ellis. 1999. Calcium absorption and kinetics are similar in 7- and 8-year-old Mexican-American and Caucasian girls despite hormonal differences. Journal of Nutrition 129(3): 666-71.

Abrams, S. A. 2006. Building bones in babies: can and should we exceed the human milk-fed infant's rate of bone calcium accretion? Nutrition Reviews 64(11): 487-94.

Abrams, S. A., P. D. Hicks and K. M. Hawthorne. 2009. Higher serum 25-hydroxyvitamin D levels in school-age children are inconsistently associated with increased calcium absorption. Journal of Clinical Endocrinology and Metabolism 94(7): 2421-7.

Ala-Houhala, M. 1985. 25-hydroxyvitamin D levels during breast-feeding with or without maternal or infantile supplementation of vitamin D. Journal of Pediatric Gastroenterology and Nutrition 4(2): 220-6.

Ala-Houhala, M., T. Koskinen, M. Koskinen and J. K. Visakorpi. 1988. Double blind study on the need for vitamin D supplementation in prepubertal children. Acta Paediatrica Scandinavica 77(1): 89-93.

Alevizaki, C. C., D. G. Ikkos and P. Singhelakis. 1973. Progressive decrease of true intestinal calcium absorption with age in normal man. Journal of Nuclear Medicine 14(10): 760-2.

Alfaham, M., S. Woodhead, G. Pask and D. Davies. 1995. Vitamin D deficiency: a concern in pregnant Asian women. British Journal of Nutrition 73(6): 881-7.

Ambroszkiewicz, J., W. Klemarczyk, J. Gajewska, M. Chelchowska and T. Laskowska-Klita. 2007. Serum concentration of biochemical bone turnover markers in vegetarian children. Advances in Medical Science 52: 279-82.

Ames, S. K., B. M. Gorham and S. A. Abrams. 1999. Effects of high compared with low calcium intake on calcium absorption and incorporation of iron by red blood cells in small children. American Journal of Clinical Nutrition 70(1): 44-8.

Andersen, R., C. Molgaard, L. T. Skovgaard, C. Brot, K. D. Cashman, E. Chabros, J. Charzewska, A. Flynn, J. Jakobsen, M. Karkkainen, M. Kiely, C. Lamberg-Allardt, O. Moreiras, A. M. Natri, M. O'Brien, M. Rogalska-Niedzwiedz and L. Ovesen. 2005. Teenage girls and elderly women living in northern Europe have low winter vitamin D status. European Journal of Clinical Nutrition 59(4): 533-41.

Anderson, P. H., R. K. Sawyer, A. J. Moore, B. K. May, P. D. O'Loughlin and H. A. Morris. 2008. Vitamin D depletion induces RANKL-mediated osteoclastogenesis and bone loss in a rodent model. Journal of Bone and Mineral Research 23(11): 1789-97.

Atkinson, S. A., B. P. Alston-Mills, B. Lonnerdal, M. C. Neville and M. P. Thompson. 1995. Major minerals and ionic constituents of human and bovine milk. In Handbook of Milk Composition, edited by R. J. Jensen. San Diego, CA: Academic Press. Pp. 593-619.

Avenell, A. and H. H. Handoll. 2004. Nutritional supplementation for hip fracture aftercare in the elderly. Cochrane Database System Review (1): CD001880.

Avenell, A., W. J. Gillespie, L. D. Gillespie and D. O'Connell. 2009. Vitamin D and vitamin D analogues for preventing fractures associated with involutional and post-menopausal osteoporosis. Cochrane Database System Review (2): CD000227.

Avioli, L. V., J. E. McDonald and S. W. Lee. 1965. The influence of age on the intestinal absorption of 47-Ca absorption in post-menopausal osteoporosis. Journal of Clinical Investigation 44(12): 1960-7.

Basile, L. A., S. N. Taylor, C. L. Wagner, R. L. Horst and B. W. Hollis. 2006. The effect of high-dose vitamin D supplementation on serum vitamin D levels and milk calcium concentration in lactating women and their infants. Breastfeeding Medicine 1(1): 27-35.

Bergink, A. P., A. G. Uitterlinden, J. P. Van Leeuwen, C. J. Buurman, A. Hofman, J. A. Verhaar and H. A. Pols. 2009. Vitamin D status, bone mineral density, and the development of radiographic osteoarthritis of the knee: The Rotterdam Study. Journal of Clinical Rheumatology 15(5): 230-7.

Biancuzzo, R. M., A. Young, D. Bibuld, M. H. Cai, M. R. Winter, E. K. Klein, A. Ameri, R. Reitz, W. Salameh, T. C. Chen and M. F. Holick. 2010. Fortification of orange juice with vitamin D(2) or vitamin D(3) is as effective as an oral supplement in maintaining vitamin D status in adults. American Journal of Clinical Nutrition 91(6): 1621-6.

Brannon, P. M., E. A. Yetley, R. L. Bailey and M. F. Picciano. 2008. Vitamin D and health in the 21st century: an update. Proceedings of a conference held September 2007 in Bethesda, Maryland, USA. American Journal of Clinical Nutrition 88(2): 483S-592S.

Bullamore, J. R., R. Wilkinson, J. C. Gallagher, B. E. Nordin and D. H. Marshall. 1970. Effect of age on calcium absorption. Lancet 2(7672): 535-7.

Bunout, D., G. Barrera, L. Leiva, V. Gattas, M. P. de la Maza, M. Avendano and S. Hirsch. 2006. Effects of vitamin D supplementation and exercise training on physical performance in Chilean vitamin D deficient elderly subjects. Experimental Gerontology 41(8): 746-52.

Burleigh, E., J. McColl and J. Potter. 2007. Does vitamin D stop inpatients falling? A randomised controlled trial. Age Ageing 36(5): 507-13.

Cancela, L., N. Le Boulch and L. Miravet. 1986. Relationship between the vitamin D content of maternal milk and the vitamin D status of nursing women and breast-fed infants. Journal of Endocrinology 110(1): 43-50.

Carter, G. D., J. L. Berry, E. Gunter, G. Jones, J. C. Jones, H. L. Makin, S. Sufi and M. J. Wheeler. 2010. Proficiency testing of 25-hydroxyvitamin D (25-OHD) assays. Journal of Steroid Biochemistry and Molecular Biology 121(1-2): 176-9.

Cashman, K. D., T. R. Hill, A. J. Lucey, N. Taylor, K. M. Seamans, S. Muldowney, A. P. Fitzgerald, A. Flynn, M. S. Barnes, G. Horigan, M. P. Bonham, E. M. Duffy, J. J. Strain, J. M. Wallace and M. Kiely. 2008. Estimation of the dietary requirement for vitamin D in healthy adults. American Journal of Clinical Nutrition 88(6): 1535-42.

Cashman, K. D., J. M. Wallace, G. Horigan, T. R. Hill, M. S. Barnes, A. J. Lucey, M. P. Bonham, N. Taylor, E. M. Duffy, K. Seamans, S. Muldowney, A. P. Fitzgerald, A. Flynn, J. J. Strain and M. Kiely. 2009. Estimation of the dietary requirement for vitamin D in free-living adults ≥64 y of age. American Journal of Clinical Nutrition 89(5): 1366-74.

Cauley, J. A., A. Z. Lacroix, L. Wu, M. Horwitz, M. E. Danielson, D. C. Bauer, J. S. Lee, R. D. Jackson, J. A. Robbins, C. Wu, F. Z. Stanczyk, M. S. LeBoff, J. Wactawski-Wende, G. Sarto, J. Ockene and S. R. Cummings. 2008. Serum 25-hydroxyvitamin D concentrations and risk for hip fractures. Annals of Internal Medicine 149(4): 242-50.

Cauley, J. A., N. Parimi, K. E. Ensrud, D. C. Bauer, P. M. Cawthon, S. R. Cummings, A. R. Hoffman, J. M. Shikany, E. Barrett-Connor and E. Orwoll. 2010. Serum 25 hydroxyvitamin D and the risk of hip and non-spine fractures in older men. Journal of Bone and Mineral Research 25(3): 545.

Chantry, C. J., P. Auinger and R. S. Byrd. 2004. Lactation among adolescent mothers and subsequent bone mineral density. Archives of Pediatrics and Adolescent Medicine 158(7): 650-6.

Chapuy, M. C., M. E. Arlot, F. Duboeuf, J. Brun, B. Crouzet, S. Arnaud, P. D. Delmas and P. J. Meunier. 1992. Vitamin D_3 and calcium to prevent hip fractures in the elderly women. New England Journal of Medicine 327(23): 1637-42.

Chung M., E. M. Balk, M. Brendel, S. Ip, J. Lau, J. Lee, A. Lichtenstein, K. Patel, G. Raman, A. Tatsioni, T. Terasawa and T. A. Trikalinos. 2009. Vitamin D and calcium: a systematic review of health outcomes. Evidence Report No. 183. (Prepared by the Tufts Evidence-based Practice Center under Contract No. HHSA 290-2007-10055-I.) AHRQ Publication No. 09-E015. Rockville, MD: Agency for Healthcare Research and Quality.

Cranney A., T. Horsley, S. O'Donnell, H. A. Weiler, L. Puil, D. S. Ooi, S. A. Atkinson, L. M. Ward, D. Moher, D. A. Hanley, M. Fang, F. Yazdi, C. Garritty, M. Sampson, N. Barrowman, A. Tsertsvadze and V. Mamaladze. 2007. Effectiveness and safety of vitamin D in relation to bone health. Evidence Report/Technology Assessment No. 158. (Prepared by the University of Ottawa Evidence-based Practice Center (UO-EPC) under Contract No. 290-02-0021.) AHRQ Publication No. 07-E013. Rockville, MD: Agency for Healthcare Research and Quality.

Cross, N. A., L. S. Hillman, S. H. Allen, G. F. Krause and N. E. Vieira. 1995. Calcium homeostasis and bone metabolism during pregnancy, lactation, and postweaning: a longitudinal study. American Journal of Clinical Nutrition 61(3): 514-23.

Dawson-Hughes, B., G. E. Dallal, E. A. Krall, S. Harris, L. J. Sokoll and G. Falconer. 1991. Effect of vitamin D supplementation on wintertime and overall bone loss in healthy postmenopausal women. Annals of Internal Medicine 115(7): 505-12.

Delvin, E. E., B. L. Salle, F. H. Glorieux, P. Adeleine and L. S. David. 1986. Vitamin D supplementation during pregnancy: effect on neonatal calcium homeostasis. Journal of Pediatrics 109(2): 328-34.

Dewey, K. G., D. A. Finley and B. Lonnerdal. 1984. Breast milk volume and composition during late lactation (7-20 months). Journal of Pediatric Gastroenterology and Nutrition 3(5): 713-20.

Ensrud, K. E., B. C. Taylor, M. L. Paudel, J. A. Cauley, P. M. Cawthon, S. R. Cummings, H. A. Fink, E. Barrett-Connor, J. M. Zmuda, J. M. Shikany and E. S. Orwoll. 2009. Serum 25-hydroxyvitamin D levels and rate of hip bone loss in older men. Journal of Clinical Endocrinology and Metabolism 94(8): 2773-80.

Fairweather-Tait, S., A. Prentice, K. G. Heumann, L. M. Jarjou, D. M. Stirling, S. G. Wharf and J. R. Turnlund. 1995. Effect of calcium supplements and stage of lactation on the calcium absorption efficiency of lactating women accustomed to low calcium intakes. American Journal of Clinical Nutrition 62(6): 1188-92.

Fleet, J. C., C. Gliniak, Z. Zhang, Y. Xue, K. B. Smith, R. McCreedy and S. A. Adedokun. 2008. Serum metabolite profiles and target tissue gene expression define the effect of cholecalciferol intake on calcium metabolism in rats and mice. Journal of Nutrition 138(6): 1114-20.

Fomon, S. J. and S. E. Nelson. 1993. Calcium, phosphorus, magnesium, and sulfur. In Nutrition of Normal Infants, edited by S. J. Fomon. St. Louis: Mosby-Year Book, Inc. Pp. 192-216.

Gallagher, J. C., B. L. Riggs, J. Eisman, A. Hamstra, S. B. Arnaud and H. F. DeLuca. 1979. Intestinal calcium absorption and serum vitamin D metabolites in normal subjects and osteoporotic patients: effect of age and dietary calcium. Journal of Clinical Investigation 64(3): 729-36.

Gartner, L. M., J. Morton, R. A. Lawrence, A. J. Naylor, D. O'Hare, R. J. Schanler and A. I. Eidelman. 2005. Breastfeeding and the use of human milk. Pediatrics 115(2): 496-506.

Ghannam, N. N., M. M. Hammami, S. M. Bakheet and B. A. Khan. 1999. Bone mineral density of the spine and femur in healthy Saudi females: relation to vitamin D status, pregnancy, and lactation. Calcified Tissue International 65(1): 23-8.

Grant, A. M., A. Avenell, M. K. Campbell, A. M. McDonald, G. S. MacLennan, G. C. McPherson, F. H. Anderson, C. Cooper, R. M. Francis, C. Donaldson, W. J. Gillespie, C. M. Robinson, D. J. Torgerson and W. A. Wallace. 2005. Oral vitamin D_3 and calcium for secondary prevention of low-trauma fractures in elderly people (Randomised Evaluation of Calcium Or vitamin D, RECORD): a randomised placebo-controlled trial. Lancet 365(9471): 1621-8.

Greer, F. R., J. E. Searcy, R. S. Levin, J. J. Steichen, P. S. Steichen-Asche and R. C. Tsang. 1982. Bone mineral content and serum 25-hydroxyvitamin D concentrations in breast-fed infants with and without supplemental vitamin D: one-year follow-up. Journal of Pediatrics 100(6): 919-22.

Greer, F. R. and S. Marshall. 1989. Bone mineral content, serum vitamin D metabolite concentrations, and ultraviolet B light exposure in infants fed human milk with and without vitamin D_2 supplements. Journal of Pediatrics 114(2): 204-12.

Harris, S. S. and B. Dawson-Hughes. 2002. Plasma vitamin D and 25OHD responses of young and old men to supplementation with vitamin D3. Journal of the American College of Nutrition 21(4): 357-62.

Harwood, R. H., O. Sahota, K. Gaynor, T. Masud and D. J. Hosking. 2004. A randomised, controlled comparison of different calcium and vitamin D supplementation regimens in elderly women after hip fracture: The Nottingham Neck of Femur (NONOF) Study. Age and Ageing 33(1): 45-51.

Heaney, R. P., K. M. Davies, T. C. Chen, M. F. Holick and M. J. Barger-Lux. 2003. Human serum 25-hydroxycholecalciferol response to extended oral dosing with cholecalciferol. American Journal of Clinical Nutrition 77(1): 204-10.

Holick, M. F., R. M. Biancuzzo, T. C. Chen, E. K. Klein, A. Young, D. Bibuld, R. Reitz, W. Salameh, A. Ameri and A. D. Tannenbaum. 2008. Vitamin D_2 is as effective as vitamin D_3 in maintaining circulating concentrations of 25-hydroxyvitamin D. Journal of Clinical Endocrinology and Metabolism 93(3): 677-81.

Hollis, B. W. and C. L. Wagner. 2004. Vitamin D requirements during lactation: high-dose maternal supplementation as therapy to prevent hypovitaminosis D for both the mother and the nursing infant. American Journal of Clinical Nutrition 80(Suppl 6): 1752S-8S.

Honkanen, R., E. Alhava, M. Parviainen, S. Talasniemi and R. Monkkonen. 1990. The necessity and safety of calcium and vitamin D in the elderly. Journal of the American Geriatrics Society 38(8): 862-6.

Hunt, C. D. and L. K. Johnson. 2007. Calcium requirements: new estimations for men and women by cross–sectional statistical analyses of calcium balance data from metabolic studies. American Journal of Clinical Nutrition 86(4): 1054-63.

IOM (Institute of Medicine). 1991. Nutrition During Lactation. Washington, DC: National Academy Press.

IOM. 1997. Dietary Reference Intakes for Calcium, Phosphorus, Magnesium, Vitamin D, and Fluoride. Washington, DC: National Academy Press.

Jackson, R. D., A. Z. LaCroix, M. Gass, R. B. Wallace, J. Robbins, C. E. Lewis, T. Bassford, S. A. Beresford, H. R. Black, P. Blanchette, D. E. Bonds, R. L. Brunner, R. G. Brzyski, B. Caan, J. A. Cauley, R. T. Chlebowski, S. R. Cummings, I. Granek, J. Hays, G. Heiss, S. L. Hendrix, B. V. Howard, J. Hsia, F. A. Hubbell, K. C. Johnson, H. Judd, J. M. Kotchen, L. H. Kuller, R. D. Langer, N. L. Lasser, M. C. Limacher, S. Ludlam, J. E. Manson, K. L. Margolis, J. McGowan, J. K. Ockene, M. J. O'Sullivan, L. Phillips, R. L. Prentice, G. E. Sarto, M. L. Stefanick, L. Van Horn, J. Wactawski-Wende, E. Whitlock, G. L. Anderson, A. R. Assaf and D. Barad. 2006. Calcium plus vitamin D supplementation and the risk of fractures. New England Journal of Medicine 354(7): 669-83.

Jarjou, L. M., A. Prentice, Y. Sawo, M. A. Laskey, J. Bennett, G. R. Goldberg and T. J. Cole. 2006. Randomized, placebo-controlled, calcium supplementation study in pregnant Gambian women: effects on breast-milk calcium concentrations and infant birth weight, growth, and bone mineral accretion in the first year of life. American Journal of Clinical Nutrition 83(3): 657-66.

Jarjou, L. M., M. A. Laskey, Y. Sawo, G. R. Goldberg, T. J. Cole and A. Prentice. 2010. Effect of calcium supplementation in pregnancy on maternal bone outcomes in women with a low calcium intake. American Journal of Clinical Nutrition 92(2): 450-7.

Javaid, M. K., S. R. Crozier, N. C. Harvey, C. R. Gale, E. M. Dennison, B. J. Boucher, N. K. Arden, K. M. Godfrey and C. Cooper. 2006. Maternal vitamin D status during pregnancy and childhood bone mass at age 9 years: a longitudinal study. Lancet 367(9504): 36-43.

Kalkwarf, H. J., B. L. Specker, J. E. Heubi, N. E. Vieira and A. L. Yergey. 1996. Intestinal calcium absorption of women during lactation and after weaning. American Journal of Clinical Nutrition 63(4): 526-31.

Kalkwarf, H. J., B. L. Specker, D. C. Bianchi, J. Ranz and M. Ho. 1997. The effect of calcium supplementation on bone density during lactation and after weaning. New England Journal of Medicine 337(8): 523-8.

Kalkwarf, H. J. 1999. Hormonal and dietary regulation of changes in bone density during lactation and after weaning in women. Journal of Mammary Gland Biology and Neoplasia 4(3): 319-29.

Kent, G. N., R. I. Price, D. H. Gutteridge, M. Smith, J. R. Allen, C. I. Bhagat, M. P. Barnes, C. J. Hickling, R. W. Retallack, S. G. Wilson and et al. 1990. Human lactation: forearm trabecular bone loss, increased bone turnover, and renal conservation of calcium and inorganic phosphate with recovery of bone mass following weaning. Journal of Bone and Mineral Research 5(4): 361-9.

Khosla, S., S. Amin and E. Orwoll. 2008. Osteoporosis in men. Endocrine Reviews 29(4): 441-64.

Koo, W. W., J. C. Walters, J. Esterlitz, R. J. Levine, A. J. Bush and B. Sibai. 1999. Maternal calcium supplementation and fetal bone mineralization. Obstetrics and Gynecology 94(4): 577-82.

Kovacs, C. S. and H. M. Kronenberg. 1997. Maternal-fetal calcium and bone metabolism during pregnancy, puerperium, and lactation. Endocrine Reviews 18(6): 832-72.

Larsen, E. R., L. Mosekilde and A. Foldspang. 2004. Vitamin D and calcium supplementation prevents osteoporotic fractures in elderly community dwelling residents: a pragmatic population-based 3-year intervention study. Journal of Bone and Mineral Research 19(3): 370-8.

Laskey, M. A., A. Prentice, L. A. Hanratty, L. M. Jarjou, B. Dibba, S. R. Beavan and T. J. Cole. 1998. Bone changes after 3 mo of lactation: influence of calcium intake, breast-milk output, and vitamin D-receptor genotype. American Journal of Clinical Nutrition 67(4): 685-92.

Law, M., H. Withers, J. Morris and F. Anderson. 2006. Vitamin D supplementation and the prevention of fractures and falls: results of a randomised trial in elderly people in residential accommodation. Age and Ageing 35(5): 482-6.

Li-Ng, M., J. F. Aloia, S. Pollack, B. A. Cunha, M. Mikhail, J. Yeh and N. Berbari. 2009. A randomized controlled trial of vitamin D_3 supplementation for the prevention of symptomatic upper respiratory tract infections. Epidemiology and Infection 137(10): 1396-404.

Lips, P., W. C. Graafmans, M. E. Ooms, P. D. Bezemer and L. M. Bouter. 1996. Vitamin D supplementation and fracture incidence in elderly persons. A randomized, placebo-controlled clinical trial. Annals of Internal Medicine 124(4): 400-6.

Looker, A. C. and M. E. Mussolino. 2008. Serum 25-hydroxyvitamin D and hip fracture risk in older U.S. white adults. Journal of Bone and Mineral Research 23(1): 143-50.

Lynch, M. F., I. J. Griffin, K. M. Hawthorne, Z. Chen, M. Hamzo and S. A. Abrams. 2007. Calcium balance in 1-4-y-old children. American Journal of Clinical Nutrition 85(3): 750-4.

Lyons, R. A., A. Johansen, S. Brophy, R. G. Newcombe, C. J. Phillips, B. Lervy, R. Evans, K. Wareham and M. D. Stone. 2007. Preventing fractures among older people living in institutional care: a pragmatic randomised double blind placebo controlled trial of vitamin D supplementation. Osteoporosis International 18(6): 811-8.

Melhus, H., G. Snellman, R. Gedeborg, L. Byberg, L. Berglund, H. Mallmin, P. Hellman, R. Blomhoff, E. Hagstrom, J. Arnlov and K. Michaelsson. 2010. Plasma 25-hydroxyvitamin D levels and fracture risk in a community-based cohort of elderly men in Sweden. Journal of Clinical Endocrinology and Metabolism 95(6): 2637-45.

Meyer, H. E., G. B. Smedshaug, E. Kvaavik, J. A. Falch, A. Tverdal and J. I. Pedersen. 2002. Can vitamin D supplementation reduce the risk of fracture in the elderly? A randomized controlled trial. Journal of Bone and Mineral Research 17(4): 709-15.

Millen, A. E., J. Wactawski-Wende, M. Pettinger, M. L. Melamed, F. A. Tylavsky, S. Liu, J. Robbins, A. Z. LaCroix, M. S. LeBoff and R. D. Jackson. 2010. Predictors of serum 25-hydroxyvitamin D concentrations among postmenopausal women: the Women's Health Initiative Calcium plus Vitamin D clinical trial. American Journal of Clinical Nutrition 91(5): 1324-35.

Mimouni, F., B. Campaigne, M. Neylan and R. C. Tsang. 1993. Bone mineralization in the first year of life in infants fed human milk, cow-milk formula, or soy-based formula. Journal of Pediatrics 122(3): 348-54.

Nelson, M. L., J. M. Blum, B. W. Hollis, C. Rosen and S. S. Sullivan. 2009. Supplements of 20 microg/d cholecalciferol optimized serum 25-hydroxyvitamin D concentrations in 80% of premenopausal women in winter. Journal of Nutrition 139(3): 540-6.

NOF (National Osteoporosis Foundation). 2008. Clinician's Guide to Prevention and Treatment of Osteoporosis. Washington, DC: National Osteoporosis Foundation.

O'Brien, K. O., M. S. Nathanson, J. Mancini and F. R. Witter. 2003. Calcium absorption is significantly higher in adolescents during pregnancy than in the early postpartum period. American Journal of Clinical Nutrition 78(6): 1188-93.

Okonofua, F., R. K. Menon, S. Houlder, M. Thomas, D. Robinson, S. O'Brien and P. Dandona. 1987. Calcium, vitamin D and parathyroid hormone relationships in pregnant Caucasian and Asian women and their neonates. Annals of Clinical Biochemistry 24(Pt 1): 22-8.

Orwoll, E. S., S. K. Oviatt, M. R. McClung, L. J. Deftos and G. Sexton. 1990. The rate of bone mineral loss in normal men and the effects of calcium and cholecalciferol supplementation. Annals of Internal Medicine 112(1): 29-34.

Peacock, M., G. Liu, M. Carey, R. McClintock, W. Ambrosius, S. Hui and C. C. Johnston. 2000. Effect of calcium or 25OH vitamin D_3 dietary supplementation on bone loss at the hip in men and women over the age of 60. Journal of Clinical Endocrinology and Metabolism 85(9): 3011-9.

Polatti, F., E. Capuzzo, F. Viazzo, R. Colleoni and C. Klersy. 1999. Bone mineral changes during and after lactation. Obstetrics and Gynecology 94(1): 52-6.

Porthouse, J., S. Cockayne, C. King, L. Saxon, E. Steele, T. Aspray, M. Baverstock, Y. Birks, J. Dumville, R. Francis, C. Iglesias, S. Puffer, A. Sutcliffe, I. Watt and D. J. Torgerson. 2005. Randomised controlled trial of calcium and supplementation with cholecalciferol (vitamin D_3) for prevention of fractures in primary care. British Medical Journal 330(7498): 1003.

Prentice, A., L. M. Jarjou, T. J. Cole, D. M. Stirling, B. Dibba and S. Fairweather-Tait. 1995. Calcium requirements of lactating Gambian mothers: effects of a calcium supplement on breast-milk calcium concentration, maternal bone mineral content, and urinary calcium excretion. American Journal of Clinical Nutrition 62(1): 58-67.

Prentice, A., L. Yan, L. M. Jarjou, B. Dibba, M. A. Laskey, D. M. Stirling and S. Fairweather-Tait. 1997. Vitamin D status does not influence the breast-milk calcium concentration of lactating mothers accustomed to a low calcium intake. Acta Paediatrica 86(9): 1006-8.

Priemel, M., C. von Domarus, T. O. Klatte, S. Kessler, J. Schlie, S. Meier, N. Proksch, F. Pastor, C. Netter, T. Streichert, K. Puschel and M. Amling. 2010. Bone mineralization defects and vitamin D deficiency: histomorphometric analysis of iliac crest bone biopsies and circulating 25-hydroxyvitamin D in 675 patients. Journal of Bone and Mineral Research 25(2): 305-12.

Prince, R. L., A. Devine, S. S. Dhaliwal and I. M. Dick. 2006. Effects of calcium supplementation on clinical fracture and bone structure: results of a 5-year, double-blind, placebo-controlled trial in elderly women. Archives of Internal Medicine 166(8): 869-75.

Rajakumar, K., J. D. Fernstrom, M. F. Holick, J. E. Janosky and S. L. Greenspan. 2008. Vitamin D status and response to Vitamin D(3) in obese vs. non-obese African American children. Obesity (Silver Spring) 16(1): 90-5.

Rothberg, A. D., J. M. Pettifor, D. F. Cohen, E. W. Sonnendecker and F. P. Ross. 1982. Maternal-infant vitamin D relationships during breast-feeding. Journal of Pediatrics 101(4): 500-3.

Saadi, H. F., A. Dawodu, B. O. Afandi, R. Zayed, S. Benedict and N. Nagelkerke. 2007. Efficacy of daily and monthly high-dose calciferol in vitamin D-deficient nulliparous and lactating women. American Journal of Clinical Nutrition 85(6): 1565-71.

Sanders, K. M., A. L. Stuart, E. J. Williamson, J. A. Simpson, M. A. Kotowicz, D. Young and G. C. Nicholson. 2010. Annual high-dose oral vitamin D and falls and fractures in older women: a randomized controlled trial. Journal of the American Medical Association 303(18): 1815-22.

Schou, A. J., C. Heuck and O. D. Wolthers. 2003. A randomized, controlled lower leg growth study of vitamin D supplementation to healthy children during the winter season. Annals of Human Biology 30(2): 214-9.

Smith, H., F. Anderson, H. Raphael, P. Maslin, S. Crozier and C. Cooper. 2007. Effect of annual intramuscular vitamin D on fracture risk in elderly men and women—a population-based, randomized, double-blind, placebo-controlled trial. Rheumatology 46(12): 1852-7.

Smith, S. M., K. K. Gardner, J. Locke and S. R. Zwart. 2009. Vitamin D supplementation during Antarctic winter. American Journal of Clinical Nutrition 89(4): 1092-8.

Sowers, M. 1996. Pregnancy and lactation as risk factors for subsequent bone loss and osteoporosis. Journal of Bone and Mineral Research 11(8): 1052-60.

Sowers, M., D. Zhang, B. W. Hollis, B. Shapiro, C. A. Janney, M. Crutchfield, M. A. Schork, F. Stanczyk and J. Randolph. 1998. Role of calciotrophic hormones in calcium mobilization of lactation. American Journal of Clinical Nutrition 67(2): 284-91.

Specker, B. L., M. L. Ho, A. Oestreich, T. A. Yin, Q. M. Shui, X. C. Chen and R. C. Tsang. 1992. Prospective study of vitamin D supplementation and rickets in China. Journal of Pediatrics 120(5): 733-9.

Specker, B. L., A. Beck, H. Kalkwarf and M. Ho. 1997. Randomized trial of varying mineral intake on total body bone mineral accretion during the first year of life. Pediatrics 99(6): E12.

Takeuchi, A., T. Okano, N. Tsugawa, Y. Tasaka, T. Kobayashi, S. Kodama and T. Matsuo. 1989. Effects of ergocalciferol supplementation on the concentration of vitamin D and its metabolites in human milk. Journal of Nutrition 119(11): 1639-46.

Tang, B. M., G. D. Eslick, C. Nowson, C. Smith and A. Bensoussan. 2007. Use of calcium or calcium in combination with vitamin D supplementation to prevent fractures and bone loss in people aged 50 years and older: a meta-analysis. Lancet 370(9588): 657-66.

Trivedi, D. P., R. Doll and K. T. Khaw. 2003. Effect of four monthly oral vitamin D3 (cholecalciferol) supplementation on fractures and mortality in men and women living in the community: randomised double blind controlled trial. British Medical Journal 326(7387): 469.

Tsai, K. S., H. Heath, 3rd, R. Kumar and B. L. Riggs. 1984. Impaired vitamin D metabolism with aging in women. Possible role in pathogenesis of senile osteoporosis. Journal of Clinical Investigation 73(6): 1668-72.

Van Der Klis, F. R., J. H. Jonxis, J. J. Van Doormaal, P. Sikkens, A. E. Saleh and F. A. Muskiet. 1996. Changes in vitamin-D metabolites and parathyroid hormone in plasma following cholecalciferol administration to pre- and postmenopausal women in the Netherlands in early spring and to postmenopausal women in Curacao. British Journal of Nutrition 75(4): 637-46.

van Schoor, N. M., M. Visser, S. M. Pluijm, N. Kuchuk, J. H. Smit and P. Lips. 2008. Vitamin D deficiency as a risk factor for osteoporotic fractures. Bone 42(2): 260-6.

Vatanparast, H., D. A. Bailey, A. D. Baxter-Jones and S. J. Whiting. 2010. Calcium requirements for bone growth in Canadian boys and girls during adolescence. British Journal of Nutrition: 1-6.

Viljakainen, H. T., A. M. Natri, M. Karkkainen, M. M. Huttunen, A. Palssa, J. Jakobsen, K. D. Cashman, C. Molgaard and C. Lamberg-Allardt. 2006. A positive dose–response effect of vitamin D supplementation on site-specific bone mineral augmentation in adolescent girls: a double-blinded randomized placebo-controlled 1-year intervention. Journal of Bone and Mineral Research 21(6): 836-44.

Viljakainen, H. T., M. Vaisanen, V. Kemi, T. Rikkonen, H. Kroger, E. K. Laitinen, H. Rita and C. Lamberg-Allardt. 2009. Wintertime vitamin D supplementation inhibits seasonal variation of calcitropic hormones and maintains bone turnover in healthy men. Journal of Bone and Mineral Research 24(2): 346-52.

Viljakainen, H. T., E. Saarnio, T. Hytinantti, M. Miettinen, H. Surcel, O. Makitie, S. Andersson, K. Laitinen and C. Lamberg-Allardt. 2010. Maternal vitamin D status determines bone variables in the newborn. Journal of Clinical Endocrinology and Metabolism 95(4): 1749-57.

Wagner, C. L., T. C. Hulsey, D. Fanning, M. Ebeling and B. W. Hollis. 2006. High-dose vitamin D_3 supplementation in a cohort of breastfeeding mothers and their infants: a 6-month follow-up pilot study. Breastfeeding Medicine 1(2): 59-70.

Widdowson, E. M. 1965. Absorption and excretion of fat, nitrogen, and minerals from "filled" milks by babies one week old. Lancet 2(7422): 1099-105.

6

Tolerable Upper Intake Levels: Calcium and Vitamin D

The Tolerable Upper Intake Level (UL) is not a recommended intake. Rather, it is intended to specify the level above which the risk for harm begins to increase, and is defined as the highest average daily intake of a nutrient that is likely to pose no risk of adverse health effects for nearly all persons in the general population. As intake increases above the UL, the potential risk for adverse effects increases. In short, the UL is a reference value intended to guide policy-makers and scientists charged with ensuring a safe food supply and protecting the health of the U.S. and Canadian populations. It applies to intakes on a chronic basis among free-living persons. Those responsible for determining the appropriate dosages of nutrients to be studied in carefully controlled experimental trials conducted in clinical or community settings have the opportunity to bring other considerations into play when deciding on the acceptable levels of nutrients that are appropriate for subjects taking part in such studies. ULs are not designed to address experimental protocols in which safety monitoring occurs.

This chapter is organized to include hazard identification (indicator review and selection) and hazard characterization (intake–response assessment and reference value specification), the first two steps of the general risk assessment approach for Dietary Reference Intake (DRI) development. Therefore, compared with the discussions presented in the two chapters on reference values for adequacy (Chapters 4 and 5), the discussions for ULs are contained in a single chapter. This chapter addresses adverse effects of excess intakes of calcium and vitamin D. Although adverse effects are also associated with deficiencies of calcium and vitamin D, those concerns are incorporated into the previous discussions focused on establishing reference values for adequacy.

There are often ethical issues associated with conducting clinical trials designed to study the adverse effects of substances that can limit the types of data available for DRI development. For this reason, the derivation of ULs for DRI purposes necessarily relies more heavily on observational data and information derived from animal models than does the approach for the determination of levels of intake for nutritional adequacy. Thus, the emphasis on causality and strength of evidence needed for establishing reference values for adequacy is difficult to apply to the derivation of ULs.

At the outset, it is important to distinguish between the relatively "acute" toxic effects of excess intake and the "chronic" adverse effects of high levels of intake that may manifest in other ways including disease risk. When the ULs for calcium and vitamin D were originally established in 1997, it was noted that the available data were limited relative to adverse outcomes and dose–response relationships (IOM, 1997). In that report, adverse effects from excess intakes of calcium and vitamin D were considered primarily in terms of acute toxicity, which was defined as the condition of hypercalcemia or, in some cases, hypercalciuria with or without hypercalcemia.

The conditions associated with the intoxication syndrome for calcium and vitamin D are informative, but avoiding acute toxicity is not the ideal basis for a UL, a reference value with the larger purpose of public health protection over a life time of chronic intake. Although information concerning chronic excess intakes remains limited, data have emerged recently that may warrant caution about the levels of vitamin D that are consumed and raise questions about the long-term effects of high intakes that are less than those associated with toxicity and that may result in an increase in serum 25-hydroxyvitamin D (25OHD) levels into upper ranges previously considered physiological. Caution may also be warranted in comparing the effects at these high physiological levels of 25OHD achieved through supplementation versus sun exposure, and further research is needed to clarify the relative adverse effects of different sources of vitamin D.

The model developed for UL derivation was summarized in 1998 (IOM, 1998), and it acknowledged that the lack of data would affect the ability to derive precise estimates. Specifically: "Several judgments must be made regarding the uncertainties and thus the uncertainty factor (UF) associated with extrapolating from the observed data to the general population." Although a number of reports describe the underlying basis for uncertainty factors (Zielhuis and van der Kreek, 1979; Dourson and Stara, 1983), the strength of the evidence supporting the use of a specific UL undoubtedly varies. The summary of the 2007 workshop focused on enhancing DRI development (IOM, 2008) and pointed out the need for uncertainty fac-

---

BOX 6-1
Potential Indicators of Adverse Outcomes for
Excess Intake of Calcium and Vitamin D

Calcium
- Hypercalcemia
- Hypercalciuria
- Vascular and soft tissue calcification
- Nephrolithiasis (kidney stones)
- Prostate cancer
- Interactions with iron and zinc
- Constipation

Vitamin D
- Intoxication and related hypercalcemia and hypercalciuria
- Serum calcium
- Measures in infants: retarded growth, hypercalcemia
- Emerging evidence for all-cause mortality, cancer, cardiovascular risk, falls and fractures

---

tors, but also indicated that the scientific judgment involved should be described. In developing ULs for calcium and vitamin D, the limited nature of the data resulted in the committee using UFs to adjust for uncertainties in the data. These were necessarily qualitative adjustments rather than quantitative adjustments. As suggested repeatedly during the 2007 workshop on DRIs (IOM, 2008), an educated guess for a reference value is more useful to stakeholders than the failure to set a reference value in the face of uncertainty.

Discussions related to calcium ULs are provided first, and then vitamin D ULs are considered. At the start, the committee identified potential indicators to assess adverse effects for excess intakes of calcium and vitamin D based on the available literature, as described below. The potential indicators considered are presented in Box 6-1.

CALCIUM UPPER LEVELS: REVIEW OF POTENTIAL INDICATORS AND SELECTION OF INDICATORS

Excess calcium intake from foods alone is difficult if not impossible to achieve. Rather, excess intakes are more likely to be associated with the use of calcium supplements. However, the potential indicators for the adverse outcomes of excessive calcium intake are not characterized by a robust data set that clearly provides a basis for a dose–response relationship. The measures available are confounded by a range of variables including other dietary factors and pre-existing disease conditions.

The "classic" toxicity state of hypercalcemia is seen with either calcium or vitamin D excess, although it appears that the symptoms of hypercalcemia are manifested at relatively lower intake of calcium compared with vitamin D, for which high intakes are required to reach a toxic state. In the discussions below, hypercalcemia, as well as, hypercalciuria is described first as general conditions associated with the toxicity of either nutrient, followed by a discussion of adverse outcomes associated with excess calcium intake.

The Toxic Condition of Hypercalcemia and Hypercalciuria

Hypercalcemia occurs when serum calcium levels are 10.5 mg/dL (also expressed as 2.63 mmol/L) or greater depending on normative laboratory values. It can be induced by excess intake of calcium or vitamin D, but it is more commonly caused by conditions such as malignancy and primary hyperparathyroidism (Moe, 2008). Clinical signs and symptoms of hypercalcemia may vary depending on the magnitude of the hypercalcemia and the rapidity of its elevation; they often include anorexia, weight loss, polyuria, heart arrhythmias, fatigue, and soft tissue calcifications (Jones, 2008). When serum calcium levels rise above 12 mg/dL, the kidney's ability to reabsorb calcium is often limited; in turn, hypercalciuria can occur, particularly with increased calcium or vitamin D intake. Hypercalciuria is present when urinary excretion of calcium exceeds 250 mg/day in women or 275-300 mg/day in men. Often, urinary calcium excretion is expressed as the ratio of calcium to creatinine excreted in 24 hours (milligrams of calcium per milligram of creatinine). Values above 0.3 mg/mg creatinine are considered to be within the hypercalcuric range.

Hypercalcemia, in addition to leading to hypercalciuria, can cause renal insufficiency, vascular and soft tissue calcification including calcinosis leading to nephrocalcinosis, and nephrolithiasis. Nephrolithiasis, often referred to as kidney stones, can also be caused by hypercalciuria. Hypercalciuria may occur in the absence of hypercalcemia and is related to either hyperabsorption of calcium in the gut or a renal leak whereby calcium excretion is enhanced. Both etiologies can lead to nephrocalcinosis.

In the North American population, as many as 30 percent of persons ages 60 years or older have some degree of renal insufficiency (Coresch et al., 2005; Szczech et al., 2009). Decreased renal functioning may make persons more sensitive or susceptible to the effects of excess calcium or vitamin D intake. Urinary calcium excretion decreases in older adults, although it is not clear the extent to which this may be due to decreased calcium intake as compared to decreased renal function. However, if due to decreased renal function, older persons may be at higher risk for adverse effects derived from excess intakes. Moreover, decreased renal function simultaneously increases cardiovascular disease (CVD) risk and impairs calciuric responses and calcium and phosphate homeostasis. Likewise, those using thiazide-based diuretics—a sizeable proportion of older adults—are more readily challenged by excess calcium and vitamin D due to reduction in calcium excretion from the kidney (Medarov, 2009).

Excess Calcium and Hypercalcemia Leading to Renal Insufficiency

Prior to the introduction of histamine-2 blockers and proton pump inhibitors, liquid formulations that contained high calcium levels and absorbable alkali were used to treat gastric and duodenal ulcers. High intake of these formulations, however, caused a variety of adverse effects including hypercalcemia and renal failure. The syndrome became known as "milk-alkali syndrome" or MAS (Hardt and Rivers, 1923; Burnett et al., 1949) and was originally associated with men with peptic ulcer disease. In this context, hypercalcemia causes emesis and natriuresis, which result in significant drops in extracellular blood volume. This contraction worsens the hypercalcemia. Decreases in blood volume also induce an alkalotic state that causes an increase in proximal tubular bicarbonate resorption. Also, high serum calcium levels worsen the alkalosis through suppression of parathyroid hormone (PTH), which physiologically enhances bicarbonate excretion. Although the availability of absorbable alkali in the diet may enhance the alkalotic state, it is not the major pathogenic factor in MAS.

Recently, Patel and Goldfarb (2010) suggested renaming MAS as "calcium-alkali syndrome" to better reflect the current understanding of the disorder, which now has shifted to be more prevalent in other groups including postmenopausal women. The earlier MAS presented with hyperphosphatemia after prolonged ingestion of phosphorus-containing milk with cream (Patel and Goldfarb, 2010). In contrast, the modern version of the syndrome is associated with hypophosphatemia or low-normal serum phosphorus levels as a result of the phosphorus-binding properties of calcium carbonate. The hypophosphatemia is more pronounced in elderly patients or those with eating disorders, who tend to have relatively low consumption of protein and therefore phosphorus (Picolos et al., 2005; Felsenfeld and Levine, 2006; Medarov, 2009). Confounding this, however, is the chronic renal insufficiency that often accompanies MAS; in that case, serum phosphorus levels may be normal or high. Available case reports tend to provide only serum calcium levels and do not specify calcium intakes per se, or serum phosphate, associated with the condition.

As shown in Table 6-1, a number of recent case reports have been iden-

TABLE 6-1 Case Reports of Calcium-Alkali Syndrome

Reference	Patient Gender/Age (years)	Calcium Carbonate Intake (mg/day)	Duration	Serum Calcium Level (mmol/L) mg/dL	Creatinine Level (μmol/L) mg/dL
Javed et al., 2007	Male/70	> 1,000	1 year	(3.43) 13.7	(344.8) 3.9
Nabhan et al., 2004	Female/61	1,500 + 600 IU vitamin D	Several years	(6.43) 25.7	(106.1) 1.2
Caruso et al., 2007	Male/60	> 2,000 + 800 IU vitamin D	NR	(3.08) 12.3	(530.4) 6.0
Gordon et al., 2005	Female/35	3,000	1 month	(2.64) 10.6	(190.0) 2.1
Shah et al., 2007	Female/47	3,000 + 200 IU vitamin D	NR	(4.13) 16.5	(362.4) 4.1
Kaklamanos and Perros, 2007	Female/76	5,500	2 years	(3.45) 13.8	(124.0) 1.4
Grubb et al., 2009	Female/51	7,200	NR	(5.70) 22.8	(185.6) 2.1
Ulett et al., 2010	Male/46	> 7,500	NR	(3.98) 15.9	(406.6) 4.6
Irriza-Ali et al., 2008	Case 1: Female/48 Case 2: Male/74 Case 3: Male/51	Case 1: ~ 8,000 Case 2: ~ 18,000 Case 3: ~ 44,000	Case 1: 19 years Case 2: several weeks Case 3: NR	Case 1: (3.25) 13.0 Case 2: (3.31) 13.2 Case 3: (2.97) 11.9	Case 1: (737) 8.3 Case 2: (245) 2.8 Case 3: (1,013) 11.5
Jousten and Guffens, 2008	Male/66	~ 10,000	Several months	(4.15) 16.6	(459.7) 5.2
Bailey et al., 2008	Female/40	~ 11,000	NR	(4.71) 18.8	(164.0) 1.9
Waked et al., 2009	Male/81	~ 12,500	NR	(3.65) 13.8	(733.7) 8.3

NOTE: To convert mmol/L to mg/dL, multiply by 0.25; IU = International Units; NR = not reported.

tified for calcium-alkali syndrome. For these individuals, a calcium intake of 3,000 mg/day was associated with the onset of hypercalcemia. However, in every case except one, all outcomes were found in individuals with impaired renal function and high serum creatinine levels. The one exception (Nabhan et al., 2004) was a patient who was using hydrochlorothiazide as a diuretic and was hypoparathyroid. Although these data cannot be applied directly to the normal, free-living population, they are informative and indicate that calcium levels of 3,000 mg/day are problematic for these compromised persons.

Patel and Goldfarb (2010) suggested that the incidence of calcium-alkali syndrome is growing as a result of the widespread use of over-the-counter calcium and vitamin D supplements, particularly among older persons. The basis for the suggestion is that while healthy younger adults rely on the bone reservoir to buffer excess calcium, the net flux of calcium is out of the bone for older persons, thereby making the bone less functional as a reservoir. These older persons are more susceptible to the syndrome when they begin taking supplemental calcium. Patel and Goldfarb (2010) also noted that the excess ingestion of calcium with or without vitamin D is an integral feature of this syndrome, making it potentially relevant to the consideration of upper levels of calcium intake.

Excess Calcium and Soft Tissue Calcification

Associated with Hypercalcemia

Calcification of soft tissues—calcinosis—occurs as a result of long-standing hypercalcemia, increased serum phosphate levels, or local abnormality in the affected tissues. Clinically, the condition is linked to metabolic disorders such as hyperparathyroidism, sarcoidosis, or connective tissue disease such as scleroderma.[1]

Calcification of kidney tissues, or nephrocalcinosis, results in symptoms similar to those of renal dysfunction, ranging from painful and frequent urination to nausea, vomiting, and swelling. Although nephrocalcinosis has been reported to be induced by calcium intake in rats (Peterson et al., 1996), no data link calcium intake or the use of calcium supplements in humans to the onset of nephrocalcinosis. Nephrocalcinosis may be associated with calcium nephrolithiasis under particular conditions (Vervaet et al., 2009).

Relative to hypercalcemia and calcification of vascular tissue, there is

---

[1]Soft tissue calcifications are more severe in hypocalcemic disorders such as hypoparathyroidism and renal failure, but in such cases it is the associated hyperphosphatemia that is causing the calcifications.

experimental evidence in humans and laboratory animals indicating that hypercalcemia can lead to vascular calcification in the setting of renal insufficiency as a result of elevated calcium and phosphate concentrations (Reynolds et al., 2004; Yang et al., 2004; Cozzolino et al., 2005). However, this has not been demonstrated clinically.

Associated with Calcium Supplements

Calcification of vascular tissues has been reported with high calcium intake (Goodman et al., 2000; Asmus et al., 2005; Block et al., 2005; Raggi et al., 2005); however, the reports are based on individuals with compromised kidney function. No link has been clearly established for a general population.

Bolland et al. (2008), in a recent randomized, placebo-controlled trial, found that cardiovascular events may be slightly more prevalent in older women on calcium supplementation. Reid and Bolland (2008), in a subsequent companion publication, suggested among other possibilities that vascular calcification may be relevant to their finding of an upward trend in cardiovascular event rates in healthy postmenopausal women supplemented with calcium. These findings were contrary to the purported benefits of calcium supplementation and CVD.

A more recent meta-analysis conducted by Bolland et al. (2010) examined 11 randomized controlled trials of calcium supplements in 12,000 older patients and found that there was a 30 percent increased risk of heart attack independent of age, gender, and type of supplement. Although this report is of concern, there are several relevant limitations. The studies included are small, the event frequency is low, and most outcomes have confidence intervals (CIs) that overlap. Moreover, cardiovascular events were not a primary outcome, the events may not have been well adjudicated, and renal function was not considered as a covariate. Many of the studies supplemented with 1,000 to 1,200 mg of calcium per day and did not report the total calcium intake (supplement plus diet). The events may therefore be associated with intakes higher than the supplemented dose, perhaps 2,000 mg of calcium per day or more, as reported, for example, by Jackson et al. (2006). Under these circumstances, it is difficult to conclude that calcium intakes per se in the range of 1,000 to 1,200 mg/day can be associated with cardiovascular events. In addition, some questions remain as to whether the addition of this amount of calcium to a baseline diet as a calcium supplement may have adverse consequences.

Excess Calcium and Nephrolithiasis (Kidney Stones)

More than 12 percent of men and 6 percent of women in the general population will develop kidney stones (Stamatelou et al., 2003). The morbidity of kidney stones is not limited to the pain of stone passage; stones increase the risk of renal and urinary tract infections as well as renal insufficiency. A contributing factor in stone formation is hypercalciuria from any cause; another is hyperabsorption of calcium from the gut. Hypercalciuria increases the risk for nephrolithiasis (Pak and Holt, 1976). Hypercalciuria can be present in the absence of hypercalcemia and may reflect routine excretion of excess calcium intake.

Incidence rates for kidney stones vary by age and gender. The rates are highest in men, rising after age 20, peaking between 40 and 60 years, and then beginning to decline (Johnson et al., 1979; Hiatt et al., 1982; Curhan et al., 1993). For women, incidence rates seem to be higher in the late 20s, decreasing by age 50, and then remaining relatively constant (Johnson et al., 1979; Hiatt et al., 1982; Curhan et al., 1997, 2004).

Although calcium is present in approximately 80 percent of kidney stones (Coe et al., 1992), the role of calcium and other nutrients, acting alone or in concert as risk factors, is not completely understood and may be a function of physiological context. Various dietary and non-dietary factors are associated with stone formation, making data difficult to interpret. Rodent models that have been used to explore the effect of dietary factors on the propensity to form calcium oxalate and calcium phosphate stones suggest that the role of supplemental calcium in determining risk for nephrolithiasis varies by interaction with a given dietary component. One study in rats compared renal oxalate crystallization relative to the consumption of calcium-supplemented or oxalate-rich diets as well as control diets. The study found that rats fed the calcium-supplemented diet had enhanced calcium and oxalate accumulation as well as crystallization in renal tissues, even though urinary oxalate and citrate excretion was not significantly different in rats fed the control diet (Mourad et al., 2006). In this study, measures of renal function, including glomerular filtration rate, fractional excretion of urea, and fractional reabsorption of water and magnesium were not affected by the calcium-supplemented diet, and calciuria was only slightly increased.

Nephrolithiasis in Adults

Recently, a study using data from the Women's Health Initiative (WHI) trial, which recruited more than 36,000 post-menopausal women ages 50 to 79 years (mean age 62 years), reported findings on the incidence of kidney stones (Jackson et al., 2006). Participants were randomly assigned to receive a placebo or 1,000 mg of elemental calcium (calcium carbonate) per day with 400 International Units (IU) of vitamin D_3. The primary outcome focus was fractures and measures of bone density. Mean baseline intake of calcium was approximately 1,100 mg/day and the supplement added another 1,000 mg/day, for a total average calcium intake of about

2,100 mg/day for the experimental group. The mean baseline intake for vitamin D was about 365 IU/day, which, when combined with the vitamin D supplement, resulted in an approximate vitamin D intake of 765 IU/day for the experimental group. The rate of adherence (defined as use of 80 percent or more of the assigned study supplements) ranged from 60 to 63 percent during the first 3 years of follow-up, with an additional 13 to 21 percent of the participants taking at least half of their study pills. At the end of the trial, 76 percent were still taking the study supplements, and 59 percent were taking 80 percent or more of the supplements.

Among the healthy postmenopausal women in the WHI study, the doses of calcium and vitamin D resulted in an increased risk (17 percent) of kidney stones. Kidney stones were reported by 449 women in the supplemented group, compared with 381 women in the placebo group. With respect to the intention to treat, the reported hazard ratio (HR) was 1.17 (95% CI: 1.02–1.34). Although this study did not focus on calcium intake alone, the total vitamin D intakes were around 800 IU/day, a level that is not associated with either hypercalcemia or hypercalciuria. Therefore, it is reasonable to consider the possibility that total calcium intake of 2,100 mg per day were associated with increased kidney stones in this population. Although the kidney stone events were not adjudicated specifically, adjudication problems should be randomly distributed and thus not a contributing factor to the outcome.

The WHI reflects a large, well-designed cohort study. There is also a report from a small, short trial (covering 4 years) of 236 elderly women with a baseline calcium intake of 800 mg/day and with calcium supplementation of 1,600 mg/day for 1 year (total calcium intake of approximately 2,400 mg/day) (Riggs et al., 1998). In this study, 50 percent of subjects receiving supplemental calcium and 8 percent of placebo controls had urinary calcium levels exceeding 350 mg/day, but no subjects in the calcium group experienced nephrolithiasis, nephrocalcinosis, or a decrease in glomerular filtration rate. Other smaller trials among older subjects have shed little light on the issue of nephrolithiasis and calcium intake, either because the doses were relatively low or because subjects were recruited on the basis of having had previous incidence of kidney stones (Levine et al., 1994; Williams et al., 2001; Borghi et al., 2002).

Curhan et al. (1997) examined the risk for kidney stones in women 34 to 59 years of age, using data from the Nurses' Health Study (NHS), a notably younger group of subjects than those included in the WHI study. They reported an inverse association between calcium intake from foods, but a positive relationship between risk and intake of calcium from supplements (Curhan et al., 1997). In a 2004 study, Curhan and colleagues (Curhan et al., 2004) prospectively examined data again from the NHS for an 8-year period relative to dietary factors and the risk for kidney stones in women 27 to 44 years of age. In this analysis, the inverse relationship between calcium intake from foods and the risk of kidney stone formation remained, but there was no apparent relationship between supplement use and risk. In a study of 50,000 men 40 to 75 years of age (Curhan et al., 1993), the same relationship was evident: reduced risk with increased intake of calcium from food sources, but no association with use of calcium supplements.

The suggested discrepancy between the risks from food sources of calcium and from calcium supplements may in part be due to the timing of the supplement intake (Curhan et al., 2007). Calcium present in the food will bind oxalate, a known contributor to kidney stone formation, and prevent its absorption. If taken between meals, the calcium would have less opportunity to bind oxalate, and so oxalate absorption would be increased. These observations suggest that taking calcium supplements with meals should reduce the formation of kidney stones, but this has not been tested.

Overall, the data indicate that the calcium content of foods does not cause stone formation, but may be protective against it. On the other hand, calcium supplements are emerging as a concern based on observational data, at least for some groups under certain circumstances. Further, individuals with a history of kidney stones are at increased risk if they obtain their calcium from supplements rather than food sources. There is, however, limited evidence from small, short-term trials suggesting that supplemental calcium in moderate doses may not increase risk for stone recurrence. The most important evidence to date is from the WHI trial (Jackson et al., 2006), which indicated that a mean calcium intake from foods and supplements that totaled about 2,150 mg/day—plus a vitamin D supplement of 400 IU/day, a level low enough to avoid potential confounding effects for adverse events given the mean total vitamin D intake of approximately 750 IU/day—resulted in a 17 percent increased incidence of kidney stones among postmenopausal women, regardless of whether the subjects had experienced previous clinical events related to urinary calculi formation.

Nephrolithiasis in Children

Hypercalciuria, as a secondary outcome to high calcium intake, can occur in children as well as in adults. However, the incidence of kidney stones in children is rare. There is limited evidence concerning high calcium intakes in young children relative to calcium excretion. In a study of children ages 1 to 6 years and designed to test the effects of 1,800 mg/day total calcium (supplementation adjusted on the basis of dietary calcium questionnaire), the calcium intake of 1,800 mg/day calcium did not cause urinary calcium/creatinine ratios to differ significantly from those of placebo controls (Markowitz et al., 2004).

A study by Sargent et al. (1999) provides information relevant to infants and calcium excretion. This study supplemented the formula of full-term infants with calcium glycerophosphate, providing 1,800 mg of calcium (and 1,390 mg of phosphate) per liter of formula. The mean calcium intake for infants receiving the supplemented formula was more than 4 times that of children in control groups at months 4 and 9, with a mean calcium intake of 1,563 ± 703 mg/day at 9 months. Although the focus of the study was lead absorption, the data demonstrated that total calcium intakes of about 1,550 to 1,750 mg/day did not affect urinary calcium excretion. The data are somewhat limited in that younger infants were not studied; further, the contribution from solid foods in older infants was not clearly tracked. With these limitations, the authors' conclusion that this level of intake probably would not increase the likelihood of nephrolithiasis is reasonable.

Excess Calcium and Prostate Cancer

The vast majority of the data relating to prostate cancer and calcium intake are derived from observational studies, and the ability to sort the effect of dairy products from that of calcium is challenging. Some observational data suggest a role for dairy products as a risk factor for prostate cancer (Tominaga and Kuroishi, 1997; Grant, 1999). A recent case–control study examined associations between dairy products and dietary calcium and prostate cancer risk among men ages 35 to 84 years with a histological diagnosis of prostate cancer (Raimondi et al., 2010). Intake of dairy products, in particular milk consumption, was associated with a two-fold increased risk for prostate cancer, whereas consumption of other dairy products (cheese, yogurt, and cream) suggested no association for increased risk. Total calcium intake was not significantly associated with risk for prostate cancer ($p = 0.09$).

Other observational studies evaluating associations between milk or dairy product intake and overall risk for prostate cancer have suggested that supplemental calcium intake may be a stronger risk factor for prostate cancer than calcium from foods, particularly for aggressive prostate cancer with high mortality. Studies of associations between calcium supplement use and risk for incident prostate cancer provide mixed results. A small case–control study assessed men ages 40 to 64 years with newly diagnosed prostate cancer for multivitamin and supplement use by questionnaire (Kristal et al., 1999). Although about a third of both cases and controls reported using multivitamins, only 5 percent reported taking calcium supplements. No association was found between calcium supplement use and risk for incident prostate cancer in this relatively young and low-risk population. A prospective study of male participants ages 50-74 years from the Cancer Prevention Study II examined associations between calcium and dairy product intake and risk for incident prostate cancer (Rodriguez et al., 2003). This analysis of 65,321 men found a small increase in overall prostate cancer risk for calcium intakes of 2,000 mg/day and higher compared with intakes less than 700 mg/day. High calcium intake (≥ 2,000 mg/day), however, was significantly associated with risk for advanced prostate cancer. When calcium supplements (≥ 500 mg/day) were analyzed, controlled for total calcium intake, a weak association was found for prostate cancer risk. Dairy product intake was not associated with risk for prostate cancer. The report from the World Cancer Research Fund/American Institute for Cancer Research (WCRF/AICR, 2007) concluded that the relationship between prostate cancer and milk and dairy product intake is inconsistent from both cohort and case–control studies, and there is limited evidence suggesting that milk and dairy products are a cause of prostate cancer. A food-use questionnaire administered at baseline to participants in the Alpha-Tocopherol, Beta-Carotene Cancer Prevention (ATBC) Study explored associations between intake of certain foods and nutrients and risk for incident prostate cancer in a large cohort of male smokers ages 50 to 69 years. This study analyzed intake of calcium and dairy foods and found no associations with development of prostate cancer (Chan et al., 2000). In a longitudinal follow-up of this cohort, Mitrou et al. (2007) found a graded positive association between increasing total calcium intake and total prostate cancer risk. A prospective study of male participants ages 40 to 75 years from the Health Professionals Follow-Up Study (HPFS) examined whether calcium and fructose intake were risk factors for prostate cancer (Giovannucci et al., 1998). Calcium intake exceeding 2,000 mg/day was found to be associated with higher risk for total, advanced, and metastatic prostate cancer. Further, supplemental calcium intake above 900 mg/day was associated with metastatic prostate cancer risk at all levels of total calcium intake. In a follow-up analysis of this cohort, Giovannucci et al. (2006a) found a significantly increased risk for advanced prostate cancer associated with increasing total calcium intake and for fatal prostate cancer associated with supplemental calcium intakes of 401 mg/day and above. The WCRF/AICR (2007) concluded that there is a probable association between diets high in calcium and prostate cancer.

In the case of intervention studies, one randomized controlled multicenter clinical trial based on 672 men (mean age 61.8 years) living in the United States examined risk for prostate cancer from supplemental calcium intake. Participants received either 3 g of calcium carbonate or placebo daily for 4 years and were followed for up to 12 years for prostate cancer diagnosis (Baron et al., 2005). Over the entire study period, risk for prostate cancer was lower in the calcium-supplemented group than in controls (relative risk [RR] = 0.83; 95% CI: 0.52–1.32) but was not statistically significant. For specific years in the study, increase in prostate cancer risk was statistically significant between baseline and year 6 (RR = 0.52; 95% CI: 0.28–0.98) and between years 2 and 6 (RR = 0.44; 95% CI: 0.21–0.94).

No significant differences were found for total calcium intake and prostate cancer risk.

The 2009 analysis from the Agency for Healthcare Research and Quality (Chung et al., 2009; hereafter referred to as AHRQ-Tufts) examined 12 cohort studies that reported on the association between calcium intake and the risk of prostate cancer (Schuurman et al., 1999; Chan et al., 2001; Rodriguez et al., 2003; Baron et al., 2005; Tseng et al., 2005; Giovannucci et al., 2006a; Koh et al., 2006; Mitrou et al., 2007; Park et al., 2007a,b; Rohrmann et al., 2007; Kurahashi et al., 2008). One of the studies also provided a post hoc analysis of a randomized controlled trial on calcium supplementation. The incidence of prostate cancer in these studies ranged from 0.008 to 0.10. Most of the studies were conducted in Europe or North America, and one study was conducted in Japan. The mean age of the subjects ranged from 53 to 67 years, but did include men 51 to 70 years of age. No study specifically targeted men older than 70 years of age. Total calcium intake ranged from less than 500 mg/day to at least 2,000 mg/day. The time between dietary assessment and the diagnosis of prostate cancer varied from 1 to 17 years. AHRQ-Tufts rated the studies for methodological quality as follows: four studies were rated A, seven studies were rated B, and one study was rated C. The studies included participants in the age range of 51 to 70 years. Seven studies did not find an association between calcium intake and the risk of prostate cancer (Baron et al., 2005; Koh et al., 2006; Mitrou et al., 2007; Park et al., 2007a,b; Kurahashi et al., 2008). The remaining five studies found that the risk was higher in the groups that took more calcium compared with those that took a lower amount; the higher amount ranged from 921 to at least 2,000 mg of calcium per day.

Overall, data in this area are at best emerging. Although observational studies suggest that total calcium intake of 2,000 mg/day or higher may be associated with increased risk for prostate cancer and particularly with advanced and metastatic cancer, these data are not sufficiently robust to serve as an indicator for a UL. The one available trial was negative. The observations, however, are notable for levels of intake that are less than those that produce hypercalcemia and hypercalciuria.

Excess Calcium and Nutrient Interactions: Iron and Zinc

Despite the absence of clinically or functionally significant depletion of relevant mineral nutrients, calcium interaction with other minerals in the diet has been considered a potential risk related to high calcium intakes. The 1997 DRI report (IOM, 1997) specifically called for increased study in this area. However, data remain limited.

With respect to iron, Ilich-Ernst et al. (1998) carried out a placebo-controlled randomized trial assessing the effects of calcium supplementation on bone mass in adolescent girls ages 8 to 13 years ($n = 354$). A secondary analysis at year 4 of this 7-year trial found that girls in the supplemented group achieved a total calcium (food plus supplements) intake of 1,500 mg/day. When assessed for interactions between calcium and iron, measures of iron status—hemoglobin, hematocrit, and corpuscular indexes—were not significantly different from those of girls in the placebo group who reached a calcium intake of 800 mg/day. Ames et al. (1999) found no effect of a calcium intake of approximately 1,200 mg/day compared with 500 mg/day for 5 weeks on iron absorption in children 3 to 5 years of age.

With respect to zinc, McKenna et al. (1997) conducted a calcium and zinc balance study on a subset ($n = 26$) of participants in a longitudinal clinical trial of the effects of calcium supplementation on bone mass in girls with a mean age of 11 years. Trial participants received either 1,000 mg/day of supplemental calcium or a placebo. Mean calcium intake reached 847 ± 287 and 821 ± 224 mg/day from diet for placebo and intervention groups, respectively, at 6 months. With the additional supplement, the mean calcium intake in the intervention group exceeded 1,700 mg/day. The results of the balance study found no effect in the intervention group from intake of approximately 1,700 mg of calcium per day on net zinc absorption, zinc excretion, or zinc balance compared with intakes of approximately 800 mg/day in the placebo group.

Taken together, the studies suggest that calcium intakes of 1,500 to 1,700 mg/day do not interfere with iron or zinc absorption in adolescent girls. However, as calcium intakes among this age group could be higher than those studied, there is little evidence to shed light on the larger issue.

Excessive Calcium and Constipation

Calcium supplement intake has long been associated with constipation. In fact approximately 1 of every 10 participants in the WHI calcium–vitamin D supplementation trial reported moderate to severe constipation (Jackson et al., 2006). If a food source of calcium is the problem, the constipation is likely due to the components of dairy products (Anthoni et al., 2009) rather than to the calcium in food. Calcium supplements, which are regarded as "binding," can cause side effects for some people, such as constipation and gas (Jackson et al., 2006; Prince et al., 2006), which varies greatly from person to person. Usually the constipation is alleviated by increasing intakes of water or fiber-rich foods, or by trying another form of supplement (calcium citrate may be less constipating than calcium carbonate, for example). Although such conditions warrant attention, the utility of constipation as an indicator for DRI development is doubtful.

Selection of Indicator for Calcium UL

The risk assessment framework, as described in Chapter 1, specifies that, in the case of ULs, the available data pertaining to adverse effects be first examined for evidence of a benchmark intake (BI). Alternatively, either a no observed adverse effect level (NOAEL) or a lowest observed adverse effect level (LOAEL) is considered. In the case of calcium, limited new information has become available since 1997. The indicators selected are calcium excretion for younger age groups, and kidney stone formation for older age groups. The calcium excretion data provide information for a group for which no data were available in 1997. The newer data on kidney stone formation form a basis for a UL that is more akin to conditions experienced by the normal, healthy population than is calcium-alkali syndrome, although the cautions expressed by Patel and Goldfarb (2010) concerning the vulnerability of older persons to calcium-alkali syndrome with the use of calcium supplements are worthy of note.

The available data could not offer a BI or be used to estimate a dose–response relationship. The basis for the ULs is a NOAEL for infants and a LOAEL for adults, as described further below for specific life stage groups.

CALCIUM UPPER LEVELS: INTAKE-RESPONSE ASSESSMENT AND SPECIFICATION OF UPPER LEVELS

The ULs for calcium established for the DRI life stage groups are shown in Table 6-2. These values suggest that the levels of intake regarded as consistent with a UL are relatively close to the levels of intake considered to be appropriate for nutritional adequacy.

ULs for Infants 0 to 12 Months of Age

Infants 0 to 6 Months of Age	
	UL 1,000 mg/day Calcium
Infants 6 to 12 Months of Age	
	UL 1,500 mg/day Calcium

In the previous 1997 DRI report (IOM, 1997), a UL for calcium for infants was not specified owing to lack of data. The 1997 report noted a small, randomized trial of 81 infants (103 at baseline, ages 2.5 to 5.0 months at entry) designed to examine the tolerance of calcium-supplemented infant formula through 9 months of age (Dalton et al., 1997). The data, as analyzed in 1997 (IOM, 1997), indicated only that infants fed calcium at up to approximately 1,750 mg/day experienced no adverse effect on iron status.

TABLE 6-2 Calcium Tolerable Upper Intake Levels (UL) by Life Stage

Life Stage Group	UL
Infants	
0 to 6 mo	1,000 mg
6 to 12 mo	1,500 mg
Children	
1–3 y	2,500 mg
4–8 y	2,500 mg
Males	
9–13 y	3,000 mg
14–18 y	3,000 mg
19–30 y	2,500 mg
31–50 y	2,500 mg
51–70 y	2,000 mg
> 70 y	2,000 mg
Females	
9–13 y	3,000 mg
14–18 y	3,000 mg
19–30 y	2,500 mg
31–50 y	2,500 mg
51–70 y	2,000 mg
> 70 y	2,000 mg
Pregnancy	
14–18 y	3,000 mg
19–30 y	2,500 mg
31–50 y	2,500 mg
Lactation	
14–18 y	3,000 mg
19–30 y	2,500 mg
31–50 y	2,500 mg

Using these same data, Sargent et al. (1999) later reported on calcium excretion measures, and this measure serves as the UL indicator for infants. This 1999 report has provided the ability to estimate a NOAEL for calcium intake for infants based on calcium excretion. Within the confines of the limitations of the data, they suggest that infants can tolerate approximately 1,750 mg of calcium per day with no noted adverse effects. A NOAEL of 1,750 mg/day is therefore established for infants on this basis.

Infants 0 to 6 Months of Age

The presumed sensitivity of the young infant to excess intakes of any substance, as well as the lack of direct evidence to clarify the nature of adverse effects for this group, warrants a cautious approach. Quantitative factors relative to metabolic differences between younger infants and older infants in terms of handling excess calcium cannot be derived based on the literature, and little is available to inform the scientific judgment for public health protection except body weight. According to the Centers for Disease Control and Prevention (CDC) growth charts,[2] infants should increase their weight between birth and 3 months of age from about 7.0 pounds (3.5 kg) to 13.0 pounds (6 kg), and then to about 17.5 pounds (8 kg) by 6 months of life. The NOAEL of 1,750 mg/day—which is derived from one study within the age range of 3 to 9 months (Sargent et al., 1999)—is reduced by an uncertainty factor of 2 to adjust for this weight difference and rounded to 1,000 mg of calcium per day to serve as the UL for this life stage group. This is admittedly a cautious approach but, by establishing a UL for infants, their safety is more readily ensured than would be the case in the absence of a UL, and the value is reasonable in view of the available data and current biological understandings. The 1997 IOM report on calcium DRIs did not establish a UL for infants (IOM, 1997).

Infants 6 to 12 Months of Age

The NOAEL of 1,750 mg/day is a reasonable starting point for the UL for older infants. Consistent with general principles of human physiology and toxicology, the committee considered that an infant's capacity to handle excess nutritional substances is increased with increased body size. Presumably in the case of calcium, which is a critical requirement during these periods of bone development, the infant's ability to tolerate higher levels of intake is greater as the infant grows and develops skeletal structure. Therefore, the NOAEL of 1,750 mg/day is not unreasonable as the basis for a UL. However, given the paucity of data, a slight uncertainty correction is warranted, and the UL is set at 1,500 mg/day for infants 7 to 12 months of age. No UL for this age group was established in 1997 (IOM, 1997).

ULs for Children and Adolescents 1 Through 18 Years

Children 1 Through 3 Years of Age	
Children 4 Through 8 Years of Age	
	UL 2,500 mg/day Calcium
Children 9 Through 13 Years of Age	
Adolescents 14 Through 18 Years of Age	
	UL 3,000 mg/day Calcium

---

[2]Available online at http://www.cdc.gov/growthcharts/ (accessed July 19, 2010).

New data on adverse outcomes due to excess calcium intake among children and adolescents—specifically data that would identify a NOAEL or LOAEL—have not emerged since the last DRI report on calcium in 1997 (IOM, 1997). At that time, it was noted that the safety of excess calcium intake in children and adolescents had not been studied. A UL of 2,500 mg of calcium per day was established in 1997 for all children and adolescents in these life stage groups, largely on the basis of the UL established for adults (i.e., 2,500 mg/day) (IOM, 1997).

There is currently no evidence that the 1997 level is too low to provide public health protection for this group; further, when compared with the new UL set for infants, the level of 2,500 mg of calcium per day is a reasonable increase given the expected increases in body weight and metabolic capacities, especially for younger children between the ages of 1 and 8 years.

However, for older children it is also appropriate to take into account the likely increases in tolerated intakes as metabolic demands increase and the pubertal growth spurt associated with bone accretions sets in, primarily between 9 and 18 years of age. Again, there are no data to allow quantitative uncertainty factors to be developed to mathematically correct for the likelihood of increased capacities during the bone growth spurt, but to do so in some fashion is consistent with a general toxicological approach. An added level of 500 mg/day is reasonable, resulting in a UL of 3,000 mg of calcium per day for children 9 to 13 years of age and adolescents 14 to 18 years of age.

The UL for children 1 through 8 years of age is the same as that established for these life stage groups in 1997 (IOM, 1997). However, the UL has been increased by 500 mg/day for older children and adolescents compared with 1997 (IOM, 1997). This is based on a biologically reasonable adjustment intended to take into account increased need and therefore increased capacity to tolerate a slight increase in a UL value.

ULs for Adults 19 or More Years of Age

Adults 19 Through 30 Years of Age	
Adults 31 Through 50 Years of Age	
	UL 2,500 mg/day Calcium
Adults 51 Through 70 Years of Age	
Adults >70 Years of Age	
	UL 2,000 mg/day Calcium

The onset of hypercalcemia is clearly an adverse outcome. However, it was not selected as an indicator for ULs for adults because it reflects an extreme pathological condition, and the ability to consider other adverse events associated with sustained, high levels of intake has emerged. Specifically, kidney stone formation is an adverse outcome, notably among post-menopausal women. Although there is also evidence related to calcium-alkali syndrome among adults, most of the data relate to those with compromised kidney function. Vascular calcification in postmenopausal women has emerged as an interesting hypothesis, but available data are conflicting, and threshold levels for intake are unknown. Evidence related to prostate cancer, although concerning, was too confounded to allow this disease risk to serve as an indicator for establishing ULs for calcium intake. Further, neither constipation nor nutrient interactions were associated with data to suggest that these outcomes would serve as indicators for UL development.

Given the size and quality of the WHI trial, its outcome relative to the incidence of kidney stones (Jackson et al., 2006) results in the selection of kidney stones as the indicator for adults for DRI purposes. The levels of calcium intake that may cause kidney stones within a normal population cannot be specified with certainty and are known to be variable depending upon a number of factors, including baseline renal function, pre-existing disease conditions, and interactions with drugs. Based on the findings of Jackson et al. (2006), and with the understanding that the data are derived from women between the ages of 50 and 79 years, there is a concern for kidney stone risk at total calcium intakes of approximately 2,000 mg/day. Underpinning the concern is the recognition that intakes of calcium from food do not readily result in excess intakes and are not associated with adverse effects; rather, the adverse effects appear to be a function of calcium supplementation added to baseline intake. The level of 2,000 mg of calcium per day is established as the LOAEL for adults, including men, more than 50 years of age. The very limited data available for adults 19 to 50 years of age do not allow the specification of a LOAEL or NOAEL for this younger group and the UL for this group is derived from considerations used for the UL for persons above 50 years of age. For this reason the ULs for older adults are discussed first below, followed by adults 19 to 50 years of age.

Adults 51 Years of Age and Older

The committee considered the option of applying an uncertainty factor to lower the LOAEL, given the limited data. However, the unknowns surrounding the precision of the LOAEL coupled with the observation that the LOAEL is very close to intakes that are considered adequate and recommended, caused the committee to conclude that, until there are better data related to calcium intakes from supplements and the incidence of kidney stones or other relevant health outcomes, establishing a UL of 2,000 mg of calcium per day is justified and provides a reasonable degree of public health protection without overly restricting the intake of calcium (notably from calcium supplements) for both men and women. There is no apparent reason to conclude that men in this age group are more sensitive than women. Although one 1993 observational study does not support the potential for increased kidney stone formation with supplement use among men, public health protection warrants caution for this older group. Moreover, the value of 2,000 mg of calcium per day is also somewhat below the 3,000 mg/day associated with calcium-alkali syndrome among persons with waning kidney function, the only other potential indicator with an estimate of threshold levels for effect.

The new UL of 2,000 mg of calcium per day for persons 51 to 70 years of age and for persons more than 70 years of age is lower than the 1997 UL of 2,500 mg/day for these groups (IOM, 1997). The newer data related to kidney stone formation are the primary basis for the new UL. It is extremely difficult to reach the UL on the basis of food sources of calcium. Rather, the excess intake comes about from the use of calcium supplements. Special considerations about the use of high level calcium supplements and the timing of supplement intake are discussed in Chapter 8.

Adults 19 Through 50 Years of Age

Although the LOAEL (which is also the UL, as described above) for older adults more than 50 years of age is established at 2,000 mg/day, it can only serve as a starting point for UL consideration for adults 19 to 50 years of age given the observations that kidney stone formation in younger adults does not appear to be driven by calcium supplement use, and, as a rule, calcium supplement use is not as prevalent among younger adults. However, kidney stone formation is notable among younger persons; as discussed previously, the incident rate is actually higher among younger adults than among older adults. Given the UL of 3,000 mg/day for calcium set for adolescents up to the age of 18 years (based on high rate of bone accretion) as well as the likelihood that younger adults are able to tolerate higher maximal levels of calcium than other adults for whom kidney function may be slowly decreasing, an interpolation approach is used to establish a UL of 2,500 mg/day for adults 19 to 30 and 31 to 50 years of age, based on the mid-point between the UL of 2,000 mg of calcium per day set for persons more than 50 years of age and the UL of 3,000 mg/day set for adolescents 14 to 18 years of age. Further, concerns about the timing of calcium supplement intake would still be relevant to this group and are discussed in Chapter 8.

ULs for Pregnancy and Lactation

Pregnant or Lactating 14 Through 18 Years of Age
UL 3,000 mg/day Calcium
Pregnant or Lactating 19 Through 30 Years of Age
Pregnant or Lactating 31 Through 50 Years of Age
UL 2,500 mg/day Calcium

Hypercalciuria is often present during normal pregnancy as a consequence of the doubling of intestinal calcium absorption that occurs, and pregnancy itself increases the risk of kidney stones. Consequently, excess intakes of calcium during pregnancy will aggravate hypercalciuria and possibly increase the risk of kidney stones. During lactation, the serum calcium (both ionized and albumin-corrected total calcium) level rises and usually remains within the normal range (although hypercalcemia can occur during normal lactation), and urinary excretion of calcium is reduced to the low-normal range or below. Consequently, higher intakes of calcium during lactation could potentially increase the risk of hypercalcemia. However, there is no evidence to suggest that the risk manifests itself at intakes lower than the UL for non-pregnant or non-lactating women, although it is acknowledged that relevant studies have not been rigorously carried out for pregnancy and lactation. Given that available evidence suggests that requirements for calcium among pregnant and lactating females are similar to those of non-pregnant and non-lactating females, and lacking data to suggest a basis for a different UL, the ULs for calcium for pregnancy and lactation have been kept the same as those for their non-pregnant and non-lactating counterparts.

VITAMIN D UPPER LEVELS: REVIEW OF POTENTIAL INDICATORS AND SELECTION OF INDICATORS

Few studies have been designed to specifically evaluate the safety of vitamin D intake, and there is not general agreement about the intake levels at which vitamin D may cause harm. A recent National Institutes of Health conference highlighted the lack of knowledge about mechanisms of action and toxic forms of the vitamin as well as the many limitations in the available evidence. Conference participants noted that available randomized controlled trials designed to illuminate health benefits likely underestimate the true potential for risk because: (1) for ethical reasons, adverse outcomes are secondary outcomes, (2) studies are of relatively short duration, (3) adverse outcomes are not always adequately monitored or completely reported, and (4) adverse outcomes generally lack adequate statistical power for detection (Brannon et al., 2008). Further, inclusion and exclusion criteria prevent persons at greatest risk from being study participants (Yetley et al., 2009).

Over the years, excess intake of vitamin D has been considered in the context of "intoxication" or "hypervitaminosis D"; as such, the condition is perhaps best regarded as a relatively acute response. Symptoms can appear in less than 4 weeks of continual excess ingestion. The hallmark of vitamin D intoxication is hypercalcemia, which is associated with a rise in serum 25OHD levels. The conditions of hypercalcemia and hypercalciuria were described previously in the section on calcium. Vitamin D intoxication generally presents with non-specific symptoms that may vary and often include anorexia, weight loss, polyuria, and heart arrhythmias (Jones, 2008). The condition eventually leads to vascular and tissue calcification with subsequent renal and cardiovascular damage.

Although data about vitamin D intoxication are informative, avoiding this relatively acute toxicity is not the intended purpose of a UL. Rather, the UL reflects a long-term level of intake that will not cause harm to the normal, free-living population. The 2007 AHRQ analysis (Cranney et al., 2007; hereafter referred to as AHRQ-Ottawa) concluded that few adverse outcomes could be identified for intakes "above current recommended levels," but it raised concerns about potential previously unrecognized adverse effects, including an increased risk of pancreatic cancer. The later AHRQ-Tufts analysis further identified all-cause mortality as an emerging concern, but the authors also pointed to the dearth of data.

Unfortunately, as pointed out in the earlier IOM report on DRIs for vitamin D, there continues to be a large uncertainty about the progressive health effects for regular ingestion of even moderately high amounts of vitamin D over several decades (IOM, 1997). Most available evidence is based on short-term exposures (less than 6 months). Generalization to long-term exposures—as would occur during a lifetime—is challenging. Also, most evidence is derived from adult populations with few data specific to children or vulnerable groups. For the purposes of an overview of the literature concerning adverse effects of excess vitamin D, the effects related to vitamin D intoxication (hypervitaminosis D) are discussed first and are based on a paper prepared for the committee by Hector DeLuca (DeLuca, 2009). They can provide a starting point for UL considerations. The emerging concerns about the adverse effects at higher intakes that are less than those associated with the toxicity are discussed next and are examined in the context of the appropriateness of introducing caution into the specification of ULs for vitamin D.

Vitamin D Intoxication and Related Hypercalcemia

Etiology and Effects of Vitamin D Intoxication

Increased serum 25OHD levels and resulting hypercalcemia are the hallmarks of vitamin D toxicity (Jones, 2008). Although intakes of either vitamin D_2 or vitamin D_3 can cause toxicity, there is evidence that higher levels of vitamin D_2 can be tolerated (Hunt et al., 1972; Stephenson and Peiris, 2009). Similarly, in laboratory animal experiments, vitamin D_3 has been reported to be more toxic (Roborgh and de Man, 1960).

The hypercalcemia that occurs from a rise in serum 25OHD level is due to increased bone resorption (Jones, 2008). In the early stages of intoxication, hypercalcemia may be modest and the renal glomerular filtration rate (GFR) remains stable. As bone resorption continues, however, the increasing blood levels of calcium lead to suppression of PTH production. The function and activity of the parathyroid–kidney–bone axis have thus emerged as contributors to the "set point" for toxicity of excess vitamin D and calcium. Decreased renal function simultaneously increases CVD risk and impairs calciuric responses and calcium phosphate homeostasis. Thus, elderly people represent a high-risk group for both extant CVD and impaired parathyroid–kidney–bone interactions that preserve normal calcium–phosphate homeostasis. Eventually, there is a loss of urinary concentrating mechanisms of the kidney tubule as well as a decrease in GFR (Towler, 2009). Hypercalciuria results from the hypercalcemia and the disruption of normal reabsorption processes of the renal tubules (IOM, 1997). As renal function declines (as occurs in disease and, to a lesser extent, with aging), there is additional loss of homeostatic control of serum calcium and phosphorus levels. Failure of the kidney and cardiovascular system is likely the ultimate cause of death in vitamin D intoxication. The prolonged ingestion of excess amounts of vitamin D and the accompanying hypercalcemia can cause metastatic calcification of soft tissues (IOM, 1997). Calcification of vascular tissue has long been known to be associated with vitamin D toxicity (Taussig, 1966; Bajwa et al., 1971; Kamio et al., 1979). Major perturbations in calcium–phosphate homeostasis may increase the risk of CVD, related in part to arterial calcium deposition (Hruska et al., 2009). The hypothesis that excess vitamin D intake may be associated with kidney stone formation is not supported by the available data.

Animal models of vitamin D toxicity reveal symptoms that are almost identical to those described for humans and have provided useful information (Shephard and DeLuca, 1980; Littledike and Horst, 1982a,b;

Tryfonidou et al., 2003; Harmeyer and Schlumbohm, 2004). Rats, in particular, have been used to study vitamin D toxicity. The form of vitamin D that rises exponentially in plasma following overdose is 25OHD, not calcitriol (Vieth, 1990; Jones, 2008; Stephenson and Peiris, 2009). Shephard and DeLuca (1980) administered graded doses of either vitamin D_3 or calcitriol to rats for a 2-week period. The results indicated that frank toxicity was achieved at 650 nmol of vitamin D_3 per day or 50,000 IU/kg body weight, producing a blood 25OHD level of 1,607 nmol/L, while calcitriol levels were markedly reduced. These results support 25OHD and not calcitriol as the likely toxicant. In fact, in most species, vitamin D intoxication is accompanied by a *decrease* in plasma calcitriol level (Hughes et al., 1977; Shephard and DeLuca, 1980; Harrington and Page, 1983). Nonetheless, a case has been made that the "free" calcitriol level in the plasma—that is, the metabolite displaced from the plasma transport protein, vitamin D binding protein, by other accumulating metabolites—increases in vitamin D intoxication (Vieth, 2007; Jones, 2008). Overall, however, the accumulating 25OHD appears to be the critical factor in triggering the intoxication.

Serum 25OHD Concentrations as Indicative of Toxicity

In the absence of well-controlled studies, the serum 25OHD level representing the vitamin D toxicity threshold in humans is not readily defined. Similarly, the vitamin D intakes required to trigger toxicity symptoms are not precisely known. Moreover, even though the physiological changes that occur with vitamin D toxicity are correlated to serum 25OHD levels, they may not be precisely aligned (Towler, 2009) and may vary from subject to subject and among sub-populations. Appendix G summarizes a number of human vitamin D toxicity case studies gathered from the scientific literature from early in the 20th century to the present. Some of these reports originated from a time before vitamin D metabolism was discovered and hence lack confirmation that the causative agent was vitamin D overdose. Table 6-3 contains case reports from the past 35 years in which the data are supported by vitamin D dose administered, serum calcium levels, and serum 25OHD levels. Also provided are data from several month-long studies with a range of vitamin D supplements in which fully documented vitamin D intoxication was not identified. It is concluded that occasional reports of hypercalcemia in these studies are not related to vitamin D.

As shown in Table 6-3, the literature contains evidence that a range of vitamin D supplements from 800 to 300,000 IU/day have been used for periods ranging from months to years. Doses below 10,000 IU/day are not usually associated with toxicity, whereas doses equal to or above 50,000 IU/day for several weeks or months are frequently associated with toxic side effects including documented hypercalcemia.

TABLE 6-3 Case Reports of Vitamin D Intoxication: Intake and Plasma Measures

Vitamin D Intake (IU/day)	Duration	Serum Calcium (mg/dL)	Serum 25OHD (nmol/L)	Serum Creatinine (µmol/L)	Urinary Calcium (mmol/L GFR)	Reference
Vitamin D supplementation studies without documented hypercalcemia							
800	4–6 mo	NCa[a]	60–105[b]	—	—	Byrne et al., 1995[e]
1,800	3 mo	NCa	65, 80[c]	—	—	Byrne et al., 1995[e]
1,800	3 mo	NCa	57–86	82.4–3.8	—	Honkanen et al., 1990[f]
2,000	6 mo	NCa	—	—	—	Johnson et al., 1980[g]
10,000	4 wk	—	105[d]	—	—	Stamp et al., 1977
10,000	10 wk	—	110[d]	—	—	Davie et al., 1982
20,000	4 wk	—	150[d]	—	—	Stamp et al., 1977
Vitamin D supplementation studies reporting hypercalcemia							
50,000	6 wk	15.0	320	388	—	Schwartzman and Franck, 1987
50,000	15 y	12.5	560	—	—	Davies and Adams, 1978
100,000	10 y	12.8	865	215	0.508	Selby et al., 1995
200,000	2 y	15.1	1,202	207	—	Selby et al., 1995
300,000	6 y	13.2	1,692	184	0.432	Rizzoli et al., 1994
300,000	3 wk	11.3	800	339	0.065	Rizzoli et al., 1994
Accidental vitamin D intoxication							
~ 1,131,840; vitamin D overdose	—	15.0	1,171	265	—	Klontz and Acheson, 2007

TABLE 6-3 Continued

~ 1,700,000; vitamin D poisoning	—	15.3	1,555	442	—	Vieth et al., 2002
~ 9,000,000; vitamin D overdose	—	11.3	> 375	159	—	Chiricone et al., 2003
~ 18,000,000; vitamin D overdose	—	15.3	> 375	329	—	Chiricone et al., 2003
Vitamin D poisoning	—	13.8–18.4 ($n = 11$)	847–1,652	—	—	Pettifor et al., 1995
Overfortification of milk	—	13.1 ($n = 35$)	560	—	—	Blank et al., 1995
Reference levels	—	8.6–10.6	20–100 (10)	18–150	< 0.045	Blank et al., 1995
			25–200 (9)			Haddad, 1980

NOTE: IU = International Units; GFR = glomerular filtration rate; mo = month(s); wk = week(s); y = year(s).

[a]NCa = normocalcemic.
[b]Five studies; $n = 188$.
[c]Two studies; $n = 55$.
[d]Indicates extrapolation from graphic data.
[e]Byrne et al. (1995) reported that 3 of 449 subjects had hypercalcemia, but 2 were deemed to be non–vitamin D related.
[f]Honkanen et al. (1990) measured serum 25OHD levels but observed no side effects of the vitamin D or calcium supplements.
[g]Johnson et al. (1980) reported that 2 of 63 subjects developed hypercalcemia but provided no details of the 2 subjects and did not measure serum 25OHD levels in their study protocol.

DeLuca (2009) concluded that, overall, the toxicity of hypercalcemia becomes evident at vitamin D intakes above 25,000 IU/day, corresponding to a serum 25OHD level of about 500 nmol/L. Hathcock et al. (2007), following an analysis of more than 20 publications, concluded that there was no association between harm and intakes of 10,000 IU/day. Although toxic effects associated with 400 IU/day seem implausible,[3] the diverse range of intakes and serum 25OHD levels is notable. Most reports suggest that the toxicity threshold is between 10,000 and 40,000 IU of vitamin D per day. Also, most do not identify toxicity until serum 25OHD levels of 500 to 600

---

[3]It is noted that Adams and Lee (1997) reported toxicity at a serum 25OHD level of 160 nmol/L, but this is based on a single patient with an elevated urinary calcium level that was corrected by withdrawing a vitamin D supplement of 1,200 IU/day.

nmol/L or higher are reached; frank toxicity has been associated with a serum 25OHD level of 750 nmol/L (Jones, 2008; Deluca, 2009).

There have been no reports of vitamin D intoxication by ultraviolet B light alone (Webb et al., 1989). Davie et al. (1982), using high-performance liquid chromatographic analysis, found that skin irradiation reached a plateau after 5 to 6 weeks of exposure and achieved a plasma $25OHD_3$ level of no more than 45 nmol/L. In a study of healthy men ($n = 26$) who had just completed a summer of extended outdoor activity, Barger-Lux and Heaney (2002) found that the median serum 25OHD level was 122 nmol/L in late summer and decreased to 74 nmol/L by late winter. Binkley et al. (2007) found that among subjects ($n = 93$) with habitually high sun exposure (~ 29 hours/week), the mean serum 25OHD level was 79 nmol/L, with the highest reported level of 155 nmol/L. In a study of subjects ($n = 50$) who used a tanning bed on a regular basis (at least once a week), serum 25OHD levels were 90 percent higher in tanners than in controls ($n = 106$) (115.5 ± 8.0 nmol/L vs. 60.3 ± 3.0 nmol/L) (Tangpricha et al., 2004).

Conclusion

Clearly, there are a number of variables that may affect the onset of toxic symptoms in the face of excess vitamin D intake. There has been a paucity of longer-term studies that have investigated the effects of doses over 10,000 IU or the maintenance of serum 25OHD levels above 250 nmol/L. What the data do suggest is that it would be unlikely to observe symptoms of toxicity at daily intakes below 10,000 IU, while it is possible that daily intakes above 10,000 IU could be associated with toxicity. In any case, such short-term findings related to the extreme conditions of toxicity are not the ideal basis for setting ULs for the general population, which apply to long-term (essentially lifetime) exposures. Thus, additional considerations were evaluated, as discussed next.

Excess Vitamin D and Serum Calcium

The 1997 IOM report on DRIs for vitamin D used the effect of vitamin D intake on serum calcium level in humans as the basis for developing ULs for vitamin D (IOM, 1997). The work of Johnson et al. (1980) and most notably that of Narang et al. (1984) were taken into account. In the Narang et al. (1984) study, serum calcium levels in humans (with and without tuberculosis) were measured as a function of daily vitamin D doses of 400, 800, 1,200, 2,400, and 3,800 IU for 3 months. Thirty healthy men and women ranging in age from 21 to 60 years and without tuberculosis were included in the study. Hypercalcemia with vitamin D supplementation was reported in 63 percent of the patients with active tuberculosis, consistent with the known effect of granulomatous diseases on enhancement of 1α-hydroxylase activity. In the 30 subjects reported to be normal, statistically significant increases in serum calcium level were observed with vitamin D doses of 2,400 and 3,800 IU/day; however, only at the dose of 3,800 IU/day did the serum calcium level exceed the upper limits of normal (i.e., 10.5 mg/dL). Moreover, there were only five subjects in the highest dose group, the duration of the effect was not reported, and the heterogeneity within that subgroup was reflected by the large standard error.

Although increased serum calcium levels are of concern, the Narang et al. (1984) study is likely too small to allow any conclusions to be drawn beyond the potential risk of hypercalcemia during vitamin D supplementation in patients with tuberculosis. More recently, Aloia et al. (2008) conducted a 6-month dose–response study using 138 white and African American adults to determine the intake of vitamin D_3 needed to achieve a targeted plasma 25OHD level. Doses of vitamin D varied but reached means of $3,915 \pm 840$ IU/day for blacks and $3,040 \pm 1,136$ IU/day for whites. No patient presented with a serum calcium level above 265 mmol/L (or 10.6 mg/dL).

Excess Vitamin D and Measures in Infants

Jeans and Stearns (1938) found a retarded linear growth rate in 35 infants up to 45 weeks of age who received daily doses of 1,800 to 4,500 IU of vitamin D as supplements (without regard to sun exposure), for a minimum of 6 months, compared with infants receiving supplemental doses of 340 IU/day or less. Fomon et al. (1966), in a similar study, explored the effects of vitamin D on linear growth in infants ($n = 13$) ingesting 1,380 to 2,170 IU/day (mean = 1,775 IU/day) of vitamin D from fortified evaporated milk formulas as the only source of vitamin D, compared with infants receiving 350 to 550 IU/day ($n = 11$) from another batch of formula. No effect was found in infants who were enrolled in the study from the first 9 days after birth up to 6 months of age. Newer data to better elucidate the relationship between vitamin D and retarded linear growth in infants have not emerged in recent years.

Reports in Britain in the 1950s, when foods were being liberally fortified with vitamin D, indicated an unusually large number of cases of "idiopathic hypercalcemia" (British Paediatric Association, 1956). Given the number of foods fortified at the time, the British Paediatric Association (1956) estimated an intake of about 4,000 IU of vitamin D per day for an infant who consumed a typical diet of milk (1.5 pints), cereal (1 ounce), and cod liver oil (1 teaspoon). The outbreak of idiopathic hypercalcemia that took place was attributed to vitamin D supplementation, but the cause cannot be determined with certainty. Survey data apparently reported a marked decline in hypercalcemia in infants, from 7.2 cases per month in a 1953 to 1955 survey, to 3.0 cases per month in a 1960 to 1961 survey (British Paediatric Association, 1956, 1964). This change occurred at the time new guidelines were introduced for fortification of food products with vitamin D. Data from the British Paediatric Association (1956) and Bransby et al. (1964) also suggested that the estimated total vitamin D intake in infants at the 75th percentile declined from 4,000 IU/day to a range of 724 to 1,343 IU/day between the two surveys.

Other Adverse Effects of Excess Vitamin D: Mortality, Chronic Disease, Falls and Fractures

The committee reviewed the evidence emerging from observational/association studies and a limited number of clinical trials related to vitamin D intake and a diverse set of health outcomes, ranging from breast cancer to falls and fractures. The purpose was not to determine that certain levels of intake definitively cause harm, but rather to decide whether the emerging data were sufficiently compelling to warrant caution relative to vitamin D intakes and associated serum 25OHD concentrations that may be less than those associated with the more widely known acute toxicity but still associated with adverse effects that may occur as a result of chronic intake. The potential adverse effects are considered in alphabetical order.

All-Cause Mortality

All-cause mortality data emerging from the examination of national survey data as well as observational studies suggest adverse effects at serum 25OHD levels much lower than those associated with the toxicity demonstrated by hypervitaminosis D. The AHRQ-Tufts analysis identified four cohort studies (Sambrook et al., 2004, 2006; Visser et al., 2006; Jia et al., 2007; Melamed et al., 2008) that focused on the relationship between serum 25OHD level and all-cause mortality. In general, these studies, as expected, indicated that low serum 25OHD levels akin to deficiency states (< 30 nmol/L) are associated with an increased risk of mortality. Further, as serum 25OHD levels increase—up to a point—mortality is lowered.[4] However, some, but not all, of the studies have observed a troubling U-shaped (or perhaps more appropriately a reverse-J-shaped) relationship. For example, Jia et al. (2007) found a statistically significant trend between increasing serum 25OHD levels and lower odds ratios for all-cause

---

[4]Note: The studies adjusted for lifestyle factors linked with poor vitamin D nutriture and other factors; not unexpectedly the relationship became weaker, reflecting some confounding factors.

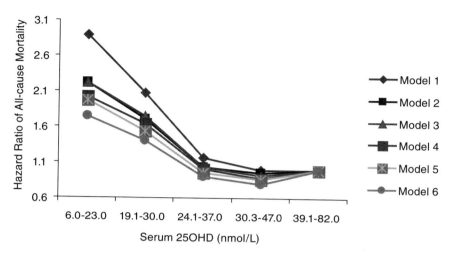

FIGURE 6-1 Hazard ratios of risk of death according to baseline serum 25OHD level (subjects with serum 25OHD levels 39.1–82.0 nmol/L are the referent category).
NOTE: Model 1 is adjusted for age and gender; model 2 is adjusted for model 1 and taking five or more kinds of medicine and self-perceived health status; model 3 is adjusted for model 2 and having heart problem and/or diabetes at baseline; model 4 is adjusted for model 3 and sunlight exposure (i.e., season of blood sampling, sunbathing, and outdoor physical activity); model 5 is adjusted for model 3 and use of a supplement containing vitamin D; model 6 is adjusted for model 3 and variables in models 4 and 5.
SOURCE: Jia et al. (2007).

mortality ($p = 0.03$); however, a U-shaped or reverse-J-shaped relationship between serum 25OHD level and mortality was observed, with the lowest mortality at serum 25OHD levels below 50 nmol/L (see Figure 6-1). Visser et al. (2006) showed a similar pattern, with reduced mortality associated with higher than deficiency levels, but increased mortality at the highest blood 25OHD levels (see Figure 6-2). Melamed et al. (2008), using data from the Third National Health and Nutrition Examination Survey (NHANES III), also suggested a U-shaped or reverse-J-shaped risk curve with increasing risk at about 75 nmol/L (see Figure 6-3). The similar patterns emerging in these studies are of concern and are suggestive of at least a reverse-J-shaped curve, if not precisely a U-shaped curve for risk relative to serum 25OHD levels and all-cause mortality. Of note, Sambrook et al. (2004, 2006) found no relationship between mortality and the log of serum 25OHD levels in a sample ($n = 842$) of frail, institutionalized persons, most

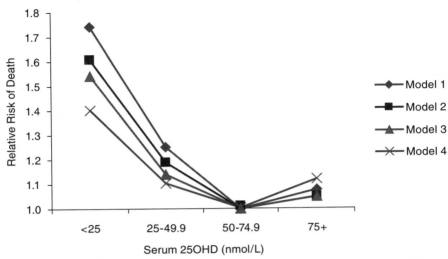

FIGURE 6-2 Risk of death in elderly people according to baseline serum 25OHD level in the Longitudinal Aging Study (subjects with serum 25OHD levels of 50.0–74.9 nmol/L are the referent category).
NOTE: Model 1 is adjusted for gender, age, and education; model 2 is adjusted for model 1 and for chronic disease, serum creatinine concentration, cognitive status, and depressive symptoms; model 3 is adjusted for model 2 and for lifestyle variables including body mass index, smoking status, alcohol consumption, and physical activity; model 4 is adjusted for model 3 and for frailty indicators: mobility performance, low serum albumin concentration, and low serum total cholesterol concentration.
SOURCE: Visser et al. (2006).

over the age of 80 years. Also, the committee identified another cohort study not included in the AHRQ-Tufts report (Semba et al., 2009) that did not observe a U-shaped relationship, but the highest exposure category in this Italian cohort was approximately 64 nmol/L. In addition to these published observational studies, a preliminary analysis of NHANES III data limited to data on non-Hispanic blacks with follow-up as of December 31, 2006, also saw a U-shaped relationship, although the suggested increase in risk was seen at a lower serum 25OHD concentration of approximately 60 nmol/L.[5]

Turning to evidence from vitamin D supplementation trials, AHRQ-Tufts calculated an overall relative risk (RR) for all-cause mortality of 0.97 (95% CI: 0.92–1.02), with no evidence of between-study heterogeneity. The doses studied included 400 and 880 IU of supplemental vitamin D per day,

_____

[5]Personal communication, R. Durazo-Arvizu, Loyola University, Maywood, IL, May 28, 2010.

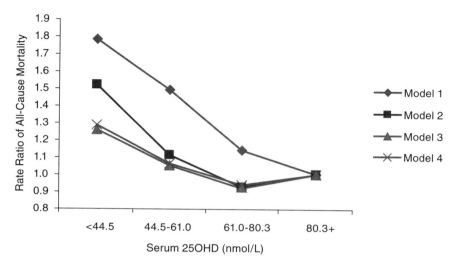

FIGURE 6-3 Rate ratios of all-cause mortality by serum 25OHD level in NHANES III (subjects with serum 25OHD levels above 80.3 nmol/L are the referent category). NOTE: Model 1 is unadjusted; model 2 is adjusted for age, gender, race, and season; model 3 is adjusted for age, gender, race, season, hypertension, history of prior cardiovascular disease, diabetes, smoking, high-density lipoprotein cholesterol, total cholesterol, use of cholesterol medications, estimated glomerular filtration rate categories, serum albumin, log (albumin-creatinine ratio), log (C-reactive protein), body mass index, physical activity level, vitamin D supplementation, and low socioeconomic status; model 3 is adjusted for age, gender, race, season, cigarette use, body mass index, log (C-reactive protein), serum albumin, physical activity level, vitamin D supplementation, and low socioeconomic status.
SOURCE: Melamed et al. (2008).

and one trial that gave a supplement of 100,000 IU every 3 months, which is roughly equivalent to 1,100/day.

Because the trials did not evaluate particularly high doses and as observational studies are subject to confounding, one cannot interpret conclusively whether or not this U-shaped relationship is real or causal. However, the data are clearly suggestive of a U-shaped or reverse-J-shaped risk curve between serum 25OHD level and all-cause mortality; increases in risk are suggested at thresholds in the range of 75 to 120 nmol/L for the white population, with lower levels for the black population.

Cancer

Breast cancer   A study from the randomized, double-blind, placebo-controlled WHI trial (Chlebowski et al., 2008) indicated overall that daily supplementation with 1,000 mg of elemental calcium combined with 400 IU of vitamin D_3 had no effect on breast cancer incidence. However, through a stratified analysis, the data demonstrated an increased risk of breast cancer for women who were already consuming 600 IU of vitamin D per day at baseline, to which a supplement of 400 IU/day was added ($P_{interaction}$ = 0.003). Serum 25OHD measures were analyzed by quintile and the highest quintile was 67.6 nmol/L and above.

Pancreatic cancer Some, but not all, observational studies suggest that higher serum 25OHD levels are associated with an increased risk of pancreatic cancer. Beginning with negative studies, Skinner et al. (2006) examined two large cohort populations—the HPFS and the NHS—for associations between pancreatic cancer incidence and vitamin D intake from diet and supplements. Another study of the HPFS cohort examined associations between serum 25OHD level and total cancer mortality or digestive (including pancreatic) cancer incidence (Giovannucci et al., 2006b). Both studies found reduced risk for pancreatic cancer incidence: in one instance associated with higher vitamin D intake ($\geq$ 600 IU/day) (Skinner et al., 2006) and in the other based on a predicted serum 25OHD level (as described by the authors) for which RR was calculated for incremental increases in serum 25OHD level of 25 nmol/L (Giovannucci et al., 2006b).

In contrast, an initial study from Stolzenberg-Solomon et al. (2006), using a nested case–control protocol to evaluate associations between vitamin D nutriture and incidence of pancreatic cancer in subjects from the ATBC Study, found a positive association between higher serum 25OHD levels (highest quintile at 83.2 nmol/L) and risk for pancreatic cancer. In a subsequent nested case–control analysis of a cohort from the Prostate, Lung, Colorectal, and Ovarian (PLCO) Cancer Screening Trial, the same investigators found no association between higher serum 25OHD level and increased pancreatic cancer risk as an outcome (Stolzenberg-Solomon, 2009). The difference between the study populations included living at a northern latitude, positive smoking history, and gender (male) in the ATBC Study compared with a mixed gender U.S. population that was controlled for smoking history in the PLCO Cancer Screening Trial.

To address the dissimilarity in results from individual large cohort studies, Stolzenberg-Solomon et al. (2010) conducted a pooled nested case–control analysis of participants from several cohorts (the ATBC Study, CLUE, the Cancer Prevention Study II Nutrition Cohort, the New York University Women's Health Study, the PLCO Cancer Screening Trial, and the Shanghai Women's and Men's Health Studies) to determine associations between serum 25OHD levels pre-diagnosis and risk for incident pancreatic cancer. This large-scale pooled analysis (n = 2,285) found a statistically significant two-fold increased risk for pancreatic cancer in participants with serum 25OHD levels at or above 100 nmol/L compared with those with levels between 50 to 75 nmol. Further, the association was strongest for whites, participants in northern latitudes (> 35°N), and participants whose blood was collected in summer months. Thus, a pooled analysis of large cohort studies suggests an association for increased risk of pancreatic cancer with serum 25OHD levels greater than 100 nmol/L that is not consistently seen in analyses of individual large cohorts.

Prostate cancer   Regarding prostate cancer, Tuohimaa et al. (2004) found a higher risk of prostate cancer for those with serum 25OHD levels above 80 nmol/L. The subjects were 67 men, mostly from Norway. Although another study from Finland (Tuohimaa et al., 2004) also found an association between serum 25OHD levels and prostate cancer at levels above 80 nmol/L, a study conducted by Faupel-Badger et al. (2007) also in Finland did not find a relationship.

Cardiovascular Risk

Although Linden (1974) observed that myocardial infarct patients in Norway were more likely than matched controls to have consumed vitamin D in excess (greater than 1,200 IU/day), two later studies (Schmidt-Gayk et al., 1977; Vik et al., 1979) failed to confirm these results. Melamed et al. (2008) examined data from 3,439 persons in the NHANES 2001 to 2004 surveys to determine the relationship between serum 25OHD level and peripheral arterial disease (defined as an ankle-brachial index < 0.9). The researchers noted that there was a lower risk of CVD mortality in men and women at levels of 75 to 122 nmol/L, but a higher risk of CVD mortality in women at levels above 125 nmol/L. Recently, Ginde et al. (2009), in a prospective cohort analysis of NHANES III data (1988 to 1994) on serum 25OHD levels in adults ages 65 years and older (n = 3,408) over a median 7.3-year follow-up, examined CVD mortality. Analysis of fully adjusted data indicated an inverse relationship between CVD mortality and baseline serum 25OHD level of 50.0 to 74.9 nmol/L. Risk began to increase at approximately 75 nmol/L and then it declined after 100 nmol/L.

Analyses from the Framingham Offspring Study (Wang et al., 2008), which followed 1,739 participants (mean age 59 years) with an average follow-up at 5.4 years, found a significant relationship between low serum 25OHD levels and incident cardiovascular risk. During a mean follow-up of 5.4 years, 120 individuals developed a first cardiovascular event; vitamin D deficiency as defined in the study (serum 25OHD level < 37.5 nmol/L) was associated with increased risk for cardiovascular events. However, a closer look at the individuals with the highest serum 25OHD levels suggests that there was no additional reduction in risk with 25OHD levels above 75 nmol/L and even that the dose–response relationship may be U-shaped or reverse-J-shaped, with increased risk not only at low but also at the higher levels of serum 25OHD (i.e., > 75 nmol/L).

Fiscella and Franks (2010) conducted a retrospective cohort analysis also based on NHANES III data. They examined serum 25OHD levels and CVD mortality in participants ages 18 years and older (n = 15,363). Analysis of fully adjusted data showed a U-shaped risk profile for CVD mortality, as reported by others. Without consideration of vitamin D status, after adjusting for age, gender, season, and region, non-Hispanic blacks had a 38 percent higher cardiovascular mortality than whites. Adjusting for low serum 25OHD levels reduced the racial difference in risk by about 60 percent (to 23 percent). Including both low serum 25OHD level and poverty level reduced the racial difference in risk to 1.0, suggesting that low serum 25OHD level and poverty capture much of the racial disparity in cardiovascular mortality in blacks compared with whites; however, it must be recognized that the low serum 25OHD level may be a marker for other factors (obesity, inactivity, etc.). Additionally, a cross-sectional study conducted by Freedman et al. (2010) reported a positive association between serum 25OHD level and calcified atherosclerotic plaque in the aorta and carotid arteries of African Americans.

Falls and Fractures

In a recent trial of 2,256 community-dwelling women 70 years of age and older residing in Australia and presenting with high risk of fracture, the women were treated with 500,000 IU of vitamin D annually for 3 to 5 years (Sanders et al., 2010). Sanders et al. (2010) reported that "... participants receiving annual high-dose oral cholecalciferol experienced 15% more falls and 26% more fractures than the placebo group. Women not only experienced excess fractures after more frequent falls but also experienced more fractures that were not associated with a fall. A post hoc analysis found that the increased likelihood of falls in the vitamin D group was exacerbated in the 3-month period immediately following the annual dose and a similar temporal trend was observed for fractures. An increased risk (albeit, not significant because of smaller numbers) of falls and fracture in the vitamin D group was apparent for each year of the intervention. The results were similar after adjustment for baseline calcium intake...."

The non-physiological nature of a large one-time dose cannot be readily extrapolated to the situation in which smaller daily doses are provided. However, in view of a number of studies in the literature (e.g., Trivedi et al., 2003) in which large bolus doses have been given without apparent adverse effect, the results of the study by Sanders et al. (2010) are unexpected, but not readily dismissed. The study is notable because the adverse effect was demonstrated as a result of the intervention (which was primarily for safety) as well as through a measure of interest, serum 25OHD concentration. The median serum 25OHD concentration 1 month after dose for study participants was 120 nmol/L. By 3 months, the median value was approximately 90 nmol/L. One other study (Smith et al., 2007) also reported an increase in fracture associated with vitamin D treatment. Participants were 75 years of age or older (4,354 men and 5,086 women) and received an annual injection of 300,000 IU as ergocalciferol or placebo. In men, treatment had no effect on fractures. However, women treated with vitamin D had increased risk of fractures classified as non-vertebral (HR = 1.21), hip/femur (HR = 1.80), and hip/femur/wrist/forearm (HR = 1.59). No effect on falls was observed; however, falls were a secondary outcome and ascertainment was based on 6-month recall. Baseline serum 25OHD levels and changes in serum 25OHD levels were very similar to the results from Sanders et al. (2010). Another common feature was that calcium supplements were not given.

A recent study reported by Cauley et al. (2009) indicated that in contrast to white and American Indian women, black women and possibly Asian women appeared to be at greater risk of fracture with higher serum 25OHD levels (≥ 75 nmol/L).

Conclusion

Despite the limitations of the evidence, there is a notable congruence across different health indicators—all-cause mortality, some cancers, CVD risk, fractures and falls—for adverse outcomes associated with serum 25OHD levels ranging from about 75 to 120 nmol/L. The U-shaped curve, or possibly a reverse-J-shaped curve, for risk does indeed emerge, with adverse effects reported at either end of the serum 25OHD concentration span. Data for associated intakes of vitamin D are limited.

The committee's approach was to consider whether it was reasonable to use these findings as a basis for adjusting data on the toxicity of vitamin D, discussed above. In doing so, it was aware of recent criticisms related to taking into account these so-called U-shaped serum 25OHD response curves for elucidating levels of vitamin D that may cause adverse effects (e.g., Grant, 2010). However, although these data may be characterized as emerging and in need of further study before firm conclusions can be made, they are not reflective of flawed studies nor are they readily dismissed by other literature. Further, in the absence of data to demonstrate benefit at such serum 25OHD levels, a cautious approach is justified and appropriate given the purpose of the UL. In the committee's view, these emerging relationships do not have to be definitively proven in order to justify a cautious approach that is most likely to ensure safety, and in the absence of data to demonstrate benefit from the higher intake level or higher

DIETARY REFERENCE INTAKES FOR CALCIUM AND VITAMIN D

serum 25OHD levels, these signals can be taken into account. Focusing exclusively on vitamin D acute toxicity for the purposes of establishing a UL and ignoring the emerging data related to other adverse events is not in the best interests of public health.

Selection of Indicator for the UL: Vitamin D

The best available data set for establishing a UL for vitamin D is associated with the onset of hypercalcemia and related toxicity. This indicator is selected as the basis for the UL for all age groups except infants, with the caveat that while it serves as a starting point, it is to be subject to adjustment for uncertainty. The adjustment is based on: (1) the recognition of the goal of public health protection, which suggests that avoiding hypervitaminosis D is, of course, desirable, but not necessarily sufficient; and (2) the emerging data concerning other adverse effects at intakes lower than those associated with acute toxicity and at serum 25OHD levels previously considered to be at the high end of physiological values. Taken as a whole, the body of evidence suggests that there is reason to proceed cautiously in assuming that higher levels of vitamin D intake below those expected to cause hypervitaminosis D are harmless, especially in the absence of data to demonstrate benefit at such intake levels. For infants, the long-standing measures related to retarded linear growth serve as the indicator for the UL.

The available data could not offer a BI or be used to estimate a dose–response relationship. The basis for the ULs is a NOAEL as described further below for specific life stage groups.

VITAMIN D UPPER LEVELS: INTAKE-RESPONSE ASSESSMENT AND SPECIFICATION OF UPPER LEVELS

The ULs established for vitamin D are shown in Table 6-4 by life stage group. The ULs for infants are discussed first. This is followed by a discussion of ULs for adults rather than children and adolescents because the UL for adults is used to extrapolate or scale a UL value for children and adolescents. A discussion of ULs during pregnancy and lactation follows.

ULs for Infants 0 to 12 Months of Age

Infants 0 to 6 Months of Age	
	UL 1,000 IU (25 µg)/day Vitamin D
Infants 6 to 12 Months of Age	
	UL 1,500 IU (38 µg)/day Vitamin D

TABLE 6-4 Vitamin D Tolerable Upper Intake Levels (UL) by Life Stage

Life Stage Group	UL
Infants	
0 to 6 mo	1,000 IU (25 µg)
6 to 12 mo	1,500 IU (38 µg)
Children	
1–3 y	2,500 IU (63 µg)
4–8 y	3,000 IU (75 µg)
Males	
9–13 y	4,000 IU (100 µg)
14–18 y	4,000 IU (100 µg)
19–30 y	4,000 IU (100 µg)
31–50 y	4,000 IU (100 µg)
51–70 y	4,000 IU (100 µg)
> 70 y	4,000 IU (100 µg)
Females	
9–13 y	4,000 IU (100 µg)
14–18 y	4,000 IU (100 µg)
19–30 y	4,000 IU (100 µg)
31–50 y	4,000 IU (100 µg)
51–70 y	4,000 IU (100 µg)
> 70 y	4,000 IU (100 µg)
Pregnancy	
14–18 y	4,000 IU (100 µg)
19–30 y	4,000 IU (100 µg)
31–50 y	4,000 IU (100 µg)
Lactation	
14–18 y	4,000 IU (100 µg)
19–30 y	4,000 IU (100 µg)
31–50 y	4,000 IU (100 µg)

NOTE: IU = International Unit.

The work of Fomon et al. (1966) forms the starting point for these life stage group, as it did in the 1997 IOM report (IOM, 1997). Given the small sample size used in the study, the NOAEL for infants is based on the mean intake in this study rather than the high end of the range. The NOAEL was rounded to 1,800 IU/day from 1,775 IU/day. The British Paediatric Association (1956) data and data reported by Bransby et al. (1964) suggested that hypercalcemia could be present at intakes of 4,000 IU/day, but appeared to decline at intakes between 700 and 1,300 IU/day, lending some support to the NOAEL of 1,800 IU/day as reasonable. However, considerable uncertainty surrounds this estimate, and newer data have not emerged regarding vitamin D intake and hypercalcemia in infants. Stearns (1968) commented that Fomon et al. (1966) did not study the infants long enough, because the greatest differences in the Jeans and Stearns (1938) study appeared after 6 months. Also, a report from 1959 (Graham, 1959) suggested that a serum calcium level obtained from a study in Glasgow of infants with hypercalcemia ages 3 weeks to 11 months was associated with an estimated vitamin D intake of 1,320 IU/day. Overall, on balance, 1,800 IU/day is reasonable as a NOAEL and offers an appropriate starting point.

Infants 0 to 6 Months of Age

The first order of importance is to protect young infants, and the intake of 1,800 IU/day may not be entirely protective of such young infants. As the UL can reasonably be considered to affect all non-growth retarded infants at greater than 37 weeks gestational age at birth, and given the current practice to begin vitamin D supplementation within days of birth (Wagner and Greer, 2008), it is necessary to ensure an absence of toxicity in infants as small as 2,500 to 3,000 grams who would meet this definition. As such, applying an uncertainty factor of 0.5 and rounding would reasonably give a level of 1,000 IU/day, which is also about 400 IU/kg body weight per day, a dose that can reasonably be considered an upper safety level on a body weight basis. This UL is the same as the UL established in 1997 (IOM, 1997).

Infants 6 to 12 Months of Age

Consistent with general principles of toxicology, the committee considered that an infant's capacity to handle excess substances such as vitamin D is likely increased with increased body size, organ maturation, and growth needs. Therefore, for older infants it is reasonable to consider a higher UL than for younger infants, although available data are inadequate for quantitative risk assessment. Also, the endpoint is acknowledged to be relatively insensitive. The UL for infants 6 to 12 months of age is increased by 500 IU/day from that established for infants 0 to 6 months of age, to a value of 1,500 IU/day. This reflects a more cautious approach than would be taken if the UL were doubled and is consistent with public health protection. This UL is slightly greater than the UL for vitamin D established for this life stage group in 1997, but is consistent with the toxicological principles that older infants are likely to have greater tolerances than younger infants (IOM, 1997).

ULs for Adults 19 or More Years of Age

Adults 19 Through 30 Years of Age
Adults 31 Through 50 Years of Age
Adults 51 Through 70 Years of Age
Adults >70 Years of Age

UL 4,000 IU (100 µg)/day Vitamin D

The indicator of hypercalcemia for vitamin D toxicity is the starting point for the UL for adults. This condition is at an extreme end of an adverse outcome continuum and it may be appropriate to consider instead as a starting point for other measures, such as hypercalciuria. However, interpretation of measures such as hypercalciuria as a predictor of adverse outcomes is unclear. Therefore, the best available option as an indicator is hypercalcemia. In this case, an intake value of 10,000 IU/day reflects a NOAEL. This NOAEL is initially adjusted for uncertainty to establish a UL of 4,000 IU/day, as described below.

Initially, it should be noted that evidence pertaining to the levels of 25OHD in serum that are associated with adverse effects is less well established than that associated with benefit, and the available literature suggests considerable variability. As shown above in Table 6-3, frank toxicity has been reported to have occurred within a wide range of serum 25OHD levels, from as low as 60 nmol/L (Byrne et al., 1995) to values above 1,500 nmol/L (Rizzoli et al., 1994; Pettifor et al., 1995; Vieth et al., 2002), although the majority of available reports of toxicity involve serum 25OHD values above 350 nmol/L. The variability in the toxicity data may mean that toxicity can be affected by numerous mitigating factors or perhaps may be a function of the diversity in the nature of the available case reports. Reports on maximal sun exposure also described previously (Barger-Lux and Heaney, 2002; Binkley et al., 2007) suggest that serum 25OHD levels under these circumstances generally remain below 125 to 150 nmol/L, although the populations studied are not diverse and generally include younger men. The emerging data related to all-cause mortality, chronic disease risk, and falls would appear to suggest that adverse events may occur with serum 25OHD levels of approximately 75 nmol/L or above (Visser et al., 2006; Ginde et al., 2009), but ranging up to approximately 125 nmol/L (Melamed et al., 2008). The vagaries of serum 25OHD measures in general, the sparse data available, and the uncertainty as to the nature of the adverse effects preclude strong conclusions. On the basis of available reports, the committee considered that serum 25OHD levels above approximately 125 to 150 nmol/L should be avoided. Given the conclusion derived in Chapter 5 that bone health benefit is achieved by 97.5 percent of the population at 50 nmol/L, there is a range of serum 25OHD levels between 50 and 150 nmol/L that remains undescribed. The adjustment to the starting point of 10,000 IU/day reflects first data concerning adverse effects related to all-cause mortality, falls and fractures, and CVD risk, which, taken as a total body of evidence, provide reason for caution, as described earlier. More specifically, the evidence from the studies that focused on all-cause mortality, chronic disease, falls and fractures suggested that serum 25OHD levels between 75 nmol/L and approximately 120 nmol/L were associated with the adverse effect. There is considerable uncertainty surrounding such values, and—using information on the serum levels achieved during maximal sun exposure and to avoid being unnecessarily restrictive given the uncertainties—the committee determined that for the purposes of the UL, concern would be for levels above approximately 125 to 150 nmol/L.

Further, there are emerging data concerning the possible differences in adverse event response for African Americans and perhaps other dark-skinned population groups. The cross–sectional study from Freedman et al. (2010) reported a positive association between serum 25OHD levels and calcified atherosclerotic plaque in the aorta and carotid arteries of African Americans, and preliminary reports from NHANES suggest that the risk for all-cause mortality among non-Hispanic blacks compared with whites occurs at a lower serum 25OHD level (60 vs. 75 nmol/L).[6] These data are limited, are not necessarily consistent with other findings, and may eventually be explained by factors other than serum 25OHD levels, but they are concerning. Although data on race and ethnic differences are much too sparse to justify providing different ULs for different racial or ethnic groups, they can be incorporated as a source of uncertainty.

To determine an adjustment from the starting point of 10,000 IU/day as a NOAEL taking into account the uncertainties introduced by reports concerning all-cause mortality and other chronic disease outcomes as well as the possibility that blacks in the North American population may experience adverse effects at lower serum 25OHD concentrations than whites, the committee considered the work of Heaney et al. (2003). As suggested by the study, vitamin D intakes of 5,000 IU/day achieved serum 25OHD levels that range between 100 and 150 nmol/L, but do not surpass 150 nmol/L after 160 days of administration. Almost no other studies have assessed the safety of long-term maintenance of serum 25OHD levels in this range in relation to chronic disease risk and all-cause mortality, so the information about the increases in serum levels is useful for the purposes of establishing a UL. Given the uncertainties surrounding the data and the reliance on a

---

[6]Personal communication, R. Durazo-Arvizu, Loyola University, Maywood, IL, May 28, 2010.

single report, the UL is set 20 percent below the level identified by Heaney et al. (i.e., 5,000 IU), specifically at 4,000 IU/day.

This value is greater than that set in 1997 by the previous IOM committee. A UL of 4,000 IU/day is still, however, a reference value that reflects the interest in providing public health protection, especially when existing data do not support benefit above such intakes. Intake values in the range of 4,000 IU/day would not appear to cause serum 25OHD levels to exceed 125 to 150 nmol/L,[7] a concentration which is at the high end of the range of serum levels associated with nadir risk of outcomes such as all-cause mortality.

ULs for Children and Adolescents 1 Through 18 Years of Age

Children 1 Through 3 Years of Age
UL 2,500 IU (63 µg)/day Vitamin D
Children 4 Through 8 Years of Age
UL 3,000 IU (75 µg)/day Vitamin D
Children 9 Through 13 Years of Age
Adolescents 14 Through 18 Years of Age
UL 4,000 IU (100 µg)/day Vitamin D

No specific data are available for age groups other than adults and infants. In 1997 it was determined that increased rates of bone formation in toddlers, children, and adolescents suggested that the adult UL is appropriate for these age groups (IOM, 1997). The present committee chose to scale down the adult UL for younger children—to 2,500 IU/day for 1- to 3-year-olds and 3,000 IU/day for 4- to 8-year-olds—so as to be more consistent with concepts of graded tolerances with maturity. Although the simulated dose–response relationship between vitamin D intake and serum 25OHD level described in Chapter 5 is not affected by age, the data available did not include any children younger than 6 years old. There is no quantitative basis for such scaling, but it reflects a cautious and prudent approach given current biological understandings. Children and adolescents between 9 and 18 years of age have ULs that are the same as that for adults. All the UL values for children are slightly higher than the values provided in 1997 (IOM, 1997).

---

[7]Use of the regression model developed to estimate the vitamin D intakes needed to achieve a specific level of 25OHD in serum is not appropriate for this situation, in that the model was derived using data based on minimal sun exposure and did not anticipate estimations of such high levels of intake. However, the use of the related equations suggests that 4,000 IU/day results in a mean serum 25OHD concentration of 91 nmol/L and an upper level of 105 nmol/L.

ULs for Pregnancy and Lactation

Pregnant or Lactating 14 Through 18 Years of Age
Pregnant or Lactating 19 Through 30 Years of Age
Pregnant or Lactating 31 Through 50 Years of Age
UL 4,000 IU (100 µg)/day Vitamin D

The available data do not indicate a basis for deriving a UL for pregnant and lactating women or adolescents that is different from those for their non-pregnant and non-lactating counterparts.

REFERENCES

Adams, J. S. and G. Lee. 1997. Gains in bone mineral density with resolution of vitamin D intoxication. Annals of Internal Medicine 127(3): 203-6.

Aloia, J. F., M. Patel, R. Dimaano, M. Li-Ng, S. A. Talwar, M. Mikhail, S. Pollack and J. K. Yeh. 2008. Vitamin D intake to attain a desired serum 25-hydroxyvitamin D concentration. American Journal of Clinical Nutrition 87(6): 1952-8.

Ames, S. K., B. M. Gorham and S. A. Abrams. 1999. Effects of high compared with low calcium intake on calcium absorption and incorporation of iron by red blood cells in small children. American Journal of Clinical Nutrition 70(1): 44-8.

Anthoni, S., E. Savilahti, H. Rautelin and K. L. Kolho. 2009. Milk protein IgG and IgA: the association with milk-induced gastrointestinal symptoms in adults. World Journal of Gastroenterology 15(39): 4915-8.

Asmus, H. G., J. Braun, R. Krause, R. Brunkhorst, H. Holzer, W. Schulz, H. H. Neumayer, P. Raggi and J. Bommer. 2005. Two year comparison of sevelamer and calcium carbonate effects on cardiovascular calcification and bone density. Nephrology, Dialysis, Transplantation 20(8): 1653-61.

Bailey, C. S., J. J. Weiner, O. M. Gibby and M. D. Penney. 2008. Excessive calcium ingestion leading to milk-alkali syndrome. Annals of Clinical Biochemistry 45(Pt 5): 527-9.

Bajwa, G. S., L. M. Morrison and B. H. Ershoff. 1971. Induction of aortic and coronary atheroarteriosclerosis in rats fed a hypervitaminosis D, cholesterol-containing diet. Proceedings of the Society for Experimental Biology and Medicine 138(3): 975-82.

Barger-Lux, M. J. and R. P. Heaney. 2002. Effects of above average summer sun exposure on serum 25-hydroxyvitamin D and calcium absorption. Journal of Clinical Endocrinology and Metabolism 87(11): 4952-6.

Baron, J. A., M. Beach, K. Wallace, M. V. Grau, R. S. Sandler, J. S. Mandel, D. Heber and E. R. Greenberg. 2005. Risk of prostate cancer in a randomized clinical trial of calcium supplementation. Cancer Epidemiology, Biomarkers & Prevention 14(3): 586-9.

Binkley, N., R. Novotny, D. Krueger, T. Kawahara, Y. G. Daida, G. Lensmeyer, B. W. Hollis and M. K. Drezner. 2007. Low vitamin D status despite abundant sun exposure. Journal of Clinical Endocrinology and Metabolism 92(6): 2130-5.

Blank, S., K. S. Scanlon, T. H. Sinks, S. Lett and H. Falk. 1995. An outbreak of hypervitaminosis D associated with the overfortification of milk from a home-delivery dairy. American Journal of Public Health 85(5): 656-9.

Block, G. A., D. M. Spiegel, J. Ehrlich, R. Mehta, J. Lindbergh, A. Dreisbach and P. Raggi. 2005. Effects of sevelamer and calcium on coronary artery calcification in patients new to hemodialysis. Kidney International 68(4): 1815-24.

Bolland, M. J., P. A. Barber, R. N. Doughty, B. Mason, A. Horne, R. Ames, G. D. Gamble, A. Grey and I. R. Reid. 2008. Vascular events in healthy older women receiving calcium supplementation: randomised controlled trial. British Medical Journal 336(7638): 262-6.

Bolland, M. J., A. Avenell, J. A. Baron, A. Grey, G. S. MacLennan, G. D. Gamble and I. R. Reid. 2010. Effect of calcium supplements on risk of myocardial infarction and cardiovascular events: meta-analysis. British Medical Journal 341: 3691-9.

Borghi, L., T. Schianchi, T. Meschi, A. Guerra, F. Allegri, U. Maggiore and A. Novarini. 2002. Comparison of two diets for the prevention of recurrent stones in idiopathic hypercalciuria. New England Journal of Medicine 346(2): 77-84.

Brannon, P. M., E. A. Yetley, R. L. Bailey and M. F. Picciano. 2008. Vitamin D and health in the 21st century: an update. Proceedings of a conference held September 2007 in Bethesda, Maryland, USA. American Journal of Clinical Nutrition 88(2): 483S-592S.

Bransby, E. R., W. T. Berry and D. M. Taylor. 1964. Study of the vitamin-D intakes of infants in 1960. British Medical Journal 1(5399): 1661-3.

British Paediatric Association. 1956. Hypercalcaemia in infants and vitamin D. British Medical Journal 2(4985): 149.

British Paediatric Association. 1964. Infantile hypercalcaemia, nutritional rickets, and infantile scurvy in Great Britain. British Medical Journal 1(5399): 1659-61.

Burnett, C. H., R. R. Commons and et al. 1949. Hypercalcemia without hypercalcuria or hypophosphatemia, calcinosis, and renal insufficiency; a syndrome following prolonged intake of milk and alkali. New England Journal of Medicine 240(20): 787-94.

Byrne, P. M., R. Freaney and M. J. McKenna. 1995. Vitamin D supplementation in the elderly: review of safety and effectiveness of different regimes. Calcified Tissue International 56(6): 518-20.

Caruso, J. B., R. M. Patel, K. Julka and D. C. Parish. 2007. Health-behavior induced disease: return of the milk-alkali syndrome. Journal of General Internal Medicine 22(7): 1053-5.

Cauley, J., et al. 2009. Serum 25 hydroxyvitamin (OH)D and fracture risk in multi-ethnic women: The Women's Health Initiative (WHI). Presented at ASBMR 31st Annual Meeting. Denver, CO.

Chan, J. M., P. Pietinen, M. Virtanen, N. Malila, J. Tangrea, D. Albanes and J. Virtamo. 2000. Diet and prostate cancer risk in a cohort of smokers, with a specific focus on calcium and phosphorus (Finland). Cancer Causes and Control 11(9): 859-67.

Chan, J. M., M. J. Stampfer, J. Ma, P. H. Gann, J. M. Gaziano and E. L. Giovannucci. 2001. Dairy products, calcium, and prostate cancer risk in the Physicians' Health Study. American Journal of Clinical Nutrition 74(4): 549-54.

Chiricone, D., N. G. De Santo and M. Cirillo. 2003. Unusual cases of chronic intoxication by vitamin D. Journal of Nephrology 16(6): 917-21.

Chlebowski, R. T., K. C. Johnson, C. Kooperberg, M. Pettinger, J. Wactawski-Wende, T. Rohan, J. Rossouw, D. Lane, M. J. O'Sullivan, S. Yasmeen, R. A. Hiatt, J. M. Shikany, M. Vitolins, J. Khandekar and F. A. Hubbell. 2008. Calcium plus vitamin D supplementation and the risk of breast cancer. Journal of the National Cancer Institute 100(22): 1581-91.

Chung M., E. M. Balk, S. Brendel, S. Ip, J. Lau, J. Lee, A. Lichtenstein, K. Patel, G. Raman, A. Tatsioni, T. Terasawa and T. A. Trikalinos. 2009. Vitamin D and calcium: a systematic review of health outcomes. Evidence Report No. 183. (Prepared by the Tufts Evidence-based Practice Center under Contract No. HHSA 290-2007-10055-I.) AHRQ Publication No. 09-E015. Rockville, MD: Agency for Healthcare Research and Quality.

Coe, F. L., J. H. Parks and D. R. Webb. 1992. Stone-forming potential of milk or calcium-fortified orange juice in idiopathic hypercalciuric adults. Kidney International 41(1): 139-42.

Coresh, J., D. Byrd-Holt, B. C. Astor, J. P. Briggs, P. W. Eggers, D. A. Lacher and T. H. Hostetter. 2005. Chronic kidney disease awareness, prevalence, and trends among U.S. adults, 1999 to 2000. Journal of the American Society of Nephrology 16(1): 180-8.

Cozzolino, M., D. Brancaccio, M. Gallieni and E. Slatopolsky. 2005. Pathogenesis of vascular calcification in chronic kidney disease. Kidney International 68(2): 429-36.

Cranney A., T. Horsley, S. O'Donnell, H. A. Weiler, L. Puil, D. S. Ooi, S. A. Atkinson, L. M. Ward, D. Moher, D. A. Hanley, M. Fang, F. Yazdi, C. Garritty, M. Sampson, N. Barrowman, A. Tsertsvadze and V. Mamaladze. 2007. Effectiveness and safety of vitamin D in relation to bone health. Evidence Report/Technology Assessment No. 158. (Prepared by the University of Ottawa Evidence-based Practice Center (UO-EPC) under Contract No. 290-02-0021.) AHRQ Publication No. 07-E013. Rockville, MD: Agency for Healthcare Research and Quality.

Curhan, G. C., W. C. Willett, E. B. Rimm and M. J. Stampfer. 1993. A prospective study of dietary calcium and other nutrients and the risk of symptomatic kidney stones. New England Journal of Medicine 328(12): 833-8.

Curhan, G. C., W. C. Willett, F. E. Speizer, D. Speigelman and M. J. Stampfer. 1997. Comparison of dietary calcium with supplemental calcium and other nutrients as factors affecting the risk for kidney stones in women. Annals of Internal Medicine 126(7): 497-504.

Curhan, G. C., W. C. Willett, E. L. Knight and M. J. Stampfer. 2004. Dietary factors and the risk of incident kidney stones in younger women: Nurses' Health Study II. Archives of Internal Medicine 164(8): 885-91.

Curhan, G. C. 2007. Epidemiology of stone disease. Urologic Clinics of North America 34(3): 287-93.

Dalton, M. A., J. D. Sargent, G. T. O'Connor, E. M. Olmstead and R. Z. Klein. 1997. Calcium and phosphorus supplementation of iron-fortified infant formula: no effect on iron status of healthy full-term infants. American Journal of Clinical Nutrition 65(4): 921-6.

Davie, M. W., D. E. Lawson, C. Emberson, J. L. Barnes, G. E. Roberts and N. D. Barnes. 1982. Vitamin D from skin: contribution to vitamin D status compared with oral vitamin D in normal and anticonvulsant-treated subjects. Clinical Science 63(5): 461-72.

Davies, M. and P. H. Adams. 1978. The continuing risk of vitamin-D intoxication. Lancet 2(8090): 621-3.

Deluca, H. F. 2009. Vitamin D toxicity. Paper prepared for the Committee to Review Dietary Reference Intakes for Vitamin D and Calcium. Washington, DC.

Dourson, M. L. and J. F. Stara. 1983. Regulatory history and experimental support of uncertainty (safety) factors. Regulatory Toxicology and Pharmacology 3(3): 224-38.

Faupel-Badger, J. M., L. Diaw, D. Albanes, J. Virtamo, K. Woodson and J. A. Tangrea. 2007. Lack of association between serum levels of 25-hydroxyvitamin D and the subsequent risk of prostate cancer in Finnish men. Cancer Epidemiology, Biomarkers & Prevention 16(12): 2784-6.

Felsenfeld, A. J. and B. S. Levine. 2006. Milk alkali syndrome and the dynamics of calcium homeostasis. Clinical Journal of the American Society of Nephrology 1(4): 641-54.

Fiscella, K. and P. Franks. 2010. Vitamin D, race, and cardiovascular mortality: findings from a national US sample. Annals of Family Medicine 8(1): 11-8.

Fomon, S. J., M. K. Younoszai and L. N. Thomas. 1966. Influence of vitamin D on linear growth of normal full-term infants. Journal of Nutrition 88(3): 345-50.

Freedman, B. I., L. E. Wagenknecht, K. G. Hairston, D. W. Bowden, J. J. Carr, R. C. Hightower, E. J. Gordon, J. Xu, C. D. Langefeld and J. Divers. 2010. Vitamin D, adiposity, and calcified atherosclerotic plaque in African-Americans. Journal of Clinical Endocrinology and Metabolism 95(3): 1076.

Ginde, A. A., R. Scragg, R. S. Schwartz and C. A. Camargo, Jr. 2009. Prospective study of serum 25-hydroxyvitamin D level, cardiovascular disease mortality, and all-cause mortality in older U.S. adults. Journal of the American Geriatrics Society 57(9): 1595-603.

Giovannucci, E., E. B. Rimm, A. Wolk, A. Ascherio, M. J. Stampfer, G. A. Colditz and W. C. Willett. 1998. Calcium and fructose intake in relation to risk of prostate cancer. Cancer Research 58(3): 442-7.

Giovannucci, E., Y. Liu, M. J. Stampfer and W. C. Willett. 2006a. A prospective study of calcium intake and incident and fatal prostate cancer. Cancer Epidemiology, Biomarkers & Prevention 15(2): 203-10.

Giovannucci, E., Y. Liu and W. C. Willett. 2006b. Cancer incidence and mortality and vitamin D in black and white male health professionals. Cancer Epidemiology, Biomarkers & Prevention 15(12): 2467-72.

Goodman, W. G., J. Goldin, B. D. Kuizon, C. Yoon, B. Gales, D. Sider, Y. Wang, J. Chung, A. Emerick, L. Greaser, R. M. Elashoff and I. B. Salusky. 2000. Coronary-artery calcification in young adults with end-stage renal disease who are undergoing dialysis. New England Journal of Medicine 342(20): 1478-83.

Gordon, M. V., L. P. McMahon and P. S. Hamblin. 2005. Life-threatening milk-alkali syndrome resulting from antacid ingestion during pregnancy. Medical Journal of Australia 182(7): 350-1.

Graham, S. 1959. Idiopathic hypercalcemia. Postgraduate Medicine 25(1): 67-72.

Grant, W. B. 1999. An ecologic study of dietary links to prostate cancer. Alternative Medicine Review 4(3): 162-9.

Grant, W. B. 2010. Critique of the U-shaped serum 25-hydroxyvitamin D level-disease response relation. Dermato-Endocrinology 1(6): 289.

Grubb, M., K. Gaurav and M. Panda. 2009. Milk-alkali syndrome in a middle-aged woman after ingesting large doses of calcium carbonate: a case report. Cases Journal 2: 8198.

Haddad, J. G. 1980. Competitive protein-binding radioassays for 25-OH-D; clinical applications. In Vitamin D, Volume 2, edited by Norman. New York: Marcel Dekker, Inc. Pp. 587.

Hardt, L. L. and A. B. Rivers. 1923. Toxic manifestations following the alkaline treatment of peptic ulcer. Archives of Internal Medicine 31(2): 171-80.

Harmeyer, J. and C. Schlumbohm. 2004. Effects of pharmacological doses of vitamin D_3 on mineral balance and profiles of plasma vitamin D_3 metabolites in horses. Journal of Steroid Biochemistry and Molecular Biology 89-90(1-5): 595-600.

Harrington, D. D. and E. H. Page. 1983. Acute vitamin D_3 toxicosis in horses: case reports and experimental studies of the comparative toxicity of vitamins D_2 and D_3. Journal of the American Veterinary Medical Association 182(12): 1358-69.

Hathcock, J. N., A. Shao, R. Vieth and R. Heaney. 2007. Risk assessment for vitamin D. American Journal of Clinical Nutrition 85(1): 6-18.

Heaney, R. P., K. M. Davies, T. C. Chen, M. F. Holick and M. J. Barger-Lux. 2003. Human serum 25-hydroxycholecalciferol response to extended oral dosing with cholecalciferol. American Journal of Clinical Nutrition 77(1): 204-10.

Hiatt, R. A., L. G. Dales, G. D. Friedman and E. M. Hunkeler. 1982. Frequency of urolithiasis in a prepaid medical care program. American Journal of Epidemiology 115(2): 255-65.

Honkanen, R., E. Alhava, M. Parviainen, S. Talasniemi and R. Monkkonen. 1990. The necessity and safety of calcium and vitamin D in the elderly. Journal of the American Geriatrics Society 38(8): 862-6.

Hruska, K. A., S. Mathew, R. J. Lund, I. Memon and G. Saab. 2009. The pathogenesis of vascular calcification in the chronic kidney disease mineral bone disorder: the links between bone and the vasculature. Seminars in Nephrology 29(2): 156-65.

Hughes, M. R., D. J. Baylink, W. A. Gonnerman, S. U. Toverud, W. K. Ramp and M. R. Haussler. 1977. Influence of dietary vitamin D_3 on the circulating concentration of its active metabolites in the chick and rat. Endocrinology 100(3): 799-806.

Hunt, R. D., F. G. Garcia and R. J. Walsh. 1972. A comparison of the toxicity of ergocalciferol and cholecalciferol in rhesus monkeys (Macaca mulatta). Journal of Nutrition 102(8): 975-86.

Ilich-Ernst, J. Z., A. A. McKenna, N. E. Badenhop, A. C. Clairmont, M. B. Andon, R. W. Nahhas, P. Goel and V. Matkovic. 1998. Iron status, menarche, and calcium supplementation in adolescent girls. American Journal of Clinical Nutrition 68(4): 880-7.

IOM (Institute of Medicine). 1997. Dietary Reference Intakes for Calcium, Phosphorus, Magnesium, Vitamin D, and Fluoride. Washington, DC: National Academy Press.

IOM. 1998. Dietary Reference Intakes: A Risk Assessment Model for Establishing Upper Intake Levels for Nutrients. Washington, DC: National Academy Press.

IOM. 2008. The Development of DRIs 1994-2004: Lessons Learned and New Challenges: Workshop Summary. Washington, DC: The National Academies Press.

Irtiza-Ali, A., S. Waldek, E. Lamerton, A. Pennell and P. A. Kalra. 2008. Milk alkali syndrome associated with excessive ingestion of Rennie: case reports. Journal of Renal Care 34(2): 64-7.

Jackson, R. D., A. Z. LaCroix, M. Gass, R. B. Wallace, J. Robbins, C. E. Lewis, T. Bassford, S. A. Beresford, H. R. Black, P. Blanchette, D. E. Bonds, R. L. Brunner, R. G. Brzyski, B. Caan, J. A. Cauley, R. T. Chlebowski, S. R. Cummings, I. Granek, J. Hays, G. Heiss, S. L. Hendrix, B. V. Howard, J. Hsia, F. A. Hubbell, K. C. Johnson, H. Judd, J. M. Kotchen, L. H. Kuller, R. D. Langer, N. L. Lasser, M. C. Limacher, S. Ludlam, J. E. Manson, K. L. Margolis, J. McGowan, J. K. Ockene, M. J. O'Sullivan, L. Phillips, R. L. Prentice, G. E. Sarto, M. L. Stefanick, L. Van Horn, J. Wactawski-Wende, E. Whitlock, G. L. Anderson, A. R. Assaf and D. Barad. 2006. Calcium plus vitamin D supplementation and the risk of fractures. New England Journal of Medicine 354(7): 669-83.

Javed, R. A., M. A. Rafiq, K. Marrero and J. Vieira. 2007. Milk-alkali syndrome: a reverberation of the past. Singapore Medical Journal 48(4): 359-60.

Jeans, P. C. and G. Stearns. 1938. The effect of vitamin D on linear growth in infancy: II. The effect of intakes above 1,800 U.S.P. units daily. Journal of Pediatrics 13(5): 730-40.

Jia, X., L. S. Aucott and G. McNeill. 2007. Nutritional status and subsequent all-cause mortality in men and women aged 75 years or over living in the community. British Journal of Nutrition 98(3): 593-9.

Johnson, C. M., D. M. Wilson, W. M. O'Fallon, R. S. Malek and L. T. Kurland. 1979. Renal stone epidemiology: a 25-year study in Rochester, Minnesota. Kidney International 16(5): 624-31.

Johnson, K. R., J. Jobber and B. J. Stonawski. 1980. Prophylactic vitamin D in the elderly. Age and Ageing 9(2): 121-7.

Jones, G. 2008. Pharmacokinetics of vitamin D toxicity. American Journal of Clinical Nutrition 88(2): 582S-6S.

Jousten, E. and P. Guffens. 2008. Milk-alkali syndrome caused by ingestion of antacid tablets. Acta Clinica Belgica 63(2): 103-6.

Kaklamanos, M. and P. Perros. 2007. Milk alkali syndrome without the milk. British Medical Journal 335(7616): 397-8.

Kamio, A., T. Taguchi, M. Shiraishi, K. Shitama, K. Fukushima and S. Takebayashi. 1979. Vitamin D sclerosis in rats. Acta Pathologica Japonica 29(4): 545-62.

Klontz, K. C. and D. W. Acheson. 2007. Dietary supplement-induced vitamin D intoxication. New England Journal of Medicine 357(3): 308-9.

Koh, K. A., H. D. Sesso, R. S. Paffenbarger, Jr. and I. M. Lee. 2006. Dairy products, calcium and prostate cancer risk. British Journal of Cancer 95(11): 1582-5.

Kristal, A. R., J. L. Stanford, J. H. Cohen, K. Wicklund and R. E. Patterson. 1999. Vitamin and mineral supplement use is associated with reduced risk of prostate cancer. Cancer Epidemiology, Biomarkers & Prevention 8(10): 887-92.

Kurahashi, N., M. Inoue, M. Iwasaki, S. Sasazuki and A. S. Tsugane. 2008. Dairy product, saturated fatty acid, and calcium intake and prostate cancer in a prospective cohort of Japanese men. Cancer Epidemiology, Biomarkers and Prevention 17(4): 930-7.

Levine, B. S., J. S. Rodman, S. Wienerman, R. S. Bockman, J. M. Lane and D. S. Chapman. 1994. Effect of calcium citrate supplementation on urinary calcium oxalate saturation in female stone formers: implications for prevention of osteoporosis. American Journal of Clinical Nutrition 60(4): 592-6.

Linden, V. 1974. Vitamin D and myocardial infarction. British Medical Journal 3(5932): 647-50.

Littledike, E. T. and R. L. Horst. 1982a. Vitamin D_3 toxicity in dairy cows. Journal of Dairy Science 65(5): 749-59.

Littledike, E. T. and R. L. Horst. 1982b. Metabolism of vitamin D_3 in nephrectomized pigs given pharmacological amounts of vitamin D_3. Endocrinology 111(6): 2008-13.

Markowitz, M. E., M. Sinnett and J. F. Rosen. 2004. A randomized trial of calcium supplementation for childhood lead poisoning. Pediatrics 113(1 Pt 1): e34-9.

McKenna, A. A., J. Z. Ilich, M. B. Andon, C. Wang and V. Matkovic. 1997. Zinc balance in adolescent females consuming a low- or high-calcium diet. American Journal of Clinical Nutrition 65(5): 1460-4.

Medarov, B. I. 2009. Milk-alkali syndrome. Mayo Clinic Proceedings 84(3): 261-7.

Melamed, M. L., E. D. Michos, W. Post and B. Astor. 2008. 25-hydroxyvitamin D levels and the risk of mortality in the general population. Archives of Internal Medicine 168(15): 1629-37.

Mitrou, P. N., D. Albanes, S. J. Weinstein, P. Pietinen, P. R. Taylor, J. Virtamo and M. F. Leitzmann. 2007. A prospective study of dietary calcium, dairy products and prostate cancer risk (Finland). International Journal of Cancer 120(11): 2466-73.

Moe, S. M. 2008. Disorders involving calcium, phosphorus, and magnesium. Primary Care; Clinics in Office Practice 35(2): 215-37, v-vi.

Mourad, B., N. Fadwa, T. Mounir, E. Abdelhamid, N. Mohamed Fadhel and S. Rachid. 2006. Influence of hypercalcic and/or hyperoxalic diet on calcium oxalate renal stone formation in rats. Scandinavian Journal of Urology and Nephrology 40(3): 187-91.

Nabhan, F. A., G. W. Sizemore and P. M. Camacho. 2004. Milk-alkali syndrome from ingestion of calcium carbonate in a patient with hypoparathyroidism. Endocrine Practice 10(4): 372-5.

Narang, N. K., R. C. Gupta and M. K. Jain. 1984. Role of vitamin D in pulmonary tuberculosis. Journal of the Association of Physicians of India 32(2): 185-8.

Pak, C. Y. and K. Holt. 1976. Nucleation and growth of brushite and calcium oxalate in urine of stone-formers. Metabolism 25(6): 665-73.

Park, S. Y., S. P. Murphy, L. R. Wilkens, A. M. Nomura, B. E. Henderson and L. N. Kolonel. 2007a. Calcium and vitamin D intake and risk of colorectal cancer: the Multiethnic Cohort Study. American Journal of Epidemiology 165(7): 784-93.

Park, S. Y., S. P. Murphy, L. R. Wilkens, D. O. Stram, B. E. Henderson and L. N. Kolonel. 2007b. Calcium, vitamin D, and dairy product intake and prostate cancer risk: the Multiethnic Cohort Study. American Journal of Epidemiology 166(11): 1259-69.

Patel, A. M. and S. Goldfarb. 2010. Got calcium? Welcome to the calcium-alkali syndrome. Journal of the American Society of Nephrology 21(9): 1440-3.

Peterson, C. A., D. H. Baker and J. W. Erdman, Jr. 1996. Diet-induced nephrocalcinosis in female rats is irreversible and is induced primarily before the completion of adolescence. Journal of Nutrition 126(1): 259-65.

Pettifor, J. M., D. D. Bikle, M. Cavaleros, D. Zachen, M. C. Kamdar and F. P. Ross. 1995. Serum levels of free 1,25-dihydroxyvitamin D in vitamin D toxicity. Annals of Internal Medicine 122(7): 511-3.

Picolos, M. K., V. R. Lavis and P. R. Orlander. 2005. Milk-alkali syndrome is a major cause of hypercalcaemia among non-end-stage renal disease (non-ESRD) inpatients. Clinical Endocrinology 63(5): 566-76.

Prince, R. L., A. Devine, S. S. Dhaliwal and I. M. Dick. 2006. Effects of calcium supplementation on clinical fracture and bone structure: results of a 5-year, double-blind, placebo-controlled trial in elderly women. Archives of Internal Medicine 166(8): 869-75.

Raggi, P., G. James, S. K. Burke, J. Bommer, S. Chasan-Taber, H. Holzer, J. Braun and G. M. Chertow. 2005. Decrease in thoracic vertebral bone attenuation with calcium-based phosphate binders in hemodialysis. Journal of Bone and Mineral Research 20(5): 764-72.

Raimondi, S., J. B. Mabrouk, B. Shatenstein, P. Maisonneuve and P. Ghadirian. 2010. Diet and prostate cancer risk with specific focus on dairy products and dietary calcium: a case–control study. Prostate 70(10):1054-65.

Reid, I. R. and M. J. Bolland. 2008. Calcium supplementation and vascular disease. Climacteric 11(4): 280-6.

Reynolds, J. L., A. J. Joannides, J. N. Skepper, R. McNair, L. J. Schurgers, D. Proudfoot, W. Jahnen-Dechent, P. L. Weissberg and C. M. Shanahan. 2004. Human vascular smooth muscle cells undergo vesicle-mediated calcification in response to changes in extracellular calcium and phosphate concentrations: a potential mechanism for accelerated vascular calcification in ESRD. Journal of the American Society of Nephrology 15(11): 2857-67.

Riggs, B. L., W. M. O'Fallon, J. Muhs, M. K. O'Connor, R. Kumar and L. J. Melton, 3rd. 1998. Long-term effects of calcium supplementation on serum parathyroid hormone level, bone turnover, and bone loss in elderly women. Journal of Bone and Mineral Research 13(2): 168-74.

Rizzoli, R., C. Stoermann, P. Ammann and J. P. Bonjour. 1994. Hypercalcemia and hyper-osteolysis in vitamin D intoxication: effects of clodronate therapy. Bone 15(2): 193-8.

Roborgh, J. R. and T. de Man. 1960. The hypercalcemic activity of dihydrotachysterol-2 and dihydrotachysterol-3 and of the vitamins D_2 and D_3 after intravenous injection of the aqueous preparations. 2. Comparative experiments on rats. Biochemical Pharmacology 3: 277-82.

Rodriguez, C., M. L. McCullough, A. M. Mondul, E. J. Jacobs, D. Fakhrabadi-Shokoohi, E. L. Giovannucci, M. J. Thun and E. E. Calle. 2003. Calcium, dairy products, and risk of prostate cancer in a prospective cohort of United States men. Cancer Epidemiology, Biomarkers & Prevention 12(7): 597-603.

Rohrmann, S., E. A. Platz, C. J. Kavanaugh, L. Thuita, S. C. Hoffman and K. J. Helzlsouer. 2007. Meat and dairy consumption and subsequent risk of prostate cancer in a US cohort study. Cancer Causes and Control 18(1): 41-50.

Sambrook, P. N., J. S. Chen, L. M. March, I. D. Cameron, R. G. Cumming, S. R. Lord, J. Schwarz and M. J. Seibel. 2004. Serum parathyroid hormone is associated with increased mortality independent of 25-hydroxy vitamin d status, bone mass, and renal function in the frail and very old: a cohort study. Journal of Clinical Endocrinology and Metabolism 89(11): 5477-81.

Sambrook, P. N., C. J. Chen, L. March, I. D. Cameron, R. G. Cumming, S. R. Lord, J. M. Simpson and M. J. Seibel. 2006. High bone turnover is an independent predictor of mortality in the frail elderly. Journal of Bone and Mineral Research 21(4): 549-55.

Sanders, K. M., A. L. Stuart, E. J. Williamson, J. A. Simpson, M. A. Kotowicz, D. Young and G. C. Nicholson. 2010. Annual high-dose oral vitamin D and falls and fractures in older women: a randomized controlled trial. Journal of the American Medical Association 303(18): 1815-22.

Sargent, J. D., M. A. Dalton, G. T. O'Connor, E. M. Olmstead and R. Z. Klein. 1999. Randomized trial of calcium glycerophosphate-supplemented infant formula to prevent lead absorption. American Journal of Clinical Nutrition 69(6): 1224-30.

Schmidt-Gayk, H., J. Goossen, F. Lendle and D. Seidel. 1977. Serum 25-hydroxycalciferol in myocardial infarction. Atherosclerosis 26(1): 55-8.

Schuurman, A. G., P. A. van den Brandt, E. Dorant and R. A. Goldbohm. 1999. Animal products, calcium and protein and prostate cancer risk in The Netherlands Cohort Study. British Journal of Cancer 80(7): 1107-13.

Schwartzman, M. S. and W. A. Franck. 1987. Vitamin D toxicity complicating the treatment of senile, postmenopausal, and glucocorticoid-induced osteoporosis. Four case reports and a critical commentary on the use of vitamin D in these disorders. American Journal of Medicine 82(2): 224-30.

Selby, P. L., M. Davies, J. S. Marks and E. B. Mawer. 1995. Vitamin D intoxication causes hypercalcaemia by increased bone resorption which responds to pamidronate. Clinical Endocrinology 43(5): 531-6.

Semba, R. D., D. K. Houston, L. Ferrucci, A. R. Cappola, K. Sun, J. M. Guralnik and L. P. Fried. 2009. Low serum 25-hydroxyvitamin D concentrations are associated with greater all-cause mortality in older community-dwelling women. Nutrition Research 29(8): 525-30.

Shah, B. K., S. Gowda, H. Prabhu, J. Vieira and H. C. Mahaseth. 2007. Modern milk alkali syndrome—a preventable serious condition. New Zealand Medical Journal 120(1262): U2734.

Shephard, R. M. and H. F. Deluca. 1980. Plasma concentrations of vitamin D_3 and its metabolites in the rat as influenced by vitamin D_3 or 25-hydroxyvitamin D_3 intakes. Archives of Biochemistry and Biophysics 202(1): 43-53.

Skinner, H. G., D. S. Michaud, E. Giovannucci, W. C. Willett, G. A. Colditz and C. S. Fuchs. 2006. Vitamin D intake and the risk for pancreatic cancer in two cohort studies. Cancer Epidemiology, Biomarkers & Prevention 15(9): 1688-95.

Smith, H., F. Anderson, H. Raphael, P. Maslin, S. Crozier and C. Cooper. 2007. Effect of annual intramuscular vitamin D on fracture risk in elderly men and women—a population-based, randomized, double-blind, placebo-controlled trial. Rheumatology 46(12): 1852-7.

Stamatelou, K. K., M. E. Francis, C. A. Jones, L. M. Nyberg and G. C. Curhan. 2003. Time trends in reported prevalence of kidney stones in the United States: 1976-1994. Kidney International 63(5): 1817-23.

Stamp, T. C., J. G. Haddad and C. A. Twigg. 1977. Comparison of oral 25-hydroxycholecalciferol, vitamin D, and ultraviolet light as determinants of circulating 25-hydroxyvitamin D. Lancet 1(8026): 1341-3.

Stearns, G. 1968. Fifty years of experience in nutrition and a look to the future: III. Early studies of vitamin D requirement during growth. American Journal of Public Health and the Nations Health 58(11): 2027-35.

Stephenson, D. W. and A. N. Peiris. 2009. The lack of vitamin D toxicity with megadose of daily ergocalciferol (D2) therapy: a case report and literature review. Southern Medical Journal 102(7): 765-8.

Stolzenberg-Solomon, R. Z., R. Vieth, A. Azad, P. Pietinen, P. R. Taylor, J. Virtamo and D. Albanes. 2006. A prospective nested case–control study of vitamin D status and pancreatic cancer risk in male smokers. Cancer Research 66(20): 10213-9.

Stolzenberg-Solomon, R. Z. 2009. Vitamin D and pancreatic cancer. Annals of Epidemiology 19(2): 89-95.

Stolzenberg-Solomon, R. Z., E. J. Jacobs, A. A. Arslan, D. Qi, A. V. Patel, K. J. Helzlsouer, S. J. Weinstein, M. L. McCullough, M. P. Purdue, X. O. Shu, K. Snyder, J. Virtamo, L. R. Wilkins, K. Yu, A. Zeleniuch-Jacquotte, W. Zheng, D. Albanes, Q. Cai, C. Harvey, R. Hayes, S. Clipp, R. L. Horst, L. Irish, K. Koenig, L. Le Marchand and L. N. Kolonel. 2010. Circulating 25-hydroxyvitamin D and risk of pancreatic cancer: Cohort Consortium Vitamin D Pooling Project of Rarer Cancers. American Journal of Epidemiology 172(1): 81-93.

Szczech, L. A., W. Harmon, T. H. Hostetter, P. E. Klotman, N. R. Powe, J. R. Sedor, P. Smedberg and J. Himmelfarb. 2009. World Kidney Day 2009: problems and challenges in the emerging epidemic of kidney disease. Journal of the American Society of Nephrology 20(3): 453-5.

Tangpricha, V., A. Turner, C. Spina, S. Decastro, T. C. Chen and M. F. Holick. 2004. Tanning is associated with optimal vitamin D status (serum 25-hydroxyvitamin D concentration) and higher bone mineral density. American Journal of Clinical Nutrition 80(6): 1645-9.

Taussig, H. B. 1966. Possible injury to the cardiovascular system from vitamin D. Annals of Internal Medicine 65(6): 1195-200.

Tominaga, S. and T. Kuroishi. 1997. An ecological study on diet/nutrition and cancer in Japan. International Journal of Cancer (Suppl 10): 2-6.

Towler, D. 2009. Adverse health effects of excessive vitamin D and calcium intake: considerations relevant to cardiovascular disease and nephrocalcinosis. A white paper commissioned for the Committee to Review Dietary Reference Intakes for Vitamin D and Calcium. Washington, DC.

Trivedi, D. P., R. Doll and K. T. Khaw. 2003. Effect of four monthly oral vitamin D_3 (cholecalciferol) supplementation on fractures and mortality in men and women living in the community: randomised double blind controlled trial. British Medical Journal 326(7387): 469.

Tryfonidou, M. A., M. A. Oosterlaken-Dijksterhuis, J. A. Mol, T. S. van den Ingh, W. E. van den Brom and H. A. Hazewinkel. 2003. 24-hydroxylase: potential key regulator in hypervitaminosis D_3 in growing dogs. American Journal of Physiology, Endocrinology, and Metabolism 284(3): E505-13.

Tseng, M., R. A. Breslow, B. I. Graubard and R. G. Ziegler. 2005. Dairy, calcium, and vitamin D intakes and prostate cancer risk in the National Health and Nutrition Examination Epidemiologic Follow-up Study cohort. American Journal of Clinical Nutrition 81(5): 1147-54.

Tuohimaa, P., L. Tenkanen, M. Ahonen, S. Lumme, E. Jellum, G. Hallmans, P. Stattin, S. Harvei, T. Hakulinen, T. Luostarinen, J. Dillner, M. Lehtinen and M. Hakama. 2004. Both high and low levels of blood vitamin D are associated with a higher prostate cancer risk: a longitudinal, nested case–control study in the Nordic countries. International Journal of Cancer 108(1): 104-8.

Ulett, K., B. Wells and R. Centor. 2010. Hypercalcemia and acute renal failure in milk-alkali syndrome: a case report. Journal of Hospital Medicine 5(2): E18-20.

Vervaet, B. A., A. Verhulst, P. C. D'Haese and M. E. De Broe. 2009. Nephrocalcinosis: new insights into mechanisms and consequences. Nephrology, Dialysis, Transplantation 24(7): 2030-5.

Vieth, R. 1990. The mechanisms of vitamin D toxicity. Bone and Mineral 11(3): 267-72.

Vieth, R., T. R. Pinto, B. S. Reen and M. M. Wong. 2002. Vitamin D poisoning by table sugar. Lancet 359(9307): 672.

Vieth, R. 2007. Vitamin D toxicity, policy, and science. Journal of Bone and Mineral Research 22(Suppl 2): V64-8.

Vik, B., K. Try, D. S. Thelle and O. H. Forde. 1979. Tromso Heart Study: vitamin D metabolism and myocardial infarction. British Medical Journal 2(6183): 176.

Visser, M., D. J. Deeg, M. T. Puts, J. C. Seidell and P. Lips. 2006. Low serum concentrations of 25-hydroxyvitamin D in older persons and the risk of nursing home admission. American Journal of Clinical Nutrition 84(3): 616-22; quiz 671-2.

Wagner, C. L. and F. R. Greer. 2008. Prevention of rickets and vitamin D deficiency in infants, children, and adolescents. Pediatrics 122(5): 1142-52.

Waked, A., A. Geara and B. El-Imad. 2009. Hypercalcemia, metabolic alkalosis and renal failure secondary to calcium bicarbonate intake for osteoporosis prevention—"modern" milk alkali syndrome: a case report. Cases Journal 2: 6188.

Wang, T. J., M. J. Pencina, S. L. Booth, P. F. Jacques, E. Ingelsson, K. Lanier, E. J. Benjamin, R. B. D'Agostino, M. Wolf and R. S. Vasan. 2008. Vitamin D deficiency and risk of cardiovascular disease. Circulation 117(4): 503-11.

WCRF (World Cancer Research Fund)/AICR (American Institute for Cancer Research). 2007. Food, Nutrition, Physical Activity, and the Prevention of Cancer: A Global Perspective. Washington, DC: AICR.

Webb, A. R., B. R. DeCosta and M. F. Holick. 1989. Sunlight regulates the cutaneous production of vitamin D_3 by causing its photodegradation. Journal of Clinical Endocrinology and Metabolism 68(5): 882-7.

Williams, C. P., D. F. Child, P. R. Hudson, G. K. Davies, M. G. Davies, R. John, P. S. Anandaram and A. R. De Bolla. 2001. Why oral calcium supplements may reduce renal stone disease: report of a clinical pilot study. Journal of Clinical Pathology 54(1): 54-62.

Yang, H., G. Curinga and C. M. Giachelli. 2004. Elevated extracellular calcium levels induce smooth muscle cell matrix mineralization in vitro. Kidney International 66(6): 2293-9.

Yetley, E. A., D. Brule, M. C. Cheney, C. D. Davis, K. A. Esslinger, P. W. Fischer, K. E. Friedl, L. S. Greene-Finestone, P. M. Guenther, D. M. Klurfeld, M. R. L'Abbe, K. Y. McMurry, P. E. Starke-Reed and P. R. Trumbo. 2009. Dietary reference intakes for vitamin D: justification for a review of the 1997 values. American Journal of Clinical Nutrition 89(3): 719-27.

Zielhuis, R. L. and F. W. van der Kreek. 1979. Calculation of a safety factor in setting health based permissible levels for occupational exposure. II. Comparison of extrapolated and published permissible levels. International Archives of Occupational and Environmental Health 42(3-4): 203-15.

7

Dietary Intake Assessment

Conducting an intake assessment—after the available scientific data have allowed the estimation of reference values (see Chapters 5 and 6)—is one of the hallmarks of nutrient risk assessment. Estimates of population intake (i.e., "exposure") are obtained, and these are examined in view of the estimated reference values. When information is available, consideration of biochemical and clinical measures of nutriture is a useful adjunct to the intake assessment and can provide important information about the adequacy of intake as well as excess intake.

In the case of the United States and Canada, data from national government surveys form the basis for the intake assessment. In this chapter, the national surveys are described first. Then information about calcium intake is presented, followed by information about vitamin D intake and serum 25-hydroxyvitamin D (25OHD) concentrations. In this report, the term "dietary intake" includes the intake of foods and supplements and is also referred to as "total intake."

THE NATIONAL SURVEYS AND APPROACH USED

Nutrient intake data for the intake assessment are available through the websites for the national surveys in each country. The U.S. survey data are reported on the basis of Dietary Reference Intake (DRI) life stage groups and are divided by males and females rather than combined. In the case of intake estimates, Canadian data are reported for children ages 1 to 3 and 4 to 8 years without distinction by gender, but they are reported on the basis of males and females for the older groups. Serum 25OHD levels for Canadians are collected for persons between the ages of 6 and 79 years. However, in arranging these data from survey age/sex groups into the DRI life stage groups, sample sizes did not allow adequate representation for children less than 9 years of age. Therefore, the data were used to construct values for the DRI life stage groups only between ages 9 to 79 years for Canadians. In addition, neither country reports data for infants 0 to 12 months of age or for pregnant and lactating women; sample sizes for these groups are too low in the surveys to provide nationally representative estimates.

United States: The National Health and Nutrition Examination Survey

Information about the U.S. National Health and Nutrition Examination Survey (NHANES) is available from the survey's main website,[1] and is therefore only summarized here. In the 1960s, the U.S. government initiated the National Health Examination Survey to assess the health status of individuals ages 6 months through 74 years. Nutritional intake was added as a survey component in the 1970s, beginning with the first NHANES, known as NHANES I (1971 to 1974). NHANES II covered the time period 1976 to 1980, and NHANES IIII encompassed 1988 to 1994. NHANES has reflected a continuous and standardized data collection based on a representative sample of the U.S. population and provides critical diet and health measures for federal program planning and policy making. The survey relies on the gold standard for dietary intake measures, two or more 24-hour dietary recalls per person (IOM, 2000). The U.S. Department of Agriculture's (USDA's) food composition database has provided the sources of information that allow the estimates of food intake collected in the NHANES to be translated into quantitative nutrient intake (Bodner-Montville et al., 2006; Briefel, 2006).

In 1999, the survey became a continuous program that has a changing focus on a variety of health and nutrition measurements to meet emerging needs;[2] the survey data are reported on the basis of 2-year periods. The survey now examines a nationally representative sample of about 5,000 persons each year. These persons are located in counties across the country, 15 of which are visited each year.[3] The NHANES and related food intake surveys conducted by the USDA were integrated in 2002; at that time, the

---

[1]Available online at http://www.cdc.gov/nchs/nhanes.htm (accessed July 23, 2010).

[2]Available online at http://www.cdc.gov/nchs/nhanes/about_nhanes.htm (accessed July 23, 2010).

[3]Available online at http://www.cdc.gov/nchs/nhanes/about_nhanes.htm (accessed July 23, 2010).

dietary reports from the integrated survey became known as What We Eat in America (WWEIA). For this report data for the 2003 to 2004 and 2005 to 2006 period were used because the data for the 2007 and 2008 period did not become available until after the committee had completed its deliberations. Calcium intake has been estimated since NHANES I. Intakes for vitamin D were first published in 2009 and currently are available for the 2003–2006 survey period. The NHANES is said to "follow the sun" in that the survey is generally conducted in the southern states during the winter months and in the northern states in the summer months.

The NHANES is unique in that it collects and tracks both total intake and health measures in a national sample of Americans, and provides an important aspect of the nation's health monitoring system. As would be expected, total intake estimates are limited by survey respondents' abilities to accurately report foods and amounts consumed and by the accuracy, specificity, and timeliness of the food composition databases linked to foods reported in the survey. Respondents are also prone to under-reporting intake (IOM, 2000). Issues related to estimation of usual intake from WWEIA-NHANES have been reviewed by others (Dwyer et al., 2003), including the challenges of updating food composition tables and addressing the under-reporting of intake amounts by participants.

In the case of nutrient intake data for the United States, calcium and vitamin D intake estimates from the WWEIA report series[4] have formed the basis of an expanded analysis conducted and made available by the National Cancer Institute (NCI) of the National Institutes of Health. The NCI analysis was used in this report, as described below.

Intake Estimates for Calcium and Vitamin D

The USDA has produced the Vitamin D Addendum to the USDA Food and Nutrient Database for Dietary Studies 3.0,[5] and in turn WWEIA reported the vitamin D intake from foods as well as calcium intake from foods.[6] The expanded analysis carried out by NCI has allowed the incorporation of estimates of intake from dietary supplements collected as part of the NHANES but not included in the WWEIA reports, thereby providing an estimate of total calcium and vitamin D intake. Calcium intake data were available for the entire period 2003 to 2006 for the United States. However, although the USDA released vitamin D intake data for the 2003 to 2006

---

[4]Available online at http://www.ars.usda.gov/Services/docs.htm?docid=13793 (accessed July 23, 2010).

[5]Available online at http://www.ars.usda.gov/Services/docs.htm?docid=18807 (accessed July 23, 2010).

[6]Available online at http://www.ars.usda.gov/Services/docs.htm?docid=18349 (accessed July 23, 2010).

period in July 2010, vitamin D intake data at the time of the NCI analysis were available only for 2005 to 2006. Therefore, the calcium and vitamin D intake data used in this report reflect overlapping, but not identical, time periods.

Given that there is considerable interest in estimates of total calcium intake and total vitamin D intake from all sources (i.e., foods and supplements), and data on total intake provide the best basis for DRI assessments, the committee relied on the expanded analysis of the NHANES data conducted by NCI and reported by Bailey et al. (2010).[7] Detailed information provided to the committee by NCI staff appears in Appendix H. The related methodologies have been described in detail by Bailey et al. (2010) and provide the opportunity to take into account sources of calcium and vitamin D from supplements.

As described in Bailey et al. (2010), the intake estimates for calcium and vitamin D derived through the NCI method will vary slightly (i.e., by less than 1 percent) from those that appear in the WWEIA. This is because the NCI method uses supplement intake as a covariate in the model for nutrient intake from foods, and because—relative to obtaining usual intake percentiles—a shrinkage estimator approach was incorporated into the analysis rather than a Monte Carlo approach.

Serum 25OHD Concentrations

Measures of serum 25OHD concentrations among survey participants are relevant to the process of a dietary intake assessment in that, whenever possible, the assessment should consider biological parameters thereby basing the assessment on the totality of the evidence and not on intake from foods and supplements alone (IOM, 2000). Also, intake from foods and supplements can often be under-reported by survey participants (IOM, 2000). Analysis of serum 25OHD concentrations has been a component of the NHANES survey since NHANES III. The laboratory methodologies are described on the related website.[8] In 2009, the Centers for Disease Control and Prevention (CDC) posted an Analytical Note[9] regarding the analysis of serum 25OHD levels. Users were cautioned about making direct comparisons between values from NHANES 2000 to 2006 and values obtained in NHANES III. Further, it was noted that serum 25OHD data from the 2000 to 2006 surveys were likely affected by drifts in the assay performance

---

[7]In addition, the study authors provided tables of intakes arrayed for percentile groupings. These have been made available in the Institute of Medicine public access file available at http://www8.nationalacademies.org/cp/.

[8]Available online at http://www.cdc.gov/nchs/data/nhanes/nhanes_09_10/labcompf.pdf (accessed July 23, 2010).

[9]Available online at http://www.cdc.gov/nchs/nhanes.htm (accessed July 23, 2010).

(method bias and imprecision) over time. For this reason, the committee used serum 25OHD levels that had been adjusted for this assay drift and posted on the agency's website. This assay drift was discussed in Chapter 3.

Canada: Canadian Health Measures Survey and Canadian Community Health Survey

Data relevant to the Canadian intake of calcium and vitamin D from foods, as well as measures of serum 25OHD concentrations[10] for a representative sample of Canadians, are available from national surveys conducted by the Government of Canada. These are described below.

Intake Estimates for Calcium and Vitamin D

The Canadian Community Health Survey (CCHS) began in 2000, with the goal of providing population-level information on health determinants, health status, and health system utilization.[11] The survey series is a joint effort among Health Canada, Statistics Canada, and the Canadian Institute for Health Information. The CCHS, a nationally representative cross–sectional survey, that operated on a 2-year data collection cycle from 2000 to 2007, and now operates on an ongoing basis, comprises two types of surveys. The first is a general health survey that takes place in the first year of the cycle (i.e., Cycle 1.1, 2.1, etc.). It samples approximately 130,000 Canadians and provides information at the level of regional health units within each province. The second is a focused topic survey that until 2007 took place in the second year of each cycle (i.e., Cycle 1.2, 2.2, etc.), and now takes place every 3 years. It samples approximately 35,000 Canadians, providing information at the national and provincial levels. The focused topic for CCHS 2004 was a food consumption survey and was designed to estimate the distribution of usual total intake in terms of foods, food groups, dietary supplements, nutrients, and eating patterns among a representative sample of Canadians at the national and provincial levels using the same 24-hour recall methodology used in the NHANES. The data from CCHS 2004 were disseminated in three separate releases between 2005 and 2008 (and revised February 2009). The data reflect nutrient intakes from foods only; information on the quantitative contributions from supplement use is not available at this time, but data on the frequency of general supplement use have been collected. Survey methodologies are described

---

[10] These measures reflect plasma 25OHD concentrations in the case of the Canadian survey data, but for the purposes of this report they are described as serum 25OHD concentrations.
[11] Available online at http://www.hc-sc.gc.ca/fn-an/surveill/index-eng.php (accessed July 23, 2010).

online.[12] The food composition data used to estimate the nutrient values of the foods consumed are provided by the Canadian Nutrient File (CNF). This database reports the average nutritional values for foods available in Canada. According to the CNF documentation,[13] many of the data in the CNF have been derived from the USDA data base because these foods are available on the Canadian market. Canadian modifications included in the CNF consist of levels of fortification and regulatory standards specific to Canada and certain foods that are unique to the Canadian food supply.

Serum 25OHD Concentrations

Serum 25OHD concentrations have been measured and reported as part of the Canadian Health Measures Survey (CHMS). The CHMS, which was initiated in 2007, collects blood and urine for analysis and also carries out direct physical measurements of blood pressure, height, and weight. Those surveyed are persons 6 through 79 years of age and reflect approximately 97 percent of the population. Participants are those living in privately occupied dwellings in the 10 provinces and the 3 territories; persons living on Indian (First Nation) reserves or Crown land, as well as residents of institutions are excluded. Descriptions of sampling, data sources, error detection, quality evaluation, and laboratory methods can be found online.[14] The currently available data are from the 2007 to 2009 time period and can be accessed online.[15]

Approach Used

An earlier IOM committee addressed applications of the DRIs in dietary assessment and described statistical approaches to estimating the prevalence of inadequate intakes, specifically the probability approach and a shortcut to the probability approach called the Estimated Average Requirement (EAR) cut-point method (IOM, 2000). These approaches are based on a distribution of usual intakes, and by definition the prevalence of inadequate intakes for a group is the *proportion* of the group with intakes below the median requirement (or EAR). The 2000 IOM report also points out that it is inappropriate to compare usual nutrient intakes with the

---

[12]Available online at http://www.statcan.gc.ca/cgi-bin/imdb/p2SV.pl?Function=getSurvey &SDDS=5049&lang=en&db=imdb&adm=8&dis=2#a2 (accessed July 23, 2010).

[13]Available online at http://www.hc-sc.gc.ca/fn-an/nutrition/fiche-nutri-data/user_guide _d_utilisation02-eng.php (accessed July 23, 2010).

[14]Available online at http://www.statcan.gc.ca/cgi-bin/imdb/p2SV.pl?Function=getSurvey &SDDS=5071&lang=en&db=imdb&adm=8&dis=2#b3 (accessed July 23, 2010).

[15]Available online at http://www.statcan.gc.ca/pub/82-623-x/2010002/part-partie1-eng. htm (accessed July 23, 2010).

Recommended Dietary Allowance (RDA), because this approach will lead to estimates of inadequacy that are too large.

Based on the 2000 IOM report cited above (IOM, 2000), whenever possible, the assessment of apparent dietary adequacy should consider relevant biological parameters. In the case of vitamin D, an important biological parameter reflective of dietary exposure—serum 25OHD concentrations—was available and could be compared to values that the committee estimated to be approximately equivalent to an EAR or an RDA. However, the existing statistical models provided in the 2000 IOM report (IOM, 2000) address only dietary intake data and do not provide a basis for considering a biological parameter such as serum measures in order to specify the prevalence of inadequate intakes in population groups. Further, the apparent discrepancy between the intake data for vitamin D, as described below, and the biological parameter was also concerning and decreased the confidence in the appropriateness of estimating prevalence of inadequacy based on a distribution of vitamin D intakes. Therefore, a descriptive rather than an analytical approach is used for the vitamin D intake assessment.

CALCIUM INTAKE

As presented in Chapters 5 and 6, the Estimated Average Requirements (EARs), Recommended Dietary Allowances (RDAs), Adequate Intakes (AIs), and Tolerable Upper Intake Levels (ULs) for calcium are summarized in Table 7-1. The intake assessment takes into account these reference values.

U.S. Calcium Intake

Estimated calcium intakes from food sources only, by intake percentile groups, are shown as bar graphs in Figure 7-1. The prevalence of dietary inadequacy for a group can be estimated by the proportion of the group with intakes less than the EAR (IOM, 2000). The 5th percentile of intake for children 1 to 3 years of age is approximately equal to their EAR of 500 mg/day, implying a low prevalence of inadequacy (less than 5 percent). However, for all other age and gender groups of children, the prevalence is at least 25 percent, because intake at the 25th percentile is below the EAR. For adults, the prevalence of inadequacy from food sources alone is high.

As shown in Figure 7-2, the addition of information about calcium intake from supplements to the data set, thereby allowing an estimate of total intake, appears to impact primarily women over 50 years of age. All life stage groups show a slight increase when supplements are taken into account, but women 51 to 70 years of age demonstrate an estimated median total calcium intake (i.e., from foods plus supplements) of 1,044 mg/

TABLE 7-1 Calcium Dietary Reference Intakes by Life Stage (amount/day)

Life Stage Group	AI	EAR	RDA	UL
Infants				
0 to 6 mo	200 mg	—	—	1,000 mg
6 to 12 mo	260 mg	—	—	1,500 mg
Children				
1–3 y	—	500 mg	700 mg	2,500 mg
4–8 y	—	800 mg	1,000 mg	2,500 mg
Males				
9–13 y	—	1,100 mg	1,300 mg	3,000 mg
14–18 y	—	1,100 mg	1,300 mg	3,000 mg
19–30 y	—	800 mg	1,000 mg	2,500 mg
31–50 y	—	800 mg	1,000 mg	2,500 mg
51–70 y	—	800 mg	1,000 mg	2,000 mg
> 70 y	—	1,000 mg	1,200 mg	2,000 mg
Females				
9–13 y	—	1,100 mg	1,300 mg	3,000 mg
14–18 y	—	1,100 mg	1,300 mg	3,000 mg
19–30 y	—	800 mg	1,000 mg	2,500 mg
31–50 y	—	800 mg	1,000 mg	2,500 mg
51–70 y	—	1,000 mg	1,200 mg	2,000 mg
> 70 y	—	1,000 mg	1,200 mg	2,000 mg
Pregnancy				
14–18 y	—	1,100 mg	1,300 mg	3,000 mg
19–30 y	—	800 mg	1,000 mg	2,500 mg
31–50 y	—	800 mg	1,000 mg	2,500 mg
Lactation				
14–18 y	—	1,100 mg	1,300 mg	3,000 mg
19–30 y	—	800 mg	1,000 mg	2,500 mg
31–50 y	—	800 mg	1,000 mg	2,500 mg

NOTE: AI = Adequate Intake; EAR = Estimated Average Requirement; RDA = Recommended Dietary Allowance; UL = Tolerable Upper Intake Level.

day compared with 755 mg/day from foods alone, while median intake for women more than 70 years of age was 983 mg/day compared to 706 mg/day without supplements. Thus, when intake from supplements is considered, the prevalence of dietary inadequacy for older women is approximately 50 percent (i.e., intake at the 50th percentile is approximately equal to the EAR of 1,000 mg/day calcium in Figure 7-2, Panel B).

Total calcium intakes at the 95th percentile are below the UL of 2,000 mg of calcium per day for most of the adult life stage groups, implying that less than 5 percent are at risk of excessive intake. The exception is older women, who have estimated total calcium intakes at the 95th percentile of 2,364 mg/day for those 51 to 70 years of age, and 2, 298 mg/day for those more than 70 years of age, so more than 5 percent are at risk of excessive

Panel A:
Persons 1–18 y

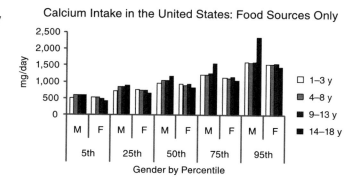

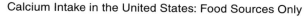

Panel B:
Persons 19+ y

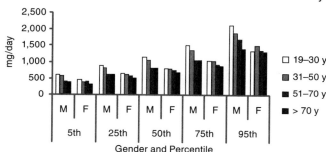

FIGURE 7-1 Estimated calcium intakes in the United States from food sources only, by intake percentile groups, age, and gender.
NOTE: F = female; M = male; y = years.
SOURCE: NHANES 2003–2006 as analyzed by Bailey et al. (2010). Data used to create figure can be found in Appendix H.

intakes. By contrast, the 95th percentile of calcium consumption from food sources alone are 1,353 and 1,337 mg/day for these two life stage groups, respectively.

Canadian Calcium Intake

Estimates of calcium intake from foods for Canadians appear to be similar to those reported for the United States, although the median intake drops at a younger age for men, at the 31- to 50-year life stage as compared to the 51- to 70-year life stage in the United States (Figure 7-3). Overall, estimated intakes of calcium from foods in Canada appear to be slightly lower than those reported for the United States. Although differences in survey

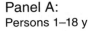

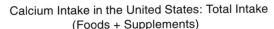

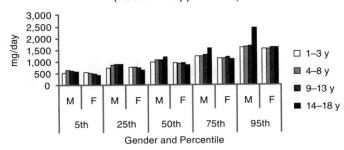

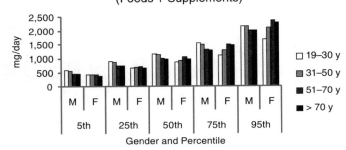

FIGURE 7-2 Estimated total calcium intakes in the United States from food and supplements, by intake percentile groups, age, and gender.
NOTE: F = female; M = male; y = years.
SOURCE: NHANES 2003–2006 as analyzed by Bailey et al. (2010). Data used to create figure can be found in Appendix H.

methodologies could be responsible for some of the difference, the surveys use very similar methodologies and work to ensure uniformity as much as possible. A more likely possibility is that the differences are attributable to food fortification practices. In Canada, calcium may only be added to a limited number of foods. Flour, cornmeal, plant-based beverages, and orange juice may be fortified with calcium, but not breakfast cereals and bread. However, discretionary fortification with calcium is widespread in the United States and can encompass breakfast cereals, breads, and an array of beverages.

At the time of this study, only intake data for foods were available for Canadians; estimates of total calcium intake (i.e., foods plus supplements)

Panel A:
Persons 1–18 y

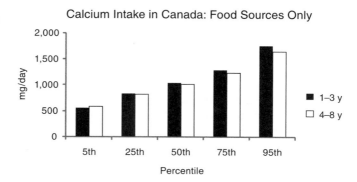

Panel B:
Persons 19–30 y

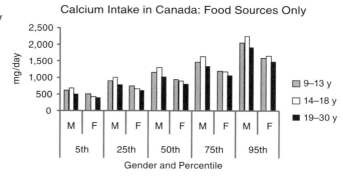

Panel C:
Persons 31+ y

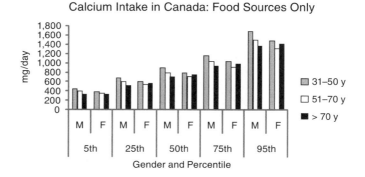

FIGURE 7-3 Estimated calcium intakes in Canada from food sources only, by intake percentile groups, age, and gender.
NOTE: F = female; M = male; y = years.
SOURCE: Statistics Canada, Canadian Community Health Survey (CCHS), Cycle 2.2, Nutrition 2004. Data used to create figure can be found in Appendix H.

had not yet been compiled. After the completion of the study, information on total intake was published (Garriguet, 2010).

VITAMIN D INTAKE AND SERUM 25OHD CONCENTRATIONS

The EARs, RDAs, AIs, and ULs for vitamin D as presented earlier in Chapters 5 and 6 are relevant to the intake assessment discussions and are shown in Table 7-2.

Considerations about the adequacy of vitamin D intake must be interpreted in view of the fact that these reference values assume that no vitamin D is contributed to the human body by sun exposure. Given the unknowns concerning the contribution from sunlight as well as the inability to recommend an acceptable level of sun exposure, this assumption was necessary. However, it confounds interpretation of the intake assessment. If persons are obtaining some vitamin D from sun exposure, they are less likely to be at risk for inadequacy if their intakes are below the reference value. Although the extent to which this may be the case cannot be determined, a concomitant examination of serum 25OHD levels can assist in better describing the assessment. Moreover, as mentioned earlier, it is an appropriate component of the assessment of dietary adequacy (foods and supplements) because, whenever possible, the assessment should consider biological parameters (IOM, 2000).

U.S. Vitamin D Intakes and Serum 25OHD Concentrations

Figure 7-4 shows U.S. vitamin D intake from foods alone. Median vitamin D intake levels for males ranged from 272 to 396 International Units (IU)/day depending upon life stage group. For females, median vitamin D intakes spanned between 160 and 260 IU/day. When intake from supplements is considered to provide total intakes (Figure 7-5), all life stage groups for both male and female Americans show a slight increase in values. The most marked increase is among older women, as was the case for calcium. For women 51 to 70 years of age, median intake of vitamin D from both food and supplements increases to 308 IU/day, compared with vitamin D intake from foods alone, at 140 IU/day. For women more than 70 years of age, the increase in median intake associated with supplement use is an additional 196 IU/day (356 IU with supplements vs. 160 IUs from foods alone).

As shown in Figure 7-5, the 95th percentiles for total vitamin D (foods plus supplements) for males and females range between 568 and 940 IU/day, with both this high and low value found among the female life stage

TABLE 7-2 Vitamin D Dietary Reference Intakes by Life Stage (amount/ day)

Life Stage Group	AI	EAR	RDA	UL
Infants				
0 to 6 mo	400 IU (10 µg)	—	—	1,000 IU (25 µg)
6 to 12 mo	400 IU (10 µg)	—	—	1,500 IU (38 µg)
Children				
1–3 y	—	400 IU (10 µg)	600 IU (15 µg)	2,500 IU (63 µg)
4–8 y	—	400 IU (10 µg)	600 IU (15 µg)	3,000 IU (75 µg)
Males				
9–13 y	—	400 IU (10 µg)	600 IU (15 µg)	4,000 IU (100 µg)
14–18 y	—	400 IU (10 µg)	600 IU (15 µg)	4,000 IU (100 µg)
19–30 y	—	400 IU (10 µg)	600 IU (15 µg)	4,000 IU (100 µg)
31–50 y	—	400 IU (10 µg)	600 IU (15 µg)	4,000 IU (100 µg)
51–70 y	—	400 IU (10 µg)	600 IU (15 µg)	4,000 IU (100 µg)
> 70 y	—	400 IU (10 µg)	800 IU (20 µg)	4,000 IU (100 µg)
Females				
9–13 y	—	400 IU (10 µg)	600 IU (15 µg)	4,000 IU (100 µg)
14–18 y	—	400 IU (10 µg)	600 IU (15 µg)	4,000 IU (100 µg)
19–30 y	—	400 IU (10 µg)	600 IU (15 µg)	4,000 IU (100 µg)
31–50 y	—	400 IU (10 µg)	600 IU (15 µg)	4,000 IU (100 µg)
51–70 y	—	400 IU (10 µg)	600 IU (15 µg)	4,000 IU (100 µg)
> 70 y	—	400 IU (10 µg)	800 IU (20 µg)	4,000 IU (100 µg)
Pregnancy				
14–18 y	—	400 IU (10 µg)	600 IU (15 µg)	4,000 IU (100 µg)
19–30 y	—	400 IU (10 µg)	600 IU (15 µg)	4,000 IU (100 µg)
31–50 y	—	400 IU (10 µg)	600 IU (15 µg)	4,000 IU (100 µg)
Lactation				
14–18 y	—	400 IU (10 µg)	600 IU (15 µg)	4,000 IU (100 µg)
19–30 y	—	400 IU (10 µg)	600 IU (15 µg)	4,000 IU (100 µg)
31–50 y	—	400 IU (10 µg)	600 IU (15 µg)	4,000 IU (100 µg)

NOTE: AI = Adequate Intake; EAR = Estimated Average Requirement; IU = International Units; RDA = Recommended Dietary Allowance; UL = Tolerable Upper Intake Level.

groups. Persons in the 95th percentile for total intake did not appear to exceed the UL for their group.

The comparison between vitamin D intake estimates and serum 25OHD concentrations is worthy of note, but it is important to recognize that this comparison, although interesting, is somewhat problematic because the only possible comparison is based on group means, rather than on data linked to individuals. Moreover, as pointed out previously (IOM, 2000; Dwyer et al., 2003), estimates of intake tend to reflect an underestimation. With these caveats, the comparison is presented in Table 7-3. Shown are the average intakes for the various life stage groups, along with the average serum 25OHD levels for those life stage groups. For this table, serum 25OHD concentration data from the 2005 to 2006 surveys were used rather

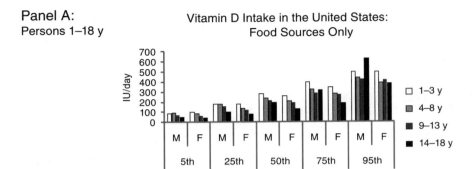

Panel A:
Persons 1–18 y

Panel B:
Persons 19+ y

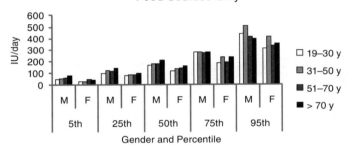

FIGURE 7-4 Estimated vitamin D intakes in the United States from food sources only, by intake percentile groups, age, and gender.
NOTE: F = female; IU = International Units; M = male; y = years.
SOURCE: NHANES 2005–2006 as analyzed by Bailey et al. (2010). Data used to create figure can be found in Appendix H.

than those from the 2003 to 2006 data set because intake estimates for total vitamin D (i.e., the NCI method) are currently available only for the 2005 to 2006 data.

Assuming that a serum 25OHD level of 40 nmol/L is consistent with a desirable median intake,[16] the comparison would suggest that, on average,

---

[16] As discussed in Chapter 5, measures of 27.5 nmol/L in children, and 30 nmol/L in adults remain a level below which frank deficiency including rickets and osteomalacia may be expected to occur. The vitamin D-related bone health needs of approximately one-half of the population may be expected to be met at serum 25OHD concentrations between 30 and 40 nmol/L; most of the remaining members of the population are likely to have vitamin D needs met when serum concentrations between 40 and 50 nmol/L are achieved. Failure to achieve such serum concentrations place persons at greater risk for less than desirable bone

Panel A:
Persons 1–18 y

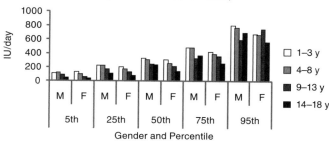

Panel B:
Persons 19+ y

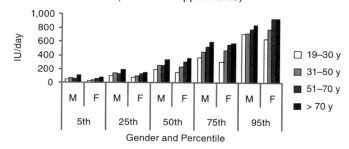

FIGURE 7-5 Estimated total vitamin D intakes in the United States from food and supplements, by intake percentile groups, age, and gender.
NOTE: F = female; IU = International Units; M = male; y = years.
SOURCE: NHANES 2005–2006 as analyzed by Bailey et al. (2010). Data used to create figure can be found in Appendix H.

persons may be experiencing intakes below the reference values, but are exhibiting serum 25OHD levels above 40 nmol/L. In fact, all are above the 50 nmol/L concentration, the level associated with the RDA. There is an additional factor to consider in this comparison, in that the NHANES data are generally collected during the summer months in the northern regions of the United States and in the winter months in the southern regions; this introduces the variable of sun exposure into the comparison in that it decreases the likelihood that individuals surveyed will be experiencing low levels of sun exposure. As an informal conceptual check, it is

---

health as manifested by, depending upon age, rates of bone accretion, bone mineral density, and fractures.

TABLE 7-3 Mean Vitamin D Intake and Mean Serum 25OHD Concentrations for the United States, 2005–2006, by Life Stage Groups

Life Stage Group (years)	Vitamin D Intake (IU/day) Food Alone[a]	Total Intake[b]	Serum 25OHD Levels (nmol/L) Mean[c]	Adjusted for Sun Exposure (Reduced by 1/3)
Males				
1–3	288 ± 8	364 ± 16	71.1 ± 2.0	47
4–8	256 ± 12	372 ± 16	70.5 ± 2.0	47
9–13	228 ± 8	300 ± 28	65.9 ± 2.2	44
14–18	244 ± 16	276 ± 20	60.1 ± 1.9	40
19–30	204 ± 12	264 ± 16	57.9 ± 2.0	38
31–50	216 ± 12	316 ± 12	58.5 ± 1.1	39
51–70	204 ± 12	352 ± 16	57.3 ± 1.8	38
> 70	224 ± 16	428 ± 28	58.9 ± 1.3	39
Females				
1–3	276 ± 16	336 ± 16	71.4 ± 1.9	47
4–8	220 ± 12	316 ± 24	70.5 ± 2.1	47
9–13	212 ± 24	308 ± 40	59.1 ± 1.6	39
14–18	152 ± 8	200 ± 20	57.6 ± 1.9	38
19–30	144 ± 12	232 ± 12	62.7 ± 2.8	41
31–50	176 ± 12	308 ± 20	57.6 ± 1.7	38
51–70	156 ± 16	404 ± 40	57.2 ± 1.5	38
> 70	180 ± 8	400 ± 20	56.5 ± 1.8	37

NOTE: IU = International Units; SE = standard error.
[a]Data are mean ± SE for foods only.
[b]Data are mean ± SE for total intake: foods and dietary supplements.
[c]Data are mean ± SE.
SOURCE: NHANES, 2005–2006; Bailey et al., 2010.

possible to adjust these data so as to roughly simulate a reduction in serum 25OHD levels consistent with the difference between the summer zenith and the winter nadir. Specifically, if the estimate that there is a one-third difference in serum 25OHD levels between the winter nadir and summer zenith as described in Chapter 3 is applied to this comparison, reducing these serum 25OHD levels by one-third results in a range of serum 25OHD levels from a low of 37 nmol/L (women > 70 years) to a high of 47 nmol/L (found in four life stage groups), which are still very close to, and in many cases above, a 40 nmol/L concentration consistent with an estimated average required intake. Given the observation made in Chapter 5 that the seasonal decline during the winter may differ between those with high and low initial baseline values, the correction applied using a 30 percent reduction may overestimate the decline in those at lower baseline 25OHD levels below 50 nmol/L. Moreover, this adjustment is excessive because for those persons living in the southern United States, their serum 25OHD measures were taken generally during the winter, not summer, months; the one-third reduction is therefore an over-correction in this case. However, because it is not possible using the data available to the committee to distinguish between values taken in the summer in northern areas and in the winter in southern areas, the adjustment cannot be further refined.

Although serum 25OHD levels from the 2005 to 2006 period in the United States are the data used for Table 7-3 because total intake data are available only for 2005 to 2006, serum 25OHD levels are available for the 2003 to 2006 data set, the two most current surveys, which, when combined, provide a larger data set. For comparison, these are shown in Table 7-4 and appear to reflect values very similar to those reported for 2005 to 2006 alone. No effort has been made to consider vitamin D intake for this period (2003 to 2006) because only data from the WWEIA are available for 2003 to 2006, which would not provide information on total intake (foods plus supplements).

TABLE 7-4 Mean Serum 25OHD Concentrations for the United States, 2003–2006, by Life Stage Group

Life Stage Group (years)	Mean Serum 25OHD Concentration (nmol/L ± SE)
Males	
1–3	71.8 ± 1.4
4–8	70.6 ± 1.2
9–13	64.7 ± 1.4
14–18	60.3 ± 1.4
19–30	57.2 ± 1.3
31–50	59.3 ± 1.1
51–70	59.9 ± 1.2
> 70	59.1 ± 1.0
Females	
1–3	70.4 ± 1.2
4–8	69.3 ± 1.4
9–13	58.9 ± 1.1
14–18	59.9 ± 1.7
19–30	62.2 ± 1.9
31–50	58.1 ± 1.2
51–70	57.6 ± 1.1
> 70	57.4 ± 1.1

NOTE: SE = standard error.
SOURCE: NHANES, 2003–2006.

Canadian Vitamin D Intakes and Serum 25OHD Concentrations

As previously mentioned, the available Canadian survey data provided information on vitamin D intake from foods alone; quantified information on vitamin D supplement intake among Canadians, and thus on total intake from foods and supplements, was not available at the time of the study. Figure 7-6 outlines the estimated intakes of vitamin D from foods alone, which overall tend to be slightly higher than those reported for the United States. Median vitamin D intakes ranged from a low of 176 IU/day (women 51 to 70 years) to a high of 264 IU/day (boys 9 to 13 years). Similar to the U.S. population, persons in the 95th percentile of intake of vitamin D from foods would be expected to be considerably below the UL for their life stage.

Comparison between mean intakes of vitamin D and mean serum 25OHD concentrations for Canadians is problematic. For Canada, intake estimates are provided for the survey year 2004 based on the CCHS, whereas the serum 25OHD concentrations available reflect data from the 2007 to 2009 CHMS. The mean serum 25OHD levels for Canadians are shown in Table 7-5, and no effort has been made to compare these with intake estimates. As a general matter, average serum 25OHD concentrations of Canadians are above both the 40 and 50 nmol/L concentration levels. Although average intakes of vitamin D among Canadians from foods alone (i.e., not taking into account supplements) are less than the EAR, measures of serum 25OHD levels are well above the 40 nmol/L level consistent with the EAR. Again, as described earlier, the ability to interpret the prevalence of inadequacy based on serum 25OHD concentrations using the methodology as established in the 2000 IOM report (IOM, 2000) is unclear.

DIFFERENCES BETWEEN THE UNITED STATES AND CANADA: NATIONAL SURVEY DATA FOR CALCIUM AND VITAMIN D

All total intake estimates are subject to uncertainties owing to a variety of factors that affect estimates of food intake, ranging from the depth and nature of the probing carried out to obtain the information on food consumption to the ability of persons to accurately recall and estimate their food intake. Overall, the nature and approach of the national surveys in the United States and Canada are notably similar, which suggest that the small differences seen in intake estimates for calcium and vitamin D may reflect true differences in intake.

With respect to vitamin D intake from foods alone, to the extent a comparison is appropriate given that they reflect different periods—2004 for Canada and 2005 to 2006 for the United States—Canadian intakes of

Panel A:
Persons 1–18 y

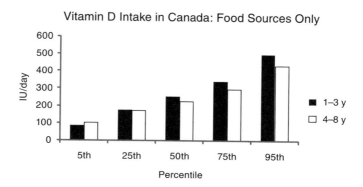

Panel B:
Persons 19–30 y

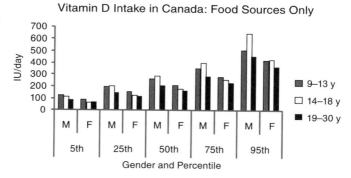

Panel C:
Persons 31+ y

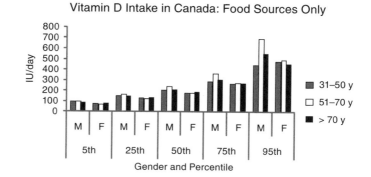

FIGURE 7-6 Estimated vitamin D intakes in Canada from food sources only, by intake percentile groups, age, and gender.

NOTE: F = female; IU = International Units; M = male; y = years.

SOURCE: Statistics Canada, Canadian Community Health Survey (CCHS), Cycle 2.2, Nutrition 2004. Data used to create figure can be found in Appendix H.

TABLE 7-5 Serum 25OHD Levels for Canadians by Percentile Group, Age, and Gender

Life Stage Group (years)	Mean Serum 25OHD Level (nmol/L) (Confidence Interval)
Males	
9–13	73.4 (69.7–77.2)
14–18	65.2 (57.2–73.1)
19–30	62.5 (53.3–71.7)
31–50	61.6 (57.0–66.2)
51–70	69.2 (65.4–73.1)
71–79	73.7 (67.1–80.3)
Females	
9–13	69.5 (63.6–75.5)
14–18	68.6 (63.0–74.2)
19–30	72.5 (67.2–77.9)
31–50	67.1 (63.7–70.4)
51–70	68.9 (66.3–71.5)
71–79	77.8 (72.6–83.0)

SOURCE: Statistics Canada, Canadian Health Measures Survey (CHMS), Cycle 1, 2007–2009.

vitamin D from food sources are somewhat more than those in the United States. This may be due to the Canadian food supply having mandatory fortification of margarine with vitamin D in addition to fortification of milk.

Further, differences in serum 25OHD concentrations between the United States and Canada are evident. The estimates for Canadians are consistently higher than those for the United States. Although differences in the food supply may account for some of these differences, it is noted that the analyses for the Canadian data are based on the use of the "Liaison" kit,[17] whereas the U.S. data are derived from the "DiaSorin RIA" kit.[18] Direct comparison of the two kits within the CHMS laboratory at Health Canada indicates a 6 to 9 percent difference, with the Liaison measuring values higher than the RIA kit.[19] Other researchers have also performed comparisons with various outcomes. The differences may be laboratory-specific because Wagner et al. (2009) found no difference, although data from Carter et al. (2010) suggest a 5 percent bias, with the RIA kit giving higher values. It is notable that the serum 25OHD levels in Canada are not lower than those in the United States, as would be predicted if higher latitudes were responsible for reduced serum 25OHD levels.

Finally, Appendix I contains information about the proportion of per-

[17]DiaSorin Liaison (Stillwater, MN).
[18]DiaSorin Radio-immunoassay (RIA) (Stillwater, MN).
[19]Personal communication, S. Brooks, Health Canada, August 9, 2010.

sons in both countries above or below designated levels of serum 25OHD. These data are included as information for the users of this report and have been provided by the U.S. Centers for Disease Control and Prevention and by Statistics Canada. However, these data were not reviewed by the committee given that the analyses did not take place until after the close of the committee deliberations.

SUMMARY

The intake assessment conducted in this report suggests that calcium remains a nutrient of public health concern in some population groups. Girls 9 to 18 years of age, who have a fairly high requirement for calcium, are clearly falling below desirable intake estimates in both countries when only food sources of calcium are considered, as are women over the age of 50 years. On the other hand, available data from the United States on the total intake of calcium when dietary supplements are considered, suggests that older women on average, at least in the United States, have added to their calcium intakes through supplement use. For girls, the increase in intake that might be attributable to supplement use is small. No life stage groups exceeded the UL for calcium when foods alone were considered. However, when supplement use was taken into account (United States only), those women consuming at the 95th percentile of calcium intake appeared to be at risk for exceeding the UL. This suggests that there may be value in underscoring the need for older girls to modestly increase intake of calcium, and in emphasizing that for older women high intakes from supplements may be concerning.

Due to the desirability of considering biological parameters for intake assessments whenever possible (IOM, 2000), the vitamin D assessment presented some challenges. Although median vitamin D intakes from foods in both countries for all life stage groups were below the EAR of 400 IU/day, these data and any future intake analyses conducted using the IOM methodology (IOM, 2000) should be considered in light of the corresponding serum 25OHD concentrations. However, specific prevalence estimates based on serum values are not provided here because the appropriate application of the IOM methodology outlined in 2000 (IOM, 2000), which is focused on use of dietary intake estimates, is currently unclear and may not be appropriate for use with serum values.

Average serum 25OHD concentrations from the NHANES were well above the 40 nmol/L established as consistent with an intake equivalent to the EAR, although a number of North Americans have serum values below 40 nmol/L. All average values were above 50 nmol/L, the level consistent with an intake equivalent to the RDA. When the U.S. data were "adjusted" to simulate conditions more consistent with winter months, at least in the more northern parts of the United States, mean serum 25OHD levels hovered around 40 nmol/L, consistent with an EAR intake. Further, this adjustment over-corrects because for persons living in southern parts of the United States—where NHANES generally is conducted during the winter months—their serum 25OHD levels are already reflective of winter and are not appropriately corrected from a summer level to a winter level. In the case of data for Canada from the CHMS, the mean serum 25OHD levels for all life stage groups are at or above 60 nmol/L. The fact that they are higher than those for the U.S. population may be in part a function of differences in the assay methods used, although this is not clearly established. If it is assumed that the Canadian values would be 8 percent lower if analyzed using the same methodology that was used in the U.S. survey, then they would then be quite similar to those for the United States, leaving open the question of whether the latitude difference between the two countries has a meaningful impact on serum 25OHD levels.

REFERENCES

Bailey, R. L., K. W. Dodd, J. A. Goldman, J. J. Gahche, J. T. Dwyer, A. J. Moshfegh, C. T. Sempos and M. F. Picciano. 2010. Estimation of total usual calcium and vitamin D intake in the United States. Journal of Nutrition 140(4): 817-22.

Bodner-Montville, J., J. K. C. Ahuja, L. A. Ingwersen, E. S. Haggerty, C. W. Enns and B. P. Perloff. 2006. USDA Food and Nutrient Database for Dietary Studies: Released on the web. Journal of Food Composition and Analysis 19(Suppl 1): S100-7.

Briefel, R. R. 2006. Nutrition monitoring in the United States. In Present Knowledge in Nutrition, 9th Edition, Volume II, edited by B. A. Bowman and R. M. Russell. Washington, DC: ILSI. Pp. 838-58.

Carter, G. D., J. L. Berry, E. Gunter, G. Jones, J. C. Jones, H. L. Makin, S. Sufi and M. J. Wheeler. 2010. Proficiency testing of 25-hydroxyvitamin D (25-OHD) assays. Journal of Steroid Biochemistry and Molecular Biology 121(1-2): 176-9.

Dwyer, J., M. F. Picciano and D. J. Raiten. 2003. Estimation of usual intakes: what we eat in America-NHANES. Journal of Nutrition 133(2): 609S-23S.

Garriguet, D. 2010. Combining nutrient intake from food/beverages and vitamin/mineral supplements. Health Reports, Statistics Canada, Catalogue no. 82-003-XPE 21(4): 1-15.

IOM (Institute of Medicine). 2000. Dietary Reference Intakes: Applications in Dietary Assessment. Washington, DC: National Academy Press.

Wagner, D., H. E. C. Hanwell and R. Vieth. 2009. An evaluation of automated methods for measurement of serum 25-hydroxyvitamin D. Clinical Biochemistry 42(15): 1549-56.

8

Implications and Special Concerns

The last step in the risk assessment process is the step of so-called risk characterization. Its intent is to highlight the nature of the "risks" or public health problems that are relevant to the use of Dietary Reference Intakes (DRIs) and to alert users of the DRI reference values to implications of the assessors' work and to related special issues. This chapter reflects the risk characterization step of the risk assessment approach and is organized to provide: a brief summary of the assessment; discussions about the implications of the committee's work for stakeholders; and discussions to highlight population segments and conditions of interest relative to calcium and vitamin D nutriture.

SUMMARY OF ASSESSMENT

The new DRIs establish, for the first time, an Estimated Average Requirement (EAR) and a Recommended Dietary Allowance (RDA) for calcium and vitamin D. Previously, the DRIs for these nutrients reflected Adequate Intakes (AIs). The ability to set EARs and RDAs rather than AIs enhances the utility of the reference values for national planning and assessment activities. It is important to recognize that these values are intended for the North American population, and also that the requirement for each nutrient is based on the assumption that the requirement for the other nutrient is being met.

Considerable effort was made to ensure that an array of indicators was examined as a possible basis for setting requirements, as well as upper levels of intake. The intent was to fully and objectively examine the scientific basis for the suggested benefit before drawing conclusions. Despite the many claims of benefit surrounding vitamin D in particular, the evidence did not support a basis for a causal relationship between vitamin D and many of the numerous health outcomes purported to be affected by vitamin D intake. Although the current interest in vitamin D as a nutrient with broad and expanded benefits is understandable, it is not supported by the available evidence. The established function of vitamin D remains that of ensuring bone health, for which causal evidence across the life stages exists and has grown since the 1997 DRIs were established (IOM, 1997). The conclusion that there is not sufficient evidence to establish a relationship between vitamin D and health outcomes other than bone health does not mean that future research will not reveal a compelling relationship between vitamin D and another health outcome. The question is open as to whether other relationships may be revealed in the future.

Of great concern recently have been the reports of widespread vitamin D deficiency in the North American population. Based on this committee's work and as discussed below, the concern is not well founded. In fact, the cut-point values used to define deficiency, or as some have suggested, "insufficiency," have not been established systematically using data from studies of good quality. Nor have values to be used for such determinations been agreed upon by consensus within the scientific community. When higher cut-point values are used compared with those used in the past, they necessarily result in a larger proportion of the population falling below the cut-point value and thereby defined as deficient. This, in turn, leads to higher estimations of the prevalence of deficiency among the population and possibly to unnecessary intervention incorporating high-dose supplementation in the health care of individuals. National survey data suggest that the serum 25-hydroxyvitamin D (25OHD) levels in the North American population generally exceed the levels identified in this report as sufficient for bone health, underscoring the inability to conclude that there are significant levels of deficiency in the population.

Specifically in terms of the new DRIs and challenges for calcium and vitamin D nutriture, several points can be highlighted, within the context of the limitations of estimates of dietary intake, which tend to be underestimates of actual consumption. First, for calcium, adolescent girls continue to be a group at risk for low intakes from food sources. Older women use calcium supplements in greater proportion, and some may be at risk for excess intake as a result of the use of high-dose supplements. If supplements are needed to ensure adequate calcium intake, it would appear that lower dose supplements should be considered. Many older women have baseline calcium intakes that are close to or just below requirements, and therefore the practice of calcium supplementation at high levels may be unnecessary. This is a special concern for calcium supplement use given the possibility that total intakes (diet plus supplements) above 2,000 mg/ day may increase the risk for kidney stones, and demonstrate no increase in benefits relative to bone health. There is also some limited evidence that the long-term use of calcium supplements may increase the risk for cardiovascular disease. Although no attempt was made to compare systematically the data used for the North American population that is the subject of this report with data from other countries focused on persons who are genetically and environmentally different from those in the United States and Canada, it should be recognized that calcium requirements may be subject to a variety of factors that have not yet been fully elucidated and so therefore cannot yet be integrated into DRI reviews.

For vitamin D, the challenges introduced by issues of sun exposure cannot be ignored. This nutrient is unique in that it functions as a pro-hormone, and the body has the capacity to synthesize the nutrient if sun exposure is adequate. However, concerns about skin cancer risk preclude making recommendations about sun exposure; in any case, there are a number of unknowns surrounding the effects of sun exposure on vitamin D synthesis. At this time, the only solution when DRIs are to be set for vitamin D is to proceed on the basis of an assumption of minimal sun exposure and set a reference value assuming that all of the vitamin D must come from the diet. Moreover, the possibility of risk for persons typically of concern because of reduced synthesis of vitamin D, such as persons with dark skin or older persons in institutions, is minimized given the assumption of minimal sun exposure for the DRIs.

One unknown in the process of DRI development for vitamin D is the degree to which waning kidney function with aging may be relevant. It appears that increasing serum 25OHD levels do not typically increase calcitriol levels in aging persons with mild renal insufficiency, and a dietary strategy to address the concern is not evident.

Although ensuring adequacy is important, there is now an emerging issue of excess vitamin D intakes. A congruence of diverse data on health outcomes ranging from all-cause mortality to cardiovascular risk suggests that adverse health outcomes may be associated with vitamin D intakes that are much lower than those classically associated with hypervitaminosis D and that appear to occur at serum 25OHD levels achievable through current levels of supplement use.

IMPLICATIONS

The extensive review of the data required to conduct this study and to determine DRIs for calcium and vitamin D that are consistent with existing scientific understandings has answered many questions. But, the process has also identified or left unanswered other questions due to the limitations of the available evidence. Because uncertainties exist in the knowledge base related to the role of vitamin D and calcium in health outcomes, it is important to acknowledge that there are uncertainties surrounding these reference values for calcium and vitamin D. The development of any reference value should be viewed as a work in progress, which may be subject to change if there are significant changes in the science base.

Further, an important aspect of DRI development is its grounding in public health applications and the concept of distributions of risk. This approach may appear strange to some and may be disconcerting to those with a clinical orientation who are familiar with the medical model in which the goal is to treat the patient in the most efficacious manner to enhance a positive outcome. The interpretation and use of data in the case of DRI development are within the context of the relevant probability distributions of risk; the DRI task focuses on median requirements and the description of risk, whereas the medical model is based on maximizing effects that ensure beneficial outcomes for all persons. This report, therefore in contrast to a medical model approach, determines dose–response relationships by assessing the level at which 50 percent of the population's needs are met (the EAR) and the level at which approximately 97.5 percent of the population are likely to have their needs met (the RDA). The distribution of dose–response effects is highly relevant to DRI development, compared with information about a maximizing effect for benefit. A difficulty the committee too often faced was studies that included only a placebo or baseline low dose coupled with a relatively large, single supplemental dose, as these are relatively uninformative for DRI development.

Discussions below call attention to the uncertainties surrounding the DRI values for calcium and vitamin D and also highlight important conclusions that stem from the process of developing these DRIs. In addition, given that this report is the first effort to develop DRIs since the 2007 IOM workshop that explored lessons learned and new challenges and outlined the risk assessment approach for DRI development (IOM, 2008; Taylor, 2008), comments are offered about the process. Specific research recommendations for the future development of DRIs related to calcium and vitamin D are presented in Chapter 9.

Assumption of Minimal Sun Exposure

The committee's assumption of minimal sun exposure is a markedly cautious approach given that the vast majority of North Americans appear to obtain at least some vitamin D from inadvertent or deliberate sun exposure. Currently, there is a lack of information about whether certain levels of sun exposure may be experienced without increased risk of cancer and whether such exposure would be consistent with a contribution of vitamin

D useful to the body. Therefore, at this time, recommendations concerning sun exposure relative to vitamin D requirements cannot and should not be offered; there are no options other than to base dietary recommendations on the assumption of minimal sun exposure. The evidence to indicate that the synthesis of vitamin D from sun exposure is subject to a feedback loop that precludes toxicity from sun exposure is reassuring and, when coupled with the checks and balances introduced into the DRI development process, makes it very unlikely that consumption of the DRI levels of vitamin D, even if combined with high levels of sun exposure, will be problematic to the general population.

However, given that many North Americans appear to obtain at least some vitamin D from inadvertent or deliberate sun exposure, there are implications for the interpretation of intake levels of the vitamin. In short, the intake data for vitamin D cannot stand alone as a basis for public health action on a national population level. Such considerations are consistent with the 2000 IOM report on applications of DRIs in dietary assessment (IOM, 2000), which states: "Whenever possible, the assessment of apparent dietary adequacy should consider biological parameters such as anthropometry, ... biochemical indices, ... diagnoses, ... clinical status, and other factors as well as diet. Dietary adequacy should be assessed and diet plans formulated based on the totality of the evidence, not on dietary intake data alone." In short, for policy making and decisions about the adequacy of the food supply for the general population at the national level, vitamin D must be considered in the context of measures of serum 25OHD, an established biomarker of exposure from endogenous synthesis as well as diet, including supplements. Although the reported estimates of vitamin D intake appear to be less than needed to meet requirements, the serum 25OHD data available—when coupled with the committee's assessment of serum 25OHD levels consistent with EAR and RDA values—suggest that average requirements are being met for the DRI age groups nationally in both countries. That is, although mean total intakes of vitamin D generally are lower than the estimated median requirement (the EAR), the available clinical measures do not suggest widespread deficiency states. This underscores the possibility that sun exposure is contributing generally to the maintenance of adequate serum 25OHD concentrations.

Uncertainties

As discussed in the preceding chapters, there are limited data for many topics of interest in setting DRI values for calcium and vitamin D. Overall, the uncertainties surrounding the DRI values for calcium are less than those for vitamin D, because the evidence base is considerably larger for calcium, and the physiology and metabolism of calcium are better understood. The following key issues were identified by the committee as introducing uncertainty into the DRI values for calcium and vitamin D, as based on bone health outcomes:

- The tendency for study protocols to administer a combination of calcium and vitamin D, reducing the opportunity to ascertain the effects of each nutrient independently;
- The lack of data examining the responses and health outcomes due to graded doses of calcium or vitamin D intake so as to elucidate dose–response relationships;
- The interaction between calcium and vitamin D to the extent that it would appear that adequate calcium intake greatly diminishes the need for vitamin D relative to bone health outcomes;
- The unique situation in which a nutrient (vitamin D) physiologically serves as a prohormone introduced a myriad of variables and feedback loops related to its health effects;
- The paucity of data and resulting uncertainty concerning sun exposure that confound interpretation of the dose–response relationship between intakes of vitamin D and various health outcomes. This, coupled with the apparent contribution of sun exposure to overall vitamin D nutriture in North American populations, leads to an inability to characterize and integrate sun exposure with intake recommendations as much as may be appropriate, given the concern for skin cancer risk reduction, which must be paramount. Thus, for individuals who do not follow recommendations to avoid sun exposure, the uncertainty of the DRI values is greater than for those who do;
- The lack of clarity concerning the validity of the serum 25OHD measure as a biomarker of effect;
- The variability surrounding measures of serum 25OHD concentrations as a result of different methodologies used;
- A number of findings suggesting a strong role for metabolic adaptations and controls in the case of vitamin D, which complicates estimations of nutrient requirements. These include: the non-linear response of serum 25OHD level to vitamin D intake, which, in turn, suggests that it requires proportionately more vitamin D to continue to increase serum 25OHD levels after a certain serum 25OHD level is reached; the observation that seasonal declines in serum 25OHD level are greater if a person begins the winter season with a higher compared with a lower serum 25OHD level; and the lack of effect of age and body size (other than adiposity) on serum 25OHD levels;

- The limited number of long-term clinical trials related to calcium and vitamin D intakes and health outcomes; and
- The need to set ULs based on limited data in order to ensure public health protection.

An important question that will undoubtedly be asked given this committee's report, is: Why is it that so much information about the positive effects of vitamin D on outcomes such as cancer, diabetes, and immunity is said to exist and is reported almost daily in the press, but this committee found no basis to support these causal relationships? The short answer is that a systematic examination of the evidence, using established guidelines for measuring the strength and quality of studies, revealed that the claimed benefits based on the associations of low or high intakes of vitamin D on non-skeletal health outcomes could not be supported by the studies—the evidence was inconsistent and/or conflicting or did not demonstrate causality. In addition, some effects were not related to setting nutritional requirements for vitamin D. This conclusion, however, does not preclude pursuing investigation of causal relationships.

Moreover, a related question that will be asked is: With the advent of newer studies, why is there still so much uncertainty? At least one reason is that most studies were not designed to seek data maximally useful for DRI development, which is well described by others (Yetley et al., 2009). DRI development fundamentally requires elucidation of dose–response relationships and benefits from data of high quality obtained in randomized controlled trials. In making its conclusions about potential indicators other than bone health, the committee noted the findings previously specified by an IOM committee tasked with examining the evolution of evidence for nutrient and disease relationships (IOM, 2002). That committee concluded that evidence about relationships between specific nutrients and a disease or health outcome typically remains elusive for a number of reasons (IOM, 2002). These include the following:

- Although preliminary evidence, usually from mechanistic studies, experimental animal studies, and observational studies in humans, can generate exciting new hypotheses about nutrient–health relationships, evidence from these studies has limitations. For instance, even in well-designed, large-scale observational studies, it is difficult to isolate the effects of a single nutrient under investigation from the confounding effects of other nutrients and from non-nutrient factors.
- Scientific advances in understanding relationships between specific nutrients and health outcomes do not necessarily emerge

within a short time, and progress is often erratic. Some gaps are filled, while others are created.

- The etiology of disease–health relationships, especially in the case of chronic disease, is commonly multi-factorial. Even if diet has a prominent role, it is extremely unlikely that a single nutrient is directly responsible for a chronic disease or, conversely, that addition of a single nutrient will eliminate disease risk. It is possible that a focus on specific nutrients as risk factors for diseases in relatively homogeneous or diseased populations can lead to a number of spurious associations.

- Clinical trials, which are generally considered to provide the strongest evidence about the effects of nutrient intake on subsequent disease and health, are complex, expensive, and time-consuming, especially for chronic diseases that develop over decades and are influenced by a host of genetic, physiological, and environmental factors that may also affect risk.

The committee found all of the above findings to be the case for non-skeletal health outcomes for vitamin D, as the discussions of the strength, consistency, and causality of the evidence demonstrate in Chapter 4.

Finally, an important uncertainty focuses on the issue of excess intake. This is particularly true for vitamin D, which has been hypothesized to confer health benefits at relatively high levels of intake. Although the committee's decisions for the ULs made use of emerging data concerning a U-shaped (or perhaps reverse-J-shaped) curve for risk, which suggested adverse effects at levels much lower than those associated with hypervitaminosis D, the lack of data on the safety of higher intakes of vitamin D when used chronically is very concerning. Byers (2010), in a recent editorial commenting on the outcomes of a pooling study focused on vitamin D and six types of cancer in which the only association observed was a doubling of the risk for pancreatic cancer for those in the highest quintile of circulating serum 25OHD levels, offered the following observation: "We have learned some hard lessons…. and we now know that taking vitamins in supernutritional doses can cause serious harm."

Conclusions About Vitamin D Deficiency in the United States and Canada

Serum 25OHD levels have been used as a "measure of adequacy" for vitamin D, as they reflect intake from the diet coupled with the amount contributed by cutaneous synthesis. The cut-point levels of serum 25OHD intended to specify deficiency and sufficiency for the purposes of interpreting laboratory analyses and for use in clinical practice are not specifically within the charge to this committee. However, the committee notes with some concern that serum 25OHD cut-points defined as indicative of deficiency (or as reported by some, "insufficient") for vitamin D have been subject to a wide variation in specification without a systematic, evidence-based consensus development process. In order to ensure clarity, the discussion in this section expresses serum 25OHD levels in both nmol/L and ng/mL measures.

From this committee's perspective, a considerable over-estimation of the levels of vitamin D deficiency in the North American population now exists due to the use by some of cut-points for serum 25OHD levels that greatly exceed the levels identified in this report as consistent with the available data. The 1997 IOM report (IOM, 1997) specified a serum 25OHD concentration of 27.5 nmol/L (11 ng/mL) and above as an indicator of vitamin D adequacy from birth through 18 years of age, and a concentration of 30 nmol/L (12 ng/mL) and above as an indicator of vitamin D adequacy for adults. This level (27.5 nmol/L for children, and 30.0 nmol/L for adults) remains a level below which frank deficiency including rickets and osteomalacia may be expected to occur. In recent years, others have suggested different cut-point values as determinants of deficiency (or "insufficiency"). These include values ranging from less than 50 nmol/L (20 ng/mL) to values above 125 nmol/L (50 ng/mL). Based on this committee's deliberations, the vitamin D–related bone health needs of approximately one-half of the population may be expected to be met at serum 25OHD concentrations between 30 and 40 nmol/L (12 and 16 ng/mL); most of the remaining members of the population are likely to have vitamin D needs met when serum concentrations between 40 and 50 nmol/L (16 and 20 ng/mL) are achieved. Failure to achieve such serum concentrations place persons at greater risk for less than desirable bone health as manifested by, depending upon age, increased rates of bone accretion, bone mineral density, and fractures.

Use of higher than appropriate cut-points for serum 25OHD levels would be expected to artificially increase the estimates of the prevalence of vitamin D deficiency. The specification of cut-point values for serum 25OHD levels has serious ramifications not only for the conclusions about vitamin D nutriture and nutrition public policy, but also for clinical practice. At this time, there is no central body that is responsible for establishing such values for clinical use. This committee's review of data suggests that persons are at risk of deficiency at serum 25OHD levels of below 30 nmol/L (12 ng/mL). Some, but not all, persons are potentially at risk for inadequacy at serum 25OHD levels from 30 up to 50 nmol/L (12 to < 20 ng/mL). Practically all persons are sufficient at levels of 50 nmol/L (20 ng/mL) and above. Serum concentrations of 25OHD above 75 nmol/L (30 ng/mL) are not associated with increased benefit. There may be reason for concern at serum 25OHD levels above 125 nmol/L (50 ng/mL). Given the concern about high serum 25OHD levels as well as the desirability of avoiding mis-classification of vitamin D deficiency, there is a critical public health and clinical practice need for consensus cut-points for serum 25OHD. The current lack of evidence-based consensus guidelines is problematic and of concern because individuals with levels of 25OHD serum above 50 nmol/L (20 ng/mL) may at times be diagnosed as deficient and treated with high-dose supplements of vitamin D containing many times the levels of intake outlined in this report.

Decisions Regarding Levels of Calcium and Vitamin D to Be Administered in Controlled Clinical Trials

Although this report identifies upper levels of intake below which adverse effects are not expected to arise, ULs are intended to serve as a lifetime public health measure for a free-living, unmonitored population. Those responsible for determining the appropriate dosages of nutrients to be studied in carefully controlled experimental trials conducted with appropriate adverse event and safety monitoring have the opportunity to bring other considerations into play when deciding on the levels of nutrients that are acceptable and appropriate for subjects taking part and being monitored in such studies. Research using intakes higher than those specified in the ULs can be justified under a number of circumstances after careful review of the literature and through the use of appropriate study protocols. Indeed, such studies are likely to be informative to the understanding of dose–response relationships and the health benefits or risks associated with calcium and vitamin D intakes.

The DRI Development Process

As described in Chapter 1, the DRI development process has recently been subjected to a review as well as targeted discussions about the process and ways to enhance it (IOM, 2008). As an overall result of these discussions, DRI development is now placed more clearly in the context of the risk assessment approach—that is, an organizing framework for conducting evaluations with public health implications often made with evidentiary uncertainties. There is also a series of existing "gap issues"—specifically, needed methodologies and guidelines—that have been identified as important to improving and enhancing the process for developing DRIs and would benefit from targeted efforts to resolve the gaps (Taylor, 2008).

The report of this committee is the first DRI report to be completed subsequent to the 2004 to 2008 evaluation of the DRI development process. It has been structured to be consistent with the risk assessment process with the intent of enhancing its transparency, especially in the face of uncertainties. Although this committee was mindful of the identified methodological gaps for enhancing the DRI process, it was not tasked with addressing them; in any case, virtually all of the relevant issues are complex and suggest a need to convene groups of individuals with specific expertise germane to the question at hand. Because this DRI report is an initial effort to set DRI development on the path of a risk assessment approach, its experience points to the importance of addressing several gap issues. Specifically:

- The identification of dose–response relationships for calcium and vitamin D relative to health outcomes was a major challenge. The gap issue[1] (number 5-5 in Taylor, 2008) that is focused on methodologies for approximating dose–response relationships warrants attention, as it is likely that DRI efforts in the future will face the same challenges.
- With the exception of the inclusion of osteoporosis within the bone health measures, the existing data precluded the use of a chronic disease such as cancer or heart disease as an indicator for DRI development. However, had it been possible, this DRI process would have benefited from guidelines specifying what, if any, differences may apply to using chronic disease endpoints versus other types of endpoints for DRI development (gap issue number 4-4[2] in Taylor, 2008).
- In the committee's judgment, sufficient new data were available to allow the development of EARs and RDAs, and it was no longer necessary to make use of AI estimates for calcium and vitamin D, except for infants. The AI is useful in that it allows the specification of some type of a reference value for use in public health settings—which is better than the absence of any value. However, it presents challenges in public health applications (gap issue num-

---

[1]"New methodologies—many from other fields of study—are emerging and can be useful for examining and approximating dose–response relationships when available data are limited. These should be more closely examined and incorporated into the DRI process as appropriate" (Taylor, 2008).

[2]"There is considerable interest—as well as more than 10 years of experience—surrounding the inclusion of chronic disease indicators within DRI development. A variety of perspectives were put forward. There is a need for focused discussions about how to include chronic disease indicators in the DRI process, including specific approaches for addressing their confounders, identification of appropriate biomarkers, and quantifying their effects" (Taylor, 2008).

ber 4-2[3] in Taylor, 2008), because it is not entirely consistent with the statistical approach based on distributions of requirements that underpin the DRIs. Guidelines for the use of AIs would be helpful, both those that exist for other nutrients at this time as well as those that might be specified in the future.

POPULATION SEGMENTS AND CONDITIONS OF INTEREST

Adiposity

As highlighted in Chapter 3, excess adiposity or obesity—defined as a body mass index (BMI) measure of 30 mg/m^2 or higher—is associated with lower serum 25OHD concentrations (and higher parathyroid hormone levels) than found in non-obese counterparts. This would appear to be due to sequestration of 25OHD by adipose tissue, given that supplementation of obese and lean persons with vitamin D appears to result in no significant difference in response between the two groups (Jones, 2008). Moreover, a few studies of modest weight loss have found circulating 25OHD levels to increase despite no increased intake of vitamin D from diet or sun exposure (Riedt et al., 2005; Reinehr et al., 2007; Zittermann et al., 2009; Tzotzas et al., 2010), suggesting release from adipose stores with adipose depletion. Further, neither season nor ethnicity influences these biochemical parameters (Alemzadeh et al., 2008).

An important concern is whether the lower serum 25OHD levels associated with obesity have meaningful consequences for the DRI indicator of bone health. Evidence for effects of obesity on bone density is mixed. The combined influence of increased weight-bearing activity and endogenous synthesis of estrogen due to outcomes of increased adiposity has long been associated with higher bone density (Reid, 2008). In a population-based study in Finland of perimenopausal and early postmenopausal women, Pesonen et al. (2005) found that increased body weight was a strong predictor of high bone density. Likewise, Morin and Leslie (2009), in a retrospective cohort study, found a strong correlation between higher BMI category and high bone density in postmenopausal women.

Although these and other studies have suggested that total body mass contributes to bone density and would appear to support the role of increased weight-bearing activity as a factor positively influencing bone density (Prentice et al., 1991; Khosla et al., 1996; Wortsman et al., 2000; Finkelstein et al., 2002, 2008), more recent studies lead to further ques-

---

[3]"There is broad interest in addressing the AIs as a component of the DRI values, but no clear path has emerged in terms of clarifying, adapting or eliminating AIs. Nor is there agreement about directions to be taken in the future for AI development" (Taylor, 2008).

tions. The distribution of body fat may influence bone mass, such that excess intra-abdominal fat could adversely affect bone remodeling and even contribute to greater fracture risk (Premaor et al., 2010; Sukumar et al., 2011). One possibility is that intra-abdominal adipose tissue is more biologically active than subcutaneous fat, secreting cytokines and adipokines that negatively affect osteoblast and osteoclast activity (Kawai and Rosen, 2010). Moreover, both lean and fat mass contribute to weight-bearing effects. Because obesity is accompanied by increases in both lean mass and fat mass, at least in younger individuals, it is difficult to attribute the effect on bone density to fat mass as opposed to lean mass. Further, body composition changes with age, even in the obese; in turn, there may be less lean body mass in older individuals.

This complicates the ability to clarify how adiposity may affect bone health. As noted, some studies have suggested that adiposity or increased fat mass itself may be a factor in the development rather than the prevention of osteoporosis, particularly in the elderly. Zhao et al. (2007) observed that when the effect of mechanical loading from high body weight on bone density was statistically controlled, fat mass was inversely correlated with bone mineral content. Further investigation by Zhao et al. (2008) suggested that molecular signaling pathways involved in osteoblast differentiation may contribute to the previously identified effect of increased adiposity on decreased bone mineral content, although a mechanism has not been elucidated. However, this science is just emerging and it is premature to speculate on its significance or relevance to bone health and bone density.

At this time, there is the possibility that obesity, at least in older persons, may not be beneficial for bone health and may be demonstrated to be a risk factor, not an advantage, for decreased bone density and, in turn, reduced bone health. There is no evidence that increases in calcium or vitamin D nutriture beyond the requirements specified for non-obese persons can affect this purported outcome.

Persons Living at Upper Latitudes in North America

The question of the impact of latitude on vitamin D nutriture is often a topic of concern or, at least, interest. The issue, however, is set in the context of the inability to specify a safe dose of sunlight that could contribute to vitamin D synthesis while also avoiding the risk of skin cancer. There are also the recognized challenges associated with quantifying the contributions from sun exposure coupled with the limited information on the role of stored vitamin D during seasonal changes. The prevailing assumption about the effect of latitude is that ultraviolet B (UVB) penetration decreases with increasing latitude (i.e., distance from the equator) and this, in turn, causes persons living at higher latitudes in North America to experience little or no UVB exposure, making them at risk for vitamin D deficiency. This assumption may not be entirely accurate. However, the question of latitude may work in tandem with other factors, discussed below, such as limited sun exposure overall or cultural and dietary practices. This section focuses only on the issue of latitude per se.

The relationship between UVB penetration and latitude is complex and not merely a function of distance from the equator. Other factors that come into play include the reduced atmosphere at the poles (about 50 percent less than at the equator), more cloud cover at the equator than at the poles, differences in ozone cover, and the duration of sunlight in summer versus winter. Geophysical surveys have indicated that UVB penetration over 24 hours during the summer months at Canadian north latitudes equals or exceeds UVB penetration at the equator (Lubin et al., 1998), suggesting that persons living in the northern latitudes are not necessarily receiving notably less total sunlight during the year. Rather, it suggests that there may be considerable opportunity during the spring, summer, and fall months in the far north for humans to form vitamin D and store it in liver and fat. Likewise, animals living in the same region that are consumed as part of the traditional diet are also rich sources of vitamin D (Keiver et al., 1988; Kenny et al., 2004; Brunborg et al., 2006; Kuhnlein et al., 2006).

These factors help to explain why latitude alone does not appear to predict serum 25OHD concentrations in humans. In a Finnish study, healthy subjects living above the Arctic Circle (latitude 66°N) did not have lower serum 25OHD levels than subjects living in southern Finland; in fact, the group living above the Arctic Circle had higher levels. Both groups achieved mean serum 25OHD levels above 90 nmol/L during the summer, whereas the mean serum 25OHD level at the winter nadir was 56 nmol/L in the south and 68 nmol/L in those living above the Arctic Circle (Lamberg-Allardt et al., 1983).

Persons Experiencing Reduced Vitamin D Synthesis from Sun Exposure

The DRIs for vitamin D established in this report are based on the assumption of minimal sun exposure. Therefore, they are regarded as adequate for persons who may be experiencing a reduced synthesis of vitamin D from sun exposure. Assuming that some population groups may be consuming less than the current DRI values for vitamin D, the question is to what extent are these persons at risk for vitamin D deficiency, or, conversely, to what extent can inadvertent sun exposure be expected to compensate for lower intakes for these persons?

Dark Skin

As described in Chapter 3, skin pigmentation—due to melanin in the epidermal layer—can reduce the amount of vitamin D synthesized by the human body. The amount of UVB required for changes in serum 25OHD levels is partly related to the degree of skin pigmentation. Further, a number of reports through the years have indicated consistently lower serum 25OHD levels in persons identified as black compared with those identified as white (Specker et al., 1985; Harkness and Cromer, 2005; Stein et al., 2006; Armas et al., 2007; Basile et al., 2007; Bodnar et al., 2007). Looker et al. (2008), using the National Health and Nutrition Examination Surveys (NHANES) 2000 to 2004, reported lower serum 25OHD levels for non-Hispanic blacks compared with Mexican Americans and whites. Mexican Americans had serum 25OHD concentrations that were intermediate between those of non-Hispanic blacks and whites.

The question is whether the consistently lower levels of serum 25OHD for persons with dark skin pigmentation have significant health consequences. Based on the data of Looker et al. (2008), non-Hispanic blacks in the NHANES had an average serum 25OHD concentration of 40.14 nmol/L (± 0.88 nmol/L [standard error of the mean]). Given that 40 nmol/L may be reflective of an acceptable median level for serum 25OHD in serum based on this committee's work, it is difficult to suggest that this average serum 25OHD level is indicative of widespread deficiency, although such conclusions cannot be based solely on mean values. However, at least for those of African American ancestry, there are corollary data to suggest that rates of osteoporosis and bone disease are not higher among African Americans; in fact, African Americans have reduced rates of fracture and osteoporosis compared with whites (see Chapter 4). There are no data in this regard for other ethnic groups with dark skin, such as South Asians, so firm conclusions about their risk related to bone health cannot be drawn. Furthermore, it is possible that risk may be introduced or modulated by an array of variables, including cultural and ethnic practices.

Given the unknowns, dark-skinned immigrant groups who now reside in North America may present a concern, as described below. There is also a concern for dark-skinned infants and children whose overall diet may be low in calcium and who may have low serum 25OHD levels, especially if exclusively breast-fed and not otherwise supplemented (see below). The vitamin D and calcium issues related specifically to African Americans have been described earlier in Chapter 4.

South Asian and Middle Eastern immigrant groups South Asians (e.g., Indians, Pakistanis, Sri Lankans) are now residing in greater numbers in North America, and are reported to be at increased risk for vitamin D–

deficiency. This group has a significant presence in Canada and is growing in number (Statistics Canada, 2010). A recent study by Wu et al. (2009) measured vitamin D intakes and serum 25OHD levels in three different ethnic groups in southern Ontario and found that levels were significantly lower in South Asians than in Eastern Asian or European groups. Over the past few decades, there have been sporadic reports of vitamin D–deficiency rickets in Canadians, almost always in breast-fed, dark-skinned Canadians of African or Asian descent, but the total number of cases, even in a major metropolitan area like Toronto, is small (17 over a 5-year period from 1988 to 1993) (Binet and Kooh, 1996). Similar to the situation in African Americans (see Chapter 3), the lower serum 25OHD levels observed are not associated with significant rises in the rates of bone disease (osteomalacia or rickets) in the Canadian South Asian cohort. In other South Asian communities living at relatively high latitudes (> 50°N) in Europe (e.g., Scotland), there have been reports of rickets and osteomalacia dating back to the early 1970s (Ford et al., 1976; Goel et al., 1976) and suggestions that vitamin D deficiency might also be associated with higher rates of tuberculosis (Yesudian et al., 2008). Although ensuring that the DRIs are met for these groups should reduce the risk for deficiency states to the extent that their conditions mimic those from minimal sun exposure, it is considered advisable to exercise vigilance for this growing group.

Some immigrant populations or religious groups adhere to cultural practices regarding clothing that can greatly reduce exposure to sun light and exacerbate the effects of low intake of vitamin D. There is the suggestion that at least 20 percent of the body's surface must be exposed to UVB for serum 25OHD levels to increase (Specker et al., 1985; Hollis, 2005). Whether such sun exposure is a wise public health practice for any group is not the issue, only that there is a need for awareness when such cultural practices limit sun exposure.

Dark-skinned, exclusively breast-fed infants In 2000, a report was published concerning rickets among nine children from various areas of the United States (Shah et al., 2000). Eight children were described as African American, and one child was described as Hispanic. All patients were primarily breast-fed for more than 11 months, with minimal intake of dairy products and without vitamin D supplementation. Breast milk, is of course, not a source of vitamin D for infants. This report had been preceded by a 1979 report from Bachrach et al. (1979), who noted 24 cases of vitamin D–deficiency rickets in black, breast-fed infants who were otherwise healthy and had no underlying malabsorptive or renal diseases, but whose parents belonged to groups that subscribed to dietary restrictions and clothing habits that minimized their exposure to sunlight. Later, a 2001 report described a black infant who was breast-fed until 10 months of age and then weaned to a soy food beverage that was not fortified with vitamin D or calcium (Carvalho et al., 2001). The infant developed normally until about 9 months of age when the child's height and weight became severely arrested. In 2003, DeLucia et al. (2003) commented on 43 children with nutritional rickets reported from 1986 through 2002 and located in the New Haven, Connecticut area. Approximately 86 percent were of African American, Hispanic, or Middle Eastern descent. More than 93 percent of the children had been breast-fed. In this case, the authors implicated both low calcium intake as well as marginal vitamin D nutriture in rickets.

A recent 2-year survey of Canadian pediatricians found the incidence of rickets in their patients to be 2.9 per 100,000; the mean age at diagnosis was 1.4 years (range of 2 weeks to 6.3 years). Ninety-four percent of the children with rickets had been breast-fed. Additional risk factors included dark skin, living in the far north, born of mother who took no vitamin supplements, limited sun exposure, emigrated from a region where vitamin D deficiency is endemic, and delayed initiation of solid foods (Ward et al., 2007).

Vitamin D supplementation of partially or fully breast-fed infants should begin in the first week of life and provide approximately 400 IU/day, as breast milk is not a source of this nutrient for infants, and sun exposure to compensate for this cannot be adequately described but neither can it be recommended given the concerns for skin cancer. It is important to be especially vigilant regarding supplementation in the case of exclusively breast-fed, dark-skinned infants, as they appear to be at higher risk than lighter-skinned infants.

Use of Sunscreen

Sunscreen absorbs ultraviolet light and prevents it from reaching the skin. It has been reported that sunscreen with a sun protection factor (SPF) of 8 based on the UVB spectrum can decrease vitamin D synthetic capacity by 95 percent, whereas sunscreen with an SPF of 15 can reduce synthetic capacity by 98 percent (Matsuoka et al., 1987). The extent and frequency of use of sunscreen are unknown, and therefore the significance of the role that sunscreen may play in reducing the opportunity to synthesize vitamin D is unclear. Increases in serum 25OHD levels seen in summer months in national surveys conducted in both the United States and Canada would suggest either that sunscreen is not used consistently by the population as a whole or that the actual decrease in serum 25OHD level due to appropriate use of sunscreen has been overstated. Although inconsistent with advice provided by the American Academy of Dermatology[4] and the National

---

[4]Available online at http://www.aad.org/media/background/news/Releases/American_Academy_of_Dermatology_Issues_Updated_Pos/.(accessed July 28, 2010).

Council on Skin Cancer Prevention[5] for skin cancer protection, given the carcinogenic potential of UVB light, one report indicated that there is adequate vitamin D production when exposure of hands, face, arms and legs to sunlight is for an amount of time equal to about 25 percent of what it would take to develop a "mild sunburn"; after this extent of exposure, a sunscreen should be applied to prevent damage (Holick, 2003). However, this is in contrast to a recent report on mathematical models of observational data regarding the impact of seasonal sun exposure (Diffey, 2010). The effect of the use of sunscreen, as with other factors that may limit exposure, warrants vigilance. However, its use should not constitute a concern, given that the DRI values assume minimal sun exposure.

Indoor Environments and Institutionalized Older Persons

Increased urbanization and the normative condition among North Americans to work and recreate indoors cannot be quantified or addressed in terms of increased risk for vitamin D deficiency. The newly established DRI values assume minimal sun exposure, and therefore vitamin D intake need not be increased above this level for normal persons living in urban settings and spending time primarily indoors.

However, data for institutionalized, frail older persons suggest a propensity for lower serum 25OHD levels generally. Causation, however, is uncertain. It is likely that many factors contribute, such as their restriction to primarily indoor environments often coupled with inadequate total intake overall. Further, aging skin is known to be less effective in synthesizing vitamin D in part because of a decrease in skin provitamin D (7-dehydrocholesterol) levels and in part because of alterations in skin morphology (MacLaughlin and Holick, 1985). The EAR and RDA values have taken this group into consideration to the extent possible and allowed by the data. Given the unknowns, however, monitoring institutionalized elderly people for vitamin D (and calcium) nutriture is appropriate. Supplementation, however, should not be random and without cause, because excess intakes of these nutrients may have adverse consequences for this frail sub-population.

Alternative Diets or Changes in Dietary Patterns

Dairy and Animal Product Exclusion: Lactose Intolerance, Cow's Milk Food Allergy, Ovo-Vegetarianism, and Veganism

Exclusion of dairy products occurs therapeutically in those with lactose intolerance or cow's milk food allergy, and voluntarily in those who are

---

[5]Available online at http://www.skincancerprevention.org/ (accessed July 28, 2010).

vegans or non-lacto vegetarians. As noted in the recent National Institutes of Health (NIH) Consensus Statement on Lactose Intolerance (Brannon et al., 2010; Suchy et al., 2010), exclusion of dairy products, all of which are rich sources of calcium and some of which are fortified with vitamin D (e.g., fluid milks, some yogurts, and limited other dairy products [Yetley, 2008]), can be a risk factor for inadequate intakes of calcium and vitamin D. This is also true for vegans (Craig, 2009) and likely others who systematically exclude dairy foods as well as other animal products from their diets. However, as pointed out by the American Dietetic Association (American Dietetic Association and Dieticians of Canada, 2003; Craig and Mangels, 2009) as well as the Dietitians of Canada (American Dietetic Association and Dietitians of Canada, 2003), appropriately planned vegetarian diets, including total vegetarian or vegan diets, are healthful and nutritionally adequate.

The North American prevalence of lactose intolerance, a clinical syndrome characterized by diarrhea, bloating and/or flatulence following consumption of lactose, is challenging to determine because the parameters surrounding lactose intolerance, lactose malabsorption, and lactase non-persistence are not well defined, and frequent self-diagnosis occurs (Brannon et al., 2010; Suchy et al., 2010). The prevalence of cow's milk allergy reported in a systematic evidence review (Rona et al., 2007) was 0.6 to 0.9 percent by skin test, specific immunoglobulin E measurement, or food challenge test; this is lower than the self-reported prevalence of 3 percent. Similarly to lactose intolerance, individuals may perceive that they have cow's milk food allergy when they do not. With respect to vegetarians, in 2006, approximately 1.4 percent of U.S. adults and nearly 1 percent of children and adolescents 8 to 18 years of age self-reported that they were vegans, and 2.3 to 3 percent reported themselves to be vegetarians.[6] In a 2002 survey, about 4 percent of Canadian adults reported being vegetarians (American Dietetic Association and Dietitians of Canada, 2003). Although there are few data to document the consequences of poorly planned diets that exclude dairy or animal products—it is noted that Craig (2009) reported a 30 percent increased risk of fracture for vegans—it is best to assume that persons who have chosen or must follow such diets should make special efforts to ensure nutritional adequacy.

Strategies for ensuring adequate intakes of calcium and vitamin D vary depending on the reason for dietary exclusion. Using an Agency for Healthcare Research and Quality systematic evidence review as a basis (Shaukat et al., 2010; Wilt et al., 2010), an NIH Consensus Panel found that individuals with lactose intolerance or lactose malabsorption are able to tolerate up to 12 g of lactose, the equivalent of one cup of milk, in a

---

[6]Available online at http://www.vrg.org/journal/vj2006issue4/vj2006issue4poll.htm (accessed July 28, 2010).

single dose and may be able to tolerate larger amounts if consumed in smaller doses spread over the day and with other foods. Larger amounts of reduced-lactose dairy products such as certain yogurts and fluid milks as well as virtually unrestricted amounts of reduced-fat hard cheeses with very low amounts of lactose may be ingested to ensure adequate intakes of calcium. For those who avoid all dairy because of allergies or personal choice, consumption of non-dairy sources of calcium, such as low-oxalate vegetables (e.g., kale, bok choy, Chinese cabbage, broccoli, and collards), calcium-containing tofu, or fortified plant-based foods, such as cereals or fruit juice are feasible strategies to ensure adequate intakes of highly bioavailable calcium (Weaver et al., 1999). Finally, supplements of calcium are also a strategy, although care should be taken not to over-supplement.

Meeting vitamin D needs is more challenging in the absence of sun exposure. Plant foods are not natural sources of vitamin D,[7] but the marketplace in the United States is increasingly offering plant-based fortified alternatives such as cereals and juices. In addition, the Canadian food supply includes margarines fortified with vitamin D and plant-based beverages that are fortified with vitamin D and calcium. Such fortified foods can be helpful in meeting the DRIs across age groups. As with calcium, a dietary supplement of vitamin D is also an option, but total intake (foods plus supplements) should not exceed the Tolerable Upper Intake Level (UL).

Changes in Dietary Patterns of Indigenous Canadian Populations

Among the indigenous Canadian populations, switching from a traditional diet that contains vitamin D–rich foods to a westernized diet may increase the likelihood of vitamin D deficiency, especially if UVB exposure is limited or avoided. This has been underscored by a survey of Inuit living in Greenland, which reported that those consuming a westernized diet had lower serum 25OHD levels than those consuming a traditional diet (32 vs. 53 nmol/L in summer, 29 vs. 41 nmol/L in winter) (Rejnmark et al., 2004). As noted above, there is ample opportunity during the spring, summer, and fall months in the far north for animals that commonly comprise the traditional diet of indigenous groups to form vitamin D and store it in liver and fat. In turn, the blubber and liver of various arctic marine mammals (e.g., seal, narwhal, beluga, walrus) and fish (e.g., char, cisco, lake trout, loche, sculpin, whitefish) are sources of vitamin D for those who consume a traditional diet (Keiver et al., 1988; Kenny et al., 2004; Brunborg et al., 2006; Kuhnlein et al., 2006).

---

[7]Some algal supplements and mushrooms that have been processed with irradiation contain vitamin D, but not in significant amounts. Available online at http://ods.od.nih.gov/factsheets/vitamind.asp (accessed July 28, 2010).

The Canadian Health Measures Survey does not collect data on these indigenous populations living at upper northern latitudes, and overall dietary and health data for them are limited. One recent survey (Kuhnlein et al., 2008) in northern Canada found that the intakes of vitamin D differed by ethnic group. The median vitamin D intake was 200 IU/day in both Yukon First Nations[8] and Dene/Métis. However, much higher median intakes were found in older (over age 40) Inuit who consumed a traditional diet (1,000 IU/day and 680 IU/day in men and women, respectively), whereas younger Inuit had much lower intakes (328 IU/day and 372 IU/day in men and women, respectively). This research group also surveyed indigenous women of reproductive age from various communities in the Canadian Arctic and found the mean daily intakes of vitamin D to be 456 IU/day in Inuit from Qikiqtarjuaq, 364 IU/day in Inuit from 18 other communities, and 228 IU/day in a combined data set of Dene, Métis, and Yukon First Nations. Pregnant and lactating women had higher vitamin D intakes, with the highest mean intake being 816 IU/day in lactating Inuit from Qikiqtarjuaq (Berti et al., 2008). Neither of these surveys measured serum 25OHD levels.

A 1999 survey (Smith, 1999) estimated vitamin D intakes and measured serum 25OHD levels in 121 pregnant women living in the Inuvik region of the Northwest Territories. The sample included 33 whites, 51 Inuit, and 37 First Nations people. The investigator did not report whether the First Nations and Inuit mothers were consuming a traditional or a western diet; moreover, the accuracy for the measures of the vitamin D content of traditional foods is unclear. The estimated daily mean vitamin D intake of Inuit and First Nations people was 324 IU/day with supplements (136 IU/day without) compared with 532 IU with supplements (232 IU without) to whites. At the point of delivery, the plasma levels of 25OHD were lower in the First Nations and Inuit mothers and their babies than in their white counterparts. Not quite as far north, a survey of 104 pregnant women from three First Nations communities in northern Manitoba found that their serum 25OHD levels ranged from < 15 nmol/L (undetectable) to 63 nmol/L, with mean values of 18, 21, and 24 nmol/L in each of the three communities (Smith, 1999). No information was provided in that report as to whether the women were consuming a traditional or western diet. A chart review was done of all babies born in 1993 and 1994 to determine how many had been diagnosed with rickets, and a high prevalence was found. Despite similar serum 25OHD levels in all three communities,

---

[8]First Nation: A term that came into common usage in the 1970s to replace the word "Indian." Among its uses, the term "First Nations peoples" refers to the Indian peoples in Canada, both Status and non-Status. Definitions available online at http://www.ainc-inac.gc.ca/ap/tln-eng.asp (accessed July 28, 2010).

there was a marked difference in the prevalence of rickets: 85/1,000 and 55/1,000 in two communities, but none in the third. No clear explanation for the differing prevalence was obtained by the investigator (Smith, 1999).

Taken as a whole, the limited data surrounding indigenous Canadian populations suggest a basis for concern regarding vitamin D nutriture, most notably in the likelihood that typical diets are changing from traditional foods to more westernized foods. Although the assumption of minimal sun exposure underpinning the DRI values may not entirely align with this group of people who may experience considerable sun exposure in the summer, ensuring that the diet meets the DRI values should provide assurances that risk of vitamin D deficiency has been greatly reduced.

Use of Calcium Supplements

The forms and nature of calcium supplements have been discussed in Chapter 2, and their possible role in kidney stone formation as well as the emerging data regarding possible adverse cardiovascular effects have been outlined in Chapter 6. The mechanisms for differential effects of food sources and supplement forms of calcium on kidney stone formation are complex and may relate to the timing of calcium administration. Approximately 80 percent of kidney stones contain calcium combined with oxalate or, less often, phosphate (Park and Pearle, 2007). Calcium in food or in supplements taken with food is believed to bind to dietary oxalate in the digestive tract, reducing the absorption and subsequent urinary excretion of oxalate and thus risk for kidney stones (urinary oxalate may be more critical than urinary calcium with respect to calcium oxalate crystallization) (Curhan et al., 1997). When calcium supplements are not taken with food, dietary oxalate is absorbed unopposed and thus is more available for stone formation. Although dairy foods, which are the major source of calcium in much of North America, have been suggested to contain an unidentified protective compound not found in supplements (Curhan et al., 1997), this possibility has not been well studied. Obtaining sufficient calcium via dietary sources is the preferred strategy—and it remains uncertain as to whether taking calcium supplements with food may reduce the likelihood of stone formation associated with supplement use. Head-to-head comparisons of different calcium supplement formulations with respect to risk for kidney stone formation are also lacking. In any case, given the desirability of not surpassing the UL for calcium intake and given that even those not meeting their requirement for calcium are nonetheless consuming some calcium from dietary sources that range from breads to dairy products, care must be taken in selecting a calcium supplement that when combined with dietary intake does not result in a total intake above the UL. The UL for a sizable proportion of the population, including groups that commonly consume calcium supplements, is 2,000 mg/day, which is relatively close to the EAR and RDA values. For these more vulnerable groups, supplements containing amounts less than the RDA may be appropriate given that their diet is likely to contain at least some calcium. Further, until better information is available to clarify the possible link between supplement use and kidney stone formation, taking calcium supplements with foods is advisable.

Moreover, in the case of persons prone to developing kidney stones who cannot get adequate calcium from diet (e.g., due to lactose intolerance), there is limited evidence from small, short-term trials suggesting that supplemental calcium in moderate doses may not increase risk for stone recurrence (Levine et al., 1994; Williams et al., 2001; Lewandowski and Rodgers, 2004). Again, taking supplements with food is desirable.

The ULs are defined for the healthy, general population. Nonetheless, gray areas are acknowledged to exist between healthy people and those with medical conditions; for some persons in these gray areas a calcium intake as high as the UL may no longer be considered without any risk. The effect of calcium intake in situations of hypercalciuria is not fully understood, but conditions leading to hypercalciuria (which may be exacerbated by adding extra vitamin D to an already high calcium intake) may warrant a more cautious approach to ULs for calcium in the future. In older adults experiencing illness or decline, hypercalciuria may develop. For pregnant women experiencing absorptive hypercalciuria and therefore at higher risk of renal stone formation, keeping calcium intake below the UL may also be most appropriate. Similarly, as lactation drives bone resorption, urinary calcium excretion decreases, the ionized serum calcium concentration rises slightly, intravascular volume is contracted and occasionally women become hypercalcemic. Under these and similar conditions, ensuring a calcium intake below the UL may be most appropriate. Greater surveillance of urinary calcium excretion in future studies may shed more light on the relationship between higher levels of total calcium intake and risk of hypercalciuria or hypercalcemia under special conditions.

Oral Contraceptive Use

The use of ethinyl estradiol oral contraceptives (OCs) has been hypothesized to reduce bone resorption and preserve bone density in premenopausal and postmenopausal women. This concept was based on clinical and observational evidence that ethinyl estrogen–based hormone replacement therapy reduced risk for osteoporosis in postmenopausal women (Zittermann, 2000). A non-systematic review of clinical trials carried out before 1994 indicated that the evidence at that time largely supported positive effects of OCs on bone density in postmenopausal women, although a number of trials in the review showed no effects (DeCherney,

1996). Among clinical trials and observational evidence examining the effects of OCs on bone density from the past two decades, results have been mixed and, when considered in total, are inconclusive. A systematic review of 75 studies of varied design, including 11 randomized controlled trials, examined outcomes of OC use and bone density in healthy premenopausal, amenorrheic premenopausal, anorexic premenopausal, and perimenopausal women (Liu and Lebrun, 2006). A meta-analysis was not done; however, the review found good evidence for a positive effect of OCs on bone density in perimenopausal women, fair evidence for an effect in amenorrheic premenopausal women, and limited evidence for an effect in anorexic and healthy premenopausal women.

Observational studies published since Liu and Lebrun (2006) also suggest mixed results from studies on OC use and bone density that may be related to the population group studied. A small study on OC use and bone density and bone size in a young white female cohort found that OC use had a significant negative effect on bone density at the spine and heel and resulted in a non-significant decrease in hip bone density (Ruffing et al., 2007). Similarly, Hartard et al. (2007), in a cross–sectional analysis of young white women taking OCs, also suggested a negative effect of OCs on bone density. Women who had ever used OCs had significantly lower bone densities at the tibial shaft and femoral neck compared with those who had never used OCs. In premenopausal and postmenopausal women no significant difference was found between OCs users and never users in another cross–sectional study of the effects of OCs on bone density and bone markers (Allali et al., 2009).

Randomized trials of estrogen treatment with and without vitamin D and calcium supplementation suggest a positive effect on bone density in postmenopausal women. Recker et al. (1999) tested vitamin D and calcium supplementation with and without low-dose hormone replacement therapy for effectiveness in maintaining bone density in postmenopausal women more than 65 years of age. Although this study did not differentiate between hormone replacement therapy alone and therapy combined with vitamin D and calcium supplementation, it did suggest an effect of increasing bone density and bone markers in older women who received the combination therapy compared with those who received vitamin D and calcium supplementation alone. A randomized, double-blind, placebo-controlled trial of OC therapy either alone or combined with calcitriol therapy found a significant increase in bone density and reduction in bone resorption at the hip compared with OC therapy alone in postmenopausal women (ages 65 to 77 years) who had normal bone density for their age (Gallagher et al., 2001). Another prospective randomized trial in postmenopausal women (ages 53 to 79 years) treated with hormone replacement therapy alone or with calcitriol also found a significant increase in bone density, at multiple sites and total body, for the combined therapy compared with hormone replacement alone (Gutteridge et al., 2003).

Given the variability in all the study outcomes reviewed by the committee and the unresolved question of the effect of age and endogenous estrogen status on the ability of OCs to preserve bone density or prevent bone resorption, specific recommendations to address the impact of OCs with or without vitamin D and calcium supplementation for both premenopausal and postmenopausal women cannot be offered at this time.

Premature Infants

Premature infants are a clinical population and thus outside the scope of this committee's task, which is focused on the normal, healthy population. However, because premature infants are a highly vulnerable group and do raise special concerns relative to calcium and vitamin D nutriture, this group is discussed here briefly.

The minerals in human milk, especially calcium and phosphorus, do not fully meet the needs of rapidly growing premature infants who rely primarily on passive intestinal absorption of calcium, therefore "this and other factors place premature infants at high risk for nutritional rickets" (Abrams, 2005). "The recent addition of various forms of mineral salts and/or mineral fortifiers to human milk and the use of specialized preterm infant formulas with high calcium content have been reported to enhance the amount of calcium and other minerals retained from the diet, to increase the bone mineral content of the infants and to decrease the incidence of osteopenia and frank rickets in preterm infants (Schanler et al., 1988; Schanler and Abrams, 1995; Schanler, 1998)... The bioavailability of the calcium in these fortifiers may be a key aspect of their adequacy. Using a commercially available human milk fortifier, Schanler and Abrams (1995) reported that net calcium retention was 104 ± 36 mg/kg body weight per day in premature infants, a value approximating the *in utero* accretion rate during the third trimester. These retention values are well above those achieved using earlier human milk fortifiers (Schanler et al., 1988)" (Abrams, 2005).

"Of interest is that calcium absorption from both fortified human milk and specialized preterm formula averages 50 to 65 percent in many studies (Abrams et al., 1991; Bronner et al., 1992). This constancy of absorptive fraction in premature infants suggests that much of the calcium absorption by premature infants and newborn full-term infants is not vitamin D dependent..." (Abrams, 2005), which is the conclusion of a review of more than 100 balance studies by Bronner et al. (1992).

How much vitamin D is needed by premature infants is more difficult to determine. Unfortunately, there are no studies using modern isotope

TABLE 8-1 Drugs and Their Effect on Vitamin D Metabolism

Drug Name/Category	25OHD	Calcitriol	24,25-Dihydroxyvitamin D
Aluminum	Not changed	Increase/decrease	—
Anticonvulsants (phenobarbital, Dilantin, Tegretol)	Decrease	Not changed	Decrease
Antituberculosis	Decrease	Decrease	—
Bisphosphonates	Not changed	Increase/decrease/ not changed	Increase
Cimetidine	Decrease	Not changed	Not changed
Corticosteroids	Decrease/ not changed	Decrease/not changed	Not changed
Ethanol	Increase	Decrease	—
Heparin	Not changed	Decrease	Not changed
Hypolipidemic agents	Decrease/ not changed	Not changed	—
Immunosuppressives	Not changed	Not changed	—
Ketoconazole	Not changed	Decrease	Decrease
Lithium	Not changed	Not changed	—
Rifabutin (anti-HIV)	Decrease	Not changed	—
Thiazides	Increase	Decrease	Increase

NOTE: — indicates that no information has been reported; HIV = human immunodeficiency virus.
SOURCES: Hahn et al. (1972); Favus et al. (1973); Avioli (1975); Compston and Thompson (1977); Compston and Horton (1978); Bell et al. (1979); Alfrey et al. (1980); Palmer et al. (1980); Adams et al. (1981); Williams et al. (1985); Feldman (1986); Lalor et al. (1986); Lawson-Matthew et al. (1988); Dobs et al. (1991); Katz et al. (1994); Bolland et al. (2008).

techniques of the effects of vitamin D on calcium absorption in premature infants, nor could such studies be possible practically or ethically. One study with oral vitamin D intakes as low as 160 IU/day (Koo et al., 1995) and multiple studies with intakes of 200 to 400 IU/day (Cooke et al., 1990; Pittard et al., 1991; Backstrom et al., 1999a) "demonstrated adequate serum 25OHD concentrations and clinical outcomes with oral vitamin D intakes as low as 160 IU/day (Koo et al., 1995). In addition, studies have generally failed to show any clinical benefit to increasing vitamin D intake above 400 IU/day in preterm infants (Backstrom et al., 1999b)" (Abrams, 2005).

Routine measurement of serum 25OHD levels in premature infants is not supported by currently available clinical research. No studies have related serum 25OHD level in these infants to specific clinical outcomes, and extremely few data suggest a dose–response relationship between serum 25OHD levels and other outcomes. A normal level at different gestational ages or postnatal ages is not available for 25OHD in serum based on endpoints such as calcium absorption or bone mineral content. However, in the presence of a likely impairment of 25-hydroxylation, such as might be present in an infant with cholestasis, measurement of serum 25OHD level might be considered, especially to ensure a level at or above 50 nmol/L (20 ng/mL). "The effects of other formula components on mineral absorption have also been considered. A study using a triple lumen perfusion technique demonstrated that calcium absorption was greater using a solution that included a glucose polymer rather than lactose (Stathos et al., 1996). As glucose polymers are widely used in preterm formulas, this effect may be clinically important. Altering the fat blend of infant formula to more closely resemble that of human milk may also enhance mineral absorption in premature infants (Carnielli et al., 1995; Lucas et al., 1997)" (Abrams, 2005).

Interactions Between Vitamin D and Prescription Drugs

Although clinical practice and related guidelines are outside this committee's purview, it is useful to acknowledge that measures of the various forms of vitamin D can be affected by prescription drugs and related medications. A brief listing of key interactions can be found in Table 8-1.

REFERENCES

Abrams, S. A., N. V. Esteban, N. E. Vieira and A. L. Yergey. 1991. Dual tracer stable isotopic assessment of calcium absorption and endogenous fecal excretion in low birth weight infants. Pediatric Research 29(6): 615-8.

Abrams, S. A. 2005. Chapter 49: Vitamin D deficiency and calcium absorption during infancy and childhood. In Vitamin D, 2nd Edition, edited by D. Feldman, J. W. Pike and F. Glorieux. London: Elsevier Academic Press.

Adams, J. S., T. O. Wahl and B. P. Lukert. 1981. Effects of hydrochlorothiazide and dietary sodium restriction on calcium metabolism in corticosteroid treated patients. Metabolism 30(3): 217-21.

Alemzadeh, R., J. Kichler, G. Babar and M. Calhoun. 2008. Hypovitaminosis D in obese children and adolescents: relationship with adiposity, insulin sensitivity, ethnicity, and season. Metabolism 57(2): 183-91.

Alfrey, A. C., A. Hegg and P. Craswell. 1980. Metabolism and toxicity of aluminum in renal failure. American Journal of Clinical Nutrition 33(7): 1509-16.

Allali, F., L. El Mansouri, F. Abourazzak, L. Ichchou, H. Khazzani, L. Bennani, R. Abouqal and N. Hajjaj-Hassouni. 2009. The effect of past use of oral contraceptive on bone mineral density, bone biochemical markers and muscle strength in healthy pre and post menopausal women. BMC Women's Health 9: 31.

American Dietetic Association and Dietitians of Canada. 2003. Position of the American Dietetic Association and Dietitians of Canada: vegetarian diets. Canadian Journal of Dietetic Practice & Research 64(2): 62-81.

Armas, L. A., S. Dowell, M. Akhter, S. Duthuluru, C. Huerter, B. W. Hollis, R. Lund and R. P. Heaney. 2007. Ultraviolet-B radiation increases serum 25-hydroxyvitamin D levels: the effect of UVB dose and skin color. Journal of the American Academy of Dermatology 57(4): 588-93.

Avioli, L. V. 1975. Heparin-induced osteopenia: an appraisal. Advances in Experimental Medicine and Biology 52: 375-87.

Bachrach, S., J. Fisher and J. S. Parks. 1979. An outbreak of vitamin D deficiency rickets in a susceptible population. Pediatrics 64(6): 871-7.

Backstrom, M. C., R. Maki, A. L. Kuusela, H. Sievanen, A. M. Koivisto, R. S. Ikonen, T. Kouri and M. Maki. 1999a. Randomised controlled trial of vitamin D supplementation on bone density and biochemical indices in preterm infants. Archives of Disease in Childhood. Fetal and Neonatal Edition 80(3): F161-6.

Backstrom, M. C., R. Maki, A. L. Kuusela, H. Sievanen, A. M. Koivisto, M. Koskinen, R. S. Ikonen and M. Maki. 1999b. The long-term effect of early mineral, vitamin D, and breast milk intake on bone mineral status in 9- to 11-year-old children born prematurely. Journal of Pediatric Gastroenterology and Nutrition 29(5): 575-82.

Basile, L. A., S. N. Taylor, C. L. Wagner, L. Quinones and B. W. Hollis. 2007. Neonatal vitamin D status at birth at latitude 32 degrees 72': evidence of deficiency. Journal of Perinatology 27(9): 568-71.

Bell, R. D., C. Y. Pak, J. Zerwekh, D. E. Barilla and M. Vasko. 1979. Effect of phenytoin on bone and vitamin D metabolism. Annals of Neurology 5(4): 374-8.

Berti, P. R., R. Soueida and H. V. Kuhnlein. 2008. Dietary assessment of Indigenous Canadian Arctic women with a focus on pregnancy and lactation. International Journal of Circumpolar Health 67(4): 349-62.

Binet, A. and S. W. Kooh. 1996. Persistence of vitamin D-deficiency rickets in Toronto in the 1990s. Canadian Journal of Public Health. Revue Canadienne de Sante Publique 87(4): 227-30.

Bodnar, L. M., H. N. Simhan, R. W. Powers, M. P. Frank, E. Cooperstein and J. M. Roberts. 2007. High prevalence of vitamin D insufficiency in black and white pregnant women residing in the northern United States and their neonates. Journal of Nutrition 137(2): 447-52.

Bolland, M. J., A. Grey, A. M. Horne and M. G. Thomas. 2008. Osteomalacia in an HIV-infected man receiving rifabutin, a cytochrome P450 enzyme inducer: a case report. Annals of Clinical Microbiology and Antimicrobials 7: 3.

Brannon, P. M., T. O. Carpenter, J. R. Fernandez, V. Gilsanz, J. B. Gould, K. E. Hall, S. L. Hui, J. R. Lupton, J. Mennella, N. J. Miller, S. K. Osganian, D. E. Sellmeyer, F. J. Suchy and M. A. Wolf. 2010. NIH Consensus Development Conference Statement: Lactose Intolerance and Health. NIH Consensus State of the Science Statements 27(2).

Bronner, F., B. L. Salle, G. Putet, J. Rigo and J. Senterre. 1992. Net calcium absorption in premature infants: results of 103 metabolic balance studies. American Journal of Clinical Nutrition 56(6): 1037-44.

Brunborg, L. A., K. Julshamn, R. Nortvedt and L. Frøyland. 2006. Nutritional composition of blubber and meat of hooded seal (Cystophora cristata) and harp seal (Phagophilus groenlandicus) from Greenland. Food Chemistry 96(4): 524-31.

Byers, T. 2010. Anticancer vitamins du jour—the ABCED's so far. American Journal of Epidemiology 172(1): 1-3.

Carnielli, V. P., I. H. Luijendijk, J. B. van Goudoever, E. J. Sulkers, A. A. Boerlage, H. J. Degenhart and P. J. Sauer. 1995. Feeding premature newborn infants palmitic acid in amounts and stereoisomeric position similar to that of human milk: effects on fat and mineral balance. American Journal of Clinical Nutrition 61(5): 1037-42.

Carvalho, N. F., R. D. Kenney, P. H. Carrington and D. E. Hall. 2001. Severe nutritional deficiencies in toddlers resulting from health food milk alternatives. Pediatrics 107(4): E46.

Compston, J. E. and R. P. Thompson. 1977. Intestinal absorption of 25-hydroxyvitamin D and osteomalacia in primary biliary cirrhosis. Lancet 1(8014): 721-4.

Compston, J. E. and L. W. Horton. 1978. Oral 25-hydroxyvitain D_3 in treatment of osteomalacia associated with ileal resection and cholestyramine therapy. Gastroenterology 74(5 Pt 1): 900-2.

Cooke, R., B. Hollis, C. Conner, D. Watson, S. Werkman and R. Chesney. 1990. Vitamin D and mineral metabolism in the very low birth weight infant receiving 400 IU of vitamin D. Journal of Pediatrics 116(3): 423-8.

Craig, W. J. 2009. Health effects of vegan diets. American Journal of Clinical Nutrition 89(5): 1627S-33S.

Craig, W. J. and A. R. Mangels. 2009. Position of the American Dietetic Association: vegetarian diets. Journal of the American Dietetic Association 109(7): 1266-82.

Curhan, G. C., W. C. Willett, F. E. Speizer, D. Speigelman and M. J. Stampfer. 1997. Comparison of dietary calcium with supplemental calcium and other nutrients as factors affecting the risk for kidney stones in women. Annals of Internal Medicine 126(7): 497-504.

DeCherney, A. 1996. Bone-sparing properties of oral contraceptives. American Journal of Obstetrics and Gynecology 174(1 Pt 1): 15-20.

DeLucia, M. C., M. E. Mitnick and T. O. Carpenter. 2003. Nutritional rickets with normal circulating 25-hydroxyvitamin D: a call for reexamining the role of dietary calcium intake in North American infants. Journal of Clinical Endocrinology and Metabolism 88(8): 3539-45.

Diffey, B. 2010. Modelling the seasonal variation of vitamin D due to sun exposure. British Journal of Dermatology 162: 1342-8.

Dobs, A. S., M. A. Levine and S. Margolis. 1991. Effects of pravastatin, a new HMG-CoA reductase inhibitor, on vitamin D synthesis in man. Metabolism 40(5): 524-8.

Favus, M. J., D. V. Kimberg, G. N. Millar and E. Gershon. 1973. Effects of cortisone administration on the metabolism and localization of 25-hydroxycholecalciferol in the rat. Journal of Clinical Investigation 52(6): 1328-35.

Feldman, D. 1986. Ketoconazole and other imidazole derivatives as inhibitors of steroidogenesis. Endocrine Reviews 7(4): 409-20.

Finkelstein, J. S., M. L. Lee, M. Sowers, B. Ettinger, R. M. Neer, J. L. Kelsey, J. A. Cauley, M. H. Huang and G. A. Greendale. 2002. Ethnic variation in bone density in premenopausal and early perimenopausal women: effects of anthropometric and lifestyle factors. Journal of Clinical Endocrinology and Metabolism 87(7): 3057-67.

Finkelstein, J. S., S. E. Brockwell, V. Mehta, G. A. Greendale, M. R. Sowers, B. Ettinger, J. C. Lo, J. M. Johnston, J. A. Cauley, M. E. Danielson and R. M. Neer. 2008. Bone mineral density changes during the menopause transition in a multiethnic cohort of women. Journal of Clinical Endocrinology and Metabolism 93(3): 861-8.

Ford, J. A., W. V. McIntosh, R. Butterfield, M. A. Preece, J. Pietrek, W. A. Arrowsmith, M. W. Arthurton, W. Turner, J. L. O'Riordan and M. G. Dunnigan. 1976. Clinical and subclinical vitamin D deficiency in Bradford children. Archives of Disease in Childhood 51(12): 939-43.

Gallagher, J. C., S. E. Fowler, J. R. Detter and S. S. Sherman. 2001. Combination treatment with estrogen and calcitriol in the prevention of age-related bone loss. Journal of Clinical Endocrinology and Metabolism 86(8): 3618-28.

Goel, K. M., E. M. Sweet, R. W. Logan, J. M. Warren, G. C. Arneil and R. A. Shanks. 1976. Florid and subclinical rickets among immigrant children in Glasgow. Lancet 1(7970): 1141-5.

Gutteridge, D. H., M. L. Holzherr, R. W. Retallack, R. I. Price, R. K. Will, S. S. Dhaliwal, D. L. Faulkner, G. O. Stewart, B. G. Stuckey, R. L. Prince, R. A. Criddle, P. J. Drury, L. Tran, C. I. Bhagat, G. N. Kent and K. Jamrozik. 2003. A randomized trial comparing hormone replacement therapy (HRT) and HRT plus calcitriol in the treatment of postmenopausal osteoporosis with vertebral fractures: benefit of the combination on total body and hip density. Calcified Tissue International 73(1): 33-43.

Hahn, T. J., S. J. Birge, C. R. Scharp and L. V. Avioli. 1972. Phenobarbital-induced alterations in vitamin D metabolism. Journal of Clinical Investigation 51(4): 741-8.

Harkness, L. and B. Cromer. 2005. Low levels of 25-hydroxy vitamin D are associated with elevated parathyroid hormone in healthy adolescent females. Osteoporosis International 16(1): 109-13.

Hartard, M., C. Kleinmond, M. Wiseman, E. R. Weissenbacher, D. Felsenberg and R. G. Erben. 2007. Detrimental effect of oral contraceptives on parameters of bone mass and geometry in a cohort of 248 young women. Bone 40(2): 444-50.

Holick, M. F. 2003. Vitamin D: a millenium perspective. Journal of Cellular Biochemistry 88(2): 296-307.

Hollis, B. W. 2005. Circulating 25-hydroxyvitamin D levels indicative of vitamin D sufficiency: implications for establishing a new effective dietary intake recommendation for vitamin D. Journal of Nutrition 135(2): 317-22.

IOM (Institute of Medicine). 1997. Dietary Reference Intakes for Calcium, Phosphorus, Magnesium, Vitamin D, and Fluoride. Washington, DC: National Academy Press.

IOM. 2000. Dietary Reference Intakes: Applications in Dietary Assessment. Washington, DC: National Academy Press.

IOM. 2002. Evolution of Evidence for Selected Nutrient and Disease Relationships. Washington, DC: National Academy Press.

IOM. 2008. The Development of DRIs 1994-2004: Lessons Learned and New Challenges: Workshop Summary. Washington, DC: The National Academies Press.

Jones, G. 2008. Pharmacokinetics of vitamin D toxicity. American Journal of Clinical Nutrition 88(2): 582S-6S.

Katz, I., M. Li, I. Joffe, B. Stein, T. Jacobs, X. G. Liang, H. Z. Ke, W. Jee and S. Epstein. 1994. Influence of age on cyclosporin A-induced alterations in bone mineral metabolism in the rat in vivo. Journal of Bone and Mineral Research 9(1): 59-67.

Kawai, M. and C. J. Rosen. 2010. Bone: adiposity and bone accrual-still an established paradigm? National Review of Endocrinology 6(2): 63-4.

Keiver, K. M., H. H. Draper and K. Ronald. 1988. Vitamin D metabolism in the hooded seal (Cystophora cristata). Journal of Nutrition 118(3): 332-41.

Kenny, D. E., T. M. O'Hara, T. C. Chen, Z. Lu, X. Tian and M. F. Holick. 2004. Vitamin D content in Alaskan Arctic zooplankton, fishes, and marine mammals. Zoo Biology 23(1): 33-43.

Khosla, S., E. J. Atkinson, B. L. Riggs and L. J. Melton, 3rd. 1996. Relationship between body composition and bone mass in women. Journal of Bone and Mineral Research 11(6): 857-63.

Koo, W. W., S. Krug-Wispe, M. Neylan, P. Succop, A. E. Oestreich and R. C. Tsang. 1995. Effect of three levels of vitamin D intake in preterm infants receiving high mineral-containing milk. Journal of Pediatric Gastroenterology and Nutrition 21(2): 182-9.

Kuhnlein, H. V., V. Barthet, A. Farren, E. Falahi, D. Leggee, O. Receveur and P. Berti. 2006. Vitamins A, D, and E in Canadian Arctic traditional food and adult diets. Journal of Food Composition and Analysis 19(6-7): 495-506.

Kuhnlein, H. V., O. Receveur, R. Soueida and P. R. Berti. 2008. Unique patterns of dietary adequacy in three cultures of Canadian Arctic indigenous peoples. Public Health Nutrition 11(4): 349-60.

Lalor, B. C., M. W. France, D. Powell, P. H. Adams and T. B. Counihan. 1986. Bone and mineral metabolism and chronic alcohol abuse. Quarterly Journal of Medicine 59(229): 497-511.

Lamberg-Allardt, C., M. Kirjarinta and A. G. Dessypris. 1983. Serum 25-hydroxy-vitamin D, parathyroid hormone and calcium levels in adult inhabitants above the Arctic Circle in northern Finland. Annals of Clinical Research 15(4): 142-5.

Lawson-Matthew, P. J., D. F. Guilland-Cumming, A. J. Yates, R. G. Russell and J. A. Kanis. 1988. Contrasting effects of intravenous and oral etidronate on vitamin D metabolism in man. Clinical Science (London) 74(1): 101-6.

Levine, B. S., J. S. Rodman, S. Wienerman, R. S. Bockman, J. M. Lane and D. S. Chapman. 1994. Effect of calcium citrate supplementation on urinary calcium oxalate saturation in female stone formers: implications for prevention of osteoporosis. American Journal of Clinical Nutrition 60(4): 592-6.

Lewandowski, S. and A. L. Rodgers. 2004. Renal response to lithogenic and anti-lithogenic supplement challenges in a stone-free population group. Journal of Renal Nutrition 14(3): 170-9.

Liu, S. L. and C. M. Lebrun. 2006. Effect of oral contraceptives and hormone replacement therapy on bone mineral density in premenopausal and perimenopausal women: a systematic review. British Journal of Sports Medicine 40(1): 11-24.

Looker, A. C., C. M. Pfeiffer, D. A. Lacher, R. L. Schleicher, M. F. Picciano and E. A. Yetley. 2008. Serum 25-hydroxyvitamin D status of the US population: 1988-1994 compared with 2000-2004. American Journal of Clinical Nutrition 88(6): 1519-27.

Lubin, D., E. H. Jensen and H. P. Gies. 1998. Global surface ultraviolet radiation climatology from TOMS and ERBE data. Journal of Geophysical Research 103(D20): 26061-91.

Lucas, A., P. Quinlan, S. Abrams, S. Ryan, S. Meah and P. J. Lucas. 1997. Randomised controlled trial of a synthetic triglyceride milk formula for preterm infants. Archives of Disease in Childhood. Fetal and Neonatal Edition 77(3): F178-84.

MacLaughlin, J. and M. F. Holick. 1985. Aging decreases the capacity of human skin to produce vitamin D_3. Journal of Clinical Investigation 76(4): 1536-8.

Matsuoka, L. Y., L. Ide, J. Wortsman, J. A. MacLaughlin and M. F. Holick. 1987. Sunscreens suppress cutaneous vitamin D_3 synthesis. Journal of Clinical Endocrinology and Metabolism 64(6): 1165-8.

Morin, S. and W. D. Leslie. 2009. High bone mineral density is associated with high body mass index. Osteoporosis International 20(7): 1267-71.

Palmer, F. J., T. M. Sawyers and S. J. Wierzbinski. 1980. Cimetidine and hyperparathyroidism. New England Journal of Medicine 302(12): 692.

Park, S. and M. S. Pearle. 2007. Pathophysiology and management of calcium stones. Urologic Clinics of North America 34(3): 323-34.

Pesonen, J., J. Sirola, M. Tuppurainen, J. Jurvelin, E. Alhava, R. Honkanen and H. Kroger. 2005. High bone mineral density among perimenopausal women. Osteoporosis International 16(12): 1899-906.

Pittard, W. B., 3rd, K. M. Geddes, T. C. Hulsey and B. W. Hollis. 1991. How much vitamin D for neonates? American Journal of Diseases of Children 145(10): 1147-9.

Premaor, M. O., L. Pilbrow, C. Tonkin, R. A. Parker and J. Compston. 2010. Obesity and fractures in postmenopausal women. Journal of Bone and Mineral Research 25(2): 292-7.

Prentice, A., J. Shaw, M. A. Laskey, T. J. Cole and D. R. Fraser. 1991. Bone mineral content of British and rural Gambian women aged 18-80+ years. Bone and Mineral 12(3): 201-14.

Recker, R. R., K. M. Davies, R. M. Dowd and R. P. Heaney. 1999. The effect of low-dose continuous estrogen and progesterone therapy with calcium and vitamin D on bone in elderly women. A randomized, controlled trial. Annals of Internal Medicine 130(11): 897-904.

Reid, I. R. 2008. Relationships between fat and bone. Osteoporosis International 19(5): 595-606.

Reinehr, T., G. de Sousa, U. Alexy, M. Kersting and W. Andler. 2007. Vitamin D status and parathyroid hormone in obese children before and after weight loss. European Journal of Endocrinology / European Federation of Endocrine Societies 157(2): 225-32.

Rejnmark, L., M. E. Jorgensen, M. B. Pedersen, J. C. Hansen, L. Heickendorff, A. L. Lauridsen, G. Mulvad, C. Siggaard, H. Skjoldborg, T. B. Sorensen, E. B. Pedersen and L. Mosekilde. 2004. Vitamin D insufficiency in Greenlanders on a westernized fare: ethnic differences in calcitropic hormones between Greenlanders and Danes. Calcified Tissue International 74(3): 255-63.

Riedt, C. S., M. Cifuentes, T. Stahl, H. A. Chowdhury, Y. Schlussel and S. A. Shapses. 2005. Overweight postmenopausal women lose bone with moderate weight reduction and 1 g/day calcium intake. Journal of Bone and Mineral Research 20(3): 455-63.

Rona, R. J., T. Keil, C. Summers, D. Gislason, L. Zuidmeer, E. Sodergren, S. T. Sigurdardottir, T. Lindner, K. Goldhahn, J. Dahlstrom, D. McBride and C. Madsen. 2007. The prevalence of food allergy: a meta-analysis. Journal of Allergy and Clinical Immunology 120(3): 638-46.

Ruffing, J. A., J. W. Nieves, M. Zion, S. Tendy, P. Garrett, R. Lindsay and F. Cosman. 2007. The influence of lifestyle, menstrual function and oral contraceptive use on bone mass and size in female military cadets. Nutrition and Metabolism (London) 4: 17.

Schanler, R. J., S. A. Abrams and C. Garza. 1988. Mineral balance studies in very low birth weight infants fed human milk. Journal of Pediatrics 113(1 Pt 2): 230-8.

Schanler, R. J. and S. A. Abrams. 1995. Postnatal attainment of intrauterine macromineral accretion rates in low birth weight infants fed fortified human milk. Journal of Pediatrics 126(3): 441-7.

Schanler, R. J. 1998. The role of human milk fortification for premature infants. Clinics in Perinatology 25(3): 645-57, ix.

Shah, M., N. Salhab, D. Patterson and M. G. Seikaly. 2000. Nutritional rickets still afflict children in north Texas. Texas Medicine 96(6): 64-8.

Shaukat, A., M. D. Levitt, B. C. Taylor, R. MacDonald, T. A. Shamliyan, R. L. Kane and T. J. Wilt. 2010. Systematic review: effective management strategies for lactose intolerance. Annals of Internal Medicine 152(12): 797-803.

Smith, P. J. 1999. Vitamin D deficiency in three northern Manitoba communities. PhD Diss, Smith, P.J. Winnipeg, Canada, U Manitoba.

Specker, B. L., B. Valanis, V. Hertzberg, N. Edwards and R. C. Tsang. 1985. Sunshine exposure and serum 25-hydroxyvitamin D concentrations in exclusively breast-fed infants. Journal of Pediatrics 107(3): 372-6.

Stathos, T. H., R. J. Shulman, R. J. Schanler and S. A. Abrams. 1996. Effect of carbohydrates on calcium absorption in premature infants. Pediatric Research 39(4 Pt 1): 666-70.

Statistics Canada. 2010. Canadian Health Measures Survey (CHMS). Ottawa, Ontario: Health Canada.

Stein, E. M., E. M. Laing, D. B. Hall, D. B. Hausman, M. G. Kimlin, M. A. Johnson, C. M. Modlesky, A. R. Wilson and R. D. Lewis. 2006. Serum 25-hydroxyvitamin D concentrations in girls aged 4-8 y living in the southeastern United States. American Journal of Clinical Nutrition 83(1): 75-81.

Suchy, F. J., P. M. Brannon, T. O. Carpenter, J. R. Fernandez, V. Gilsanz, J. B. Gould, K. Hall, S. L. Hui, J. Lupton, J. Mennella, N. J. Miller, S. K. Osganian, D. E. Sellmeyer and M. A. Wolf. 2010. National Institutes of Health Consensus Development Conference: lactose intolerance and health. Annals of Internal Medicine 152(12): 792-6.

Sukumar, D., Y. Schlussel, C. S. Riedt, C. Gordon, T. Stahl and S. A. Shapses. 2011. Obesity alters cortical and trabecular bone density and geometry in women. Osteoporosis International 22(2): 635-45. Epub June 9, 2010.

Taylor, C. L. 2008. Framework for DRI Development: Components "Known" and Components "To Be Explored." Washington, DC.

Tzotzas, T., F. G. Papadopoulou, K. Tziomalos, S. Karras, K. Gastaris, P. Perros and G. E. Krassas. 2010. Rising serum 25-hydroxy-vitamin D levels after weight loss in obese women correlate with improvement in insulin resistance. Journal of Clinical Endocrinology and Metabolism 95(9): 4251-7.

Ward, L. M., I. Gaboury, M. Ladhani and S. Zlotkin. 2007. Vitamin D-deficiency rickets among children in Canada. Canadian Medical Association Journal 177(2): 161-6.

Weaver, C. M., W. R. Proulx and R. Heaney. 1999. Choices for achieving adequate dietary calcium with a vegetarian diet. American Journal of Clinical Nutrition 70(Suppl 3): 543S-8S.

Williams, S. E., A. G. Wardman, G. A. Taylor, M. Peacock and N. J. Cooke. 1985. Long term study of the effect of rifampicin and isoniazid on vitamin D metabolism. Tubercle 66(1): 49-54.

Williams, C. P., D. F. Child, P. R. Hudson, G. K. Davies, M. G. Davies, R. John, P. S. Anandaram and A. R. De Bolla. 2001. Why oral calcium supplements may reduce renal stone disease: report of a clinical pilot study. Journal of Clinical Pathology 54(1): 54-62.

Wilt, T. J., A. Shaukat, T. Shamliyan, B. C. Taylor, R. MacDonald, J. Tacklind, I. Rutks, S. J. Schwarzenberg, R. L. Kane and M. Levitt. 2010. Lactose intolerance and health. Evidence Report Technology Assessment (Full Report) (192): 1-410.

Wortsman, J., L. Y. Matsuoka, T. C. Chen, Z. Lu and M. F. Holick. 2000. Decreased bioavailability of vitamin D in obesity. American Journal of Clinical Nutrition 72(3): 690-3.

Wu, H., A. Gozdzik, J. L. Barta, D. Wagner, D. E. Cole, R. Vieth, E. J. Parra and S. J. Whiting. 2009. The development and evaluation of a food frequency questionnaire used in assessing vitamin D intake in a sample of healthy young Canadian adults of diverse ancestry. Nutrition Research 29(4): 255-61.

Yesudian, P. D., J. L. Berry, S. Wiles, S. Hoyle, D. B. Young, A. K. Haylett, L. E. Rhodes and P. Davies. 2008. The effect of ultraviolet B-induced vitamin D levels on host resistance to Mycobacterium tuberculosis: a pilot study in immigrant Asian adults living in the United Kingdom. Photodermatology, Photoimmunology and Photomedicine 24(2): 97-8.

Yetley, E. A. 2008. Assessing the vitamin D status of the US population. American Journal of Clinical Nutrition 88(2): 558S-64S.

Yetley, E. A., D. Brule, M. C. Cheney, C. D. Davis, K. A. Esslinger, P. W. Fischer, K. E. Friedl, L. S. Greene-Finestone, P. M. Guenther, D. M. Klurfeld, M. R. L'Abbe, K. Y. McMurry, P. E. Starke-Reed and P. R. Trumbo. 2009. Dietary reference intakes for vitamin D: justification for a review of the 1997 values. American Journal of Clinical Nutrition 89(3): 719-27.

Zhao, L. J., Y. J. Liu, P. Y. Liu, J. Hamilton, R. R. Recker and H. W. Deng. 2007. Relationship of obesity with osteoporosis. Journal of Clinical Endocrinology and Metabolism 92(5): 1640-6.

Zhao, L. J., H. Jiang, C. J. Papasian, D. Maulik, B. Drees, J. Hamilton and H. W. Deng. 2008. Correlation of obesity and osteoporosis: effect of fat mass on the determination of osteoporosis. Journal of Bone and Mineral Research 23(1): 17-29.

Zittermann, A. 2000. Decreased urinary calcium loss and lower bone turnover in young oral contraceptive users. Metabolism 49(8): 1078-82.

Zittermann, A., S. Frisch, H. K. Berthold, C. Gotting, J. Kuhn, K. Kleesiek, P. Stehle, H. Koertke and R. Koerfer. 2009. Vitamin D supplementation enhances the beneficial effects of weight loss on cardiovascular disease risk markers. American Journal of Clinical Nutrition 89(5): 1321-7.

9

Information Gaps and Research Needs

The purpose of this report is to review available data and establish science-based reference values for calcium and vitamin D, known as Dietary Reference Intakes (DRIs). The approach used has been that of risk assessment, as described in Chapter 1. This final chapter outlines information gaps and research needs identified by the committee in carrying out its charge. These gaps and research needs are also organized according to the risk assessment framework. The listings are not comprehensive, but offer the committee's perspective on the major topic areas in need of attention. These needs are targeted to academic and medical researchers, national policy makers, the public health community, industry groups, and other relevant stakeholders and funding institutions. They provide a basis for organizing and prioritizing research efforts.

The general nature of the information gaps relevant to DRI development for calcium and vitamin D are outlined in Figure 9-1.

Although the uncertainties surrounding the DRIs have been described in this report and the scientific judgments made are documented, evidence from future research designed to overcome the limitations encountered by this committee can improve the ability to determine reference values in the future. Although the committee's discussions form the basis for the identification of these research needs, other sources of research needs were noted, for example the National Institutes of Health Roundtable on Vitamin D Research Needs (Brannon et al., 2008) and the report from the Tufts Medical Center Evidence-based Practice Center (Chung et al., 2010).

Table 9-1 presents the identified research needs, which are then outlined.

514

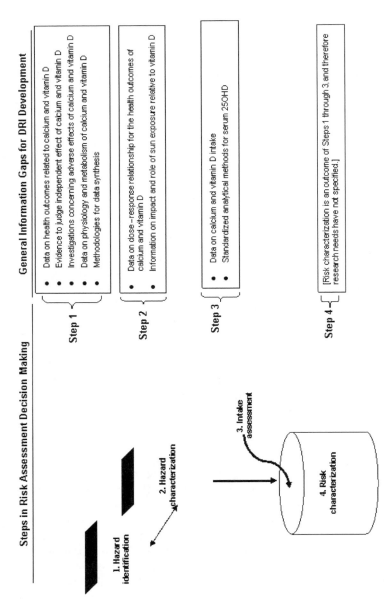

FIGURE 9-1 General nature of information gaps within the evidence base for calcium and vitamin D DRI development as related to risk assessment steps.
NOTE: 25OHD = serum 25-hydroxyvitamin D.
SOURCE: Modified from WHO, 2006.

TABLE 9-1 Vitamin D and Calcium Research Needs Organized by Risk Assessment Steps

Research Topic	Research Questions and Identified Needs
Step 1: "Hazard Identification" or Indicator Review and Selection	
Health Outcomes and Related Conditions	1. Clarify threshold effects of calcium and vitamin D on skeletal health outcomes by life stage and for different racial/ethnic groups. 2. Elucidate inter-relationship between calcium and vitamin D, and specify independent effect(s) of each. 3. Explore causal role for vitamin D in non-skeletal health. 4. Determine the appropriateness of serum 25-hydroxyvitamin D (25OHD) as a biomarker of effect. 5. Elucidate the effect of genetic variation, including that among racial/ethnic groups, and epigenetic regulation of vitamin D on developmental outcomes.
Adverse Effects, Toxicity, and Safety	1. Develop innovative methodologies to provide for identification and assessment of adverse effects of excess calcium and vitamin D. 2. Elucidate adverse effects of long-term, high-dose calcium and vitamin D. 3. Further explore nature of vitamin D toxicity.
Basic Physiology and Molecular Pathways	1. Examine the influence of calcium and phosphate on the regulation of vitamin D activation and catabolism through parathyroid hormone and fibroblast-like growth factor-23 (FGF23). 2. Clarify 25OHD distribution in body pools including storage and mobilization from adipose tissue. 3. Evaluate the nature and significance of extra-renal production of calcitriol for health outcomes. 4. Clarify the extent to which differences exist between vitamin D_2 and vitamin D_3.
Synthesizing Evidence and Research Methodology	1. Explore enhanced methodologies for data synthesis. 2. Identify approaches to weight better potential health outcomes.
Step 2: "Hazard Characterization" or Intake-Response Assessment and Specification of DRIs	
Dose–Response Relationship	1. Conduct studies to identify specific health outcomes in relation to graded and fully measured intakes of calcium and of vitamin D. 2. Clarify the influence of age, body weight, and body composition on 25OHD levels in response to intake/exposure.

Continued

TABLE 9-1 Continued

Research Topic	Research Questions and Identified Needs
Sun Exposure	1. Investigate whether a minimal-risk ultraviolet B (UVB) radiation exposure relative to skin cancer exists that also enables vitamin D production. 2. Clarify how physiological factors such as skin pigmentation, genetics age, body weight, and body composition influence vitamin D synthesis. 3. Clarify how environmental factors such as sunscreen use affect vitamin D synthesis.
	Step 3: Intake Assessment
Intake Assessment	1. Enhance dietary assessment methods for calcium and vitamin D intake, and methods for the measurement of calcium and vitamin D in foods and supplements. 2. Investigate food and supplement sources of calcium and vitamin D for bioequivalence, bioavailability, and safety. 3. Improve the standardization of assay for serum 25OHD.

STEP 1: "HAZARD IDENTIFICATION" OR INDICATOR REVIEW AND SELECTION

The committee found an overall lack of causal evidence from intervention studies for the task of identifying health outcome indicators. This was especially true for non-skeletal outcomes for vitamin D, but this was also true for skeletal outcomes, particularly in certain life stage groups. Data related to calcium were sparse for children and younger adults. Most vitamin D studies were conducted using older persons or postmenopausal women. Some available data suggested the possibility of ethnic differences in bone health, but this suggestion could not be further clarified. Very few studies explored the independent effects of calcium and vitamin D. Only limited data were available on adverse health effects. These information gaps, coupled with challenges in synthesizing disparate evidence for either calcium or vitamin D or their combination, presented challenges to DRI development. Further, lack of clarity concerning the physiology and metabolism of vitamin D was problematic as was the ability to judge the effects of vitamin D as a nutrient given its role as a prohormone.

Research Needs Related to Health Outcomes and Related Conditions

1. **Clarify threshold effects of calcium and vitamin D on skeletal health outcomes by life stage and for different racial/ethnic**

groups. Although there is a solid body of evidence related to bone health and the role of calcium and vitamin D, many data gaps remain for younger age groups and for the effect under menopausal conditions. The issue of "calcium economy" among certain groups and ethnic differences in vitamin D utilization require attention.

2. **Elucidate inter-relationship between calcium and vitamin D, and specify independent effect(s) of each.** There is a need for research protocols that examine the effects of vitamin D and calcium separately rather than as a combined administration, and which better clarify the nature of the inter-relationship. Without such data, the ability to identify requirements for calcium and for vitamin D is challenging.

3. **Explore causal role for vitamin D in non-skeletal health outcomes.** Investigation of causal relationships between vitamin D nutriture and potential non-skeletal health outcomes should undergo further research. These may include but are not limited to (no particular order): immune function and anti-inflammatory effects (especially related to obesity); total and site-specific cancers; cardiovascular disease; and diabetes. More data on the role of calcium and vitamin D, and their metabolism, during pregnancy and lactation is needed.

4. **Determine appropriateness of serum 25-hydroxyvitamin D (25OHD) as a biomarker of effect.** The ability to use the relatively accessible measure of serum 25OHD as a biomarker or surrogate is limited by a number of factors including not only its role as a prohormone, but also its variability, which is due to a number of non-nutritional factors. A better understanding of its relationship to specific health outcome would be beneficial, enhancing both the quality and quantity of research available. The measure should be studied for this purpose and also should be subject to a formal validation process.

5. **Elucidate the effect of genetic variation, including that among racial/ethnic groups, and epigenetic regulation of vitamin D on developmental outcomes.** This is an emerging field of study, which will likely prove relevant to DRI development. Studies in this area may contribute notably to an understanding of population differences related to chronic disease risk.

Research Needs Related to Adverse Effects, Toxicity, and Safety

1. **Develop innovative methodologies to provide for identification and assessment of adverse effects of excess calcium and vitamin D.** The ability to study adverse effects of calcium and vitamin D is

often limited due to ethical concerns. Creative approaches using an array of methodologies developed in other fields need to be adapted for nutritional use and incorporated into the approach for studying adverse effects of nutrients in vitro and in vivo using relevant animal models.

2. **Elucidate adverse effects of long-term, high-dose calcium and vitamin D.** The question of nutrient safety should not be a secondary aspect of study design nor can the failure to detect adverse effects as part of a study not designed for that purpose be considered an adequate assessment of safety. Dedicated studies are needed to assess adverse health effects related to long-term, high dose (although not necessarily "toxic") levels of calcium and vitamin D.

3. **Further explore the nature of vitamin D toxicity.** Although toxicity is not the most appropriate goal for setting ULs, a better understanding of the timing, doses, and mechanisms associated with vitamin D toxicity (hypervitaminosis D) would be beneficial to understanding the impact of vitamin D on the human body. Of particular import is information about the metabolic fate and dynamics of high doses of vitamin D. The identification and use of animal models (particularly large animal models) would be especially helpful. Also needed is an understanding of how weight loss in obese individuals might affect vitamin D status and adverse outcomes (e.g., bariatric surgery patients).

Research Needs Related to Basic Physiology and Molecular Pathways

1. **Examine the influence of calcium and phosphate on the regulation of vitamin D activation and catabolism through parathyroid hormone and fibroblast-like growth factor 23 (FGF23).** Identify pathways that regulate vitamin D activation and catabolism through parathyroid hormone and FGF23 in order to understand the influence of calcium and phosphate intake on vitamin D regulation.

2. **Clarify 25OHD distribution in body pools including storage and mobilization from adipose tissue.** Understanding the distribution, storage, and mobilization of 25OHD in body pools would enhance the understanding regarding relationships among exposure to vitamin D from intake or endogenous synthesis, circulation serum levels of 25OHD, and health outcomes. The role of storage compartments and factors important to the mobilization of vitamin D is noticeably lacking.

3. **Evaluate the nature and significance of extra-renal production of calcitriol for health outcomes.** Determining the significance of extra-renal production of calcitriol for health outcomes is essential

to understand whether local production of calcitriol has an impact on health outcomes. In turn, the relevance of vitamin D nutriture and serum 25OHD for such an effect should be established.

4. **Clarify the extent to which differences exist between vitamin D$_2$ and vitamin D$_3$.** Physiological responses as well as potential for differences in safety risks for the two forms of the nutrient should be further explored.

Synthesizing Evidence and Research Methodology

1. **Explore enhanced methodologies for data synthesis.** Alternative methods for synthesizing evidence from different study types and multiple parameters that consider uncertainties (including measurement error) include teleoanalysis, confidence profile predictive meta-analysis, and generalized multi-parameter evidence synthesis. In the case of calcium and vitamin D, such approaches should facilitate quantitative estimates of effect size and dose–response relationships as needed for DRI development.

2. **Identify approaches to weight better potential health outcomes.** In order to ensure the most objective and comprehensive systematic evidence reviews in the future, approaches to better weight potential health outcomes are needed.

STEP 2: "HAZARD CHARACTERIZATION" OR INTAKE-RESPONSE ASSESSMENT AND SPECIFICATION OF DIETARY REFERENCE INTAKES

The committee encountered major challenges in determining the dose–response relationships for calcium and vitamin D. Sun exposure introduced further uncertainties regarding vitamin D.

Research Related to Dose–Response Relationships

1. **Conduct studies to identify specific health outcomes in relation to graded and fully measured intakes of calcium and vitamin D.** Too few studies are specifically designed to study the effects of graded doses of calcium or vitamin D on health outcomes, both overall and as part of the same study using the same subjects and outcome measures. Further, many studies in the calcium and vitamin D area are confounded by the failure to specify or measure and thereby take into account "background" intakes of the nutrient being studied when dose–response is being explored.

2. **Clarify the influence of age, body weight, and body composition on serum 25OHD levels in response to intake/exposure.** Information about how factors such as age, body weight, and body composition affect the variability in serum 25OHD response to intake or exposure would assist in the process of establishing requirements for vitamin D. Such information is also important to ascertaining the measure's utility as a biomarker of effect and in making judgments about excess intake of the vitamin.

Research Needs Related to Sun Exposure

1. **Investigate whether a minimal-risk ultraviolet B (UVB) radiation exposure relative to skin cancer exists that also enables vitamin D production.** Whether a minimal or threshold UVB exposure level is possible to both enable subcutaneous vitamin D synthesis and avoid risk of skin cancer needs to be examined. Research should include assessment of the risk for skin cancer compared with the benefit of endogenous synthesis of vitamin D, particularly for at-risk populations.
2. **Clarify how physiological factors such as skin pigmentation, genetics, age, body weight, and body composition influence vitamin D synthesis.** Understanding how subcutaneous synthesis of vitamin D is affected by physiological factors and the impact of these factors on maintenance of serum 25OHD levels within normal physiologic ranges is important to integrating information about dietary intake and interpretation of serum 25OHD levels.
3. **Clarify how environmental factors such as sunscreen use affect vitamin D synthesis.** The impact of factors that affect endogenous vitamin D production, and notably the appropriate use of sunscreen for reducing cancer risk, needs to be determined to ascertain an appropriate risk-benefit profile for protected sun exposure as well as better elucidation of the role of sun exposure in determining vitamin D nutriture.

STEP 3: INTAKE ASSESSMENT

Although great strides have been made recently in providing intake data on calcium and notably on vitamin D, more data as well as a consistent approach to data reporting would be helpful. The committee encountered challenges in identifying standardized and consistent data on vitamin D intakes across general populations in the United States and Canada, particularly for population subgroups who may be at risk for inadequate or excessive intake. In addition, reliable data on the practice and impact of discretionary fortification on the part of food manufacturers is lacking.

1. **Enhance dietary assessment methods and comparability for calcium and vitamin D intake, and methods for the measurement of calcium and vitamin D in foods and supplements.** Methods related to dietary assessment have come far in recent years, and research in this area should continue. DRI development as it pertains to the North American population would benefit from targeted efforts to strive for comparability between the U.S. and Canadian surveys.

2. **Investigate food and supplement sources of calcium and vitamin D for bioequivalence, bioavailability, and safety.** The ability to assess whether different fortification delivery systems and food production methods affect the factors such as bioavailability or safety for both calcium and vitamin D is an important component of dietary intake assessment. Information on the practice of discretionary fortification by food manufacturers is needed.

3. **Improve the standardization of the assay for serum 25OHD.** Currently, different assays for the determination of serum 25OHD levels are in use, and they provide disparate results. In turn, reported measures are confounded by the need to understand the assay used and research reports contain results that are not readily compared. The role of standard reference materials and inter-laboratory collaboration is an important aspect of overcoming the challenges that the assay methodologies present.

RELATED RESEARCH NEED

Clinical practice was outside the scope of this committee convened to develop DRIs, which was tasked primarily with describing a distribution of requirements and upper levels of intake. However, as noted in Chapter 8, the cut-point levels of serum 25OHD intended to specify deficiency and sufficiency for the purposes of interpreting laboratory analyses and for use in clinical practice have been subject to a wide variation in specification without a systematic, evidence-based consensus development process. The importance of this specification to both the well-being of the North American population and to ensuring that the population is confident in their health and nutriture results in the committee calling attention to this research need. Its broad impact requires that it be addressed by a coalition of stakeholders under the auspices of a science-based organization such as the National Institutes of Health in conjunction with equivalent science-based organizations in Canada.

CONCLUDING REMARKS

The committee found that the greatest information gaps, and thus the most critical research needs, are related to the so-called hazard identification and hazard characterization steps in which the relationship between the nutrient and health outcomes are established. These needs for calcium and vitamin D DRI development relate to further exploring and describing both skeletal as well as non-skeletal health outcomes, long-term adverse effects of high levels of intake, and data to clarify the dose–response to intake. In the case of vitamin D, understanding the impact of sun exposure presents many challenges. Specific to the selected indicator (i.e., bone health), there is a need for more and better data related to the relatively unstudied life stage groups of children and young adults and the differences among racial/ethnic groups. Furthermore, the committee found a pressing public health need for development of consensus, science-based guidelines to establish cut-point levels for vitamin D deficiency and insufficiency.

REFERENCES

Brannon, P. M., E. A. Yetley, R. L. Bailey and M. F. Picciano. 2008. Summary of roundtable discussion on vitamin D research needs. American Journal of Clinical Nutrition 88(2): 587S-92S.

Chung, M., E. M. Balk, S. Ip, J. Lee, T. Terasawa, G. Raman, T. Trikalinos, A. H. Lichtenstein and J. Lau. 2010. Systematic review to support the development of nutrient reference intake values: challenges and solutions. American Journal of Clinical Nutrition 92(2): 273-6.

A

Acronyms, Abbreviations, and Glossary

ACRONYMS AND ABBREVIATIONS

25-hydroxyvitamin D
> In this report, 25OHD (also referred to as calcidiol or calcifediol); indicates no distinction between D_2 and D_3 forms. When relevant, forms distinguished as $25OHD_2$ and $25OHD_3$.

1,25-dihydroxyvitamin D
> In this report, calcitriol. Ercalcitriol refers to 1,25-dihydroxyvitamin D_2, but in this report, the term "calcitriol" will be used for both.

24,25-dihydroxyvitamin D
> In this report, $24,25(OH)_2D$.

AHRQ	Agency for Healthcare Research and Quality
AI	Adequate Intake
ALTM	All-laboratory trimmed mean
AMDR	Acceptable Macronutrient Distribution Range
ATBC	Alpha-Tocopherol Beta-Carotene Cancer Prevention Study
BDI	Beck Depression Inventory
BMAD	Bone mineral apparent density
BMC	Bone mineral content
BMD	Bone mineral density
BMI	Body mass index
BV	Bone volume

CCHS	Canadian Community Health Survey
CDC	Centers for Disease Control and Prevention
CG	Control group
CHMS	Canadian Health Measures Survey
CI	Confidence interval
CNF	Canadian Nutrient File
CPBA	Competitive protein binding assay
CVD	Cardiovascular disease
CYP	Cytochrome P450
DBP	Vitamin D binding protein
DEQAS	Vitamin D External Quality Assurance Scheme
DNA	Deoxyribonucleic acid
DRI	Dietary Reference Intake
DXA	Dual-energy X-ray absorptiometry
EAR	Estimated Average Requirement
EPIC	European Prospective Investigation into Cancer and Nutrition
EPIDOS	Epidémiologie de l'Ostéoporose study
FGF23	Fibroblast-like growth factor-23
FN	Femoral neck
GC	Gas chromatography
GFR	Glomerular filtration rate
HPFS	Health Professionals Follow-up Study
HR	Hazard ratio
IBD	Inflammatory bowel disease
IFN	Interferon
Ig	Immunoglobulin
IG	Intervention group
IHD	Ischemic heart disease
IL	Interleukin
IOM	Institute of Medicine
iPTH	Intact parathyroid hormone
IU	International Unit
K-MMSE	Mini-Mental State Examination for Koreans

LC	Liquid chromatography
LOAEL	Lowest-observed-adverse-effect level
LS	Lumbar spine
LSM	Least squares mean

MAS	Milk-alkali syndrome
MMSE	Mini-Mental State Examination
mo	Month(s)
mRNA	Messenger ribonucleic acid
MrOS	Osteoporotic Fractures in Men Study
MS	Mass spectrometry; Multiple sclerosis
MS/MS	Tandem mass spectrometry

NA	Not applicable
NCa	Normocalcemic
NCHS	National Center for Health Statistics
NCI	National Cancer Institute
ND	Not determined
NHANES	National Health and Nutrition Examination Survey
NHS	Nurses' Health Study
NIH	National Institutes of Health
NIST	National Institute of Standards and Technology
NOAEL	No-observed-adverse-effect level
NOD	Nonobese diabetic
NR	Not reported
NS	Not significant

OA	Osteoarthritis
OC	Oral contraceptive
OP	Osteoporosis
OR	Odds ratio
OV	Osteoid volume

PLCO	Prostate, Lung, Colorectal, and Ovarian Cancer Screening Trial
PM	Postmenopausal
POMS	Profile of Mood States
PTH	Parathyroid hormone
PTHrP	Parathyroid hormone–related protein

RA	Rheumatoid arthritis
RANK	Receptor activator for nuclear factor κ B

RCT	Randomized controlled trial
RDA	Recommended Dietary Allowance
RECORD	Randomised Evaluation of Calcium and/Or vitamin D trial
RIA	Radioimmunoassay
RNI	Recommended Nutrient Intake
RR	Relative risk
SD	Standard deviation
SE	Standard error
SEM	Standard error of the mean
SLE	Systemic lupus erythematosus
SPA	Single-photon absorptiometry
SPF	Sun protection factor
SRM	Standard Reference Material
TB	Tuberculosis; Total body
Th	T helper
TH	Total hip
Tr	Trochanter
TRPV6	Transient receptor potential cation channel, vanilloid family member 6
Tx	Treatment
UK	United Kingdom
UL	Tolerable Upper Intake Level
U.S.	United States
USDA	U.S. Department of Agriculture
UV	Ultraviolet
UVB	Ultraviolet B
VDDR	Vitamin D–dependent rickets
VDR	Vitamin D receptor
VDRE	Vitamin D–responsive element
VEGF	Vascular endothelial growth factor
WHI	Women's Health Initiative
WWEIA	What We Eat in America
wk	Week(s)
y	Year(s)

GLOSSARY

Achlorhydria
> A lack of hydrochloric acid in the digestive juices in the stomach.

Adenoma
> A benign epithelial tumor of glandular origin.

Adequate Intake
> The recommended average daily intake level of a nutrient based on observed or experimentally determined approximations or estimates of intakes that are assumed to be adequate for a group (or groups) of apparently healthy people; used when the Recommended Dietary Allowance cannot be determined.

Adipokines
> Cytokines, growth factors, and other proteins produced and secreted by adipose tissue.

Adipose tissue
> A connective tissue consisting chiefly of fat cells surrounded by reticular fibers and arranged in lobular groups or along the course of one of the smaller blood vessels.

Amenorrhea
> Abnormal suppression or absence of menstruation.

Anorexia
> The symptom of poor appetite whatever the cause.

Anorexia nervosa
> A psychophysiological disorder usually occurring in teenage women that is characterized by fear of becoming obese, a distorted self-image, a persistent aversion to food, and severe weight loss, and that is often marked by hyperactivity, self-induced vomiting, amenorrhea, and other physiological changes.

Antigen
> Any substance that stimulates an immune response in the body.

Antirachitic
> Cures or prevents rickets.

Asthma
> A chronic inflammatory disease of the airways.

Autism
> A complex developmental disability that typically appears during the first few years of life; is the result of a neurological disorder that affects the normal functioning of the brain, impacting development in the areas of social interaction and communication skills.

Biomarker

A biochemical, physiological, behavioral, or other alteration that can be measured in the body or its products that influences, predicts, or is associated with an established or possible outcome, health impairment, or disease.

Body mass index

An indirect measure of body fat calculated as the ratio of a person's body weight to the square of a person's height:

BMI (kg/m^2) = weight (kilograms)/height (meters)^2

BMI (lb/in^2) = weight (pounds)/height (inches)$^2 \times 703$

Bone mineral content

The hardness of bone results from its mineral content in the organic matrix.

Bone mineral density

A measure of bone density that reflects the strength of bones as represented by calcium content.

Calcification

Impregnation with calcium or calcium salts; hardening, as of tissue, by such impregnation.

Calcinosis

The abnormal deposition of calcium salts in a part or tissue of the body.

Calcitonin

A peptide hormone, produced by the thyroid gland in humans, that acts to lower plasma calcium and phosphate levels without augmenting calcium accretion.

Calcitriol

Another name for 1,25-dihydroxyvitamin D.

Calcium

A mineral found mainly in the hard part of bones, where it is stored; it is essential for healthy bones and is important for muscle contraction, heart action, nervous system maintenance, and normal blood clotting.

Calciuria

The presence of calcium in the urine.

Cancer

A malignant and invasive growth or tumor.

Cardiovascular disease

Any abnormal condition characterized by dysfunction of the heart and blood vessels; includes atherosclerosis (especially coronary heart disease), cerebrovascular disease, and hypertension.

Chondrocyte

A connective tissue cell that occupies a lacuna within the cartilage matrix.

Chylomicron

One of the microscopic particles of fat occurring in chyle (a digestive fluid) and in the blood, especially after a meal high in fat.

Computed tomography

Tomography used in diagnostic studies of internal bodily structures, in which computer analysis of a series of cross–sectional scans made along a single axis of a bodily structure or tissue is used to construct a three-dimensional image of that structure.

Creatinine

One of the nonprotein constituents of blood, a breakdown product of creatinine (protein used to make adenosine triphosphate). Increased quantities of serum creatinine are found in advanced stages of renal disease.

Crohn's disease

A chronic inflammatory disease of the intestines that primarily causes ulcerations (breaks in the lining) of the small and large intestines, but can affect the digestive system anywhere from the mouth to the anus.

Cut-point

A specified quantitative measure used to demarcate the presence or absence of a health-related condition; often used in interpreting measures obtained from analysis of blood (example: blood measures below "x" ng/mL indicate a deficiency state for Nutrient Y).

Cytochrome

Any of a class of iron-containing proteins important to cell respiration as catalysts of oxidation–reduction reactions.

Depression

A condition of general emotional dejection and withdrawal; sadness greater and more prolonged than that warranted by any objective reason.

Dermis

The sensitive connective tissue layer of the skin located below the epidermis, containing nerve endings, sweat and sebaceous glands, and blood and lymph vessels.

Diabetes mellitus

A group of metabolic diseases characterized by high blood sugar (glucose) levels that result from defects in insulin secretion or action, or both.

Diabetes, type 1

An autoimmune disease that occurs when T cells attack and decimate the β-cells in the pancreas that are needed to produce insulin, so that the pancreas makes too little insulin (or no insulin); there is a genetic predisposition to type 1 diabetes, and the disease tends to occur in childhood, adolescence, or early adulthood (before age 30), but it may have its clinical onset at any age.

Diabetes, type 2

Disease in which the β-cells of the pancreas produce insulin but the body is unable to use it effectively because the cells of the body are resistant to the action of insulin; also known as insulin-resistant diabetes, non-insulin-dependent diabetes, and adult-onset diabetes.

Dietary Reference Intake

A set of four distinct nutrient-based reference values that replaced the former Recommended Dietary Allowance in the United States. These include Estimated Average Requirement (EAR), Recommended Dietary Allowance (RDA), Adequate Intake (AI), and Tolerable Upper Intake Level (UL).

Dose–response assessment

Determination of the relationship between nutrient intake (dose) and some criterion of either adequacy or adverse effect.

Dual-energy X-ray absorptiometry

Means of measuring bone density with two X-ray beams with differing energy levels aimed at an individual's bones.

Emesis

The act or process of vomiting.

Endocrine

Pertaining to hormones and the glands that make and secrete them into the bloodstream through which they travel to affect distant organs.

Epidermis

The nonvascular outer protective layer of the skin, covering the dermis.

Ergosterol

A plant sterol that is converted into vitamin D by ultraviolet radiation.

Estimated Average Requirement

The average daily nutrient intake level that is estimated to meet the requirements of half of the healthy individuals in a particular life stage and gender group.

Estradiol
   The most potent naturally occurring estrogen.
Etiology
   Causes and origins of disease.

Fibroblast
   A cell ubiquitous in connective tissue that makes and secretes collagen.

Glucocorticoid
   Any of a group of steroid-like compounds, such as hydrocortisone, that are produced by the adrenal cortex, are involved in carbohydrate, protein, and fat metabolism, and are used as anti-inflammatory agents.

Hematocrit
   The percentage by volume of packed red blood cells in a given sample of blood after centrifugation.
Homeostasis
   A property of cells, tissues, and organisms that allows the maintenance and regulation of the stability and constancy needed to function properly.
Hormone
   A substance, usually a peptide or a steroid, produced by one tissue and conveyed in the bloodstream to another to effect physiological activity, such as growth or metabolism.
Hydroxyapatite
   The principal bone salt that provides the compressional strength of vertebrate bone.
Hypercalcemia
   A higher than normal level of calcium in the blood.
Hypercalciuria
   Excess calcium in the urine.
Hyperglycemia
   A high blood sugar; an elevated level specifically of the sugar glucose in the blood.
Hypertension/hypertensive
   Systolic blood pressure $\geq$ 140 mmHg or diastolic blood pressure $\geq$ 90 mmHg.
Hypophosphatemia
   Abnormally low concentrations of phosphates in the blood.

Inflammatory bowel disease

Any of several incurable and debilitating diseases of the gastrointestinal tract characterized by inflammation and obstruction of parts of the intestine.

Influenza

An acute, commonly epidemic disease occurring in several forms, caused by numerous rapidly mutating viral strains and characterized by respiratory symptoms and general prostration.

Ligand

An ion, a molecule, or a molecular group that binds to another chemical entity to form a larger complex.

LOAEL

The lowest intake (or experimental dose) of a nutrient at which an adverse effect has been identified.

Lumisterol

A naturally occurring compound that is part of the vitamin D family of steroid compounds.

Macrophage

A type of white blood cell that ingests foreign material.

Menopause

The state of an absence of menstrual periods for 12 months.

Metabolic syndrome

Also called insulin resistance syndrome and Metabolic Syndrome X. A group of conditions that increase risk of heart disease, diabetes, and stroke. The five conditions are high blood pressure, high blood sugar levels, high levels of circulating triglycerides, low levels of circulating high-density lipoprotein, and excess fat in the abdominal area.

Microsome

A small particle in the cytoplasm of a cell, typically consisting of fragmented endoplasmic reticulum to which ribosomes are attached.

Milk-alkali syndrome

Caused by the ingestion of large amounts of calcium and absorbable alkali with resulting hypercalcemia; if untreated, can lead to metastatic calcification and renal failure.

Morbidity

Illness or disease.

Mortality

A fatal outcome; death.

Multiple sclerosis

A disease in which the nerves of the central nervous system (brain and spinal cord) degenerate.

Natriuresis

Excretion of excessive amounts of sodium in the urine.

Neoplasm

A new, often uncontrolled growth of abnormal tissue; tumor.

Nephrocalcinosis

Renal lithiasis characterized by diffusely scattered foci of calcification in the kidneys.

Nephrolithiasis

Calculi in the kidneys.

NOAEL

The highest intake (or experimental dose) of a nutrient at which no adverse effect has been observed.

Nutrient

A substance (such as a chemical element or inorganic compound) that an organism needs to live and grow; a substance used in an organism's metabolism that must be taken in from its environment.

Nutriture

A state of nutrition in the body.

Osteoblast

A cell from which bone develops.

Osteoclast

A large multinucleate cell found in growing bone that resorbs bony tissue, as in the formation of canals and cavities.

Osteocyte

A branched cell imbedded in the matrix of bone tissue.

Osteogenesis

Formation and development of bony tissue.

Osteoid

Resembling bone; the bone matrix, especially before calcification.

Osteomalacia

The softening of bone, the depletion of calcium from bone; may be caused by poor dietary intake or poor absorption of calcium and other minerals needed to harden bones and can be a characteristic feature of vitamin D deficiency in adults.

Osteopenia

A condition of bone in which decreased calcification, decreased density, or reduced mass occurs.

Osteoporosis
> A condition characterized by a decrease in bone density (a decrease in bone strength that results in fragile bones); leads to abnormally porous bone that is compressible, like a sponge.

Parathyroid gland
> A gland that regulates calcium, located behind the thyroid gland in the neck, which secretes parathyroid hormone.

Parathyroid hormone
> A hormone that is made by the parathyroid gland and that is critical to calcium and phosphorus balance.

Perimenopause
> The interval in which a women's body begins its transition into menopause.

Periosteal
> Pertaining to the periosteum, the membrane covering the bones.

Phosphate
> A form of phosphoric acid; calcium phosphate makes bones and teeth hard.

Polyuria
> The excessive passage of urine, resulting in profuse urination and urinary frequency.

Preeclampsia
> A toxic condition developing in late pregnancy characterized by a sudden rise in blood pressure, generalized edema, proteinuria, severe headache, and visual disturbances that may result in eclampsia (convulsive or coma state) if untreated.

Previtamin D_3
> A short-lived intermediate form arising from exposure of provitamin D_3 (7-dehydrocholesterol) in the skin to UVB irradiation. Body heat quickly changes previtamin D_3 into vitamin D_3.

Prohormone
> An intraglandular precursor of a hormone.

Provitamin D_3 (7-dehydrocholesterol)
> A provitamin present in the skin of humans as well as the milk of mammals that becomes vitamin D_3 when exposed to ultraviolet light.

Recommended Dietary Allowance
> The average daily dietary intake level that is sufficient to meet the nutrient requirements of nearly all (97.5 percent) healthy individuals in a particular life stage and gender group.

Rheumatoid arthritis
> An autoimmune disease that causes chronic inflammation of the joints.

Rickets
> A disorder caused by a deficiency of vitamin D, calcium, or phosphate, which leads to softening and weakening of the bones and is seen most commonly in children 6 to 24 months of age.

Sarcoidosis
> A disease that results from a specific type of inflammation of tissues of the body that can appear in almost any body organ, often starting in the lungs or lymph nodes.

Scleroderma
> A pathological thickening and hardening of the skin caused by swelling and thickening of fibrous tissue.

Systemic lupus erythematosus
> A chronic, autoimmune, inflammatory disease of connective tissue that causes fever, weakness, fatigue, joint pains, and skin lesions on the face, neck, or arms.

Tachysterol
> An isomer of ergosterol that forms vitamin D_2 when irradiated with ultraviolet light.

Tolerable Upper Intake Level
> The highest average daily nutrient intake level that is likely to pose no risk of adverse effects to almost all individuals in the general population. As intake increases above the Tolerable Upper Intake Level, the potential risk of adverse effects may increase.

Transgenic
> Having genetic material (deoxyribonucleic acid) from another species.

Tuberculosis
> A highly contagious infection caused by the bacterium called *Mycobacterium tuberculosis.*

Ultraviolet
> Pertaining to electromagnetic radiation having wavelengths in the range of approximately 5 to 400 nm; shorter than visible light, but longer than X-rays.

Ultraviolet B
> Medium wavelength (280 to 320 nm) ultraviolet rays from the sun; help synthesis of vitamin D_3; the "burning" rays in the ultraviolet spectrum.

Vasodilatation

Relaxation or widening of the blood vessels; leads to a lowered blood pressure.

Vitamin D

Also referred to as calciferol; comprises a group of fat-soluble seco-sterols. The two major forms are vitamin D_2 and vitamin D_3 (both vitamin D_2 and vitamin D_3 can be synthesized commercially and may be found in dietary supplements or fortified foods; they differ only in their side chain structure).

Vitamin D_2

Also referred to as ergocalciferol; originates from plants and is found in the human diet.

Vitamin D_3

Also referred to as cholecalciferol; is synthesized in the skin of humans from 7-dehydrocholesterol and is also consumed in the diet via the intake of animal-based foods.

Vitamin D–resistant rickets

An inherited form of rickets characterized by high concentrations of phosphate in the blood due to defective renal tubular reabsorption of phosphate and subnormal absorption of dietary calcium.

Appendixes B through K are not printed in this book, but can be found on the CD at the back of the book or online at http://www.nap.edu.

Index[*]

---

[*]Appendixes B through K (pp. 537-1074) are not included in this index.

1075

in the placenta, 90, 189
in pleural fluid, 177
during preeclampsia, 189
during pregnancy, 56, 96, 174, 250–251,
　　252, 254
rheumatoid arthritis treatment, 175
rickets and osteomalacia, 49, 94
systemic lupus erythematosus treatment,
　　176
tuberculosis, 178
use of term, 78
vitamin D intoxication, 427
Calcium. *See also* Calcium balance; Serum
　　calcium
absorption. *See also* Calcium,
　　bioavailability
　adolescents, 95, 352
　African Americans, 260–261, 296
　children, 352
　dietary factors, 63–64
　fractional, 38–39
　from the gut, and increased risk for
　　nephrolithiasis, 411, 500
　impaired with rickets, 94
　as indicator of nutrient adequacy,
　　4, 129
　infants, 52, 253, 350, 503, 505
　methods of measurement, 264–265
　overview, 38–40
　during pregnancy or lactation, 242,
　　249, 250, 253, 256–257, 259,
　　277, 279, 281–282, 292, 361,
　　424
　relationship with vitamin D, 35,
　　40–41, 143, 279
　role of calcitriol, 35, 38, 39, 89, 253,
　　260, 264, 267
　and serum 25OHD, 213, 257, 259,
　　264–267, 271, 277, 284, 292,
　　366, 368, 388–389
accretion, 53–54, 269, 350, 351–353,
　　354, 503. *See also* Bone,
　　accretion
adverse effects with. *See* Adverse effects,
　　calcium; Calcium, ULs
AIs, 7, 8, 58n.4, 345, 346, 348–351. *See
　　also* Calcium balance, studies;
　　Calcium retention
autism, 183
bioaccumulation, 35, 43
bioavailability, 37, 39, 62–63, 498, 503

bone health and, 194, 292. *See also*
　　Supplements, calcium, and
　　bone health
cancer, 5, 135, 137, 139, 140, 141, 143,
　　144–145, 147, 414–416
cardiovascular disease, 148, 149
cognitive function, 186
deficiency, 35, 40, 48–50, 243–248, 254,
　　271, 386
depression, 188
diabetes, 155, 156
DRIs
　adolescents, 7, 351, 352, 354–355,
　　1104, 1108, 1114
　adults, 7, 355–361, 1104, 1108, 1114
　background of current report, 346
　children, 7, 351, 352, 353–355, 1104,
　　1108, 1114
　infants, 7, 348–351, 1104, 1108, 1114
　in IOM 1997 report, 16, 58–60, 61,
　　346, 350, 351, 404
　lactation, 7, 361, 362, 1104, 1108,
　　1114
　pregnancy, 7, 361–362, 1104, 1108,
　　1114
　summary tables, 7–8, 349, 464, 1104,
　　1108, 1114
EARs. *See also* Calcium, AIs
　and accretion/retention, 58n.4, 268,
　　272, 292
　adolescents, 7, 351, 354, 356, 357,
　　359, 1104
　adults, 7, 355, 356, 357, 359, 360–361,
　　1104
　children, 7, 351, 353, 354, 1104
　lactation, 7, 9, 349, 361, 362, 464,
　　1104
　pregnancy, 7, 9, 349, 361, 362, 464,
　　1104
　summary tables, 7, 349, 464, 1104
elemental, 37
excretion
　adolescents, 95, 352
　children, 352
　dietary factors, 63–64
　infants, 8
　during lactation, 256, 257, 282
　overview, 41–42
　postmenopausal women, 55
　during pregnancy, 189, 250
　reduction with diuretics, 407

D

Prothrombotic state, 152
Proton-pump inhibitors, 37, 407
Provitamin D. *See* 7-Dehydrocholesterol
Puberty, 8, 24, 39, 47, 262, 354. *See also*
   Adolescents
Public health considerations
  cancer, 134
  cardiovascular disease, 147
  in DRI development
    calcium, 359, 360, 421, 423, 477
    overview, 29, 293, 298, 404, 479, 482,
      488–489, 522
    vitamin D, 370, 388, 420, 440, 442,
      445, 483, 485, 488, 494

R

Race/ethnicity
  assignment of "race" in study design, 295
  breast-fed infants and vitamin D, 385,
    494–495
  calcitriol levels, 260–261
  "calcium economy," 294, 517
  calcium retention, 296, 297
  cardiovascular mortality, 438
  clothing and sun exposure, 105, 494
  fractures, 439
  limited data for DRI development, 347
  onset of breast development, 24
  relationship between serum 25OHD and
    PTH, 260–261
  research needs, 347, 516–517
  serum 25OHD levels, 101, 103, 104, 106,
    174, 260–261, 374, 431, 438,
    439, 444, 493
Radioimmunoassay (RIA), 110–111, 198
Randomised Evaluation of Calcium and/Or
    vitamin D (RECORD), 154
Recommended Dietary Allowances (RDAs)
  applicable population, 21
  background, 15
  calcium. *See* Calcium, RDAs
  defined, 3, 21, 482
  development, 3, 8, 9–10, 21
  EAR and, 2, 3, 20, 21, 23, 369
  elements, 1108–1109
  macronutrients, 1110
  throughout the life cycle. *See under specific*
    life stages
  uses, 15

  vitamin D. *See* Vitamin D, RDAs
  vitamins, 1106–1107
  water, total, 1110
Recommended Nutrient Intakes (RNIs), 15
Rectal mucosa cancer, 135
Renal function
  calcitriol formation and, 77, 84, 90, 481
  renal failure, 407, 409n.1
  renal insufficiency
    cardiovascular disease, 426
    chronic kidney disease–mineral
      disorder, 55
    hypercalcemia, 42, 406, 407–409,
      410, 425
    percent of N. Amer. population with,
      406
    renal dialysis patients, 91
    vitamin D intoxication, 88, 426
Reproductive outcomes, non-skeletal, 4,
    192–193. *See also* Preeclampsia
    and pregnancy-induced
    hypertension
Research needs
  adverse effects of vitamin D, 424–425
  background diet to calculate total level
    of intake, 346
  calcium intake and BMD, 273
  chronic diseases, 5, 486, 489
  clinical trials, 5, 12, 22, 135, 404, 486
  context, 17, 18–19
  dose–response relationships, 12, 159,
    346, 359, 360, 482, 484,
    489, 519–520. *See also* Sun
    exposure, DRI development
  ethnic/racial considerations, 347,
    516–517
  indicator review and selection, 515,
    516–519
  intake assessment, 22, 516, 520–521
  intake response–assessment, 519–520
  isolation of effects of single nutrient, 5,
    6, 11, 12, 35, 346, 485
  long-term data, 12, 425, 485, 518
  reproducibility, 26, 109
  serum 25OHD, 12, 139, 181, 517, 518,
    519, 520, 521
  summary, 513–522
  sun exposure, 12, 484, 516, 520
  vitamin D as a hormone, 12
Rheumatoid arthritis (RA), 4, 129, 174–175,
    177, 189

Summary Tables

Dietary Reference Intakes

Dietary Reference Intakes (DRIs): Estimated Average Requirements
Food and Nutrition Board, Institute of Medicine, National Academies

Life Stage Group	Calcium (mg/d)	CHO (g/kg/d)	Protein (g/d)	Vit A (μg/d)[a]	Vit C (mg/d)	Vit D (μg/d)	Vit E (mg/d)[b]	Thiamin (mg/d)	Riboflavin (mg/d)	Niacin (mg/d)[c]
Infants										
0–6 mo										
6–12 mo			1.0							
Children										
1–3 y	500	100	0.87	210	13	10	5	0.4	0.4	5
4–8 y	800	100	0.76	275	22	10	6	0.5	0.5	6
Males										
9–13 y	1,100	100	0.76	445	39	10	9	0.7	0.8	9
14–18 y	1,100	100	0.73	630	63	10	12	1.0	1.1	12
19–30 y	800	100	0.66	625	75	10	12	1.0	1.1	12
31–50 y	800	100	0.66	625	75	10	12	1.0	1.1	12
51–70 y	800	100	0.66	625	75	10	12	1.0	1.1	12
> 70 y	1,000	100	0.66	625	75	10	12	1.0	1.1	12
Females										
9–13 y	1,100	100	0.76	420	39	10	9	0.7	0.8	9
14–18 y	1,100	100	0.71	485	56	10	12	0.9	0.9	11
19–30 y	800	100	0.66	500	60	10	12	0.9	0.9	11
31–50 y	800	100	0.66	500	60	10	12	0.9	0.9	11
51–70 y	1,000	100	0.66	500	60	10	12	0.9	0.9	11
> 70 y	1,000	100	0.66	500	60	10	12	0.9	0.9	11
Pregnancy										
14–18 y	1,000	135	0.88	530	66	10	12	1.2	1.2	14
19–30 y	800	135	0.88	550	70	10	12	1.2	1.2	14
31–50 y	800	135	0.88	550	70	10	12	1.2	1.2	14
Lactation										
14–18 y	1,000	160	1.05	885	96	10	16	1.2	1.3	13
19–30 y	800	160	1.05	900	100	10	16	1.2	1.3	13
31–50 y	800	160	1.05	900	100	10	16	1.2	1.3	13

NOTE: An Estimated Average Requirement (EAR) is the average daily nutrient intake level estimated to meet the requirements of half of the healthy individuals in a group. EARs have not been established for vitamin K, pantothenic acid, biotin, choline, chromium, fluoride, manganese, or other nutrients not yet evaluated via the DRI process.

[a]As retinol activity equivalents (RAEs). 1 RAE = 1 μg retinol, 12 μg β-carotene, 24 μg α-carotene, or 24 μg β-cryptoxanthin. The RAE for dietary provitamin A carotenoids is two-fold greater than retinol equivalents (RE), whereas the RAE for preformed vitamin A is the same as RE.

[b]As α-tocopherol. α-tocopherol includes *RRR*-α-tocopherol, the only form of α-tocopherol that occurs naturally in foods, and the *2R*-stereoisomeric forms of α-tocopherol (*RRR*-, *RSR*-, *RRS*-, and *RSS*α-tocopherol) that occur in fortified foods and supplements. It does not include the *2S*-stereoisomeric forms of α-tocopherol (*SRR*-, *SSR*-, *SRS*-, and *SSS*α-tocopherol), also found in fortified foods and supplements.

Vit B$_6$ (mg/d)	Folate (µg/d)^d	Vit B$_{12}$ (µg/d)	Copper (µg/d)	Iodine (µg/d)	Iron (mg/d)	Magnesium (mg/d)	Molybdenum (µg/d)	Phosphorus (mg/d)	Selenium (µg/d)	Zinc (mg/d)
					6.9					2.5
0.4	120	0.7	260	65	3.0	65	13	380	17	2.5
0.5	160	1.0	340	65	4.1	110	17	405	23	4.0
0.8	250	1.5	540	73	5.9	200	26	1,055	35	7.0
1.1	330	2.0	685	95	7.7	340	33	1,055	45	8.5
1.1	320	2.0	700	95	6	330	34	580	45	9.4
1.1	320	2.0	700	95	6	350	34	580	45	9.4
1.4	320	2.0	700	95	6	350	34	580	45	9.4
1.4	320	2.0	700	95	6	350	34	580	45	9.4
0.8	250	1.5	540	73	5.7	200	26	1,055	35	7.0
1.0	330	2.0	685	95	7.9	300	33	1,055	45	7.3
1.1	320	2.0	700	95	8.1	255	34	580	45	6.8
1.1	320	2.0	700	95	8.1	265	34	580	45	6.8
1.3	320	2.0	700	95	5	265	34	580	45	6.8
1.3	320	2.0	700	95	5	265	34	580	45	6.8
1.6	520	2.2	785	160	23	335	40	1,055	49	10.5
1.6	520	2.2	800	160	22	290	40	580	49	9.5
1.6	520	2.2	800	160	22	300	40	580	49	9.5
1.7	450	2.4	985	209	7	300	35	1,055	59	10.9
1.7	450	2.4	1,000	209	6.5	255	36	580	59	10.4
1.7	450	2.4	1,000	209	6.5	265	36	580	59	10.4

^{c}As niacin equivalents (NE). 1 mg of niacin = 60 mg of tryptophan.

^{d}As dietary folate equivalents (DFE). 1 DFE = 1 µg food folate = 0.6 µg of folic acid from fortified food or as a supplement consumed with food = 0.5 µg of a supplement taken on an empty stomach.

SOURCES: *Dietary Reference Intakes for Calcium, Phosphorous, Magnesium, Vitamin D, and Fluoride* (1997); *Dietary Reference Intakes for Thiamin, Riboflavin, Niacin, Vitamin B$_6$, Folate, Vitamin B$_{12}$, Pantothenic Acid, Biotin, and Choline* (1998); *Dietary Reference Intakes for Vitamin C, Vitamin E, Selenium, and Carotenoids* (2000); *Dietary Reference Intakes for Vitamin A, Vitamin K, Arsenic, Boron, Chromium, Copper, Iodine, Iron, Manganese, Molybdenum, Nickel, Silicon, Vanadium, and Zinc* (2001); *Dietary Reference Intakes for Energy, Carbohydrate, Fiber, Fat, Fatty Acids, Cholesterol, Protein, and Amino Acids* (2002/2005); and *Dietary Reference Intakes for Calcium and Vitamin D* (2011). These reports may be accessed via www.nap.edu.

Dietary Reference Intakes (DRIs): Recommended Dietary Allowances and Adequate Intakes, Vitamins

Food and Nutrition Board, Institute of Medicine, National Academies

Life Stage Group	Vitamin A (μg/d)[a]	Vitamin C (mg/d)	Vitamin D (μg/d)[b,c]	Vitamin E (mg/d)[d]	Vitamin K (μg/d)	Thiamin (mg/d)
Infants						
0–6 mo	400*	40*	10*	4*	2.0*	0.2*
6–12 mo	500*	50*	10*	5*	2.5*	0.3*
Children						
1–3 y	300	15	15	6	30*	0.5
4–8 y	400	25	15	7	55*	0.6
Males						
9–13 y	600	45	15	11	60*	0.9
14–18 y	900	75	15	15	75*	1.2
19–30 y	900	90	15	15	120*	1.2
31–50 y	900	90	15	15	120*	1.2
51–70 y	900	90	15	15	120*	1.2
> 70 y	900	90	20	15	120*	1.2
Females						
9–13 y	600	45	15	11	60*	0.9
14–18 y	700	65	15	15	75*	1.0
19–30 y	700	75	15	15	90*	1.1
31–50 y	700	75	15	15	90*	1.1
51–70 y	700	75	15	15	90*	1.1
> 70 y	700	75	20	15	90*	1.1
Pregnancy						
14–18 y	750	80	15	15	75*	1.4
19–30 y	770	85	15	15	90*	1.4
31–50 y	770	85	15	15	90*	1.4
Lactation						
14–18 y	1,200	115	15	19	75*	1.4
19–30 y	1,300	120	15	19	90*	1.4
31–50 y	1,300	120	15	19	90*	1.4

NOTE: This table (taken from the DRI reports, see www.nap.edu) presents Recommended Dietary Allowances (RDAs) in **bold type** and Adequate Intakes (AIs) in ordinary type followed by an asterisk (*). An RDA is the average daily dietary intake level sufficient to meet the nutrient requirements of nearly all (97–98 percent) healthy individuals in a group. It is calculated from an Estimated Average Requirement (EAR). If sufficient scientific evidence is not available to establish an EAR, and thus calculate an RDA, an AI is usually developed. For healthy breast-fed infants, an AI is the mean intake. The AI for other life stage and gender groups is believed to cover the needs of all healthy individuals in the groups, but lack of data or uncertainty in the data prevent being able to specify with confidence the percentage of individuals covered by this intake.

[a] As retinol activity equivalents (RAEs). 1 RAE = 1 μg retinol, 12 μg β-carotene, 24 μg α-carotene, or 24 μg β-cryptoxanthin. The RAE for dietary provitamin A carotenoids is two-fold greater than retinol equivalents (REs), whereas the RAE for preformed vitamin A is the same as RE.

[b] As cholecalciferol. 1 μg cholecalciferol = 40 IU vitamin D.

[c] Under the assumption of minimal sunlight.

[d] As α-tocopherol. α-tocopherol includes *RRR*-α-tocopherol, the only form of α-tocopherol that occurs naturally in foods, and the 2*R*-stereoisomeric forms of α-tocopherol (*RRR*-, *RSR*-, *RRS*-, and *RSS*-α-tocopherol) that occur in fortified foods and supplements. It does not include the 2*S*-stereoisomeric forms of α-tocopherol (*SRR*-, *SSR*-, *SRS*-, and *SSS*-α-tocopherol), also found in fortified foods and supplements.

[e] As niacin equivalents (NE). 1 mg of niacin = 60 mg of tryptophan; 0–6 months = preformed niacin (not NE).

[f] As dietary folate equivalents (DFE). 1 DFE = 1 μg food folate = 0.6 μg of folic acid from fortified food or as a supplement consumed with food = 0.5 μg of a supplement taken on an empty stomach.

Riboflavin (mg/d)	Niacin (mg/d)[e]	Vitamin B_6 (mg/d)	Folate (µg/d)[f]	Vitamin B_{12} (µg/d)	Pantothenic Acid (mg/d)	Biotin (µg/d)	Choline (mg/d)[g]
0.3*	2*	0.1*	65*	0.4*	1.7*	5*	125*
0.4*	4*	0.3*	80*	0.5*	1.8*	6*	150*
0.5	6	0.5	150	0.9	2*	8*	200*
0.6	8	0.6	200	1.2	3*	12*	250*
0.9	12	1.0	300	1.8	4*	20*	375*
1.3	16	1.3	400	2.4	5*	25*	550*
1.3	16	1.3	400	2.4	5*	30*	550*
1.3	16	1.3	400	2.4	5*	30*	550*
1.3	16	1.7	400	2.4[h]	5*	30*	550*
1.3	16	1.7	400	2.4[h]	5*	30*	550*
0.9	12	1.0	300	1.8	4*	20*	375*
1.0	14	1.2	400[i]	2.4	5*	25*	400*
1.1	14	1.3	400[i]	2.4	5*	30*	425*
1.1	14	1.3	400[i]	2.4	5*	30*	425*
1.1	14	1.5	400	2.4[h]	5*	30*	425*
1.1	14	1.5	400	2.4[h]	5*	30*	425*
1.4	18	1.9	600[j]	2.6	6*	30*	450*
1.4	18	1.9	600[j]	2.6	6*	30*	450*
1.4	18	1.9	600[j]	2.6	6*	30*	450*
1.6	17	2.0	500	2.8	7*	35*	550*
1.6	17	2.0	500	2.8	7*	35*	550*
1.6	17	2.0	500	2.8	7*	35*	550*

[g]Although AIs have been set for choline, there are few data to assess whether a dietary supply of choline is needed at all stages of the life cycle, and it may be that the choline requirement can be met by endogenous synthesis at some of these stages.

[h]Because 10 to 30 percent of older people may malabsorb food-bound B_{12}, it is advisable for those older than 50 years to meet their RDA mainly by consuming foods fortified with B_{12} or a supplement containing B_{12}.

[i]In view of evidence linking folate intake with neural tube defects in the fetus, it is recommended that all women capable of becoming pregnant consume 400 µg from supplements or fortified foods in addition to intake of food folate from a varied diet.

[j]It is assumed that women will continue consuming 400 µg from supplements or fortified food until their pregnancy is confirmed and they enter prenatal care, which ordinarily occurs after the end of the periconceptional period—the critical time for formation of the neural tube.

SOURCES: *Dietary Reference Intakes for Calcium, Phosphorous, Magnesium, Vitamin D, and Fluoride* (1997); *Dietary Reference Intakes for Thiamin, Riboflavin, Niacin, Vitamin B_6, Folate, Vitamin B_{12}, Pantothenic Acid, Biotin, and Choline* (1998); *Dietary Reference Intakes for Vitamin C, Vitamin E, Selenium, and Carotenoids* (2000); *Dietary Reference Intakes for Vitamin A, Vitamin K, Arsenic, Boron, Chromium, Copper, Iodine, Iron, Manganese, Molybdenum, Nickel, Silicon, Vanadium, and Zinc* (2001); *Dietary Reference Intakes for Water, Potassium, Sodium, Chloride, and Sulfate* (2005); and *Dietary Reference Intakes for Calcium and Vitamin D* (2011). These reports may be accessed via www.nap.edu.

Dietary Reference Intakes (DRIs): Recommended Dietary Allowances and Adequate Intakes, Elements
Food and Nutrition Board, Institute of Medicine, National Academies

Life Stage Group	Calcium (mg/d)	Chromium (μg/d)	Copper (μg/d)	Fluoride (mg/d)	Iodine (μg/d)	Iron (mg/d)	Magnesium (mg/d)	Manganese (mg/d)
Infants								
0–6 mo	200*	0.2*	200*	0.01*	110*	0.27*	30*	0.003*
6–12 mo	260*	5.5*	220*	0.5*	130*	**11**	75*	0.6*
Children								
1–3 y	**700**	11*	**340**	0.7*	**90**	**7**	**80**	1.2*
4–8 y	**1,000**	15*	**440**	1*	**90**	**10**	**130**	1.5*
Males								
9–13 y	**1,300**	25*	**700**	2*	**120**	**8**	**240**	1.9*
14–18 y	**1,300**	35*	**890**	3*	**150**	**11**	**410**	2.2*
19–30 y	**1,000**	35*	**900**	4*	**150**	**8**	**400**	2.3*
31–50 y	**1,000**	35*	**900**	4*	**150**	**8**	**420**	2.3*
51–70 y	**1,000**	30*	**900**	4*	**150**	**8**	**420**	2.3*
> 70 y	**1,200**	30*	**900**	4*	**150**	**8**	**420**	2.3*
Females								
9–13 y	**1,300**	21*	**700**	2*	**120**	**8**	**240**	1.6*
14–18 y	**1,300**	24*	**890**	3*	**150**	**15**	**360**	1.6*
19–30 y	**1,000**	25*	**900**	3*	**150**	**18**	**310**	1.8*
31–50 y	**1,000**	25*	**900**	3*	**150**	**18**	**320**	1.8*
51–70 y	**1,200**	20*	**900**	3*	**150**	**8**	**320**	1.8*
> 70 y	**1,200**	20*	**900**	3*	**150**	**8**	**320**	1.8*
Pregnancy								
14–18 y	**1,300**	29*	**1,000**	3*	**220**	**27**	**400**	2.0*
19–30 y	**1,000**	30*	**1,000**	3*	**220**	**27**	**350**	2.0*
31–50 y	**1,000**	30*	**1,000**	3*	**220**	**27**	**360**	2.0*
Lactation								
14–18 y	**1,300**	44*	**1,300**	3*	**290**	**10**	**360**	2.6*
19–30 y	**1,000**	45*	**1,300**	3*	**290**	**9**	**310**	2.6*
31–50 y	**1,000**	45*	**1,300**	3*	**290**	**9**	**320**	2.6*

NOTE: This table (taken from the DRI reports, see www.nap.edu) presents Recommended Dietary Allowances (RDAs) in **bold type** and Adequate Intakes (AIs) in ordinary type followed by an asterisk (*). An RDA is the average daily dietary intake level sufficient to meet the nutrient requirements of nearly all (97–98 percent) healthy individuals in a group. It is calculated from an Estimated Average Requirement (EAR). If sufficient scientific evidence is not available to establish an EAR, and thus calculate an RDA, an AI is usually developed. For healthy breast-fed infants, an AI is the mean intake. The AI for other life stage and gender groups is believed to cover the needs of all healthy individuals in the groups, but lack of data or uncertainty in the data prevent being able to specify with confidence the percentage of individuals covered by this intake.

Molybdenum (μg/d)	Phosphorus (mg/d)	Selenium (μg/d)	Zinc (mg/d)	Potassium (g/d)	Sodium (g/d)	Chloride (g/d)
2*	100*	15*	2*	0.4*	0.12*	0.18*
3*	275*	20*	3	0.7*	0.37*	0.57*
17	460	20	3	3.0*	1.0*	1.5*
22	500	30	5	3.8*	1.2*	1.9*
34	1,250	40	8	4.5*	1.5*	2.3*
43	1,250	55	11	4.7*	1.5*	2.3*
45	700	55	11	4.7*	1.5*	2.3*
45	700	55	11	4.7*	1.5*	2.3*
45	700	55	11	4.7*	1.3*	2.0*
45	700	55	11	4.7*	1.2*	1.8*
34	1,250	40	8	4.5*	1.5*	2.3*
43	1,250	55	9	4.7*	1.5*	2.3*
45	700	55	8	4.7*	1.5*	2.3*
45	700	55	8	4.7*	1.5*	2.3*
45	700	55	8	4.7*	1.3*	2.0*
45	700	55	8	4.7*	1.2*	1.8*
50	1,250	60	12	4.7*	1.5*	2.3*
50	700	60	11	4.7*	1.5*	2.3*
50	700	60	11	4.7*	1.5*	2.3*
50	1,250	70	13	5.1*	1.5*	2.3*
50	700	70	12	5.1*	1.5*	2.3*
50	700	70	12	5.1*	1.5*	2.3*

SOURCES: *Dietary Reference Intakes for Calcium, Phosphorous, Magnesium, Vitamin D, and Fluoride* (1997); *Dietary Reference Intakes for Thiamin, Riboflavin, Niacin, Vitamin B$_6$, Folate, Vitamin B$_{12}$, Pantothenic Acid, Biotin, and Choline* (1998); *Dietary Reference Intakes for Vitamin C, Vitamin E, Selenium, and Carotenoids* (2000); *Dietary Reference Intakes for Vitamin A, Vitamin K, Arsenic, Boron, Chromium, Copper, Iodine, Iron, Manganese, Molybdenum, Nickel, Silicon, Vanadium, and Zinc* (2001); *Dietary Reference Intakes for Water, Potassium, Sodium, Chloride, and Sulfate* (2005); and *Dietary Reference Intakes for Calcium and Vitamin D* (2011). These reports may be accessed via www.nap.edu.

Dietary Reference Intakes (DRIs): Recommended Dietary Allowances and Adequate Intakes, Total Water and Macronutrients
Food and Nutrition Board, Institute of Medicine, National Academies

Life Stage Group	Total Water[a] (L/d)	Carbohydrate (g/d)	Total Fiber (g/d)	Fat (g/d)	Linoleic Acid (g/d)	α-Linolenic Acid (g/d)	Protein[b] (g/d)
Infants							
0–6 mo	0.7*	60*	ND	31*	4.4*	0.5*	9.1*
6–12 mo	0.8*	95*	ND	30*	4.6*	0.5*	**11.0**
Children							
1–3 y	1.3*	**130**	19*	ND[c]	7*	0.7*	**13**
4–8 y	1.7*	**130**	25*	ND	10*	0.9*	**19**
Males							
9–13 y	2.4*	**130**	31*	ND	12*	1.2*	**34**
14–18 y	3.3*	**130**	38*	ND	16*	1.6*	**52**
19–30 y	3.7*	**130**	38*	ND	17*	1.6*	**56**
31–50 y	3.7*	**130**	38*	ND	17*	1.6*	**56**
51–70 y	3.7*	**130**	30*	ND	14*	1.6*	**56**
> 70 y	3.7*	**130**	30*	ND	14*	1.6*	**56**
Females							
9–13 y	2.1*	**130**	26*	ND	10*	1.0*	**34**
14–18 y	2.3*	**130**	26*	ND	11*	1.1*	**46**
19–30 y	2.7*	**130**	25*	ND	12*	1.1*	**46**
31–50 y	2.7*	**130**	25*	ND	12*	1.1*	**46**
51–70 y	2.7*	**130**	21*	ND	11*	1.1*	**46**
> 70 y	2.7*	**130**	21*	ND	11*	1.1*	**46**
Pregnancy							
14–18 y	3.0*	**175**	28*	ND	13*	1.4*	**71**
19–30 y	3.0*	**175**	28*	ND	13*	1.4*	**71**
31–50 y	3.0*	**175**	28*	ND	13*	1.4*	**71**
Lactation							
14–18	3.8*	**210**	29*	ND	13*	1.3*	**71**
19–30 y	3.8*	**210**	29*	ND	13*	1.3*	**71**
31–50 y	3.8*	**210**	29*	ND	13*	1.3*	**71**

NOTE: This table (take from the DRI reports, see www.nap.edu) presents Recommended Dietary Allowances (RDA) in **bold type** and Adequate Intakes (AI) in ordinary type followed by an asterisk (*). An RDA is the average daily dietary intake level sufficient to meet the nutrient requirements of nearly all (97–98 percent) healthy individuals in a group. It is calculated from an Estimated Average Requirement (EAR). If sufficient scientific evidence is not available to establish an EAR, and thus calculate an RDA, an AI is usually developed. For healthy breast-fed infants, an AI is the mean intake. The AI for other life stage and gender groups is believed to cover the needs of all healthy individuals in the groups, but lack of data or uncertainty in the data prevent being able to specify with confidence the percentage of individuals covered by this intake.

[a]Total water includes all water contained in food, beverages, and drinking water.

[b]Based on g protein per kg of body weight for the reference body weight, e.g., for adults 0.8 g/kg body weight for the reference body weight.

[c]Not determined.

SOURCE: *Dietary Reference Intakes for Energy, Carbohydrate, Fiber, Fat, Fatty Acids, Cholesterol, Protein, and Amino Acids* (2002/2005) and *Dietary Reference Intakes for Water, Potassium, Sodium, Chloride, and Sulfate* (2005). The report may be accessed via www.nap.edu.

Dietary Reference Intakes (DRIs): Acceptable Macronutrient Distribution Ranges
Food and Nutrition Board, Institute of Medicine, National Academies

	Range (percent of energy)		
Macronutrient	Children, 1–3 y	Children, 4–18 y	Adults
Fat	30–40	25–35	20–35
n-6 polyunsaturated fatty acids[a] (linoleic acid)	5–10	5–10	5–10
n-3 polyunsaturated fatty acids[a] (α-linolenic acid)	0.6–1.2	0.6–1.2	0.6–1.2
Carbohydrate	45–65	45–65	45–65
Protein	5–20	10–30	10–35

[a]Approximately 10 percent of the total can come from longer-chain n-3 or n-6 fatty acids.
SOURCE: *Dietary Reference Intakes for Energy, Carbohydrate, Fiber, Fat, Fatty Acids, Cholesterol, Protein, and Amino Acids* (2002/2005). The report may be accessed via www.nap.edu.

Dietary Reference Intakes (DRIs): Additional Macronutrient Recommendations
Food and Nutrition Board, Institute of Medicine, National Academies

Macronutrient	Recommendation
Dietary cholesterol	As low as possible while consuming a nutritionally adequate diet
Trans fatty acids	As low as possible while consuming a nutritionally adequate diet
Saturated fatty acids	As low as possible while consuming a nutritionally adequate diet
Added sugars[a]	Limit to no more than 25% of total energy

[a]Not a recommended intake. A daily intake of added sugars that individuals should aim for to achieve a healthful diet was not set.
SOURCE: *Dietary Reference Intakes for Energy, Carbohydrate, Fiber, Fat, Fatty Acids, Cholesterol, Protein, and Amino Acids* (2002/2005). The report may be accessed via www.nap.edu.

Dietary Reference Intakes (DRIs): Tolerable Upper Intake Levels, Vitamins
Food and Nutrition Board, Institute of Medicine, National Academies

Life Stage Group	Vitamin A (µg/d)[a]	Vitamin C (mg/d)	Vitamin D (µg/d)	Vitamin E (mg/d)[b,c]	Vitamin K	Thiamin	Riboflavin
Infants							
0–6 mo	600	ND[e]	25	ND	ND	ND	ND
6–12 mo	600	ND	38	ND	ND	ND	ND
Children							
1–3 y	600	400	63	200	ND	ND	ND
4–8 y	900	650	75	300	ND	ND	ND
Males							
9–13 y	1,700	1,200	100	600	ND	ND	ND
14–18 y	2,800	1,800	100	800	ND	ND	ND
19–30 y	3,000	2,000	100	1,000	ND	ND	ND
31–50 y	3,000	2,000	100	1,000	ND	ND	ND
51–70 y	3,000	2,000	100	1,000	ND	ND	ND
> 70 y	3,000	2,000	100	1,000	ND	ND	ND
Females							
9–13 y	1,700	1,200	100	600	ND	ND	ND
14–18 y	2,800	1,800	100	800	ND	ND	ND
19–30 y	3,000	2,000	100	1,000	ND	ND	ND
31–50 y	3,000	2,000	100	1,000	ND	ND	ND
51–70 y	3,000	2,000	100	1,000	ND	ND	ND
> 70 y	3,000	2,000	100	1,000	ND	ND	ND
Pregnancy							
14–18 y	2,800	1,800	100	800	ND	ND	ND
19–30 y	3,000	2,000	100	1,000	ND	ND	ND
31–50 y	3,000	2,000	100	1,000	ND	ND	ND
Lactation							
14–18 y	2,800	1,800	100	800	ND	ND	ND
19–30 y	3,000	2,000	100	1,000	ND	ND	ND
31–50 y	3,000	2,000	100	1,000	ND	ND	ND

NOTE: A Tolerable Upper Intake Level (UL) is the highest level of daily nutrient intake that is likely to pose no risk of adverse health effects to almost all individuals in the general population. Unless otherwise specified, the UL represents total intake from food, water, and supplements. Due to a lack of suitable data, ULs could not be established for vitamin K, thiamin, riboflavin, vitamin B$_{12}$, pantothenic acid, biotin, and carotenoids. In the absence of a UL, extra caution may be warranted in consuming levels above recommended intakes. Members of the general population should be advised not to routinely exceed the UL. The UL is not meant to apply to individuals who are treated with the nutrient under medical supervision or to individuals with predisposing conditions that modify their sensitivity to the nutrient.

[a] As preformed vitamin A only.

[b] As α-tocopherol; applies to any form of supplemental α-tocopherol.

[c] The ULs for vitamin E, niacin, and folate apply to synthetic forms obtained from supplements, fortified foods, or a combination of the two.

Niacin (mg/d)[c]	Vitamin B_6 (mg/d)	Folate (μg/d)[c]	Vitamin B_{12}	Pantothenic Acid	Biotin	Choline (g/d)	Carotenoids[d]
ND	ND	ND	ND	ND	ND	ND	ND
ND	ND	ND	ND	ND	ND	ND	ND
10	30	300	ND	ND	ND	1.0	ND
15	40	400	ND	ND	ND	1.0	ND
20	60	600	ND	ND	ND	2.0	ND
30	80	800	ND	ND	ND	3.0	ND
35	100	1,000	ND	ND	ND	3.5	ND
35	100	1,000	ND	ND	ND	3.5	ND
35	100	1,000	ND	ND	ND	3.5	ND
35	100	1,000	ND	ND	ND	3.5	ND
20	60	600	ND	ND	ND	2.0	ND
30	80	800	ND	ND	ND	3.0	ND
35	100	1,000	ND	ND	ND	3.5	ND
35	100	1,000	ND	ND	ND	3.5	ND
35	100	1,000	ND	ND	ND	3.5	ND
35	100	1,000	ND	ND	ND	3.5	ND
30	80	800	ND	ND	ND	3.0	ND
35	100	1,000	ND	ND	ND	3.5	ND
35	100	1,000	ND	ND	ND	3.5	ND
30	80	800	ND	ND	ND	3.0	ND
35	100	1,000	ND	ND	ND	3.5	ND
35	100	1,000	ND	ND	ND	3.5	ND

[d]β-Carotene supplements are advised only to serve as a provitamin A source for individuals at risk of vitamin A deficiency.

[c]ND = Not determinable due to lack of data of adverse effects in this age group and concern with regard to lack of ability to handle excess amounts. Source of intake should be from food only to prevent high levels of intake.

SOURCES: *Dietary Reference Intakes for Calcium, Phosphorous, Magnesium, Vitamin D, and Fluoride* (1997); *Dietary Reference Intakes for Thiamin, Riboflavin, Niacin, Vitamin B₆, Folate, Vitamin B₁₂, Pantothenic Acid, Biotin, and Choline* (1998); *Dietary Reference Intakes for Vitamin C, Vitamine E, Selenium, and Carotenoids* (2000); *Dietary Reference Intakes for Vitamin A, Vitamin K, Arsenic, Boron, Chromium, Copper, Iodine, Iron, Manganese, Molybdenum, Nickel, Silicon, Vanadium, and Zinc* (2001); and *Dietary Reference Intakes for Calcium and Vitamin D* (2011). These reports may be accessed via www.nap.edu.

Dietary Reference Intakes (DRIs): Tolerable Upper Intake Levels, Elements
Food and Nutrition Board, Institute of Medicine, National Academies

Life Stage Group	Arsenic[a]	Boron (mg/d)	Calcium (mg/d)	Chromium	Copper (µg/d)	Fluoride (mg/d)	Iodine (µg/d)	Iron (mg/d)
Infants								
0–6 mo	ND[e]	ND	1,000	ND	ND	0.7	ND	40
6–12 mo	ND	ND	1,500	ND	ND	0.9	ND	40
Children								
1–3 y	ND	3	2,500	ND	1,000	1.3	200	40
4–8 y	ND	6	2,500	ND	3,000	2.2	300	40
Males								
9–13 y	ND	11	3,000	ND	5,000	10	600	40
14–18 y	ND	17	3,000	ND	8,000	10	900	45
19–30 y	ND	20	2,500	ND	10,000	10	1,100	45
31–50 y	ND	20	2,500	ND	10,000	10	1,100	45
51–70 y	ND	20	2,000	ND	10,000	10	1,100	45
> 70 y	ND	20	2,000	ND	10,000	10	1,100	45
Females								
9–13 y	ND	11	3,000	ND	5,000	10	600	40
14–18 y	ND	17	3,000	ND	8,000	10	900	45
19–30 y	ND	20	2,500	ND	10,000	10	1,100	45
31–50 y	ND	20	2,500	ND	10,000	10	1,100	45
51–70 y	ND	20	2,000	ND	10,000	10	1,100	45
> 70 y	ND	20	2,000	ND	10,000	10	1,100	45
Pregnancy								
14–18 y	ND	17	3,000	ND	8,000	10	900	45
19–30 y	ND	20	2,500	ND	10,000	10	1,100	45
61–50 y	ND	20	2,500	ND	10,000	10	1,100	45
Lactation								
14–18 y	ND	17	3,000	ND	8,000	10	900	45
19–30 y	ND	20	2,500	ND	10,000	10	1,100	45
31–50 y	ND	20	2,500	ND	10,000	10	1,100	45

NOTE: A Tolerable Upper Intake Level (UL) is the highest level of daily nutrient intake that is likely to pose no risk of adverse health effects to almost all individuals in the general population. Unless otherwise specified, the UL represents total intake from food, water, and supplements. Due to a lack of suitable data, ULs could not be established for vitamin K, thiamin, riboflavin, vitamin B_{12}, pantothenic acid, biotin, and carotenoids. In the absence of a UL, extra caution may be warranted in consuming levels above recommended intakes. Members of the general population should be advised not to routinely exceed the UL. The UL is not meant to apply to individuals who are treated with the nutrient under medical supervision or to individuals with predisposing conditions that modify their sensitivity to the nutrient.

[a]Although the UL was not determined for arsenic, there is no justification for adding arsenic to food or supplements.

[b]The ULs for magnesium represent intake from a pharmacological agent only and do not include intake from food and water.

[c]Although silicon has not been shown to cause adverse effects in humans, there is no justification for adding silicon to supplements.

Magnesium (mg/d)[b]	Manganese (mg/d)	Molybdenum (μg/d)	Nickel (mg/d)	Phosphorus (g/d)	Selenium (μg/d)	Silicon[c]	Vanadium (mg/d)[d]	Zinc (mg/d)	Sodium (g/d)	Chloride (g/d)
ND	ND	ND	ND	ND	45	ND	ND	4	ND	ND
ND	ND	ND	ND	ND	60	ND	ND	5	ND	ND
65	2	300	0.2	3	90	ND	ND	7	1.5	2.3
110	3	600	0.3	3	150	ND	ND	12	1.9	2.9
350	6	1,100	0.6	4	280	ND	ND	23	2.2	3.4
350	9	1,700	1.0	4	400	ND	ND	34	2.3	3.6
350	11	2,000	1.0	4	400	ND	1.8	40	2.3	3.6
350	11	2,000	1.0	4	400	ND	1.8	40	2.3	3.6
350	11	2,000	1.0	4	400	ND	1.8	40	2.3	3.6
350	11	2,000	1.0	3	400	ND	1.8	40	2.3	3.6
350	6	1,100	0.6	4	280	ND	ND	23	2.2	3.4
350	9	1,700	1.0	4	400	ND	ND	34	2.3	3.6
350	11	2,000	1.0	4	400	ND	1.8	40	2.3	3.6
350	11	2,000	1.0	4	400	ND	1.8	40	2.3	3.6
350	11	2,000	1.0	4	400	ND	1.8	40	2.3	3.6
350	11	2,000	1.0	3	400	ND	1.8	40	2.3	3.6
350	9	1,700	1.0	3.5	400	ND	ND	34	2.3	3.6
350	11	2,000	1.0	3.5	400	ND	ND	40	2.3	3.6
350	11	2,000	1.0	3.5	400	ND	ND	40	2.3	3.6
350	9	1,700	1.0	4	400	ND	ND	34	2.3	3.6
350	11	2,000	1.0	4	400	ND	ND	40	2.3	3.6
350	11	2,000	1.0	4	400	ND	ND	40	2.3	3.6

[d]Although vanadium in food has not been shown to cause adverse effects in humans, there is no justification for adding vanadium to food, and vanadium supplements should be used with caution. The UL is based on adverse effects in laboratory animals, and this data could be used to set a UL for adults but not children and adolescents.

[e]ND = Not determinable due to lack of data of adverse effects in this age group and concern with regard to lack of ability to handle excess amounts. Source of intake should be from food only to prevent high levels of intake.

SOURCES: *Dietary Reference Intakes for Calcium, Phosphorous, Magnesium, Vitamin D, and Fluoride* (1997); *Dietary Reference Intakes for Thiamin, Riboflavin, Niacin, Vitamin B₆, Folate, Vitamin B₁₂, Pantothenic Acid, Biotin, and Choline* (1998); *Dietary Reference Intakes for Vitamin C, Vitamin E, Selenium, and Carotenoids* (2000); *Dietary Reference Intakes for Vitamin A, Vitamin K, Arsenic, Boron, Chromium, Copper, Iodine, Iron, Manganese, Molybdenum, Nickel, Silicon, Vanadium, and Zinc* (2001); *Dietary Reference Intakes for Water, Potassium, Sodium, Chloride, and Sulfate* (2005); and *Dietary Reference Intakes for Calcium and Vitamin D* (2011). These reports may be accessed via www.nap.edu.